COVID-19: Current Status and Future Prospects

COVID-19: Current Status and Future Prospects

Editors

Peter A. Leggat
John Frean
Lucille Blumberg

MDPI • Basel • Beijing • Wuhan • Barcelona • Belgrade • Manchester • Tokyo • Cluj • Tianjin

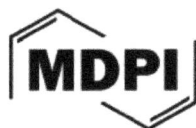

Editors

Peter A. Leggat
James Cook University
Australia

John Frean
University of the Witwatersrand
South Africa

Lucille Blumberg
National Institute for Communicable Diseases of the National Health Laboratory Service
South Africa

Editorial Office
MDPI
St. Alban-Anlage 66
4052 Basel, Switzerland

This is a reprint of articles from the Special Issue published online in the open access journal *Tropical Medicine and Infectious Disease* (ISSN 2414-6366) (available at: https://www.mdpi.com/journal/tropicalmed/special_issues/COVID_19_current_status_future_prospects).

For citation purposes, cite each article independently as indicated on the article page online and as indicated below:

LastName, A.A.; LastName, B.B.; LastName, C.C. Article Title. *Journal Name* **Year**, *Volume Number*, Page Range.

ISBN 978-3-0365-6740-2 (Hbk)
ISBN 978-3-0365-6741-9 (PDF)

© 2023 by the authors. Articles in this book are Open Access and distributed under the Creative Commons Attribution (CC BY) license, which allows users to download, copy and build upon published articles, as long as the author and publisher are properly credited, which ensures maximum dissemination and a wider impact of our publications.

The book as a whole is distributed by MDPI under the terms and conditions of the Creative Commons license CC BY-NC-ND.

Contents

About the Editors ix

Peter A. Leggat, John Frean and Lucille Blumberg
COVID-19: Current Status and Future Prospects
Reprinted from: *Trop. Med. Infect. Dis.* **2023**, *8*, 94, doi:10.3390/tropicalmed8020094 1

Syed Moinuddin Satter, Kamal Ibne Amin Chowdhury, Refah Tamanna, Zarin Abdullah, S. M. Zafor Shafique, Md Saiful Islam, et al.
COVID-19 Risk Perception and Prevention Practices among High- and Low-Density Populations in Bangladesh: A Mixed-Methods Study
Reprinted from: *Trop. Med. Infect. Dis.* **2022**, *7*, 447, doi:10.3390/tropicalmed7120447 7

Cruz S. Sebastião, Adis Cogle, Alice D'Alva Teixeira, Ana Micolo Cândido, Chissengo Tchoni, Maria João Amorim, et al.
Clinical Features Related to Severity and Mortality among COVID-19 Patients in a Pre-Vaccine Period in Luanda, Angola
Reprinted from: *Trop. Med. Infect. Dis.* **2022**, *7*, 338, doi:10.3390/tropicalmed7110338 21

Bakhtawar Chaudhry, Saiza Azhar, Shazia Jamshed, Jahanzaib Ahmed, Laiq-ur-Rehman Khan, Zahid Saeed, et al.
Factors Associated with Self-Medication during the COVID-19 Pandemic: A Cross-Sectional Study in Pakistan
Reprinted from: *Trop. Med. Infect. Dis.* **2022**, *7*, 330, doi:10.3390/tropicalmed7110330 33

Nuning Nuraini, Kamal Khairudin Sukandar, Maria Yulita Trida Tahu, Ernawati Arifin Giri-Rachman, Anggraini Barlian, Sri Harjati Suhardi, et al.
Infectious Disease Modeling with Socio-Viral Behavioral Aspects—Lessons Learned from the Spread of SARS-CoV-2 in a University
Reprinted from: *Trop. Med. Infect. Dis.* **2022**, *7*, 289, doi:10.3390/tropicalmed7100289 49

Kantarida Sripanidkulchai, Pinyo Rattanaumpawan, Winai Ratanasuwan, Nasikarn Angkasekwinai, Susan Assanasen, Peerawong Werarak, et al.
A Risk Prediction Model and Risk Score of SARS-CoV-2 Infection Following Healthcare-Related Exposure
Reprinted from: *Trop. Med. Infect. Dis.* **2022**, *7*, 248, doi:10.3390/tropicalmed7090248 73

Lan Yao, J. Carolyn Graff, Lotfi Aleya, Jiamin Ma, Yanhong Cao, Wei Wei, et al.
Mortality in Four Waves of COVID-19 Is Differently Associated with Healthcare Capacities Affected by Economic Disparities
Reprinted from: *Trop. Med. Infect. Dis.* **2022**, *7*, 241, doi:10.3390/tropicalmed7090241 87

Lorenzo H. Salamanca-Neita, Óscar Carvajal, Juan Pablo Carvajal, Maribel Forero-Castro and Nidya Alexandra Segura
Comparison of Four Real-Time Polymerase Chain Reaction Assays for the Detection of SARS-CoV-2 in Respiratory Samples from Tunja, Boyacá, Colombia
Reprinted from: *Trop. Med. Infect. Dis.* **2022**, *7*, 240, doi:10.3390/tropicalmed7090240 101

Md. Abu Sayeed, Jinnat Ferdous, Otun Saha, Shariful Islam, Shusmita Dutta Choudhury, Josefina Abedin, et al.
Transmission Dynamics and Genomic Epidemiology of Emerging Variants of SARS-CoV-2 in Bangladesh
Reprinted from: *Trop. Med. Infect. Dis.* **2022**, *7*, 197, doi:10.3390/tropicalmed7080197 113

Nsenga Ngoy, Ishata Nannie Conteh, Boniface Oyugi, Patrick Abok, Aminata Kobie, Peter Phori, et al.
Coordination and Management of COVID-19 in Africa through Health Operations and Technical Expertise Pillar: A Case Study from WHO AFRO One Year into Response
Reprinted from: *Trop. Med. Infect. Dis.* **2022**, *7*, 183, doi:10.3390/tropicalmed7080183 133

Liang En Wee, Edwin Philip Conceicao, Jean Xiang-Ying Sim, May Kyawt Aung, Aung Myat Oo, Yang Yong, et al.
Dengue and COVID-19: Managing Undifferentiated Febrile Illness during a "Twindemic"
Reprinted from: *Trop. Med. Infect. Dis.* **2022**, *7*, 68, doi:10.3390/tropicalmed7050068 147

Syed Moinuddin Satter, Taufiqur Rahman Bhuiyan, Zarin Abdullah, Marjahan Akhtar, Aklima Akter, S. M. Zafor Shafique, et al.
Transmission of SARS-CoV-2 in the Population Living in High- and Low-Density Gradient Areas in Dhaka, Bangladesh
Reprinted from: *Trop. Med. Infect. Dis.* **2022**, *7*, 53, doi:10.3390/tropicalmed7040053 157

Ganghee Chae, Aram Choi, Soyeoun Lim, Sooneun Park, Seungjun Lee, Youngick Ahn, et al.
The Effectiveness of the Use of Regdanvimab (CT-P59) in Addition to Remdesivir in Patients with Severe COVID-19: A Single Center Retrospective Study
Reprinted from: *Trop. Med. Infect. Dis.* **2022**, *7*, 51, doi:10.3390/tropicalmed7030051 171

Max Carlos Ramírez-Soto and Gutia Ortega-Cáceres
Analysis of Excess All-Cause Mortality and COVID-19 Mortality in Peru: Observational Study
Reprinted from: *Trop. Med. Infect. Dis.* **2022**, *7*, 44, doi:10.3390/tropicalmed7030044 183

Quoc-Hung Doan, Nguyen-Ngoc Tran, Manh-Hung Than, Hoang-Thanh Nguyen, Van-San Bui, Dinh-Hung Nguyen, et al.
Depression, Anxiety and Associated Factors among Frontline Hospital Healthcare Workers in the Fourth Wave of COVID-19: Empirical Findings from Vietnam
Reprinted from: *Trop. Med. Infect. Dis.* **2022**, *7*, 3, doi:10.3390/tropicalmed7010003 193

Max Carlos Ramírez-Soto, Miluska Alarcón-Arroyo, Yajaira Chilcon-Vitor, Yelibeth Chirinos-Pérez, Gabriela Quispe-Vargas, Kelly Solsol-Jacome and Elizabeth Quintana-Zavaleta
Association between Obesity and COVID-19 Mortality in Peru: An Ecological Study
Reprinted from: *Trop. Med. Infect. Dis.* **2021**, *6*, 182, doi:10.3390/tropicalmed6040182 217

Daniela Loconsole, Anna Sallustio, Francesca Centrone, Daniele Casulli, Maurizio Mario Ferrara, Antonio Sanguedolce, et al.
An Autochthonous Outbreak of the SARS-CoV-2 P.1 Variant of Concern in Southern Italy, April 2021
Reprinted from: *Trop. Med. Infect. Dis.* **2021**, *6*, 151, doi:10.3390/tropicalmed6030151 225

Alaa A. Farag, Hassan M. Hassanin, Hanan H. Soliman, Ahmad Sallam, Amany M. Sediq, Elsayed S. Abd elbaser and Khaled Elbanna
Newly Diagnosed Diabetes in Patients with COVID-19: Different Types and Short-Term Outcomes
Reprinted from: *Trop. Med. Infect. Dis.* **2021**, *6*, 142, doi:10.3390/tropicalmed6030142 233

Amin Islam, Christopher Cockcroft, Shereen Elshazly, Javeed Ahmed, Kevin Joyce, Huque Mahfuz, et al.
Coagulopathy of Dengue and COVID-19: Clinical Considerations
Reprinted from: *Trop. Med. Infect. Dis.* **2022**, *7*, 210, doi:10.3390/tropicalmed7090210 243

Jorge Aquino-Matus, Misael Uribe and Norberto Chavez-Tapia
COVID-19: Current Status in Gastrointestinal, Hepatic, and Pancreatic Diseases—A Concise Review
Reprinted from: *Trop. Med. Infect. Dis.* **2022**, 7, 187, doi:10.3390/tropicalmed7080187 261

Luis Fonte, Armando Acosta, María E. Sarmiento, Mohd Nor Norazmi, María Ginori, Yaxsier de Armas and Enrique J. Calderón
Overlapping of Pulmonary Fibrosis of Postacute COVID-19 Syndrome and Tuberculosis in the Helminth Coinfection Setting in Sub-Saharan Africa
Reprinted from: *Trop. Med. Infect. Dis.* **2022**, 7, 157, doi:10.3390/tropicalmed7080157 273

Severin Kabakama, Eveline T. Konje, Jerome Nyhalah Dinga, Colman Kishamawe, Imran Morhason-Bello, Peter Hayombe, et al.
Commentary on COVID-19 Vaccine Hesitancy in sub-Saharan Africa
Reprinted from: *Trop. Med. Infect. Dis.* **2022**, 7, 130, doi:10.3390/tropicalmed7070130 281

Shilpa Gopinath, Angela Ishak, Naveen Dhawan, Sujan Poudel, Prakriti Singh Shrestha, Prabhjeet Singh, et al.
Characteristics of COVID-19 Breakthrough Infections among Vaccinated Individuals and Associated Risk Factors: A Systematic Review
Reprinted from: *Trop. Med. Infect. Dis.* **2022**, 7, 81, doi:10.3390/tropicalmed7050081 285

Tope Oyelade, Jaber S. Alqahtani, Ahmed M. Hjazi, Amy Li, Ami Kamila and Reynie Purnama Raya
Global and Regional Prevalence and Outcomes of COVID-19 in People Living with HIV: A Systematic Review and Meta-Analysis
Reprinted from: *Trop. Med. Infect. Dis.* **2022**, 7, 22, doi:10.3390/tropicalmed7020022 311

Caterina Ledda, Claudio Costantino, Giuseppe Motta, Rosario Cunsolo, Patrizia Stracquadanio, Giuseppe Liberti, et al.
SARS-CoV-2 mRNA Vaccine Breakthrough Infections in Fully Vaccinated Healthcare Personnel: A Systematic Review
Reprinted from: *Trop. Med. Infect. Dis.* **2022**, 7, 9, doi:10.3390/tropicalmed7010009 331

About the Editors

Peter A. Leggat

Professor Peter A. Leggat, AM, ADC, is currently a professor and the Co-Director of the World Health Organization (WHO) Collaborating Centre for Vector-borne and Neglected Tropical Diseases (AUS-131), College of Public Health, Medical and Veterinary Sciences, Division of Tropical Health and Medicine, James Cook University (JCU), Australia. He served as an elected staff member on the JCU Council from 2005 to 2018. He has served on his academic board since 2018 and is currently the Deputy Chairperson. Professor Leggat has more than three decades of experience in medicine and higher education in Australia and internationally. He is a specialist in public health medicine and is also president of the International Society of Travel Medicine and the Immediate Past President of The Australasian College of Tropical Medicine. At JCU, throughout his academic career, he has been seconded for various senior academic positions. A former Fulbright scholar, Professor Leggat has published more than 500 journal papers; more than 100 chapters; and more than 35 books, directories, and proceedings.

John Frean

John Frean holds qualifications in medicine and pathology from the University of the Witwatersrand and holds postgraduate qualifications from South African, British and Australian institutions. He currently holds senior positions in the National Institute for Communicable Diseases (NICD); has a joint academic appointment in the Wits Research Institute for Malaria, University of the Witwatersrand; and is an Extraordinary Lecturer in the Faculty of Veterinary Science, University of Pretoria. His research interest is in infectious diseases, particularly tropical, parasitic and zoonotic diseases.

Lucille Blumberg

Professor Lucille Blumberg is currently a consultant at Right to Care. She focuses on creating a One Health programme within RTC, especially for rabies, and responding to health emergencies in South Africa and its surrounding region. Until 30 September 2021, she was the Deputy Director at the National Institute for Communicable Diseases (NICD) of the National Health Laboratory Service, and the founding head of the Division of Public Health Surveillance and Response. She is currently a medical consultant for the Division for Outbreak Preparedness and Response (incudes the Travel Medicine Unit) and for the Centre for Emerging, Zoonotic and Parasitic Diseases, where her major focus is on malaria, rabies, viral haemorrhagic fevers, zoonotic diseases and travel-related infections. She has worked on a number of outbreaks, including rabies, avian influenza, cholera, typhoid and the LuJo virus. She is a medical graduate of the University of the Witwatersrand; an associate professor in the Department of Medical Microbiology at the University of Stellenbosch; and a lecturer in the Faculty of Veterinary Medicine. University of Pretoria, South Africa. She has specialist qualifications in clinical microbiology, travel medicine and infectious diseases.

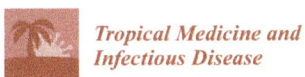

Editorial

COVID-19: Current Status and Future Prospects

Peter A. Leggat [1,2,3,*], John Frean [4] and Lucille Blumberg [4,5]

[1] World Health Organization Collaborating Centre for Vector-Borne and Neglected Tropical Diseases, College of Public Health, Medical and Veterinary Sciences, James Cook University, Townsville, QLD 4811, Australia
[2] School of Medicine, College of Medicine, Nursing and Health Sciences, University of Galway, H91 TK33 Galway, Ireland
[3] School of Public Health, Faculty of Health Sciences, University of the Witwatersrand, Johannesburg 2000, South Africa
[4] Centre for Emerging Zoonotic and Parasitic Diseases, National Institute for Communicable Diseases, Johannesburg 2131, South Africa
[5] Right to Care South Africa, Faculty of Veterinary Science University of Pretoria, Pretoria 0002, South Africa
* Correspondence: peter.leggat@jcu.edu.au; Tel.: +61-7-4781-6108

This second Special Issue in a series of Special Issues in *Tropical Medicine and Infectious Disease* looks at recent global research on the current Coronavirus (COVID-19) Pandemic. The disease is caused by a novel virus: severe acute respiratory syndrome coronavirus 2 (SARS-CoV-2) [1,2]. The International Committee on Taxonomy of Viruses (ICTV) named the virus SARS-CoV-2, as it is genetically related to the coronavirus responsible for the SARS outbreak of 2003 [2]. While related, the two viruses are quite different in their behaviour. At the time of submission for publication (9 January 2023), COVID-19, named by the World Health Organization (WHO) on 11 February 2020, caused more than 657 million cases and over 6.6 million deaths with over 430,000 new cases within the past 24 h [2].

The COVID-19 pandemic greatly affected the capacity of health systems in providing essential health care [1], but in response, there has been a remarkable and timely development of vaccines and laboratory tests, including rapid antigen tests. There has been a rigorous application and promotion of public health measures in many countries around the world. As of 6 January 2023, there have been more than 13 billion vaccine doses of COVID-19 vaccines administered [2], although there remains a question concerning how equitable their distribution is. Our knowledge has expanded on the pathogenesis and treatment of COVID-19 and experience gained within different countries, and this is reflected in the enormous number of scientific papers generated, including those in this Special Issue. There have been 24 papers published upon peer review acceptance in this Special Issue, including 17 research papers [3–19], 2 review papers [20,21], 1 opinion piece [22], 1 commentary [23], and 3 systematic reviews [24–26]. Each paper in this Special Issue contributes to our understanding of COVID-19.

The contributions of these 17 research papers can be summarized as follows. The first of the research papers aimed to explore the risk perception and prevention practices of coronavirus disease 2019 (COVID-19) among people living in high- and low-population density areas in Dhaka, Bangladesh. Interestingly, findings showed that participants were not concerned about COVID-19 and believed that coronavirus would not have a devastating impact on Bangladeshis; thus, they were reluctant to follow prevention measures and undergo testing [3]. The second study investigated the clinical features of severity and mortality among COVID-19 patients in Luanda, Angola. Fever (46%), cough (47%), gastrointestinal symptoms (26.7%), and asthenia (26.7%) were the most common symptoms. About 64.4% of the patients presented coexistent disorders, including hypertension (42%), diabetes (17%), and chronic renal diseases (6%) [4]. The third study assessed the characteristics, practices, and associated factors of self-medication (SM) by the public during the COVID-19 pandemic in Sargodha, Pakistan. Consciousness and understanding about the possible adverse effects of SM must be established and validated at a continuous level; in addition, at the commercial level, collaboration from pharmacists in not selling products (especially prescription-only medicines) without a certified prescription must be developed and implemented [5]. The fourth of these constructed a compartmental model with a time-dependent transmission rate that incorporates two sources of infection. The model was applied to the COVID-19 spread data from a university environment, namely, the Institut Teknologi Bandung, Indonesia, during its early reopening stage, with a constant number of students. The results show a significant fit between the rendered model and the recorded cases of infections [6]. The fifth of these analyzed the COVID-19 contact tracing dataset from 15 July to 31 December 2021 using multiple logistic regression analyses, considering exposure details, demographics, and vaccination history. Having symptoms, unprotected exposure, lower education level, and receiving low-potency vaccines increased the risk of laboratory-confirmed COVID-19 following healthcare-related exposure events. [7]. In the sixth of these, the cases and deaths for the four waves of COVID-19 in 119 countries and regions (CRs) were collected. They compared the mortality across CRs where populations experience different economic and healthcare disparities. The clinical outcomes in developing countries became worse along with the expansion of the pandemic [8]. The purpose of the seventh of these was to compare four commercial RT-qPCR assays with respect to their ability to detect the SARS-CoV2 virus from nasopharyngeal swab samples referred to Laboratorio Carvajal IPS, SAS in Tunja, Boyacá, Colombia. GeneFinderTM COVID-19 Plus RealAmp (GF-TM) and Berlin-modified protocols offer the best sensitivity and specificity, with similar results in comparison to the gold standard Berlin protocol [9]. The eighth of these explored the epidemiology of emerging variants of SARS-CoV-2 that circulated in Bangladesh from December 2020 to September 2021, representing the second and third waves. A rapid growth in the number of variants identified across Bangladesh showed virus adaptation and a lack of strict quarantine, prompting periodic genomic surveillance to foresee the spread of new variants, if any, and to take preventive measures as soon as possible [10]. The ninth was a document review of the health operations and technical expertise (HOTE) pillar coordination meetings' minutes, reports, policy, and strategy documents of the activities and outcomes and feedback on updates on the HOTE pillar given at regular intervals to the regional incident management support team of the World Health Organization regional office for Africa. The coordination mechanism appeared to be robust; some challenges included the duplication of coordination efforts, communication, documentation, and information management [11]. The tenth of these was the use of a triage strategy of routine COVID-19 testing for febrile patients with viral prodromes. All febrile patients with viral prodromes and no epidemiologic risk for COVID-19 were first admitted to a designated ward for COVID-19 testing. During successive COVID-19 pandemic waves in a dengue-endemic country, coinfection with dengue and COVID-19 was uncommon. [12]. The eleventh of these was a descriptive longitudinal study conducted for determining the community transmission of SARS-CoV-2 in high- and low-density areas in Dhaka city. No differences in the seropositivity rates depending on the population gradient were observed [13]. The twelfth study was conducted to determine the effectiveness of the combined use of remdesivir and regdanvimab in patients with severe COVID-19. In patients with severe COVID-19, clinical outcomes can be improved by administering regdanvimab in addition to remdesivir [14]. In the thirteenth study, the authors compared excess all-cause mortality and COVID-19 mortality in 25 Peruvian regions to determine whether most excess deaths in 2020 were attributable to COVID-19. Most excess deaths in Peru are related to COVID-19 [15]. The fourteenth study aimed to assess the magnitude of and factors associated with depression and anxiety among Vietnamese frontline hospital healthcare workers in the fourth wave of COVID-19. There was a relatively high prevalence among Vietnamese hospital healthcare workers exhibiting symptoms of depression and anxiety during the ongoing pandemic [16]. The fifteenth study explored the association between body mass index (BMI), the prevalence of overweight and obesity, and the COVID-19 mortality rates in 25 Peruvian regions, adjusted for confounding factors, using multiple linear regression. As obesity prevalence increases, COVID-19 mortality rates increase in the Peruvian population $\geq$ 15 years [17]. The sixteenth study reported on an autochthonous outbreak of SARS-CoV-2 P.1 variant infections in southern Italy in seven subjects who had not travelled to endemic areas or outside the Apulia region. The circulation of variants of concern highlights the importance of strictly monitoring the spread of SARS-CoV-2 variants using genomic surveillance and by investigating local outbreaks [18]. The goal of the last study was to determine the frequency of newly diagnosed diabetes mellitus (DM) and its different types among COVID-19 patients and to check the glycemic control in diabetic cases for three months. COVID-19 patients with newly diagnosed diabetes had a high risk of mortality [19].

There were two review papers in this Special Issue. The first of these was a review examining the coagulopathy of dengue and COVID-19, particularly looking at clinical considerations [20]. The objective of the second review was to describe the intimate relationship between the gastrointestinal tract, including the liver and pancreas, and the pathogenesis, clinical course, and outcomes of the COVID-19 pandemic. Patients with gastrointestinal autoimmune diseases require close follow-up visits and may need modifications in immunosuppression. Acute pancreatitis is a rare manifestation of COVID-19, but it must be considered in patients with abdominal pain. [21]. There are two other papers in this Special Issue. The first is an opinion piece examining the possible consequences of the overlapping of pulmonary fibrosis secondary to COVID-19 and tuberculosis in the setting of sub-Saharan Africa, the region of the world with the highest prevalence of helminth infection [22]. The second was a commentary on COVID-19 vaccine hesitancy in sub-Saharan Africa. The authors' overarching opinions were that political influences, religious beliefs, and low perceived risk exist in sub-Saharan Africa, and they collectively contribute to COVID-19 vaccine hesitancy [23]. There are also three systematic reviews. The first of these sought to assess breakthrough SARS-CoV-2 infections in vaccinated individuals by variant distribution and to identify common risk associations. It was found that continued mitigation approaches (e.g., wearing masks and social distancing) are warranted even in fully vaccinated individuals to prevent transmission [24]. The second systematic review aimed to assess the prevalence of people living with HIV (PLWH) among COVID-19 cases and whether HIV infection affects the risk of severe COVID-19 or related death at the global and continental level. Although there is a low prevalence of PLWH among COVID-19 cases, HIV infection may increase the severity of COVID-19 in Africa and increase the risk of death globally [25]. The last systematic review examined the risk of breakthrough infections in vaccinated individuals at a high risk of exposure, such as healthcare personnel (HCP). The authors' findings further support the published high effectiveness rates of mRNA vaccines in preventing SARS-CoV-2 infections among fully vaccinated HCP [26].

The diversity of papers, the depth of the topics, and the relative geographical reach of the authors in this Special Issue confirm the continued collective major interest in COVID-19. There are 253 contributors for the 24 papers published in this Special Issue with affiliations in Europe, Africa, North America, South America, and Asia-Pacific. This wide-ranging open access collection contributes to a much better understanding of the epidemiology, presentation, diagnosis, treatment, prevention, and control of COVID-19. As the editors of this Special Issue, we trust that you find the content valuable, as the authors are pleased to share their knowledge with an international audience.

We currently have another opportunity to update advances in this field via a third Special Issue, "COVID-19: Current Situation and Future Trends". We encourage you to publish your work in and/or propose a Special Issue for *Tropical Medicine and Infectious Disease*.

Acknowledgments: The Special Issue editors acknowledge all contributors to this Special Issue.

Conflicts of Interest: The authors declare no conflict of interest.

References

1. World Health Organization. Country and Technical Guidance—Coronavirus Disease (COVID-19). Available online: https://www.who.int/emergencies/diseases/novel-coronavirus-2019/technical-guidance (accessed on 10 January 2022).
2. World Health Organization. WHO Coronavirus Disease (COVID-19) Dashboard. Available online: https://covid19.who.int/ (accessed on 10 January 2022).
3. Satter, S.; Chowdhury, K.; Tamanna, R.; Abdullah, Z.; Shafique, S.; Islam, M.; Rimi, N.; Alam, M.; Nazneen, A.; Rahman, M.; et al. COVID-19 Risk Perception and Prevention Practices among High- and Low-Density Populations in Bangladesh: A Mixed-Methods Study. *Trop. Med. Infect. Dis.* **2022**, *7*, 447. [CrossRef]
4. Sebastião, C.; Cogle, A.; Teixeira, A.; Cândido, A.; Tchoni, C.; Amorim, M.; Loureiro, N.; Parimbelli, P.; Penha-Gonçalves, C.; Demengeot, J.; et al. Clinical Features Related to Severity and Mortality among COVID-19 Patients in a Pre-Vaccine Period in Luanda, Angola. *Trop. Med. Infect. Dis.* **2022**, *7*, 338. [CrossRef]
5. Chaudhry, B.; Azhar, S.; Jamshed, S.; Ahmed, J.; Khan, L.; Saeed, Z.; Madléna, M.; Gajdács, M.; Rasheed, A. Factors Associated with Self-Medication during the COVID-19 Pandemic: A Cross-Sectional Study in Pakistan. *Trop. Med. Infect. Dis.* **2022**, *7*, 330. [CrossRef]
6. Nuraini, N.; Sukandar, K.; Tahu, M.; Giri-Rachman, E.; Barlian, A.; Suhardi, S.; Pasaribu, U.; Yuliar, S.; Mudhakir, D.; Ariesyady, H.; et al. Infectious Disease Modeling with Socio-Viral Behavioral Aspects—Lessons Learned from the Spread of SARS-CoV-2 in a University. *Trop. Med. Infect. Dis.* **2022**, *7*, 289. [CrossRef]
7. Sripanidkulchai, K.; Rattanaumpawan, P.; Ratanasuwan, W.; Angkasekwinai, N.; Assanasen, S.; Werarak, P.; Navanukroh, O.; Phatharodom, P.; Tocharoenchok, T. A Risk Prediction Model and Risk Score of SARS-CoV-2 Infection Following Healthcare-Related Exposure. *Trop. Med. Infect. Dis.* **2022**, *7*, 248. [CrossRef]
8. Yao, L.; Graff, J.; Aleya, L.; Ma, J.; Cao, Y.; Wei, W.; Sun, S.; Wang, C.; Jiao, Y.; Gu, W.; et al. Mortality in Four Waves of COVID-19 Is Differently Associated with Healthcare Capacities Affected by Economic Disparities. *Trop. Med. Infect. Dis.* **2022**, *7*, 241. [CrossRef]
9. Salamanca-Neita, L.; Carvajal, Ó.; Carvajal, J.; Forero-Castro, M.; Segura, N. Comparison of Four Real-Time Polymerase Chain Reaction Assays for the Detection of SARS-CoV-2 in Respiratory Samples from Tunja, Boyacá, Colombia. *Trop. Med. Infect. Dis.* **2022**, *7*, 240. [CrossRef]
10. Sayeed, M.; Ferdous, J.; Saha, O.; Islam, S.; Choudhury, S.; Abedin, J.; Hassan, M.; Islam, A. Transmission Dynamics and Genomic Epidemiology of Emerging Variants of SARS-CoV-2 in Bangladesh. *Trop. Med. Infect. Dis.* **2022**, *7*, 197. [CrossRef]
11. Ngoy, N.; Conteh, I.; Oyugi, B.; Abok, P.; Kobie, A.; Phori, P.; Hamba, C.; Ejiofor, N.; Fitzwanga, K.; Appiah, J.; et al. Coordination and Management of COVID-19 in Africa through Health Operations and Technical Expertise Pillar: A Case Study from WHO AFRO One Year into Response. *Trop. Med. Infect. Dis.* **2022**, *7*, 183. [CrossRef]
12. Wee, L.; Conceicao, E.; Sim, J.; Aung, M.; Oo, A.; Yong, Y.; Arora, S.; Venkatachalam, I. Dengue and COVID-19: Managing Undifferentiated Febrile Illness during a "Twindemic". *Trop. Med. Infect. Dis.* **2022**, *7*, 68. [CrossRef]
13. Satter, S.; Bhuiyan, T.; Abdullah, Z.; Akhtar, M.; Akter, A.; Shafique, S.; Alam, M.; Chowdhury, K.; Nazneen, A.; Rimi, N.; et al. Transmission of SARS-CoV-2 in the Population Living in High- and Low-Density Gradient Areas in Dhaka, Bangladesh. *Trop. Med. Infect. Dis.* **2022**, *7*, 53. [CrossRef]
14. Chae, G.; Choi, A.; Lim, S.; Park, S.; Lee, S.; Ahn, Y.; Kim, J.; Ra, S.; Jegal, Y.; Ahn, J.; et al. The Effectiveness of the Use of Regdanvimab (CT-P59) in Addition to Remdesivir in Patients with Severe COVID-19: A Single Center Retrospective Study. *Trop. Med. Infect. Dis.* **2022**, *7*, 51. [CrossRef]
15. Ramírez-Soto, M.; Ortega-Cáceres, G. Analysis of Excess All-Cause Mortality and COVID-19 Mortality in Peru: Observational Study. *Trop. Med. Infect. Dis.* **2022**, *7*, 44. [CrossRef]
16. Doan, Q.; Tran, N.; Than, M.; Nguyen, H.; Bui, V.; Nguyen, D.; Vo, H.; Do, T.; Pham, N.; Nguyen, T.; et al. Depression, Anxiety and Associated Factors among Frontline Hospital Healthcare Workers in the Fourth Wave of COVID-19: Empirical Findings from Vietnam. *Trop. Med. Infect. Dis.* **2022**, *7*, 3. [CrossRef]
17. Ramírez-Soto, M.; Alarcón-Arroyo, M.; Chilcon-Vitor, Y.; Chirinos-Pérez, Y.; Quispe-Vargas, G.; Solsol-Jacome, K.; Quintana-Zavaleta, E. Association between Obesity and COVID-19 Mortality in Peru: An Ecological Study. *Trop. Med. Infect. Dis.* **2021**, *6*, 182. [CrossRef]
18. Loconsole, D.; Sallustio, A.; Centrone, F.; Casulli, D.; Ferrara, M.; Sanguedolce, A.; Accogli, M.; Chironna, M. An Autochthonous Outbreak of the SARS-CoV-2 P.1 Variant of Concern in Southern Italy, April 2021. *Trop. Med. Infect. Dis.* **2021**, *6*, 151. [CrossRef]
19. Farag, A.; Hassanin, H.; Soliman, H.; Sallam, A.; Sediq, A.; Abdelbaser, E.; Elbanna, K. Newly Diagnosed Diabetes in Patients with COVID-19: Different Types and Short-Term Outcomes. *Trop. Med. Infect. Dis.* **2021**, *6*, 142. [CrossRef]
20. Islam, A.; Cockcroft, C.; Elshazly, S.; Ahmed, J.; Joyce, K.; Mahfuz, H.; Islam, T.; Rashid, H.; Laher, I. Coagulopathy of Dengue and COVID-19: Clinical Considerations. *Trop. Med. Infect. Dis.* **2022**, *7*, 210. [CrossRef]
21. Aquino-Matus, J.; Uribe, M.; Chavez-Tapia, N. COVID-19: Current Status in Gastrointestinal, Hepatic, and Pancreatic Diseases; A Concise Review. *Trop. Med. Infect. Dis.* **2022**, *7*, 187. [CrossRef]
22. Fonte, L.; Acosta, A.; Sarmiento, M.; Norazmi, M.; Ginori, M.; de Armas, Y.; Calderón, E. Overlapping of Pulmonary Fibrosis of Postacute COVID-19 Syndrome and Tuberculosis in the Helminth Coinfection Setting in Sub-Saharan Africa. *Trop. Med. Infect. Dis.* **2022**, *7*, 157. [CrossRef]

23. Kabakama, S.; Konje, E.; Dinga, J.; Kishamawe, C.; Morhason-Bello, I.; Hayombe, P.; Adeyemi, O.; Chimuka, E.; Lumu, I.; Amuasi, J.; et al. Commentary on COVID-19 Vaccine Hesitancy in sub-Saharan Africa. *Trop. Med. Infect. Dis.* **2022**, *7*, 130. [CrossRef] [PubMed]
24. Gopinath, S.; Ishak, A.; Dhawan, N.; Poudel, S.; Shrestha, P.; Singh, P.; Xie, E.; Tahir, P.; Marzaban, S.; Michel, J.; et al. Characteristics of COVID-19 Breakthrough Infections among Vaccinated Individuals and Associated Risk Factors: A Systematic Review. *Trop. Med. Infect. Dis.* **2022**, *7*, 81. [CrossRef] [PubMed]
25. Oyelade, T.; Alqahtani, J.; Hjazi, A.; Li, A.; Kamila, A.; Raya, R. Global and Regional Prevalence and Outcomes of COVID-19 in People Living with HIV: A Systematic Review and Meta-Analysis. *Trop. Med. Infect. Dis.* **2022**, *7*, 22. [CrossRef] [PubMed]
26. Ledda, C.; Costantino, C.; Motta, G.; Cunsolo, R.; Stracquadanio, P.; Liberti, G.; Maltezou, H.; Rapisarda, V. SARS-CoV-2 mRNA Vaccine Breakthrough Infections in Fully Vaccinated Healthcare Personnel: A Systematic Review. *Trop. Med. Infect. Dis.* **2022**, *7*, 9. [CrossRef]

Disclaimer/Publisher's Note: The statements, opinions and data contained in all publications are solely those of the individual author(s) and contributor(s) and not of MDPI and/or the editor(s). MDPI and/or the editor(s) disclaim responsibility for any injury to people or property resulting from any ideas, methods, instructions or products referred to in the content.

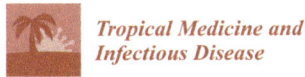

Article

COVID-19 Risk Perception and Prevention Practices among High- and Low-Density Populations in Bangladesh: A Mixed-Methods Study

Syed Moinuddin Satter [1,*,†], Kamal Ibne Amin Chowdhury [1,†], Refah Tamanna [1], Zarin Abdullah [1], S. M. Zafor Shafique [1], Md Saiful Islam [1,2], Nadia Ali Rimi [1], Muhammad Rashedul Alam [1], Arifa Nazneen [1], Mustafizur Rahman [1], Taufiqur Rahman Bhuiyan [1], Farzana Islam Khan [3], Mahbubur Rahman [3], A. S. M. Alamgir [3], Tahmina Shirin [3], Mahmudur Rahman [3,4], Firdausi Qadri [1], Meerjady Sabrina Flora [3] and Sayera Banu [1]

[1] Programme for Emerging Infections, Infectious Diseases Division, icddr,b, Dhaka 1212, Bangladesh
[2] School of Population Health, University of New South Wales, Sydney, NSW 1466, Australia
[3] Institute of Epidemiology, Disease Control and Research (IEDCR), Dhaka 1212, Bangladesh
[4] Global Health Development, EMPHNET, Dhaka 1212, Bangladesh
* Correspondence: dr.satter@icddrb.org; Tel.: +880-(0)2-2222-77001 to 10 (ext. 2590) or +880-1-7906658-68
† These authors contributed equally to this work.

Abstract: We aimed to explore coronavirus disease 2019 (COVID-19) risk perception and prevention practices among people living in high- and low-population density areas in Dhaka, Bangladesh. A total of 623 patients with confirmed COVID-19 agreed to participate in the survey. Additionally, we purposively selected 14 participants from diverse economic and occupational groups and conducted qualitative interviews for them accordingly. Approximately 70% of the respondents had low socioeconomic status. Among the 623 respondents, 146 were from low-density areas, and 477 were from high-density areas. The findings showed that study participants perceived COVID-19 as a punishment from the Almighty, especially for non-Muslims, and were not concerned about its severity. They also believed that coronavirus would not survive in hot temperatures or negatively impact Bangladeshis. This study revealed that people were reluctant to undergo COVID-19 testing. Family members hid if anyone tested positive for COVID-19 or did not adhere to institutional isolation. The findings showed that participants were not concerned about COVID-19 and believed that coronavirus would not have a devastating impact on Bangladeshis; thus, they were reluctant to follow prevention measures and undergo testing. Tailored interventions for specific targeted groups would be relevant in mitigating the prevailing misconceptions.

Keywords: socioeconomic status; risk perception; risk prevention practices; qualitative; COVID-19

Citation: Satter, S.M.; Chowdhury, K.I.A.; Tamanna, R.; Abdullah, Z.; Shafique, S.M.Z.; Islam, M.S.; Rimi, N.A.; Alam, M.R.; Nazneen, A.; Rahman, M.; et al. COVID-19 Risk Perception and Prevention Practices among High- and Low-Density Populations in Bangladesh: A Mixed-Methods Study. *Trop. Med. Infect. Dis.* **2022**, *7*, 447. https://doi.org/10.3390/tropicalmed7120447

Academic Editors: Peter A. Leggat, John Frean and Lucille Blumberg

Received: 9 November 2022
Accepted: 8 December 2022
Published: 19 December 2022

Publisher's Note: MDPI stays neutral with regard to jurisdictional claims in published maps and institutional affiliations.

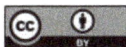

Copyright: © 2022 by the authors. Licensee MDPI, Basel, Switzerland. This article is an open access article distributed under the terms and conditions of the Creative Commons Attribution (CC BY) license (https://creativecommons.org/licenses/by/4.0/).

1. Introduction

Novel coronavirus disease 2019 (COVID-19), caused by severe acute respiratory syndrome coronavirus-2 (SARS-CoV-2), has become a global public health concern [1]. On 11 March 2020, the World Health Organization declared the COVID-19 outbreak a global pandemic [2]. As of 27 July 2022, 572 million confirmed cases of SARS-CoV-2 infection had caused 6.39 million deaths worldwide [3]. This novel virus is transmitted person-to-person via droplets and aerosols [4]. Population density [5] along with socioeconomic and cultural factors play an essential role in disease transmission and mortality [6].

Many COVID-19-affected countries have implemented various preventive measures, including national and zonal lockdowns, social distancing recommendations, isolation and quarantine of patients and contacts, guidelines for wearing facemasks, and recommendations for frequent handwashing to combat the spread of the virus [7]. South Asia's lower-middle-income countries have taken initiatives to curb the rapid transmission of the virus [8]. India enacted the "Janata curfew" on 22 March 2020, and a 21-day complete lockdown starting on 25 March 2020 [8]. The Government of Bangladesh declared a national lockdown between 26 March and 30 May 2020, in the form of general holidays [9]. The GoB restricted mass gatherings, implemented bans on passenger movement on roads, water, and rail, suspended international and domestic flights, closed schools and colleges, and shut businesses, except for critical businesses and services [9]. People were requested to stay at home and maintain social distancing [9].

Adherence to public health measures is affected by beliefs, attitudes, and risk perception [10,11]. In a study in India, it was found that 90% of the respondents had knowledge about the name and origin, mode of transmission, symptoms, and prevention control of the virus, and they maintained the recommended measures, such as staying at home, elbow sneezing, maintaining social distancing, and wearing masks. However, there was a lack of perception. Of the respondents, 33.9% perceived that eating garlic could not prevent COVID-19, and 37.9% believed that the breath-holding test could not diagnose COVID-19 [12].

In Bangladesh, the first confirmed case was reported on 8 March 2020 [8], and as of 5 October 2020, the highest reported cases (64%) and highest reported deaths (50%) were in the Dhaka division [13]. In locations with a high population density, we do not know how people perceive the risk of respiratory infection or the benefits of non-pharmaceutical interventions. This is crucial, as in Dhaka, approximately 6 lakh people live in high-density areas where almost 75% of households share one room [14,15]. Moreover, because of shared toilets and kitchens, common water sources, and a lack of education, people living in these areas are more likely to be exposed to this virus [15]. Our study aimed to explore risk perception and prevention practices among high- and low-density populations in Dhaka, Bangladesh, during the COVID-19 pandemic.

2. Materials and Methods

2.1. Study Sites, Design, and Sampling

From July to September 2020, a multidisciplinary team comprising social scientists and epidemiologists conducted a cross-sectional study in Dhaka, Bangladesh. The team selected six high-density areas and seven low-density areas of Dhaka City for evaluation. High-density areas were horizontally shared spaces, with more than five people living in a 9–12 by 6–8-foot room (according to one of our ongoing studies, PR-20005). Low-density areas were areas with high-rise buildings and apartments.

We located symptomatic and asymptomatic laboratory-confirmed index cases in the community through the "Transmission Dynamics of COVID-19 in Bangladesh" study (PR-20005). The contacts of these patients were traced for enrollment, data collection, and sample collection. If any of the cases reported having neighborhood contacts, the team validated them based on the operational definition of contacts (a person who experienced face-to-face contact within 1 m and for more than 15 min, including travel, gossip, tea stall activity, or direct physical contact) between 2 days before and 14 days after the onset of symptoms in a confirmed COVID-19 case. The team developed a list of contacts for each case and validated it using phone calls or in-person visits. For qualitative interviews, we selected participants from diverse economic and occupational groups. The influential and informative persons of selected communities (i.e., ward counselors, ward members, community leaders, members of community-based organizations, schoolteachers, and religious leaders) who kept detailed updates of ongoing activities in their communities were considered to be study participants.

We adopted the WHO First Few X Cases and Contacts (FFX) Protocol (Version: 2, Date: 10 February 2020) that guided the B1 form for our survey [16]. The team also developed, piloted, and revised the interview guidelines before administration. The field team, consisting of five social scientists, received training on the study design, data collection, participant enrollment, interviewing, recording, note-taking, and data transcription. The field team also had several years of experience working on emerging infections.

2.2. Data Collection Methods and Techniques

We asked each contact for written informed consent and enrolled those who agreed to participate in the study. Survey interviews (conducted face-to-face or by mobile phone, depending on the respondent's preference) were conducted to collect information on socioeconomic status, water safety, sanitation and hygiene (WASH) practices, and behavioral patterns related to coronavirus.

Through in-depth interviews (IDIs), we collected information on participants' perceived understanding of COVID-19 and their knowledge of transmission pathways, their infection prevention practices, perceived and real challenges in maintaining prevention practices, experiences regarding treatment facilities (if any), opinions on isolation and lockdown, the impact of social stigma due to infection (if observed or faced), and the impact of lockdown on them and their households. Each IDI lasted for an average of 60 min and was recorded using an audio recorder. One note-taker was assigned to take notes, document non-verbal responses, and ensure tape recording.

Kuppuswamy's socioeconomic scale (SES) is the most widely used scale for urban populations. We used a score of 3–29. This scale was developed based on a composite score of the family head's education, occupation, and monthly family income. It was classified as high, middle, or low SES (Table 1).

Table 1. Modified Kuppuswamy's Socioeconomic Scale [17,18].

	Score
Education	
Professional Degree	7
Graduate	6
Diploma	5
Higher Secondary Certificate	4
Secondary School Certificate	3
Primary School Certificate	2
Illiterate	1
Occupation	
Profession	10
Self-employed	6
Clerical, shop-owner, farmer	5
Skilled worker	4
Semi-skilled worker or driver	3
Unskilled worker or labor or rickshaw puller	2
Unemployed	1
Family income per month (in BDT)	
≥60,001	12
30,001–60,000	10
15,001–30,000	5
12,001–15,000	4
9001–12,000	3
3001–9000	2
≤3000	1
Socioeconomic class	
Upper/High	26–29
Upper Middle	16–25
Lower Middle	11–15
Poor	5–10
Extreme poor or Below the poverty line	0–4

2.3. Data Processing and Analysis

All categorical variables collected from the survey were summarized using frequencies and percentages. Continuous numeric variables using mean and standard deviation and variables without a normal distribution were presented as medians and interquartile ranges.

Tape-recorded discussions during the qualitative interviews were transcribed in Bengali. The accuracy and consistency of the data were ensured as the researchers cross-checked the transcripts of the interviews.

We sought assistance from Colaizzi's phenomenological analysis method [19] and analyzed the qualitative data. Two anthropologists reviewed the data separately and identified themes and sub-themes that were shared among all the authors for discussion and consensus.

2.4. Patient and Public Involvement

The study participants or associated persons were not involved in the design, conduct, reporting, or dissemination plans of this study.

2.5. Ethics Statement

The Institutional Review Board of icddr,b (PR-20066) reviewed and approved the study protocol. The Bill and Melinda Gates Foundation (BMGF) reviewed and relied on the IRB approval of icddr,b.

3. Results

3.1. Survey Results

Among the 623 respondents who participated in our survey, 146 (23%) were from low-density areas and 477 (77%) were from high-density areas. A total of 288 (46%) were males and 335 (54%) were females. The mean age was 28.54 years, with a standard deviation of 15.24. A total of 238 respondents (38%) reported having completed primary education, 180 (29%) had completed secondary education, 44 (7%) had higher secondary education, and 161 (26%) had no institutional education. A total of 157 (25%) were service holders, 97 (17%) were dependent on daily wages for their livelihood, 52 (8%) ran small-scale businesses in their locality, 34 (5%) were unemployed, 157 (25%) were housewives, and 126 (20%) were students (Table 2).

Table 2. Distribution and comparison of demographic characteristics among infected and non-infected contacts.

Characteristic	Infected Contacts, (n = 74) n (%)	Uninfected Contacts, (n = 549) n (%)	p
Density			
Low	25 (33.8)	121 (22.0)	<0.05
High	49 (66.2)	428 (78.0)	
Age, years			
<18	17 (23.0)	162 (29.5)	
18–25	22 (29.7)	105 (19.1)	>0.05
26–60	32 (43.2)	268 (48.8)	
>60	3 (4.1)	14 (2.6)	
Sex			
Male	25 (33.8)	263 (47.9)	<0.05
Female	49 (66.2)	286 (52.1)	
Education			
No education	11 (14.9)	150 (27.3)	
Primary	37 (50.0)	201 (36.6)	<0.05
Secondary	23 (31.1)	157 (28.6)	
Higher Secondary	2 (2.7)	26 (4.7)	
Graduate and above	1 (1.4)	15 (2.7)	
Occupation			
Service	19 (25.7)	138 (25.1)	
Business	6 (8.1)	46 (8.4)	>0.05
Self-employed (independent workers, employers)	9 (12.2)	88 (16.0)	

Table 2. *Cont.*

Characteristic	Infected Contacts, (n = 74) n (%)	Uninfected Contacts, (n = 549) n (%)	p
Dependent	40 (54.1)	277 (50.5)	
Religion			
Muslim	73 (99.0)	545 (99.2)	>0.05
Hindu	1 (1.0)	4 (0.8)	
Household size (median, range)	4 (1–14)	4 (1–14)	
Household size			
≤4 members	54 (73.0)	355 (64.7)	>0.05
>4 members	20 (27.0)	194 (35.3)	
No. of bedrooms (median, range)	1 (1–3)	1 (1–5)	
Average size of bedroom, sft (median, range)	120 (30–180)	120 (30–400)	
Sharing bedroom	71 (95.9)	529 (96.4)	>0.05
No. of family members sharing one bedroom (median, range)	3 (2–7)	3 (1–20)	
Average monthly income, BDT	17,939	17,846	
Average monthly expenditure, BDT	15,202	15,214	

3.1.1. Socioeconomic Status

Three families (0.5%) had high socioeconomic status, 76 (12.2%) had upper-middle socioeconomic status, 110 (17.7%) had lower status, 411 (66%) had poor socioeconomic status, and 23 (3.7%) had extremely poor socioeconomic status (Table 3).

Table 3. Distribution of SES among neighborhood contacts in low-density and high-density areas.

Characteristic	Low-Density (n = 146) n (%)	High-Density (n = 477) n (%)	p
Upper/High	3 (2.1)	0 (0.0)	
Upper Middle	28 (19.2)	48 (10.1)	
Lower Middle	29 (19.9)	81 (17.0)	<0.05
Poor	83 (56.8)	328 (68.8)	
Extremely poor or Below the poverty line	3 (2.1)	20 (4.2)	

3.1.2. Water, Sanitation, and Hygiene (WASH) Access, Behavior, and Practices

The proportion of respondents who reported the use of improved sanitation facilities was significantly higher among low-density contacts (LD vs. HD, 56% vs. 25%, $p = 0.0001$), while the perceived importance of handwashing after urination and defecation and before eating was significantly lower among low-density contacts (LD vs. HD, 43% vs. 81%, $p = 0.001$) (LD vs. HD, 51% vs. 90%, $p = 0.001$) (Table 4).

Table 4. Comparison of WASH practices among neighborhood contacts in low-density and high-density areas.

Characteristic	Low-Density (n = 146) n (%)	High-Density (n = 477) n (%)	p
Drinking water sources			
Tube-well	9 (6.2)	32 (6.7)	<0.05
Supply	118 (80.8)	424 (88.9)	
Drinks purified water	98 (67.1)	325 (68.1)	>0.05
Purification of water	77 (52.7)	206 (56.2)	>0.05
Actions are taken for purifying water			
Boil	74 (96.1)	240 (89.6)	>0.05
Use a water filter/gravel/ceramic/sand	1 (1.3)	18 (6.7)	

Table 4. Cont.

Characteristic	Low-Density (n = 146) n (%)	High-Density (n = 477) n (%)	p
Water source for drinking looks clean	143 (97.9)	442 (92.7)	>0.05
Hand washing station at home	145 (99.3)	476 (99.8)	>0.05
Hand washing duration, seconds (median, range)	20 (4–600)	20 (3–200)	
Assumption on hand washing duration (median, range)	20 (3–600)	20 (0–200)	
Use of sanitizer and soap after coming back home	141 (96.6)	460 (96.4)	>0.05
Frequency of hand washing in a day			
1–2 times	11 (13.9)	15 (3.1)	
3–4 times	35 (44.3)	119 (24.9)	<0.05
>4 times	33 (41.8)	343 (71.9)	
Assumption on occasions important for hand washing *			
Before eating	75 (51.4)	428 (89.7)	<0.05
Before feeding a child	11 (7.5)	46 (9.6)	>0.05
Before cooking /preparing/serving food	28 (19.2)	148 (31.0)	<0.05
After defecation/urination	63 (43.2)	385 (80.7)	<0.05
After cleaning a child that has defecated/changing nappies/washing diaper	12 (8.2)	23 (4.8)	>0.05
Toilet facility			
Improved sanitation facilities	82 (56.2)	118 (24.7)	<0.05
Shared sanitation facilities	64 (43.8)	353 (74.0)	
Unimproved sanitation facilities	0 (0.0)	6 (1.3)	
No. of household members/toilet (median, range)	7 (1–212)	12 (1–100)	
Frequency of cleaning toilet per day (median, range)	0 (0–7)	0 (0–2)	
Frequency of cleaning toilet per week (median, range)	2 (0–21)	2 (0–30)	
Hand washing station availability	136 (93.2)	439 (92.0)	>0.05
Soap or detergent availability	142 (97.3)	464 (97.3)	>0.05
Surface of house/floor			
Cement	79 (100.0)	456 (95.6)	>0.05
Other	0 (0.0)	21 (4.4)	
Options for cleaning floor			
Sweeping	34 (43.0)	121 (25.4)	<0.05
Mopping	44 (55.7)	355 (74.4)	
Surface of yard			
Cement	76 (96.2)	337 (70.6)	<0.05
Soil	3 (3.8)	59 (12.4)	
Options for cleaning yard			
Sweeping	61 (77.2)	380 (84.3)	<0.05
Mopping	15 (19.0)	53 (11.8)	

* multiple responses.

Cleaning their clothing after coming home from outside every day was found to be significantly higher among high-density contacts (LD vs. HD, 60% vs. 73%, $p = 0.02$), while social distancing maintained by low-density contacts was significantly higher (LD vs. HD, 70% vs. 54%, $p = 0.03$) (Table 5).

Table 5. Comparison of behavioral change of neighborhood contacts in low-density and high-density areas.

Characteristic	Low-Density ($n = 146$) n (%)	High-Density ($n = 477$) n (%)	p
Infection			
Uninfected contacts	121 (82.9)	428 (89.7)	<0.05
Infected contacts	25 (17.1)	49 (10.3)	
Frequently touch face/eyes/nose	59 (40.4)	182 (38.2)	>0.05
Practices during coughing/sneezing			
Cover face with hands/elbow before coughing or sneezing	84 (57.5)	286 (60.0)	
Cover face with tissue or handkerchief	36 (24.7)	94 (19.7)	>0.05
Nothing is done	11 (7.5)	54 (11.3)	
Others	15 (10.3)	43 (9.0)	
Mask use outside every time	128 (87.7)	422 (88.5)	>0.05
Type of mask			
Face mask/surgical single-use mask	22 (31.9)	142 (31.8)	>0.05
Cloth mask	46 (66.7)	286 (64.0)	
Frequency of cleaning mask (times/day)			
0	22 (31.9)	186 (41.6)	
1	43 (62.3)	252 (56.4)	<0.05
2	4 (5.7)	9 (2.0)	
Difficulty wearing mask	65 (44.5)	218 (45.7)	>0.05
Cleaning of outside clothes everyday	87 (59.6)	350 (73.4)	<0.05
Social distancing maintained	102 (69.9)	257 (53.9)	<0.05
Difficult behavioral changes due to SARS CoV-2			
Do not rub hands over face/eyes/nose	26 (17.8)	39 (8.2)	<0.05
Wear mask outside of home	48 (32.9)	198 (41.5)	>0.05
Cover face with elbow before coughing or sneezing	18 (12.3)	46 (9.6)	>0.05
Wash hands with soap/use sanitizer after coming home from outside	12 (8.2)	27 (5.7)	>0.05
Perceived positive behavioral change can protect from COVID-19	127 (87.0)	397 (83.2)	>0.05

3.2. Findings of Anthropological Exploration

Fourteen individuals (10 males, three females, and one transgender individual) participated in the qualitative study. Six of them were from high-density areas and eight were from low-density areas (Table 6).

Among them, seven reported running small-scale businesses in their locality; three were service holders, one was a school teacher, and one was unemployed. The other par-ticipant was a health worker who had good acceptance in the community. Moreover, among these participants, one was a ward member who had an active influence on the community through various social activities during the lockdown period. Additionally, two were social workers and community leaders. The mean age of the participants was 38 years (range, 26–48 years). Five had a graduate degree, one had received higher secondary-level education, two had received secondary education, five had received prima-ry-level education, and one did not have any institutional education. The religious back-ground of all participants was Islam.

Table 6. Socio-demographic profile of the qualitative interviewees.

Characteristics	Frequency (n)	Percentage (%)
Gender		
Male	10	71.4
Female	3	21.4
Transgender	1	7.1

Table 6. *Cont.*

Characteristics	Frequency (*n*)	Percentage (%)
Age group (years)		
21–30	5	35.7
31–40	5	35.7
41–50	4	28.6
Marital status		
Married	12	85.7
Single	2	14.3
Religion		
Islam	14	100.0
Educational level		
Illiterate	1	7.1
<Secondary	5	35.7
Secondary	2	14.3
>Secondary	6	42.9
Occupation		
Employed	6	42.9
Unemployed	1	7.1
Business	7	50.0
Place of residence		
High density	6	42.9
Low-density	8	57.1

3.3. Risk Perception

3.3.1. Beliefs in Supernatural Power

The participants shared a common belief that the Almighty had created the coronavirus. Participants with limited or no institutional education did not consider COVID-19 a disease; instead, they believed that it was a punishment from the Almighty. Participants shared a firm belief that, since Bangladesh was a Muslim country, most people living there followed the Islamic ideology and Islamic-prohibited deeds were restricted there; therefore, the virus would not infect the people of Bangladesh.

The participants also believed that the coronavirus would infect non-Muslim people. Despite using the term "non-Muslim," they specified the population as those who eat snakes, frogs, and scorpions. One participant from a low-density site or community stated that during the initial stage of COVID-19, there was a widespread belief in their community that COVID-19 would not enter a Muslim country. He also expressed that community members had a firm belief in Huzur's (the mosque's Imam) words. They did not want to maintain social distancing and protective measures following Huzur's statements, as initially, Huzur mentioned that coronavirus would not enter a Muslim country and that Muslim people would not be affected by coronavirus.

A 27-year-old male participant who was a service holder from a low-density area stated the following:

"I am not against Huzur. However, the first mistake we made was a prevailing conception that Muslim people will not be infected by corona. Those who eat snakes, frogs, and scorpions will be infected. Besides, maintaining lockdown and restrictions were hampered because people obey Huzur's words ten times more than regulation!"

The participants also perceived that coronavirus was first reported in China during the winter season. As it was summer in Bangladesh at the time of the interview, they believed that the coronavirus would not survive or be transmitted.

A 33-year-old female participant who was a social worker from a high-density area stated,

"If it could do anything, then there would have been a procession of corpses."

Those who believed that coronavirus depended on God's will were also unwilling to maintain social distancing and personal protective equipment.

3.3.2. The Reluctance to Maintain Preventive Measures

Participants conveyed that there was an indifferent tendency regarding the use of protective measures. There was a lack of adherence to preventive measures, and community members were less inclined to maintain them.

A 48-year-old male participant who ran a small business in a high-density area stated:

"I saw rural people using a bamboo-made mask for domestic cows. Why would I wear such things that are used for cows?"

People who belonged to low socioeconomic status groups and were engaged in services (those who ran a general store, shop in the bazaar, or tea stall) where they needed to deal with the general population were less inclined to wear masks.

A 45-year-old male participant who was a small-scale businessman from a low-density area mentioned:

"If I wear a mask all the time, customers do not understand properly what I was responding to them."

In low-density areas, people with low socioeconomic status are unwilling to maintain preventive measures. They perceived that as they lived from hand to mouth, God was more merciful to them, and, therefore, they would not be infected by the coronavirus.

One participant in a high-density area stated that most of her neighbors preferred to die rather than maintain preventive measures. People with low socioeconomic status in low-density areas were unwilling to maintain social distancing or follow lockdowns. Middle- and lower-middle-class people were worried that if they did not earn a livelihood, they would die of hunger.

A 45-year-old male participant who ran a small-scale business in a low-density area stated the following:

"We would rather die in corona but not out of hunger."

3.4. Perceived Reasons for Non-Adherence to Preventive Measures

3.4.1. Financial Insolvency

Participants stated that financial constraints hindered the maintenance of protective measures. One participant said that buying masks and sanitizing hands with soap were beyond their affordability. One participant from a high-density area stated that he needed to think several times before buying a mask because a mask would cost at least BDT 15 (USD 0.2), which was expensive for him.

Participants also mentioned their struggle to maintain isolation, even if their families had any patients who tested positive for COVID-19. All participants from high-density areas reported living in a single room with their families. They could not afford multiple rooms or spacious houses. Therefore, if any family members tested COVID-19-positive, they were unable to maintain isolation.

A 40-year-old male participant, a small-scale businessman from a high-density area, stated:

"I, along with my four family members, live in a single room. My neighbors as well as most of the families in our community, live in 10 feet by 10 feet single room where 6–9 members are living along."

According to the participants, community members were unwilling to undergo the COVID-19 diagnosis test because of their financial hardship.

A 26-year-old male participant who was unemployed and from a high-density area stated the following:

"As it requires 3000–4000 taka (USD 35.71–47.61) for COVID-19 test, it is impossible for the lower-middle-class people to bear these expenses."

3.4.2. Existing Rumors in the Community Regarding COVID-19

Participants opined that the prevailing rumors might increase anxiety among community members and force them to maintain preventive measures. They perceived that if they were positive for COVID-19, they would be taken away to the hospital, would not be able to return home anymore, and would be killed with injections. According to some participants (3/14), the rumor was that if they became positive, they would either be kept in isolation or taken away by the police, and the whole area would be locked down. They would be detached from their family and friends and would not be able to earn money to continue their livelihoods.

A 48-year-old male participant who ran a small-scale business from a low-density area mentioned:

> *"The most common rumor in our community is that people think if someone tested positive for COVID-19, she/he would be taken away to Dhaka Medical College hospital and killed by pushing injection. We heard people are dying in hospitals for lack of treatment, oxygen, and food, etc."*

3.5. Prevention Practices during COVID-19

Participants stated that government and non-government organizations disseminated preventive messages during the initial stage of COVID-19 and initiated restrictions, such as one-meter physical distancing and isolation. When these restrictions stopped, people became indifferent to maintaining social distancing, began roaming outdoors, and gathered for leisure time.

3.5.1. Handwashing

Participants in low-density areas stated that during the lockdown period, people became habituated to washing their hands and were used to maintaining this seriously. People panicked, and they did this out of excitement (*Hujug*). One participant said that there were arrangements for washing hands at essential points, such as the marketplace, and that people had to practice handwashing. In addition, people wash their hands after returning home from outside. However, these practices gradually faded.

3.5.2. Use of a Mask

One participant in the low-density area said that most people in his community were not inclined to wear masks unless there was a fear of police or community leaders reinforcing wearing them while going outside. He also said that some people perceived that wearing masks would spread more viruses. He opined that one of the reasons was illiteracy, and the other was religious influence. In the beginning, he noted that religious leaders told people that if they wore masks, they would be safe. However, later in mosques, *Wazz Mahfil* and *Boyan*, the *Huzurs* stated,

> *"Nothing will happen. If God gives sickness, there will be nothing to do."*

People were not inclined to wear masks initially, but later they realized this and prioritized them. A 26-year-old male participant who was unemployed and from a high-density area stated that 95% of the people were not self-conscious and less prone to wearing masks in his community. During the initial period of COVID-19, death and infection rates were broadcast on television as breaking news. Participants became tensed and panicked accordingly. However, when this briefing stopped, people started assuming that everything had returned to "normal." He also added that only a limited number of people were still concerned, as the educational institutions remained closed, and when all these opened, people started thinking that everything was as expected.

One participant in the high-density area said that in his community, most people had no educational background and were less inclined to accept the gruesomeness of the virus. He also stated that people between the ages of 40 and 50 were unwilling to maintain preventive practices. They just agreed during counseling but later did not maintain it.

3.5.3. Maintaining Social Distancing

One participant in the low-density area stated that people later realized the importance of social distancing. They were not serious about COVID-19 in the initial period and did not believe that the coronavirus would affect Bangladesh. He also added that people maintained social distancing during the lockdown period, and in some cases, they were forced to do so.

3.5.4. Not going Outside the Home

A 27-year-old male participant who was a service holder from a low-density area stated that when there was a tense situation regarding the coronavirus, people were serious about it and tended to go out less. However, because they stayed home for a long time, people started feeling uncomfortable, and the rules were not appropriately maintained.

Participants also mentioned that they used to go outside the home only during emergencies, such as buying rice, vegetables, and baby food, while wearing masks.

A 29-year-old female participant, who was a schoolteacher from a low-density area, mentioned:

"I went outside for an important purpose, not for roaming aimlessly."

3.5.5. Isolation of Infected People at Home

One participant in the low-density area stated that people belonging to the middle and lower-middle classes did not want to reveal whether they were COVID-19-positive because of an inferiority complex. He also added that the isolation of a person positive for COVID-19 was not appropriately maintained.

A participant from a high-density area who was COVID-19-positive stated that she could not maintain proper isolation during that period. She shared a bed with her husband and her four-year-old daughter. She said that she did not have any other options; she neither had her own house nor the capability to rent a house outside this area.

One participant in the high-density area shared a community incident: a ward counselor wanted to arrange a separate room for the isolation of 4–5 people who tested positive for COVID-19, but their family members would not allow them to live separately. The family members thought that the COVID-19-positive person would not be adequately cared for if they lived separately.

3.5.6. Raising Awareness, Providing Financial and other Required Support

All participants reported awareness-raising initiatives in both high- and low-density communities, such as distributing masks, setting up handwashing stations, distributing leaflets, spraying disinfectants, and raising awareness by motivating community members to maintain hygiene.

In high-density communities, several organizations such as Building Resources Across Communities (BRAC), Dushtha Sasthya Kendra (DSK), and other anonymous foreign initiatives helped people by providing food (rice, oil, and potatoes), protective equipment (masks and soaps), and financial aid so that people in the lower-middle-class could remain at home and did not need to go out to earn their livelihood. It was also reported that the solvent families of low-density communities provided food packages, including rice, oil, and onions, to their insolvent neighbors.

4. Discussion

This study explored the risk perceptions and prevention practices during the COVID-19 pandemic in low- and high-density areas. The findings showed that participants were not concerned about COVID-19 and believed that the coronavirus would not have a devastating impact on Bangladeshis. The participants highlighted that Almighty Allah would save Muslims. They also believed that Bangladesh's warm weather would create a barrier to the widespread transmission of COVID-19. Protective measures were not accepted as practical or feasible. Substantial misinformation and rumors in the community regarding government containment strategies and day-to-day dissemination of death and infection rates through authentic electronic media of the government were reported. Moreover, this study revealed that people were reluctant to undergo COVID-19 testing. Family members hid information about being COVID-19-positive and avoided complying with institutional isolation, which has the potential for household transmission.

Participants' prevention practice was influenced by their perception. They perceived that COVID-19 was a punishment from God. A study conducted in another Muslim country showed that 73.5% of Arab residents believed that COVID-19 was a dangerous disease [20]. In a study, researchers showed that people's religious and ethical beliefs affect their coping mechanisms for disease and treatment regime [21]. Researchers also showed that people usually follow their religious coping behavior (e.g., faith in God, prayer, help, and strength from God) to deal with stressful situations.

Safe water, sanitation, and hygiene are required to protect against this virus [22]. The findings showed that most respondents consumed purified water for drinking and used sanitizers and soap after returning home from outside (Table 4). This may be due to government intervention. Although evidence of the effectiveness of face masks as a prevention measure [23] is still a topic of debate, a significant proportion (88%) of our study participants mentioned that they consistently used masks outdoors (Table 5). One study suggested that early public interest in facemasks may be an essential factor in controlling the COVID-19 epidemic on a population scale. Social distancing is regarded as the most effective measure for disease mitigation [24]. Most countries have focused on social distancing based on experiences gathered from China [25]. Participants from a previous study [26] believed that social distancing and the use of facemasks could break the chain of COVID-19 spread. However, according to our study participants, protective measures such as wearing a mask, sanitizing hands with soap, and maintaining social distancing were not accepted as practical and feasible. These findings are in line with a study conducted in Nepal [27], where the authors showed that the high population density in South Asia's urban areas makes it difficult for people to maintain social distancing. A study conducted in Nepal [28] revealed a gap in knowledge regarding social distancing and quarantine; however, a positive perception of universal safety measures for COVID-19 has been reported. Another study [29] also shared participants' poor knowledge of preventive measures.

Misinformation and rumors regarding government containment strategies, lockdowns, institutional isolation, and treatment management of patients admitted to hospitals during the early period of the pandemic were prevalent in communities. Similarly, a study conducted in India [30] reported gaps in the correct perception of knowledge and the propagation of myths and misconceptions. This finding suggests the need for educational programs to address misconceptions. Other studies [31–34] have also reported misconceptions regarding this disease. This study also found that community members did not trust the government's daily announcements of deaths or infection rates. They perceived that the government announced an estimated number rather than an accurate one. Accurate information shared by the media plays a role in shaping people's perceptions of the risk of COVID-19 transmission; a lack of accessibility to this information can serve as a barrier [35]. Studies conducted in India and northern Iraq have also reported the spread of fake news on social media [12,36]. This study also revealed that due to the financial hardship and misinformation prevalent in the community, people were reluctant to undergo COVID-19 testing.

There is available evidence that individuals change their behaviors, and increasingly rely on social media influencers, especially during the pandemic situation. However, one of the limitations of this study was that it was out of scope to share the relationship between social media usage and COVID-19.

5. Conclusions

This study portrays the diverse perceptions of people belonging to different socioeconomic backgrounds. It also reveals that people's practices are influenced by their attitudes and perceptions of disease and risk. In our study, we found that those who had negative and apathetic perceptions of the disease were less likely to maintain safety measures. Moreover, religious beliefs and issues were found to play a crucial role in driving people toward new practices. Our findings suggest the need for feasible and effective health education programs that include religious leaders and could be aimed at enhancing people's disease-related knowledge, thereby helping them to perceive such diseases properly and maintain safe practices accordingly.

Author Contributions: Conceptualization, S.M.S., K.I.A.C., Z.A., T.R.B., M.R. (Mahmudur Rahman), F.Q., M.S.F. and S.B.; Methodology, S.M.S., K.I.A.C., Z.A., M.S.I. and M.S.F.; Software, K.I.A.C. and M.R.A.; Validation, K.I.A.C., S.M.Z.S., N.A.R., M.R. (Mustafizur Rahman), T.R.B., F.I.K., M.R. (Mahbubur Rahman), A.S.M.A., T.S., M.R. (Mahmudur Rahman), F.Q., M.S.F. and S.B.; Formal analysis, K.I.A.C., R.T., M.S.I. and N.A.R.; Investigation, K.I.A.C., R.T., Z.A. and A.N.; Resources, R.T. and S.M.Z.S.; Data curation, K.I.A.C., R.T., S.M.Z.S. and A.N.; Writing—original draft, S.M.S., K.I.A.C., R.T., S.M.Z.S., M.R.A. and F.Q.; Writing—review & editing, S.M.S., K.I.A.C., Z.A., M.S.I., N.A.R., A.N., M.R. (Mustafizur Rahman), T.R.B., F.I.K., M.R. (Mahbubur Rahman), A.S.M.A., T.S., M.R. (Mahmudur Rahman), F.Q., M.S.F. and S.B.; Visualization, R.T., S.M.Z.S., M.R.A., A.N. and M.R. (Mahmudur Rahman); Supervision, S.M.S., K.I.A.C., Z.A., M.R. (Mustafizur Rahman), A.S.M.A., T.S., M.R. (Mahmudur Rahman), F.Q. and S.B.; Project administration, K.I.A.C., Z.A. and S.B.; Funding acquisition, S.M.S., F.Q. and S.B. All authors have read and agreed to the published version of the manuscript.

Funding: The research was funded by the Bill and Melinda Gates Foundation (Grant number: INV-017556).

Institutional Review Board Statement: The study protocol (PR-20066) was reviewed and approved by icddr,b's Research and Ethical Review Committees.

Informed Consent Statement: Informed consent was obtained from all subjects involved in the study.

Data Availability Statement: Data cannot be shared publicly because they are confidential. Data are available from the respective department of icddr,b for researchers who meet the criteria for access to confidential data.

Acknowledgments: The authors would like to thank the Bill and Melinda Gates Foundation, the Ministry of Health and Family Welfare (MOHFW) of Bangladesh, and the Institute of Epidemiology, Disease Control and Research (IEDCR) for their continuous support. We thank all the study participants for their time and support. The authors would also like to express their sincere appreciation to the staff members of icddr,b for their dedicated work in the field and laboratory during this pandemic. icddr,b is supported by the governments of Bangladesh, Canada, Sweden, and the UK.

Conflicts of Interest: The authors declare no conflict of interest.

References

1. Wang, C.; Horby, P.W.; Hayden, F.G.; Gao, G.F. A novel coronavirus outbreak of global health concern. *Lancet* **2020**, *395*, 470–473. [CrossRef]
2. WHO. WHO Director-General's Opening Remarks at the Media Briefing on COVID-19—11 March 2020. Available online: https://www.who.int/dg/speeches/detail/who-director-general-s-opening-remarks-atthe-media-briefing-on-covid-19---11-march-2020 (accessed on 16 March 2021).
3. Worldometer. COVID-19 Coronavirus Pandemic. Available online: https://www.worldometers.info/coronavirus (accessed on 16 March 2021).
4. Haque, M. Combating COVID-19: A Coordinated Efforts of Healthcare Providers and Policy Makers with Global Participation Are Needed to Achieve the Desired Goals. *Bangladesh J. Med. Sci.* **2020**, 1–5. [CrossRef]
5. Coşkun, H.; Yıldırım, N.; Gündüz, S. The spread of COVID-19 virus through population density and wind in Turkey cities. *Sci. Total Environ.* **2021**, *751*, 141663. [CrossRef]
6. Hawkins, R.B.; Charles, E.J.; Mehaffey, J.H. Socio-economic status and COVID-19–related cases and fatalities. *Public Health* **2020**, *189*, 129–134. [CrossRef]
7. Tabari, P.; Amini, M.; Moghadami, M.; Moosavi, M. International public health responses to COVID-19 outbreak: A rapid review. *Iran. J. Med. Sci.* **2020**, *45*, 157.
8. Paul, A.; Chatterjee, S.; Bairagi, N. Prediction on COVID-19 epidemic for different countries: Focusing on South Asia under various precautionary measures. *medRxiv* **2020**. [CrossRef]

9. Kamruzzaman, M.; Sakib, S.N. Bangladesh Imposes Total Lockdown over COVID-19. Anadolu Agency. 2020. Available online: https://www.aa.com.tr/en/asia-pacific/bangladesh-imposes-total-lockdown-over-covid-19/1778272#:~{}:text=Bangladesh%20imposed%20a%20nationwide%20lockdown,and%20at%20least%2039%20infections (accessed on 16 March 2021).
10. Douedari, Y.; Alhaffar, M.; Al-Twaish, M.; Mkhallalati, H.; Alwany, R.; Ibrahim, N.B.M.; Zaseela, A.; Horanieh, N.; Abbara, A.; Howard, N. "Ten years of war! You expect people to fear a 'germ'?": A qualitative study of initial perceptions and responses to the COVID-19 pandemic among displaced communities in opposition-controlled northwest Syria. *J. Migr. Heal.* **2020**, *1–2*, 100021. [CrossRef]
11. Ferdous, M.Z.; Islam, M.S.; Sikder, M.T.; Mosaddek AS, M.; Zegarra-Valdivia, J.A.; Gozal, D. Knowledge, attitude, and practice regarding COVID-19 outbreak in Bangladesh: An online-based cross-sectional study. *PLoS ONE* **2020**, *15*, e0239254. [CrossRef]
12. Kadam, A.B.; Atre, S.R. Negative impact of social media panic during the COVID-19 outbreak in India. *J. Travel Med.* **2020**, *27*, taaa057. [CrossRef]
13. World Health Organization. COVID-19 Situation Report No. #11. 2020. Available online: https://www.who.int/docs/default-source/searo/bangladesh/covid-19-who-bangladesh-situation-reports/who-ban-covid-19-sitrep-11.pdf?sfvrsn (accessed on 28 February 2021).
14. Bangla Tribune. Dhaka Slums House More People Than Recorded in Census. Available online: https://en.banglatribune.com/others/news/72709/Dhaka-slums-house-more-people-than-recorded-in (accessed on 7 December 2022).
15. UNICEF Bangladesh. Children in Cities: Bangladesh among 10 Nations That Top the List for Rapid Urbanisation. Available online: https://www.unicef.org/bangladesh/en/children-cities%C2%A0 (accessed on 7 December 2022).
16. World Health Organization. *The First Few X Cases and Contacts (FFX) Investigation Protocol for Coronavirus Disease 2019 (COVID-19), Version 2.2. 23 February 2020*; World Health Organization: Geneva, Switzerland, 2020.
17. Bairwa, M.; Rajput, M.; Sachdeva, S. Modified Kuppuswamy's socioeconomic scale: Social researcher should include updated income criteria, 2012. *Indian J. Community Med.* **2013**, *38*, 185–186. [CrossRef]
18. Saleem, S.M.; Jan, S.S. Modified Kuppuswamy socioeconomic scale updated for the year 2019. *Indian J. Forensic Community Med.* **2019**, *6*, 1–3. [CrossRef]
19. Morrow, R.; Rodriguez, A.; King, N. Colaizzi's descriptive phenomenological method. *Psychologist* **2015**, *28*, 643–644.
20. Abdelrahman, M. Personality traits, risk perception, and protective behaviors of Arab residents of Qatar during the COVID-19 pandemic. *Int. J. Ment. Health Addiction.* **2020**, *22*, 1–2. [CrossRef]
21. Pargament, K.I.; Ensing, D.S.; Falgout, K.; Olsen, H.; Reilly, B.; Van Haitsma, K.; Warren, R. God help me:(I): Religious coping efforts as predictors of the outcomes to significant negative life events. *Am. J. Community Psychol.* **1990**, *18*, 793–824. [CrossRef]
22. World Health Organization. *Water, Sanitation, Hygiene, and Waste Management for the COVID-19 Virus: Interim Guidance, 23 April 2020*; World Health Organization: Geneva, Switzerland, 2020.
23. Feng, S.; Shen, C.; Xia, N.; Song, W.; Fan, M.; Cowling, B.J. Rational use of face masks in the COVID-19 pandemic. *Lancet Respir. Med.* **2020**, *8*, 434–436. [CrossRef]
24. Singh, R.; Adhikari, R. Age-structured impact of social distancing on the COVID-19 epidemic in India. *arXiv preprint* **2020**. [CrossRef]
25. Musinguzi, G.; Asamoah, B.O. The science of social distancing and total lock down: Does it work? Whom does it benefit? *Electron. J. Gen. Med.* **2020**, *9*, 17. [CrossRef]
26. Vadivu, T.S.; Annamuthu, P.; Suresh, A. An awareness and perception of COVID-19 among general public–a cross sectional analysis. *Int. J. Mod. Trends Sci. Technol.* **2020**, *6*, 49–53.
27. Asim, M.; Sathian, B.; Van Teijlingen, E.; Mekkodathil, A.; Subramanya, S.H.; Simkhada, P. COVID-19 pandemic: Public health implications in Nepal. *Nepal J. Epidemiol.* **2020**, *10*, 817. [CrossRef]
28. Singh, D.R.; Sunuwar, D.R.; Karki, K.; Ghimire, S.; Shrestha, N. Knowledge and perception towards universal safety precautions during early phase of the COVID-19 outbreak in Nepal. *J. Community Health* **2020**, *45*, 1116–1122. [CrossRef]
29. Jose, R.; Narendran, M.; Bindu, A.; Beevi, N.; Manju, L.; Benny, P.V. Public perception and preparedness for the pandemic COVID 19: A health belief model approach. *Clin. Epidemiol. Glob. Health* **2021**, *9*, 41–46. [CrossRef]
30. Narayana, G.; Pradeepkumar, B.; Ramaiah, J.D.; Jayasree, T.; Yadav, D.L.; Kumar, B.K. Knowledge, perception, and practices towards COVID-19 pandemic among general public of India: A cross-sectional online survey. *Curr. Med. Res. Pract.* **2020**, *10*, 153–159.
31. Islam, M.S.; Sarkar, T.; Khan, S.H.; Kamal, A.H.; Hasan, S.M.; Kabir, A.; Yeasmin, D.; Islam, M.A.; Chowdhury, K.I.; Anwar, K.S.; et al. COVID-19–related infodemic and its impact on public health: A global social media analysis. *Am. J. Trop. Med. Hyg.* **2020**, *103*, 1621. [CrossRef]
32. Menon, G.I. COVID-19: Busting Some Myths. Health and Medicine. 2020. Available online: https://indiabioscience.org/columns/indian-scenario/covid-19-busting-some-myths (accessed on 7 December 2022).
33. Dutta, S.; Acharya, S.; Shukla, S.; Acharya, N. COVID-19 Pandemic-revisiting the myths. *SSRG-IJMS.* **2020**, *7*, 7–10. [CrossRef]
34. Roy, S. Low-income countries are more immune to COVID-19: A misconception. *Indian J. Med. Sci.* **2020**, *72*, 5. [CrossRef]
35. Zegarra-Valdivia, J.; Vilca, B.N.; Guerrero, R.J. Knowledge, perception and attitudes in Regard to COVID-19 Pandemic in Peruvian Population. Available online: https://psyarxiv.com/kr9ya/ (accessed on 7 December 2022).
36. Ahmad, A.R.; Murad, H.R. The impact of social media on panic during the COVID-19 pandemic in Iraqi Kurdistan: Online questionnaire study. *J. Med. Internet Res.* **2020**, *22*, e19556. [CrossRef]

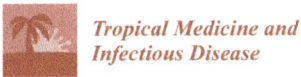 Tropical Medicine and Infectious Disease

Article

Clinical Features Related to Severity and Mortality among COVID-19 Patients in a Pre-Vaccine Period in Luanda, Angola

Cruz S. Sebastião [1,2,3], Adis Cogle [1,4], Alice D'Alva Teixeira [4], Ana Micolo Cândido [2], Chissengo Tchoni [1,4], Maria João Amorim [5,6], N'gueza Loureiro [4], Paolo Parimbelli [7], Carlos Penha-Gonçalves [5], Jocelyne Demengeot [5], Euclides Sacomboio [2,3], Manuela Mendes [7], Margarete Arrais [1,8], Joana Morais [2,9], Jocelyne Neto de Vasconcelos [1,2] and Miguel Brito [1,10,*]

1. Centro de Investigação em Saúde de Angola (CISA), Caxito, Angola
2. Instituto Nacional de Investigação em Saúde (INIS), Luanda, Angola
3. Instituto de Ciências da Saúde (ICISA), Universidade Agostinho Neto (UAN), Luanda, Angola
4. Clínica Girassol, Ministério da Saúde, Luanda, Angola
5. Instituto Gulbenkian de Ciência, 2780-156 Oeiras, Portugal
6. Católica Biomedical Research Centre, Católica Medical School, Universidade Católica Portuguesa, 1649-023 Lisbon, Portugal
7. Maternidade Lucrécia Paim, Ministério da Saúde, Luanda, Angola
8. Hospital Militar Principal, Luanda, Angola
9. Faculdade de Medicina, Universidade Agostinho Neto (UAN), Luanda, Angola
10. Health and Technology Research Center, Escola Superior de Tecnologia da Saúde de Lisboa, Instituto Politécnico de Lisboa, 1990-096 Lisbon, Portugal
* Correspondence: miguel.brito@estesl.ipl.pt

Abstract: Background: Infection due to severe acute respiratory syndrome coronavirus 2 (SARS-CoV-2) is associated with clinical features of diverse severity. Few studies investigated the severity and mortality predictors of coronavirus disease 2019 (COVID-19) in Africa. Herein, we investigated the clinical features of severity and mortality among COVID-19 patients in Luanda, Angola. Methods: This multicenter cohort study involved 101 COVID-19 patients, between December 2020 and April 2021, with clinical and laboratory data collected. Analysis was done using independent-sample t-tests and Chi-square tests. The results were deemed significant when $p < 0.05$. Results: The mean age of patients was 51 years (ranging from 18 to 80 years) and 60.4% were male. Fever (46%), cough (47%), gastrointestinal symptoms (26.7%), and asthenia (26.7%), were the most common symptoms. About 64.4% of the patients presented coexistent disorders, including hypertension (42%), diabetes (17%), and chronic renal diseases (6%). About 23% were non-severe, 77% were severe, and 10% died during hospitalization. Variations in the concentration of neutrophil, urea, creatinine, c-reactive protein, sodium, creatine kinase, and chloride were independently associated with severity and/or mortality ($p < 0.05$). Conclusion: Several factors contributed to the severity and mortality among COVID-19 patients in Angola. Further studies related to clinical features should be carried out to help clinical decision-making and follow-up of COVID-19 patients in Angola.

Keywords: SARS-CoV-2; COVID-19; clinical features; Luanda; Angola

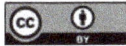

1. Introduction

At the end of 2019, the world was confronted with the emergence of cases of pneumonia of unknown etiology initially identified in Wuhan, China [1]. A new coronavirus named Severe Acute Respiratory Syndrome coronavirus 2 (SARS-CoV-2) was identified as being the causative agent of the ongoing outbreak of atypical pneumonia [2–4], and the disease was named coronavirus disease 2019 (COVID-19) [5,6]. After identifying the first cases of infection in China, the virus spread rapidly to other geographic locations worldwide acquiring pandemic dynamics and leading to an unprecedented breakdown of healthcare systems with high mortality rates among patients with arterial hypertension, diabetes mellitus, and older age [7,8]. For instance, between December 2019 and May 2022, there have been about 521 million confirmed cases including most of 6.2 million deaths, of which about 99,000 cases and 1900 deaths were reported in Angola [9].

Generally, the main clinical manifestations identified among COVID-19 patients include fever, dry cough, muscle pain, headache, nausea, vomiting, difficulty in breathing, and diarrhea [10–13]. Furthermore, while those manifestations can be mild or moderate in some patients, they can rapidly evolve into a more severe condition and death in others [14–19]. Reportedly, the progression to severe disease has predictable pathology indicators regarding hematological, biochemical, and immunological biomarkers, particularly concerning biological markers of inflammation, impaired liver and kidney function, damage to cardiac tissues and muscles, and hypercoagulation [14–19]. Indeed, the pathophysiology of SARS-CoV-2 infection is characterized by aberrant inflammatory responses that affect multiple organs of the cardiac, hepatic, and renal systems leading to unfavorable clinical outcomes [20–22].

Studies involving COVID-19 patients around the world have shown that the identification of the laboratory biomarkers of disease progression among COVID-19 patients might be crucial for clinical decision-making with a positive impact on healthcare system costs mainly in low- and middle-income countries. To the best of our knowledge, there are no published studies assessing biomarkers that could be related to the worsening of the disease or unfavorable clinical outcomes among COVID-19 patients in Luanda, the capital city, and the COVID-19 hotspot in Angola. In this study, we identify clinical features related to severity among COVID-19 patients in Angola aiming to contribute to the generation of global knowledge about the clinical effects of SARS-CoV-2 exposure and define effective management strategies for follow-up of COVID-19 patients in Angola.

2. Materials and Methods

2.1. Study Design and Setting

This was a multicenter cohort study carried out on 101 COVID-19 patients admitted to three hospitals, the Lucrecia Paim Maternity, Hospital Militar Principal, and Clínica Girassol, from December 2020 to April 2021. All health facilities are located in Luanda, Angola. All patients enrolled, have been confirmed as COVID-19 according to the diagnostic criteria established by the WHO, with positive RT-PCR detection in nasal or pharyngeal samples. The study was previously reviewed and approved by the national ethics committee of the Ministry of Health of Angola (approval no. 25/2020). The main inclusion criterion in the study was that participants had to be at least 18 years of age. Moreover, all participants were informed of the study objectives and free verbal consent was obtained from participants before being included in the study.

2.2. Sample Collection and Testing

An estimated volume of 10 mL of venous blood was collected from all participants. Of these, 5 mL of blood was placed in tubes containing ethylenediamine tetraacetic acid (EDTA) for the screening of hematological biomarkers (complete blood count or hemogram) using the Automated Hematology Analyzer SYSMEX XT-4000i (Sysmex Europe SE, Norderstedt, Germany). The other 5 mL of blood was placed in tubes with activated clot gel for serum separation and biochemical and/or immunological screening (glucose, urea, creatinine, aspartate transaminase (AST), alanine aminotransferase (ALT), lactate dehydrogenase (LDH), serum creatine kinase (SCK), alkaline phosphatase, albumin, D-Dimer, C-reactive protein (CRP), sodium, potassium, chloride, procalcitonin (PCT), interleukin-6 (IL-6)) using automatic biochemical analyzer Cobas C111 analyzer (Roche), MINI VIDAS (Biomerieux SA, Bagno A Ripoli, Italy) and Cobas E411 (Roche). In addition, we performed the quantification of IgG against SARS-CoV-2 by neutralization assays. The entire process of sample separation, as well as laboratory processing, was carried out in the hematology, biochemistry, and immunology laboratory of Instituto Nacional de Investigação em Saúde (INIS), located in Luanda—Angola. The serological assay for the detection of antibodies that recognize the SARS-CoV-2 Spike protein, by ELISA, was performed using the methodology developed by Florian Krammer [23] at the Instituto Gulbenkian de Ciência, located in Lisbon—Portugal. The baseline laboratory parameters analyzed in these COVID-19 patients were grouped into three major groups, (i) blood routine examination, (ii) serum biochemical index, and (iii) infection-related factors.

2.3. Data Sources and Processing

Medical records of all COVID-19 patients were reviewed to collect the sociodemographic (age, gender, and place of residence), clinical information (symptoms, disease severity, comorbidities, and clinical outcome), and laboratory examination results obtained through routine blood tests. The laboratory parameters were analyzed by comparing the average of the values between non-severe and severe patients, as well as between surviving and non-surviving patients. In this study, non-severe patients were those who did not report clinical manifestations but were tested with RT-PCR and included in the study for having an epidemiological link with a confirmed case of SARS-CoV-2 and also for being asymptomatic or pre-symptomatic COVID-19 patients with a high possibility to spreading the infection. On the other hand, patients who revealed any of the symptoms related to SARS-CoV-2 infection were grouped into the category of severe patients. Regarding clinical outcome, we considered surviving patients, all those who were clinically and epidemiologically discharged, while all patients who died during the hospitalization period were grouped as non-survivors.

2.4. Statistical Analysis

Statistical analyses were carried out using the SPSS v28 (IBM SPSS Statistics, Armonk, NY, USA). Descriptive data were expressed as frequencies and percentages. Independent-sample t-tests were conducted to estimate the differences of continuous data while Chi-square tests were conducted on categorical data. All reported p-values are two-tailed with a level of significance of 5%.

3. Results

3.1. Baseline Characteristics of the Studied Population

As shown in Table 1, the COVID-19 patients from Luanda, Angola, had a mean age of 51 ± 14 years, ranging from 18 to 80 years, most of the patients were male (60.4%, 61/101), and residents of urbanized areas (54.5%, 55/101). A total of 23/101 (23%) patients were non-severe, while 78/101 (77%) were classified as severe. Regarding clinical outcome, a total of 10/101 (10%) patients did not survive during hospitalization and 91/101 (90%) were discharged. The mean age of patients who did not survive was higher compared to those of patients who survived (60 ± 13 years vs. 50 ± 14 years, $p = 0.045$). The most common symptoms at onset were cough (37%), fever (36%), asthenia (27%), gastrointestinal symptoms (27%), dyspnea (19%), headache (15%), osteomyalgia (16%), and fatigue (8%). More than half of patients (64%, 65/101) had some form of the coexisting disorder, with arterial hypertension (42%, 42/101) being the most common coexisting disorder, followed by diabetes mellitus (17%, 17/101) and chronic renal disease (6%, 6/101). Statistically significant differences were observed between the presence of coexisting disorder with the severity of the disease ($p < 0.001$). The top three coexisting disorders in patients who died were arterial hypertension (60%), diabetes mellitus (20%), and chronic kidney disease (20%). Compared to the survivors, the non-survivors were over 40 years old (100%), from urbanized areas (60%), and with a coexisting disorder (90%). Furthermore, another significant difference was observed between the clinical outcome with the presence of chronic kidney disease ($p = 0.048$) or allergic rhinitis ($p = 0.002$). We also explore humoral immune responsiveness by assessing late-stage disease antibodies or Immunoglobulin G (IgG) in approximately 80% of patients (80.2%, 81/101). Immunity assessment results showed that 33% (27/81) had developed an immune response against SARS-CoV-2 and had considerable levels of IgG (mean of 1.67 ± 0.22, ranging from 1.07 to 1.99), while 67%

(54/81) had no IgG antibodies. No statistically significant difference was observed between the presence of IgG antibodies and disease severity or clinical outcome. As we expected, the presence of IgG antibodies was more frequently observed among patients with severe disease (37%, 23/78) or in patients who died (44%, 4/10), compared to non-severe patients (21%, 4/23) or patients who survived (32%, 23/91), respectively.

Table 1. Baseline characteristics related to disease severity and clinical outcome among COVID-19 patients in Luanda, Angola.

Baseline Characteristic	N (%)	Disease Severity			Clinical Outcome		
		Non-Severe	Severe	p-Value	Survivors	Non-Survivors	p-Value
Overall	101 (100%)	23 (22.8)	78 (77.2)		91 (90.1)	10 (9.90)	
Age							
Mean ± SD—yr	51.1 ± 14.2	50.4 ± 13.1	51.3 ± 14.5	0.774	50.2 ± 14.1	59.6 ± 12.5	**0.045**
Distribution—No. (%)							
<20 yr	1 (1.00)	0 (0.0)	1 (1.30)	0.826	1 (1.10)	0 (0.0)	0.161
20–40 yr	24 (23.8)	5 (21.7)	19 (24.4)		24 (26.4)	0 (0.0)	
>40 yr	76 (75.2)	18 (78.3)	58 (74.4)		66 (72.5)	10 (100)	
Gender—No. (%)							
Female	40 (39.6)	11 (47.8)	29 (37.2)	0.359	35 (38.5)	5 (50.0)	0.479
Male	61 (60.4)	12 (52.2)	49 (62.8)		56 (61.5)	5 (50.0)	
Place of residence—No. (%)							
Rural area	46 (45.5)	9 (39.1)	37 (47.4)	0.482	42 (46.2)	4 (40.0)	0.711
Urban area	55 (54.5)	14 (60.9)	41 (52.6)		49 (53.8)	6 (60.0)	
Fever on admission							
Mean (SD)	36.5 ± 0.73	36.3 ± 0.27	36.5 ± 0.81	0.268	36.5 ± 0.69	36.5 ± 1.04	0.955
Distribution of temp.—°C							
<37.5 °C	88 (87.1)	23 (100)	65 (83.3)	0.221	80 (87.9)	8 (80.0)	0.565
37.5–37.9 °C	3 (3.00)	0 (0.0)	3 (3.80)		3 (3.30)	0 (0.0)	
38.0–38.9 °C	9 (8.90)	0 (0.0)	9 (11.5)		7 (7.70)	2 (20.0)	
≥39.0 °C	1 (1.00)	0 (0.0)	1 (1.30)		1 (1.10)	0 (0.0)	
Signs and symptoms—No. (%)	78 (77.2)	0 (0.0)	78 (100)	**<0.001**	68 (74.7)	10 (100)	0.070
Fever	36 (35.6)	0 (0.0)	36 (46.2)	**<0.001**	34 (37.4)	2 (20.0)	0.277
Cough	37 (36.6)	0 (0.0)	37 (47.4)	**<0.001**	32 (35.2)	5 (50.0)	0.355
Headache	15 (14.9)	0 (0.0)	15 (19.2)	**0.023**	14 (15.4)	1 (10.0)	0.649
Fatigue	8 (7.90)	0 (0.0)	8 (10.3)	0.109	7 (7.70)	1 (10.0)	0.798
Asthenia	27 (26.7)	0 (0.0)	27 (34.6)	**<0.001**	23 (25.3)	4 (40.0)	0.318
Dyspnea	19 (18.8)	0 (0.0)	19 (24.4)	**0.009**	16 (17.6)	3 (30.0)	0.340
Osteomyalgia	16 (15.8)	0 (0.0)	16 (20.5)	**0.018**	15 (16.5)	1 (10.0)	0.594
Gastrointestinal symptoms	27 (26.7)	0 (0.0)	27 (34.6)	**<0.001**	24 (26.4)	3 (30.0)	0.806
Apathy	2 (2.00)	0 (0.0)	2 (2.60)	0.438	1 (1.10)	1 (10.0)	0.055
Anosmia	9 (8.90)	0 (0.0)	9 (11.5)	0.088	9 (9.90)	0 (0.0)	0.297
Malaise	20 (19.8)	0 (0.0)	20 (25.6)	**0.007**	16 (17.6)	4 (40.0)	0.091
Hemiplegia	1 (1.00)	0 (0.0)	1 (1.30)	0.585	0 (0.0)	1 (10.0)	**0.002**
Loss of consciousness	1 (1.00)	0 (0.0)	1 (1.30)	0.585	0 (0.0)	1 (10.0)	**0.002**
Coexisting disorder—No. (%)							
No	36 (35.6)	17 (73.9)	19 (24.4)	**<0.001**	35 (38.5)	1 (10.0)	0.074
Yes	65 (64.4)	6 (26.1)	59 (75.6)		56 (61.5)	9 (90.0)	
Disorder distribution—No. (%)							
Chronic pulmonary disease	3 (3.00)	0 (0.0)	3 (3.80)	0.438	3 (3.30)	0 (0.0)	0.636
Arterial hypertension	42 (41.6)	4 (17.4)	38 (48.7)	**0.007**	36 (39.6)	6 (60.0)	0.213
Chronic renal disease	6 (5.90)	0 (0.0)	6 (7.70)	0.170	4 (4.40)	2 (20.0)	**0.048**
Diabetes	17 (16.8)	4 (17.4)	13 (16.7)	0.935	15 (16.5)	2 (20.0)	0.778
Cancer	1 (1.00)	0 (0.0)	1 (1.30)	0.585	1 (1.10)	0 (0.0)	0.739
Immunodeficiency	1 (1.00)	0 (0.0)	1 (1.30)	0.585	1 (1.10)	0 (0.0)	0.739
Hepatitis B infection	1 (1.00)	0 (0.0)	1 (1.30)	0.585	1 (1.10)	0 (0.0)	0.739
Allergic rhinitis	1 (1.00)	0 (0.0)	1 (1.30)	0.585	0 (0.0)	1 (10.0)	**0.002**
IgG							
No	54 (66.7)	15 (78.9)	39 (62.9)	0.194	49 (68.1)	5 (55.6)	0.453
Yes	27 (33.3)	4 (21.1)	23 (37.1)		23 (31.9)	4 (44.4)	

Bold numbers mean that results were statistically significant for independent-sample t-tests ($p < 0.05$) and Chi-square tests ($p < 0.05$).

3.2. Baseline Laboratory Parameters Related to Disease Severity and Clinical Outcome

Laboratory testing results as well as the average of the laboratory parameters for patients from non-severe vs. severe disease or non-survivors vs. survivors are shown in Table 2. In terms of blood parameters, no significant differences were found between patients classified as non-severe and severe, except for neutrophils (2.40 vs. 5.48, $p = 0.035$). Regarding the biochemical indexes, we observed statistically significant increases in the mean from non-severe patients to severe patients for urea (19.2 vs. 28.1, $p = 0.017$) and CRP (1.57 vs. 7.44, $p = 0.006$), while a significant decrease was observed for sodium (136 vs. 127, $p = 0.007$). A significant increase was observed between survivors and non-survivors for urea (26.5 vs. 29.2, $p = 0.039$), while a significant decrease was observed in creatinine (1.06 vs. 0.50, $p = 0.025$), SCK (230 vs. 136, $p = 0.039$), and chloride (101 vs. 99.7, $p = 0.026$). As we expected, laboratory parameters varied according to gender and age groups. Significant variations for gender were observed with an increase from female to male in AST (31.0 to 55.9, $p < 0.001$), ALT (24.5 to 52.0, $p < 0.001$) and decrease in alkaline phosphatase (105 to 76.5, $p = 0.029$) and chloride (103 to 101, $p = 0.017$). On the other hand, significant variations for the age group were observed with an increase from patients under 40 years to over 40 years in urea (19.7 to 30.9, $p = 0.003$), SCK (155 to 287, $p = 0.024$) and D-Dimer (3.50 to 6.42, $p = 0.033$).

3.3. Treatments and Clinical Outcomes among COVID-19 Patients

The therapeutic description used among COVID-19 patients according to gender, age groups, disease severity, and clinical outcomes are described in Table 3. The most used drug groups among the COVID-19 patients analyzed in this study were antibiotics (73%, 74/101), corticosteroids (52%, 51/101), anticoagulants (43%, 43/101), antihypertensives (19%, 19/101), and analgesics (13%, 12/101). Of these therapeutic groups, only antibiotic use was statistically related to clinical outcome, with all non-surviving patients (100%, 10/10) using antibiotics compared to 70% (64/91) of surviving patients exposed to antibiotic therapy. In addition, antibiotics use was also related to disease severity ($p < 0.001$), age group ($p = 0.025$), and gender ($p = 0.015$). Corticosteroid use was related to severity ($p = 0.001$) and age group ($p = 0.002$). Similarly, the use of anticoagulants was related to severity ($p = 0.001$) and age group ($p = 0.002$). Finally, the use of antihypertensive drugs was related to the age group ($p = 0.029$). Curiously, patients treated with antimalarial were part of the group of severe, although the total number is too low to make the result statistically significant.

Table 2. Baseline laboratory parameters related to disease severity and clinical outcome among COVID-19 patients in Luanda, Angola.

Laboratory Findings	All Patients (101)		Gender			Age Group			Disease Severity			Clinical Outcome		
	N (%)	Mean ± SD	Female (Mean ± SD)	Male (Mean ± SD)	p-Value	<40 yr (Mean ± SD)	≥40 yr (Mean ± SD)	p-Value	Non-Severe (n = 23)	Severe (n = 78)	p-Value	Survivors (n = 91)	Non-Survivors (n = 10)	p-Value
Blood routine examination														
Erythrocytes, ×10^{12}/L	101 (100)	4.62 ± 3.09	4.43 ± 0.95	4.74 ± 1.11	0.140	4.94 ± 1.31	4.52 ± 0.95	0.149	4.77 ± 1.07	4.58 ± 1.06	0.455	4.67 ± 1.05	4.14 ± 1.04	0.131
Hemoglobin, g/dL	101 (100)	12.7 ± 3.09	12.1 ± 2.78	13.1 ± 3.25	0.109	13.7 ± 3.81	12.4 ± 2.77	0.113	13.1 ± 3.10	12.6 ± 3.12	0.552	12.8 ± 3.06	11.6 ± 3.37	0.238
Leukocytes, ×10^9/L	101 (100)	7.44 ± 4.13	6.94 ± 2.97	7.77 ± 4.73	0.282	6.39 ± 3.56	7.79 ± 4.26	0.111	4.57 ± 1.08	7.87 ± 4.66	0.083	6.79 ± 4.16	12.7 ± 4.62	0.079
Neutrophils, ×10^9/L	98 (97)	4.75 ± 3.40	4.43 ± 2.92	4.97 ± 3.70	0.420	4.34 ± 3.19	4.89 ± 3.47	0.472	2.40 ± 0.17	5.48 ± 4.17	0.035	4.40 ± 3.53	10.6 ± 4.60	0.385
Lymphocytes, ×10^9/L	99 (98)	1.54 ± 0.75	1.69 ± 0.71	1.44 ± 0.77	0.096	1.45 ± 0.70	1.58 ± 0.77	0.440	1.37 ± 0.47	1.61 ± 0.99	0.081	1.62 ± 0.97	1.19 ± 0.18	0.098
Eosinophil, ×10^9/L	98 (97.0)	0.12 ± 0.27	0.15 ± 0.32	0.10 ± 0.22	0.328	0.10 ± 0.14	0.13 ± 0.30	0.607	0.21 ± 0.49	0.10 ± 0.15	0.078	0.11 ± 0.27	0.21 ± 0.18	0.334
Platelets, ×10^3/mm^3	101 (100)	229 ± 122	218 ± 75.5	237 ± 144	0.391	211 ± 83.8	235 ± 132	0.292	154 ± 49.8	270 ± 155	0.212	252 ± 157	255 ± 55.2	0.215
Serum biochemical index														
Glucose, mg/dL	96 (95)	126 ± 89.3	124 ± 100	127 ± 82.9	0.896	103 ± 80.4	132 ± 91.1	0.160	117 ± 19.0	148 ± 97.0	0.739	144 ± 92.2	140 ± 95.0	0.512
Urea, mg/dL	93 (92)	28.2 ± 22.3	27.1 ± 29.3	28.9 ± 17.0	0.733	19.7 ± 10.9	30.9 ± 24.3	0.003	19.2 ± 1.95	28.1 ± 8.82	0.017	26.5 ± 9.20	29.2 ± 0.98	**0.039**
Creatinine, mg/dL	94 (93)	1.45 ± 2.99	2.16 ± 4.85	1.03 ± 0.29	0.176	0.89 ± 3.22	1.63 ± 3.42	0.074	1.03 ± 0.49	0.99 ± 0.38	0.362	1.06 ± 0.36	0.50 ± 0.00	**0.025**
AST, U/L	99 (98)	46.3 ± 38.7	31.0 ± 16.6	55.9 ± 45.1	<0.001	49.1 ± 52.6	45.5 ± 33.8	0.755	63.0 ± 32.1	34.6 ± 23.4	0.069	35.4 ± 21.5	70.6 ± 53.0	0.629
ALT, U/L	98 (97)	41.3 ± 45.1	24.5 ± 20.7	52.0 ± 52.7	<0.001	46.9 ± 54.1	40.0 ± 42.2	0.554	61.8 ± 18.1	30.7 ± 20.1	0.261	34.4 ± 20.4	43.5 ± 48.7	0.276
LDH, U/L	73 (72)	416 ± 318	379 ± 226	439 ± 364	0.388	317 ± 268	451 ± 329	0.087	291 ± 59.3	380 ± 281	0.091	297 ± 139	991 ± 309	0.114
SCK, U/L	86 (85)	261 ± 326	189 ± 182	303 ± 383	0.066	155 ± 156	287 ± 352	0.024	355 ± 168	197 ± 248	0.253	230 ± 252	136 ± 49.3	**0.039**
Alkaline phosphatase, U/L	78 (77)	87.5 ± 50.3	105 ± 62.6	76.5 ± 37.5	0.029	117 ± 82.2	79.4 ± 33.7	0.084	79.0 ± 14.1	82.6 ± 52.1	0.394	80.9 ± 50.6	92.8 ± 14.0	0.675
Albumin, g/L	82 (81)	38.3 ± 7.15	37.7 ± 7.79	38.5 ± 6.81	0.645	37.3 ± 9.21	38.5 ± 6.57	0.620	45.8 ± 2.39	35.6 ± 7.69	0.125	37.7 ± 8.27	32.0 ± 0.99	0.052
D-Dimer, g/L	37 (37)	5.47 ± 4.01	5.84 ± 3.51	5.27 ± 4.32	0.671	3.50 ± 3.57	6.42 ± 3.93	0.033	2.75 ± 4.01	4.39 ± 3.84	0.274	4.22 ± 3.98	3.4 ± 2.37	0.311
C-reactive protein, mg/L	95 (94)	7.30 ± 15.0	5.56 ± 7.33	8.36 ± 18.1	0.294	4.61 ± 7.04	8.16 ± 16.7	0.153	1.57 ± 1.05	7.44 ± 7.42	0.006	5.61 ± 6.54	15.2 ± 8.90	0.099
Sodium, mmol/L	66 (65)	129 ± 8.66	132 ± 10.4	128 ± 7.36	0.070	124 ± 11.5	130 ± 7.86	0.160	136 ± 5.10	127 ± 7.92	0.007	128 ± 8.57	131 ± 4.17	0.403
Potassium, mmol/L	60 (59)	8.78 ± 8.38	8.04 ± 9.78	9.12 ± 7.75	0.677	10.1 ± 14.1	8.54 ± 7.13	0.748	3.81 ± 0.54	9.06 ± 9.78	0.082	8.29 ± 9.59	8.07 ± 6.14	0.667
Chloride, mmol/L	65 (64)	102 ± 3.81	103 ± 3.51	101 ± 3.74	0.017	101 ± 2.82	102 ± 3.95	0.431	102 ± 1.03	100 ± 3.61	0.061	101 ± 3.55	99.7 ± 1.06	**0.026**
Infection-related factors														
PCT, ng/mL	37 (37)	0.62 ± 2.08	1.27 ± 3.78	0.38 ± 0.92	0.251	2.09 ± 4.28	0.22 ± 0.46	0.256	0.09 ± 0.02	1.04 ± 3.01	0.150	0.98 ± 2.93	0.19 ± 0.15	0.900
IL-6, ng/dL	40 (40)	136 ± 314	105 ± 259	151 ± 340	0.477	364 ± 554	60.2 ± 114	0.119	142 ± 231	191 ± 451	0.855	202 ± 441	20.3 ± 19.3	0.524

Abbreviation: AST, aspartate transaminase; ALT, alanine aminotransferase; LDH, lactate dehydrogenase; SCK, serum creatine kinase; PCT, procalcitonin; IL-6, Interleukin 6. Bold numbers mean that results were statistically significant for independent-sample t-tests ($p < 0.05$).

Table 3. Treatments related to clinical outcomes among COVID-19 patients in Luanda, Angola.

Treatment	Total (n = 101)	Gender			Age Group			Disease Severity			Clinical Outcome		
		Female (n = 40)	Male (n = 61)	p-Value	<40 yr (n = 25)	≥40 yr (n = 76)	p-Value	Non-Severe (n = 23)	Severe (n = 78)	p-Value	Survivors (n = 91)	Non-Survivors (n = 10)	p-Value
Antibiotics	74 (73.3)	24 (60.0)	50 (82.0)	**0.015**	14 (56.0)	60 (78.9)	**0.025**	7 (30.4)	67 (85.9)	**<0.001**	64 (70.3)	10 (100)	**0.044**
Corticosteroids	52 (51.5)	14 (35.0)	38 (62.3)	**0.007**	9 (36.0)	43 (56.6)	0.074	5 (21.7)	47 (60.3)	**0.001**	44 (48.4)	8 (80.0)	0.057
Anticoagulant	43 (42.6)	14 (35.0)	29 (47.5)	0.213	4 (16.0)	39 (51.3)	**0.002**	3 (13.0)	40 (51.3)	**0.001**	36 (39.6)	7 (70.0)	0.065
Antihypertensives	19 (18.8)	4 (10.0)	15 (24.6)	0.067	1 (4.00)	18 (23.7)	**0.029**	3 (13.0)	16 (20.5)	0.421	18 (19.8)	1 (10.0)	0.453
Analgesic	12 (11.9)	6 (15.0)	6 (9.80)	0.433	4 (16.0)	8 (10.5)	0.463	1 (4.30)	11 (14.1)	0.204	12 (13.2)	0 (0.0)	0.221
Antiacid	8 (7.90)	3 (7.50)	5 (8.20)	0.899	2 (8.00)	6 (7.90)	0.987	0 (0.0)	8 (10.3)	0.109	6 (6.60)	2 (20.0)	0.136
Antidiabetics	7 (6.90)	1 (2.50)	6 (9.80)	0.156	0 (0.0)	7 (9.20)	0.116	1 (4.30)	6 (7.70)	0.579	7 (7.70)	0 (0.0)	0.363
Antimalarial	5 (5.00)	1 (2.50)	4 (6.60)	0.358	2 (8.00)	3 (3.90)	0.418	0 (0.0)	5 (6.40)	0.213	4 (4.40)	1 (10.0)	0.438
Vitamins	5 (5.00)	2 (5.00)	3 (4.90)	0.985	2 (8.00)	3 (3.90)	0.418	0 (0.0)	5 (6.40)	0.213	5 (5.50)	0 (0.0)	0.447
Antiemetic	3 (3.00)	1 (2.50)	2 (3.30)	0.822	1 (4.00)	2 (2.60)	0.727	0 (0.0)	3 (3.80)	0.340	3 (3.30)	0 (0.0)	0.560

Bold numbers mean that results were statistically significant for Chi-square tests ($p < 0.05$).

4. Discussion

This extensive, multicenter cohort study was performed among patients with COVID-19 who had a definitive clinical outcome in Angola, a sub-Saharan African country, a continent for which there is a limited number of studies. In the present study, the mean age of all COVID-19 patients was 51 years, which was higher than the mean age reported by Huang et al. (49 years) [16], but lower than that reported by Chen et al. (56 years) [13], and Wang et al. (56 years) [24]. The critically ill patients were mainly older than 40 years old, male, from urbanized regions, and with comorbidities, which resemble findings already reported in Angola by our research group [25]. Furthermore, patients who have the same characteristics related to age and gender have been observed by Zhang et al., in a study conducted in China [12]. As the data are relative to the first wave of the pandemic, it reports data on the first infection of individuals, prior to re-infection or vaccine administrations. Therefore, our data on biological indicators of risk factors associated with worsening and death among COVID-19 patients are free from the confounding effects associated with viral circulating in the population, including prior immunity to the pathogen. Key signs and symptoms as well as the main comorbidities (Table 1) observed in the studied population were in line with many independent reports [12–16]. In contrast with the study carried out by Zhang et al. [12] in which no patient came forward with Rhinitis, our research presented a patient with rhinitis, which was significantly associated with unfavorable clinical outcomes (p = 0.002). Currently, we do not have a reasonable explanation of whether allergic conditions such as rhinitis could constitute an independent predictor of mortality amongst COVID-19 patients in Angola. However, additional studies of this possible relationship should be taken into consideration in future studies.

Besides men being those with the most serious disease (Table 1), it was also a group that came forward with a slight decrease in lymphocytes compared with groups of women (0.096), although it is not a statistically significant reduction (Table 2).

Liver damage among COVID-19 patients could affect the C-reactive protein concentrations that were three times higher (5.61 mg/L to 15.2 mg/L) in response to disease severity (Table 2). We observed that the adult age group above 40 years was the group that mostly used antibiotics (Table 3), which could have affected the outcome of these patients, since all patients who died had exposure to antibiotics (p = 0.044). All patients who used antimalarial in our study had severe COVID-19 although the total number is too low to make the result statistically significant, which corresponds with previous studies that have seen no benefit and even a trend toward worse clinical outcomes with the use of antimalarial in COVID-19 patients [26,27]. Recently our research team reported a 14% rate of malaria/SARS-CoV-2 coinfection in Luanda [28], which suggests that genetic peculiarities or local diseases such as vector-borne diseases (e.g., malaria, dengue, and chikungunya), might influence the course of the COVID-19 disease representing risk or protective factors for COVID-19 severity and mortality, which deserve further investigation [29]. The biological indicators used to assess responsiveness to infection in these COVID-19 patients were IgG and IL-6. The higher frequency of patients without antibodies IgG is not surprising, as patients were recruited early after disease onset, presumably without having yet developed a humoral response to infection. The increase in IgG antibodies with the severity of the disease is expected and is in accordance with the profile of the immune response to SARS-CoV-2 infection [30,31]. In agreement with our results, Marklund et al. showed that patients with severe COVID-19 seroconvert earlier and develop higher concentrations of SARS-CoV-2-specific IgG compared to patients with non-severe disease, which could improve patient outcomes [30]. Nonetheless, the rate of patients without antibodies (55.6%) who died was higher compared to patients who died despite the presence of antibodies (44.4%), which could indicate that patients who develop IgG antibodies tend to increase their chances of survival. Indeed, a previous study carried out by Corona et al. showed that treatment based on an infusion of IgG enriched with IgM and IgA seems to give a survival advantage in cases of severe infection by SARS-CoV-2 [31].

Our data show a significant difference in sodium concentration in non-severe vs. severe patients (136 mmol/L vs. 127 mmol/L, $p = 0.007$), which is in agreement with a study carried out by Guan et al. where non-severe COVID-19 patients also showed high sodium [31,32]. In our study, patients who died (131 mmol/L) had higher sodium concentrations compared to surviving patients (128 mmol/L) ($p = 0.403$), showing that a high concentration of sodium could be a protective biological factor against an unfavorable clinical outcome. It is also worth mentioning that these results show that during hospitalization, some patients could have developed a state of dehydration which could have led to disturbances in brain function, such as seizures and abnormalities in the level of consciousness. Consistently, loss of consciousness was observed among severe patients and was significantly related to the unfavorable clinical outcome ($p = 0.002$), since the patient with loss of consciousness in this study died during their hospital stay (Table 1).

Generally neglected, variations in sodium concentration could be an indicator of disease severity and have been linked to late hospitalization and significant morbidity [33]. Our results were similar to a study carried out by Albeladi et al. observed low concentrations of sodium in severely COVID-19 patients on admission [34]. A recent study carried out by Chen et al. in China showed that the SARS-CoV-2 infection has a strong association with a decrease in potassium, which was not consistent with the results of this study [35]. Measurement of sodium among severe COVID-19 patients is crucial to avoid complications related to a potassium imbalance, such as dangerous cardiac irregularities [36], once, Moreno-P et al. showed that the reduction of potassium is an indication of disease severity and need for invasive mechanical ventilation [37]. We also observed a significant relationship between the mean concentration of chlorine between surviving and non-surviving patients ($p = 0.026$), indicating that chlorine could be an extremely sensitive biological indicator of SARS-CoV-2 and that reduction could be predictive of bad outcomes. Albeladi et al., also noted that there was a significant decrease in serum chloride values at admission, although during hospitalization the levels increased significantly [34]. In agreement with our results, Petnak et al. showed that serum chloride at hospital discharge in the range of 100–108 mmol/L predicted a favorable clinical outcome [38], which was similar to the mean chlorine concentration of 102 ± 1.03 mmol/L observed among survived patients (Table 2). The reasons for this relationship between chloride concentration and mortality ($p = 0.026$) as well as biological systems with affected biological function due to variation in chlorine concentration among COVID-19 patients have not been explored. Interestingly, there was a decrease in eosinophils with disease severity but an increase in mortality, similar to that seen by Zhang et al. [12], that could also serve as an indicator of infection and mortality.

Previously undertaken studies showed advanced age might be a significant stand-alone predictor of severity and mortality between patients infected with SARS and MERS [39–41]. We confirmed that an increase in mean age has been linked to mortality among COVID-19 patients ($p = 0.045$) (Table 1). It is worth noting that all patients who have died were patients aged over 40 years, which represents a group of the largest clinical concerns that require timely intervention from the beginning of the laboratory screening to follow-up during hospitalization. Regarding biological indicators, a significant increase in the concentrations of urea ($p = 0.003$), SCK ($p = 0.024$), and D-Dimer ($p = 0.033$) were observed in the present study among the patients aged over 40 years compared to the younger patients. Nonetheless, we do not know whether these systemic disorders are caused by the fact that patients have COVID-19 or whether there are other genetic, clinical, or behavioral reasons. It is worth mentioning that, during disease progression, the D-dimer significantly increases with the platelets [11]. In this study, we observed increased clotting activity, marked by an increase in D-dimer concentrations by 1.6 times higher in severe COVID-19 patients, 1.8 times higher in patients over 40 years, and a reduction among patients who did not survive (Table 2), which was similar to study carried out by Milbrandt et al. [42] who also observed increased D-dimer in about 90% of hospitalized patients. Our findings support the hypothesis proposed by other authors that SARS-CoV-2 infection activates the coagulation cascade in ways leading to hypercoagulability [11]. On the other hand, our results do not corroborate the association between D-dimer and mortality from COVID-19, reported by Zhou et al. or by Rodelo et al. among COVID-19 patients in Wuhan and Colombia, respectively [14,43].

This study has some caveats. First, the number of participants is low. Second, the patients come from Luanda and might not represent the entire country. Thirdly, due to the limitations in laboratory resources, not all laboratory tests were performed for all patients. Finally, most patients were transferred with high disease severity to health units, and not sampled in this study. Despite these limitations, our study presents the clinical features of COVID-19 patients, explores possible biological indicators related to severity and mortality, allowing an in-depth assessment of the baseline clinical features that might be related to COVID-19 in Angola. Further investigations from a clinical and laboratory point of view must be carried out, to explore and clarify the main laboratory changes that occur during SARS-CoV-2 infection. Furthermore, the possibility of co-infection between viral and bacterial agents and its relationship with severity and clinical outcome should also be investigated in the future. It is also worth mentioning that with the emergence of numerous variants of SARS-CoV-2 with different degrees of infectivity, severity, and mortality, it would be crucial to consider the possibility of exploring the clinical differences and laboratory variations that could occur according to the different variants of SARS-CoV-2.

In conclusion, we identified several biological factors that contributed to the severity and mortality among COVID-19 patients during a period of pre-vaccine in Luanda, Angola. However, further studies related to clinical features, severity, and mortality due to SARS-CoV-2 infection should be carried out to help clinical decision-making and follow-up of COVID-19 patients in Angola.

Author Contributions: Conceptualization and methodology: C.S.S., M.J.A., C.P.-G., J.N.d.V. and M.B. Formal analysis and data curation: C.S.S., E.S. and M.B. Investigation: C.S.S., A.C., A.D.T., A.M.C., C.T., M.J.A., N.L., P.P., M.M., C.P.-G., J.D. and M.A. Supervision: C.S.S., J.N.d.V. and M.B. Project administration: C.S.S., J.M., J.N.d.V. and M.B. Writing—original draft preparation: C.S.S. Writing—review and editing: C.S.S., E.S., J.M., A.C., A.D.T., M.J.A., M.A., C.T., J.N.d.V. and M.B. All authors have read and agreed to the published version of the manuscript.

Funding: Financial support was provided by the Fundação Calouste Gulbenkian (FCG)/Camões, IP agreement nr. 2208700707/22.10.202, and Science and Technology Development Project Funding agreement 11/MESCTI/PDCT/2020 for the action entitled Building COVID-19 Response Capacity in Angola.

Institutional Review Board Statement: The study was previously reviewed and approved by the national ethics committee of the Ministry of Health of Angola (approval no. 25/2020).

Informed Consent Statement: Informed consent was obtained from all subjects involved in the study.

Data Availability Statement: Not applicable.

Acknowledgments: The authors are grateful for the participation of all Angolan COVID-19 patients enrolled in the study. We also wish to express our gratitude to the Fundação Calouste Gulbenkian (FCG) and Camões, IP, for financial assistance. Gratitude also goes to the CISA, INIS, Hospital Militar Principal, Clínica Girassol, and Lucrécia Paim Maternity, for institutional backing. We also want to recognize Anabela Mateus, Welwitschia Dias, Luzia Quipungo, Luísa Dachala, Bruno Cardoso, Celestina Gaston, Domingos Biete Alfredo, Janete António, Manuela Galangue, and Francisco Manuel for laboratory support or patient recruitment; Zinga David and António Mateus to provide administrative support; Vera Mendes and Joana Sebastião for logistical assistance.

Conflicts of Interest: The authors declare no conflict of interest.

References

1. Lu, H.; Stratton, C.W.; Tang, Y.W. Outbreak of pneumonia of unknown etiology in Wuhan, China: The mystery and the miracle. *J. Med. Virol.* **2020**, *92*, 401–402. [CrossRef] [PubMed]
2. Gorbalenya, A.E.; Baker, S.C.; Baric, R.S.; de Groot, R.J.; Drosten, C.; Gulyaeva, A.A.; Haagmans, B.L.; Lauber, C.; Leontovich, A.M.; Neuman, B.W.; et al. The species Severe acute respiratory syndrome-related coronavirus: Classifying 2019-nCoV and naming it SARS-CoV-2. *Nat. Microbiol.* **2020**, *5*, 536–544.
3. Wu, A.; Peng, Y.; Huang, B.; Ding, X.; Wang, X.; Niu, P.; Meng, J.; Zhu, Z.; Zhang, Z.; Wang, J.; et al. Genome Composition and Divergence of the Novel Coronavirus (2019-nCoV) Originating in China. *Cell Host Microbe* **2020**, *27*, 325–328. [CrossRef] [PubMed]
4. Zhou, P.; Yang, X.L.; Wang, X.G.; Hu, B.; Zhang, L.; Zhang, W.; Si, H.R.; Zhu, Y.; Li, B.; Huang, C.L.; et al. A pneumonia outbreak associated with a new coronavirus of probable bat origin. *Nature* **2020**, *579*, 270–273. [CrossRef]
5. Sohrabia, C.; Alsafib, Z.; O'Neilla, N.; Khanb, M.; Kerwanc, A.; Al-Jabirc, A.; Iosifidisa, C.; Aghad, R. World Health Organization declares global emergency: A review of the 2019 novel coronavirus (COVID-19). *Int. J. Surg.* **2020**, *76*, 71–76.
6. Adhanom Ghebreyesus, T. WHO Director-General's opening remarks at the media briefing on COVID-19-11 March 2020. *World Health Organ.* **2020**, *4*, 1–4.
7. Bulut, C.; Kato, Y. Epidemiology of COVID-19. *Turkish J. Med. Sci.* **2020**, *50*, 563–570. [CrossRef]
8. WHO Coronavirus disease (COVID-19): Situation Report–107. *World Health Organ.* **2020**, *2019*, 2633.
9. WHO Coronavirus Disease: Symptoms. *WHO*. 2022. Available online: https://covid19.who.int/ (accessed on 1 September 2022).
10. Guan, W.J.; Ni, Z.Y.; Hu, Y.; Liang, W.H.; Ou, C.Q.; He, J.X.; Liu, L.; Shan, H.; Lei, C.L.; Hui, D.S.C.; et al. Clinical Characteristics of Coronavirus Disease 2019 in China. *N. Engl. J. Med.* **2020**, *382*, 1708–1720. [CrossRef]
11. Li, T.; Lu, H.; Zhang, W. Clinical observation and management of COVID-19 patients. *Emerg. Microbes Infect.* **2020**, *9*, 687–690. [CrossRef]
12. Zhang, J.; Dong, X.; Cao, Y.; Yuan, Y.; Yang, Y.; Yan, Y.; Akdis, C.A.; Gao, Y. Clinical characteristics of 140 patients infected with SARS-CoV-2 in Wuhan, China. *Allergy Eur. J. Allergy Clin. Immunol.* **2020**, *75*, 1730–1741. [CrossRef]
13. Chen, N.; Zhou, M.; Dong, X.; Qu, J.; Gong, F.; Han, Y.; Qiu, Y.; Wang, J.; Liu, Y.; Wei, Y.; et al. Epidemiological and clinical characteristics of 99 cases of 2019 novel coronavirus pneumonia in Wuhan, China: A descriptive study. *Lancet* **2020**, *395*, 507–513. [CrossRef]
14. Zhou, F.; Yu, T.; Du, R.; Fan, G.; Liu, Y.; Liu, Z.; Xiang, J.; Wang, Y.; Song, B.; Gu, X.; et al. Clinical course and risk factors for mortality of adult inpatients with COVID-19 in Wuhan, China: A retrospective cohort study. *Lancet* **2020**, *395*, 1054–1062. [CrossRef]
15. Weiss, P.; Murdoch, D.R. Clinical course and mortality risk of severe COVID-19. *Lancet Comment* **2020**, *395*, 1014–1015. [CrossRef]
16. Huang, C.; Wang, Y.; Li, X.; Ren, L.; Zhao, J.; Hu, Y.; Zhang, L.; Fan, G.; Xu, J.; Gu, X.; et al. Clinical features of patients infected with 2019 novel coronavirus in Wuhan, China. *Lancet* **2020**, *395*, 497–506. [CrossRef]
17. Liu, L.; Huang, J.; Zhong, M.; Yuan, K.; Chen, Y. Seroprevalence of Dengue Virus among Pregnant Women in Guangdong, China. *Viral Immunol.* **2020**, *33*, 48–53. [CrossRef] [PubMed]
18. Ruan, Q.; Yang, K.; Wang, W.; Jiang, L.; Song, J. Clinical predictors of mortality due to COVID-19 based on an analysis of data of 150 patients from Wuhan, China. *Intensive Care Med.* **2020**, *46*, 846–848. [CrossRef] [PubMed]
19. Henry, B.M.; De Oliveira, M.H.S.; Benoit, S.; Plebani, M.; Lippi, G. Hematologic, biochemical and immune biomarker abnormalities associated with severe illness and mortality in coronavirus disease 2019 (COVID-19): A meta-analysis. *Clin. Chem. Lab. Med.* **2020**, *8*, 1021–1028. [CrossRef]
20. Tay, M.Z.; Poh, C.M.; Rénia, L.; MacAry, P.A.; Ng, L.F.P. The trinity of COVID-19: Immunity, inflammation and intervention. *Nat. Rev. Immunol.* **2020**, *20*, 363–374. [CrossRef]
21. Wong, C.K.; Lam, C.W.K.; Wu, A.K.L.; Ip, W.K.; Lee, N.L.S.; Chan, I.H.S.; Lit, L.C.W.; Hui, D.S.C.; Chan, M.H.M.; Chung, S.S.C.; et al. Plasma inflammatory cytokines and chemokines in severe acute respiratory syndrome. *Clin. Exp. Immunol.* **2004**, *136*, 95–103. [CrossRef]
22. Qin, C.; Zhou, L.; Hu, Z.; Zhang, S.; Yang, S.; Tao, Y.; Xie, C.; Ma, K.; Shang, K.; Wang, W.; et al. Dysregulation of immune response in patients with COVID-19 in Wuhan, China. *Clin. Infect. Dis. An Off. Publ. Infect. Dis. Soc. Am.* **2020**, *15*, 762–768. [CrossRef] [PubMed]
23. Phelan, T.; Dunne, J.; Conlon, N.; Cheallaigh, C.N.í.; Abbott, W.M.; Faba-Rodriguez, R.; Amanat, F.; Krammer, F.; Little, M.A.; Hughes, G.; et al. Dynamic Assay for Profiling Anti-SARS-CoV-2 Antibodies and Their ACE2/Spike RBD Neutralization Capacity. *Viruses* **2021**, *13*, 1371. [CrossRef] [PubMed]
24. Wang, D.; Hu, B.; Hu, C.; Zhu, F.; Liu, X.; Zhang, J.; Wang, B.; Xiang, H.; Cheng, Z.; Xiong, Y.; et al. Clinical Characteristics of 138 Hospitalized Patients With 2019 Novel Coronavirus–Infected Pneumonia in Wuhan, China. *J. Am. Med. Assoc.* **2020**, *323*, 1061. [CrossRef] [PubMed]
25. Sebastião, C.S.; Neto, Z.; Martinez, P.; Jandondo, D.; Antonio, J.; Galangue, M.; De Carvalho, M.; David, K.; Miranda, J.; Afonso, P.; et al. Sociodemographic characteristics and risk factors related to SARS-CoV-2 infection in Luanda, Angola. *PLoS ONE* **2021**, *16*, 1–10.
26. Gagnon, L.R.; Sadasivan, C.; Yogasundaram, H.; Oudit, G.Y. Review of Hydroxychloroquine Cardiotoxicity: Lessons From the COVID-19 Pandemic. *Curr. Heart Fail. Rep.* **2022**, *27*, 1–9. [CrossRef]

27. Di Stefano, L.; Ogburn, E.L.; Ram, M.; Scharfstein, D.O.; Li, T.; Khanal, P.; Baksh, S.N.; McBee, N.; Gruber, J.; Gildea, M.R.; et al. Hydroxychloroquine/chloroquine for the treatment of hospitalized patients with COVID-19: An individual participant data meta-analysis. *PLoS ONE* **2022**, *17*, e0273526. [CrossRef]
28. Sebastião, C.S.; Gaston, C.; Paixão, J.P.; Sacomboio, E.N.M.; Neto, Z.; de Vasconcelos, J.N.; Morais, J. Coinfection between SARS-CoV-2 and vector-borne diseases in Luanda, Angola. *J. Med. Virol.* **2021**, *94*, 366–371. [CrossRef]
29. Monticelli, M.; Mele, B.H.; Andreotti, G.; Cubellis, M.V.; Riccio, G. Why does SARS-CoV-2 hit in different ways? Host genetic factors can influence the acquisition or the course of COVID-19. *Eur. J. Med. Genet.* **2021**, *64*, 104227. [CrossRef]
30. Marklund, E.; Leach, S.; Axelsson, H.; Nyström, K.; Norder, H.; Bemark, M.; Angeletti, D.; Lundgren, A.; Nilsson, S.; Andersson, L.-M.; et al. Serum-IgG responses to SARS-CoV-2 after mild and severe COVID-19 infection and analysis of IgG non-responders. *PLoS ONE* **2020**, *15*, e0241104. [CrossRef]
31. Corona, A.; Richini, G.; Simoncini, S.; Zangrandi, M.; Biasini, M.; Russo, G.; Pasqua, M.; Santorsola, C.; Gregorini, C.; Giordano, C. Treating Critically Ill Patients Experiencing SARS-CoV-2 Severe Infection with Ig-M and Ig-A Enriched Ig-G Infusion. *Antibiotics* **2021**, *10*, 930. [CrossRef]
32. Guan, X.; Zhang, B.; Fu, M.; Li, M.; Yuan, X.; Zhu, Y.; Peng, J.; Guo, H.; Lu, Y. Clinical and inflammatory features based machine learning model for fatal risk prediction of hospitalized COVID-19 patients: Results from a retrospective cohort study. *Ann. Med.* **2021**, *53*, 257–266. [CrossRef] [PubMed]
33. Maklad, S.; Basiony, F. Electrolyte disturbances in patients with acute exacerbation of chronic obstructive pulmonary disease. *Sci. J. Al-Azhar Med. Fac. Girls* **2019**, *3*, 427. [CrossRef]
34. Albeladi, F.I.; Wahby Salem, I.M.; Albandar, A.A.; Almusaylim, H.A.; Albandar, A.S. Electrolyte imbalance in infectious disease patients at King Abdulaziz Hospital, Jeddah. *J. Taibah Univ. Med. Sci.* **2022**, *17*, 256–263. [CrossRef] [PubMed]
35. Chen, D.; Chen, D.; Li, X.; Song, Q.; Hu, C.; Hu, C.; Su, F.; Su, F.; Dai, J.; Dai, J.; et al. Assessment of Hypokalemia and Clinical Characteristics in Patients with Coronavirus Disease 2019 in Wenzhou, China. *JAMA Netw. Open* **2020**, *3*, 1–12. [CrossRef] [PubMed]
36. Weiner, I.D.; Wingo, C.S. Hyperkalemia: A potential silent killer. *J. Am. Soc. Nephrol.* **1998**, *9*, 1535–1543. [CrossRef]
37. Moreno, -P.O.; Leon-Ramirez, J.M.; Fuertes-Kenneally, L.; Perdiguero, M.; Andres, M.; Garcia-Navarro, M.; Ruiz-Torregrosa, P.; Boix, V.; Gil, J.; Merino, E.; et al. Hypokalemia as a sensitive biomarker of disease severity and the requirement for invasive mechanical ventilation requirement in COVID-19 pneumonia: A case series of 306 Mediterranean patients. *Int. J. Infect. Dis.* **2020**, *100*, 449–454. [CrossRef]
38. Petnak, T.; Thongprayoon, C.; Cheungpasitporn, W.; Bathini, T.; Vallabhajosyula, S.; Chewcharat, A.; Kashani, K. Serum Chloride Levels at Hospital Discharge and One-Year Mortality among Hospitalized Patients. *Med. Sci.* **2020**, *8*, 22. [CrossRef]
39. Hong, K.-H.; Choi, J.-P.; Hong, S.-H.; Lee, J.; Kwon, J.-S.; Kim, S.-M.; Park, S.Y.; Rhee, J.-Y.; Kim, B.-N.; Choi, H.J.; et al. Predictors of mortality in Middle East respiratory syndrome (MERS). *Thorax* **2018**, *73*, 286–289. [CrossRef]
40. Choi, K.W.; Chau, T.N.; Tsang, O.; Tso, E.; Chiu, M.C.; Tong, W.L.; Lee, P.O.; Ng, T.K.; Ng, W.F.; Lee, K.C.; et al. Outcomes and Prognostic Factors in 267 Patients with Severe Acute Respiratory Syndrome in Hong Kong. *Ann. Intern. Med.* **2003**, *139*, 715–724. [CrossRef]
41. Alfaraj, S.H.; Al-Tawfiq, J.A.; Assiri, A.Y.; Alzahrani, N.A.; Alanazi, A.A.; Memish, Z.A. Clinical predictors of mortality of Middle East Respiratory Syndrome Coronavirus (MERS-CoV) infection: A cohort study. *Travel Med. Infect. Dis.* **2019**, *29*, 48–50. [CrossRef]
42. Milbrandt, E.B.; Reade, M.C.; Lee, M.; Shook, S.L.; Angus, D.C.; Kong, L.; Carter, M.; Yealy, D.M.; Kellum, J.A. Prevalence and Significance of Coagulation Abnormalities in Community-Acquired Pneumonia. *Mol. Med.* **2009**, *15*, 438–445. [CrossRef] [PubMed]
43. Rodelo, J.R.; De La Rosa, G.; Valencia, M.L.; Ospina, S.; Arango, C.M.; Gómez, C.I.; García, A.; Nuñez, E.; Jaimes, F.A. D-dimer is a significant prognostic factor in patients with suspected infection and sepsis. *Am. J. Emerg. Med.* **2012**, *30*, 1991–1999. [CrossRef] [PubMed]

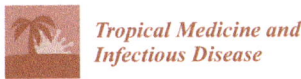 *Tropical Medicine and Infectious Disease*

Article

Factors Associated with Self-Medication during the COVID-19 Pandemic: A Cross-Sectional Study in Pakistan

Bakhtawar Chaudhry [1], Saiza Azhar [1], Shazia Jamshed [2,*], Jahanzaib Ahmed [1], Laiq-ur-Rehman Khan [1], Zahid Saeed [1], Melinda Madléna [3], Márió Gajdács [3] and Abdur Rasheed [4,*]

1. College of Pharmacy, University of Sargodha, Sargodha 40100, Pakistan
2. Department of Clinical Pharmacy and Practice, Faculty of Pharmacy, Universiti Sultan Zainal Abidin, Kuala Terengganu 21300, Malaysia
3. Department of Oral Biology and Experimental Dental Research, Faculty of Dentistry, University of Szeged, 6720 Szeged, Hungary
4. School of Public Health Dow, University of Health Sciences, Karachi 74200, Pakistan
* Correspondence: shaziajamshed@unisza.edu.my (S.J.); abdur.rasheed@duhs.edu.pk (A.R.)

Citation: Chaudhry, B.; Azhar, S.; Jamshed, S.; Ahmed, J.; Khan, L.-u.-R.; Saeed, Z.; Madléna, M.; Gajdács, M.; Rasheed, A. Factors Associated with Self-Medication during the COVID-19 Pandemic: A Cross-Sectional Study in Pakistan. *Trop. Med. Infect. Dis.* 2022, 7, 330. https://doi.org/10.3390/tropicalmed7110330

Academic Editors: Peter A. Leggat, John Frean and Lucille Blumberg

Received: 13 August 2022
Accepted: 22 October 2022
Published: 25 October 2022

Publisher's Note: MDPI stays neutral with regard to jurisdictional claims in published maps and institutional affiliations.

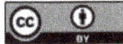

Copyright: © 2022 by the authors. Licensee MDPI, Basel, Switzerland. This article is an open access article distributed under the terms and conditions of the Creative Commons Attribution (CC BY) license (https://creativecommons.org/licenses/by/4.0/).

Abstract: Self-medication (SM) is characterized by the procurement and use of medicines by bypassing primary healthcare services and without consulting a physician, usually to manage acute symptoms of self-diagnosed illnesses. Due to the limited availability of primary healthcare services and the anxiety associated with the COVID-19 pandemic, the compulsion to SM by the public has increased considerably. The study aimed to assess the characteristics, practices, and associated factors of SM by the public during the COVID-19 pandemic in Sargodha, Pakistan. χ^2-tests and univariable analyses were conducted to explore the identification of characteristics and the potential contributing factors for SM during COVID-19, while multivariable logistic regression models were run to study the effect of variables that maintained a significant association. The study was performed during July–September 2021, with $n = 460$ questionnaires returned overall (response rate: 99.5%). The majority of respondents were males (58.7%, $n = 270$) who live in the periphery of the town (63.9%, $n = 294$), and most of the respondents belonged to the age group of 18–28 years (73.3%, $n = 339$). A large number, 46.1% ($n = 212$), of the participants were tested for COVID-19 during the pandemic, and among them, 34.3% ($n = 158$) practiced SM during the pandemic; the most common source of obtaining medicines was requesting them directly from a pharmacy (25.0%; $n = 127$). The chances of practicing SM for medical health professionals were 1.482 (p-value = 0.046) times greater than for non-medical health personnel. The likelihood of practicing SM in participants whose COVID-19 test was positive was 7.688 (p-value < 0.001) times more than who did not test for COVID-19. Allopathic medicines, acetaminophen (23.6%), azithromycin (14,9%), and cough syrups (13%), and over the counter (OTC) pharmaceuticals, vitamin oral supplements, such as Vitamin C (39.1%), folic acid (23.5%), and calcium (22.6%), were the most commonly consumed medicines and supplements, respectively; being a healthcare professional or having a COVID-test prior showed a significant association with the usage of Vitamin C ($p < 0.05$ in all cases). Respondents who mentioned unavailability of the physician and difficulty in travelling/reaching healthcare professionals were found 2.062-times (p-value = 0.004) and 1.862-times (p-value = 0.021) more likely to practice SM, respectively; SM due to fear of COVID was more common in individuals who had received COVID-tests prior ($p = 0.004$). Practices of SM were observed at alarming levels among our participants. Consciousness and understanding about the possible adverse effects of SM must be established and validated on a continuous level; in addition, on a commercial level, collaboration from pharmacists not to sell products (especially prescription-only medicines) without a certified prescription must be developed and implemented.

Keywords: self-medication; COVID-19; pandemic; over-the-counter; medicine use; Pakistan

1. Introduction

Self-medication (SM) is characterized by the procurement and use of medicines by bypassing primary healthcare services and without consulting a physician, usually to manage acute symptoms of self-diagnosed illnesses [1,2]. Based on the World Health Organization's (WHO) definition, SM is "the choice and use of drugs by any individual in order to treat their own self-identified illness or symptoms" [3]. Drugs used for SM normally include over the counter drugs (OTC), however, in some cases (when the patients acquire them from various sources) prescription-only medicines (POM) are also relevant [4]. The intention of utilizing SM may be affected by various factors, such as individual, organizational, and environmental variables [5]. Individual factors include age, income, gender, highest level of education, life satisfaction, convenience, and urgency/severity of symptoms [6]. Commercials and adverts by pharmaceutical companies via the media and the internet also have a considerable role in facilitating this practice [7]. SM incorporates purchasing drugs (both from formal and informal sources), or re-utilizing stashes (i.e., leftovers from a medicine cabinet) from past prescriptions, receiving medicines from and taking them on the counsel of relatives, neighbors, and friends [8]. SM is a global public health issue; nevertheless, the prevalence of this practice is more common in developing countries (i.e., low and middle-income countries) [9,10]. In these regions, organizational attributes, such as poor quality and availability of healthcare services, a relatively high number of individuals without health insurance, a lack of human resources, unavailability of transport services, non-professional behaviors of healthcare providers, and long turnaround times—coupled with the availability of drugs for purchase from "hawkers"—considerably increase the SM [11,12]. The lack of knowledge regarding the use of pharmaceuticals (i.e., their indications, dosage, appropriate treatment duration, and possible side effects) and mistrust towards physicians may also facilitate SM [13,14]. Although the WHO has noted that the practice of SM may remedy some minor obsessive situations at a reasonable expense, there have been reports that it might lead to the squandering of medical assets and excess pharmaceutical waste [15]. In addition, inappropriate use of pharmaceuticals carries the risk of a delayed diagnosis, an unfavorable response to medications, excess morbidity, and the emergence of multi-drug resistant (MDR) organisms in the case of antimicrobials [15–17]. The general population of Pakistan turned to self-medication and symptomatic therapy because of inadequate care for the COVID-19 infection; about 80% of the population also stockpiled drugs for use during the pandemic [18].

During the first part of 2020, the WHO cautioned the world about the rapid spread of the novel coronavirus (SARS-CoV-2), which later progressed into a global pandemic; due to the associated disease (COVID-19), an overall lockdown was set off in the greater part of the world [19]. The pandemic has caused a considerable burden on healthcare infrastructures worldwide, especially in countries where the healthcare framework was fragile to begin with [20]. In response to the limited availability of primary healthcare services and the anxiety associated with the pandemic, the compulsion to SM by the public has increased considerably, as in the eyes of many, this was the only sensible "link" to healthcare [21,22]. In parallel with the onset of the pandemic, many studies (both preclinical and clinical) have been published on the effectiveness of various drugs in the treatment and prevention of COVID-19; these included anti-malarial agents (chloroquine and hydroxychloroquine), antibiotics (azithromycin and doxycycline), antiparasitic drugs (ivermectin), decongestants (azelastine), leukotriene inhibitors (montelukast), non-steroidal anti-inflammatory drugs, and acetaminophen, alongside nutrients, such as Vitamin C and D, zinc, and calcium [23]. Although the effectiveness of most of the above mentioned therapies has largely been disproven by multicentric clinical trials, in the first and second waves of the pandemic—in combination with the rampant "infodemic" regarding COVID treatments in online media—attempts to treat COVID-19 with e.g., hydroxychloroquine in the absence of any healthcare professional consultation or prescription (as a prime example of SM) were widespread [24–26]. Due to the overlap of symptoms between COVID-19 and other viral respiratory infections (e.g., throat aches, dry cough, malaise, fever, and shortness of breath), in many regions, individuals began taking drugs without being tested for COVID-19 at all, often leading to drug shortages due to supply chain issues [27].

Since its global spread in 2020, COVID-19 has led to considerable morbidity and mortality, significant upheaval in healthcare systems worldwide, and the fear of infection has been constantly present in the lives of individuals; this has led to anxiety and tension in both medical service laborers and the overall population in numerous parts of the world [28]. These factors may have contributed to an increase in SM; thus, the present study aimed to investigate the characteristics, practices, and potential contributing factors towards the use of SM during COVID-19 in Sargodha, Pakistan. This research also explored the different types of medicines used for SM during COVID-19.

2. Materials and Methods

2.1. Study Design, Study Site and Population

A questionnaire-based cross-sectional study design was adopted to assess the characteristics, practices, and contributing factors towards SM during the COVID-19 pandemic in Sargodha, Pakistan (155 km^2, 12th largest city by population, with ~660,000 inhabitants and a literacy rate ~80%). The potential population of this study was the general population of Sargodha city and its periphery. The respondents or participants were selected through convenience and snowball sampling methods. The study was conducted between July and September 2021.

2.2. Sample Size Calculation

To establish the required sample size for our study, a sample size calculation was performed by using the Raosoft sample size calculator [29,30], based on the Formula (1) below:

$$n = N \frac{x}{(N-1)E2 + x} \quad (1)$$

where the population N was set at 20,000 (as the general population of Sargodha city was >20,000; however, in such population ranges, higher population values do not have an effect on the target sample size), x is the confidence interval of 95%, E is the margin of error set at 5%, and the expected response rate is set at 50%.

The calculated initial sample size of residents of Sargodha was 384, which was increased by 20% for added contingency (to adjust for factors such as withdrawals, missing and incomplete questionnaires), with the final sample size set at $n = 462$.

2.3. Study Instrument and Data Collection

Before the development of the research instrument, a literature search was performed to ascertain potentially relevant questions and topics; during this process, we converted the research topic into keywords, which served as the foundation of an efficient search by providing results based on any of the terms included. After a thorough search of the literature, a structured and validated questionnaire was developed as a data collection tool. The questionnaire was validated by experts and researchers and for a better understanding of the respondents, then an interviewer-administered technique was used. The questionnaire was comprised of statements and items pertaining to the following sections: (i) socio-demographic data and general questions about the participants, including whether they are healthcare professionals or their history of being COVID tested; (ii) knowledge, attitudes, and practices towards SM during the COVID-19 pandemic, types of medicines used for SM; and (iii) piotential contributing factors influencing SM. The translation and adaptation of the questionnaire were performed according to the criteria of Beaton et al. [31]. Before the main study, pilot testing was performed (involving 30 participants not included in the sample population) for the instrument to assess its face and content validity and comprehension/readability by the respondents. Using Cronbach's Alpha, the instrument's internal consistency and reliability were evaluated; the resultant value ($\alpha = 0.710$) showed acceptable reliability in questionnaire-based research. Based on the experiences from the pilot testing of the questionnaire, various minor changes have been made in the wording of the paper questionnaire to produce the final instrument (Supplementary Material S1). The final instrument was then administered by the interviewer, which meant that the principal researcher approached each participant personally, and the interviewer gave the respondent feedback or repeated the question or available options (if an invalid one was given) to obtain an appropriate response. Each participant was explained the nature of the study and asked their responses. If any query arose at that time, the principal researcher clarified the doubts and proceeded with data collection.

2.4. Inclusion and Exclusion Criteria

The participants included in this study were willing adults (between 18 and 60 years of age) without having any communication problems, either due to illness or some other reason. Adults who could not participate without a caretaker or guardian, and people approached who were unwilling to participate were excluded.

2.5. Statistical Analysis

Data analysis—including descriptive statistics (frequencies, means, and percentages) and all inferential statistical analyses were performed using SPSS (Statistical Package for Social Sciences) version 24 (SPSS Inc., Chicago, IL, USA). χ^2-tests and univariable analyses were conducted to explore the identification of characteristics and the potential contributing factors for self-medication during COVID-19. Multivariable logistic regression models were run to study the effects of variables that maintained a significant association. Results are presented as odds ratios (OR) and 95% confidence intervals (CI); p-values ≤ 0.05 were considered statistically significant.

2.6. Ethical Considerations

The study was conducted in accordance with the Declaration of Helsinki and national and institutional ethical standards. Study approval for the study protocol was obtained from the Advanced Studies and Research Board of the University of Sargodha (Ref number: SU/Acad/1723). All participants were informed of the nature and aims of the study and the data collected; all willing participants of the study signed an informed consent form. The confidentiality and anonymity of the participants were protected throughout the study.

3. Results

3.1. Socio-demographic Characteristics of the Participants

Out of the 462 questionnaires, n = 460 questionnaires were returned completely filled out, resulting in a response rate of 99.5%. The socio-demographic characteristics of the study participants are summarized in Table 1; participants were invited to add their age in years, but later it was binned to groups. The majority of respondents were males (58.7%, n = 270) who lived in the periphery of the town (63.9%, n = 245), and most of the respondents belonged to the age group of 18–28 years (73.3%, n = 339). Only 46.1% (n = 212) of the participants were tested for COVID-19 during the pandemic. Almost half (46.5%, n = 214) of the respondents were working in the healthcare field.

Table 1. Demographic characteristics and general information of participants.

Demographic Characteristics	Category	n, %
Age (Years)	18–28	339 (73.3)
	29–38	61 (13.5)
	39–48	32 (7.0)
	49–58	28 (6.2)
Gender	Male	270 (58.7)
	Female	190 (41.3)

Table 1. Cont.

Demographic Characteristics	Category	n, %
Marital Status	Single	307 (66.7)
	Married	142 (30.9)
	Divorced	10 (2.4)
Area of Residence	Sargodha	166 (36.1)
	Peripheral part of the city	294 (63.9)
Healthcare-Professional	Yes	215 (46.7)
	No	245 (53.3)
Tested for COVID-19	Yes (the result was positive)	34 (7.2)
	Yes (the result was negative)	178 (38.7)
	No	248 (53.9)

3.2. Characteristics of SM during the COVID-19 Pandemic

Table 2 presents our main findings regarding the practices of SM in our study population. Overall, 34.3% ($n = 158$) of participants self-medicated during the COVID-19 pandemic. The most common sources of drugs for SM were from requesting them directly from a pharmacy (25.0%). A significant association was observed between responses to SM, being employed in the healthcare profession ($p = 0.046$), and being tested for COVID-19 ($p < 0.001$). The types of medicines (allopathic vs. others and OTC and POM vs. POM only) used for SM were associated with area of residence and COVID-testing ($p < 0.001$). The majority of the respondents, about 65.9% ($n = 304$), were aware of the possible adverse effects of the SM drug taken, there was a significant association found with being employed in the healthcare profession ($p < 0.001$) and being tested for COVID-19 ($p = 0.004$).

3.3. Types of Medicines Used as SM during the COVID-19 Pandemic

The types of medicines used as SM and the associated correlates with their use were summarized in Table 3. The use of herbal medicines as SM was prevalent among respondents: 51.7% of participants never used any herbal medicines, while 20.0 % used Senna Makhi Kehwa; their use was significantly associated with area of residence ($p < 0.001$), being affiliated with the medical profession ($p < 0.001$) and undergoing a test for COVID-19 ($p < 0.017$). Among allopathic medicines, the most commonly used drugs were acetaminophen (23.6 %), azithromycin (14,9 %), and cough syrups (13.0 %), all drugs associated with the SM for the prevention and treatment of COVID infections during lockdowns; area of residence, being a healthcare professional, or having a COVID-test were important correlates. The most commonly consumed supplements during COVID-19 in our sample were vitamins (Vitamin C: 39.1%, folic acid: 23.5%, and calcium: 22.6%); area of residence, being a healthcare professional, or having a COVID-test showed significant correlation ($p < 0.001$) with the use of these supplements to boost immunity against COVID.

3.4. Possible Contributing Factors and Reasons Associated with SM during the COVID-19 Pandemic

Potential contributing factors for SM were identified based on the literature review of factors shown to increase SM, and an expert consensus of a group of public health specialists. Reported reasons and contributing factors associated with SM in our sample are shown in Table 4. While previously existing SM habits (7.3%) were also noted, the main reasons for SM were identified, i.e., the unavailability (13.9%) and difficulty in travelling/reaching healthcare professionals (12%), which may have led to preventive SM. SM associated with unavailability of a physician was more common in the peripheral parts of the city ($p = 0.010$), while SM due to difficulty in travelling/reaching healthcare professionals was more common in individuals who had received COVID-tests prior ($p = 0.030$).

Table 2. Characteristics of SM during the COVID-19 pandemic.

Descriptors			p-Values					
Variables	Categories	n, %	Age	Gender	Marital Status	Area of Residence	Medical Health Professional	Tested for COVID 19
Did you practice SM?	Yes No	158 (34.3) 302 (65.7)	0.042	0.212	0.52	0.194	0.046	<0.001
Types of medicines used	Allopathic Herbal Both None	71 (15.4) 104 (22.6) 69 (15.0) 216 (47.0)	N/A	0.892	N/A	<0.001	0.05	<0.001
Did you use POM during SM?	Yes No	99 (21.5) 361 (78.5)	0.072	0.344	0.004	0.002	0.001	<0.001
Sources of medicines	From a prescription for a family member	48 (9.5)	N/A	0.798	0.255	0.147	0.294	0.02
	From a prescription for a friend	39 (7.7)	N/A	0.186	0.356	0.956	0.939	<0.001
	Requested directly from pharmacy	127 (25.0)	0.725	0.744	0.829	0.054	0.11	0.004
	Drugs from family members	53 (10.5)	N/A	0.248	0.219	0.593	0.034	0.235
	Drugs from friends	18 (3.5)	N/A	0.093	0.803	0.816	0.842	0.1
	Other	222 (43.8)	0.186	0.748	0.053	0.001	0.373	<0.001
Were you aware of the possible side effects of the SM drugs?	Yes No	304 (65.9) 156 (34.1)	0.899	0.57	0.005	0.306	<0.001	0.004
Did you receive information regarding the possible side effects of the SM drugs?	No Yes, from a physician Yes, from a family member Yes, from a colleague Yes, from the internet Yes, from other sources	104 (22.6) 60 (13) 100 (21.7) 23 (5.0) 62 (13.5) 111 (24.2)	N/A	<0.001	0.049	<0.001	<0.001	0.001
Have you felt improvement in your symptoms due to above mentioned medicines/substances?	Yes No	284 (61.7) 176 (38.3)	0.021	0.456	0.027	0.738	<0.001	0.036
Have you felt improvement in your symptoms due to above mentioned medicines/substances?	Yes No	259 (56.3) 201 (43.7)	0.04	0.022	0.41	0.019	<0.001	0.006
Does pharmacist demand for a prescription when you visit to buy medicines?	Yes No	259 (56.3) 201 (43.7)	0.04	0.022	0.41	0.019	<0.001	0.006

p values ≤ 0.05 were presented in **boldface**; POM: prescription-only medicine.

Table 3. Medicines used as SM during the COVID-19 pandemic.

Variables	Descriptions			p-Values				
	Categories	n, %	Age	Gender	Marital Status	Area of Residence	Healthcare Professional	Tested for COVID-19
Herbal medicines	Senna Makhi Kehwa	92 (20.0)	0.619	0.166	0.667	<0.001	<0.001	0.017
	Homeopathic medicine	79 (17.2)						
	None	238 (51.7)						
	Other	51 (11.1)						
Allopathic medicines	Azithromycin	110 (14.9)	0.468	**0.006**	0.195	0.371	**<0.001**	0.152
	Dexamethasone	54 (7.3)	N/A	0.331	0.429	0.856	0.347	**0.001**
	Hydroxychloroquine	81 (11.0)	**0.004**	0.108	0.645	0.059	**<0.001**	**<0.001**
	Ivermectin	13 (1.8)	0.375	0.833	0.186	0.055	**0.005**	**0.050**
	Acetaminophen	174 (23.6)	0.376	0.980	0.430	**0.049**	0.139	0.949
	Aspirin	45 (6.1)	**0.033**	0.652	**0.001**	0.065	0.212	0.587
	Stool softeners	42 (5.7)	0.312	0.153	0.387	0.354	0.156	0.652
	Cough syrups	96 (13)	0.600	0.5.37	0.177	**0.002**	**0.003**	0.102
	Unknown	121 (16.6)	0.905	0.387	**0.006**	0.813	**<0.001**	**<0.001**
Supplements	Vitamin D	47 (10.2)	0.190	0.451	0.307	0.347	**0.030**	0.318
	Vitamin C	180 (39.1)	0.772	**0.039**	0.618	**<0.001**	**0.004**	**<0.001**
	Folic acid	108 (23.5)	0.147	**0.032**	0.378	0.233	0.097	0.122
	Calcium	104 (22.6)	0.365	0.115	0.673	0.603	0.719	0.128
	Other	114 (24.8)	0.417	0.675	0.432	**0.005**	**<0.001**	**<0.001**

p values ≤ 0.05 were presented in **boldface**.

Table 4. Contributing factors and reasons associated with SM during the COVID-19 pandemic.

Variables	Categories	n, %	Age	Gender	Area of Residence	Healthcare Professional	Tested for COVID-19
Reasons for SM	Already existing habits	40 (7.3)	N/A	0.619	0.873	0.231	0.153
	Unavailability of the physician	76 (13.9)	0.096	0.506	**0.010**	0.713	0.710
	Financial issues	39 (7.1)	N/A	0.016	0.984	0.680	0.680
	Difficulty in travelling/reaching healthcare professionals	66 (12.0)	N/A	0.091	0.920	0.170	**0.030**
	Lack of effectiveness of medicines prescribed by physician	58 (10.6)	N/A	0.399	0.540	0.758	0.594
	Fear of contracting the virus	41 (7.5)	N/A	0.177	0.825	0.969	0.784
	Bad experience with physician	44 (8.0)	N/A	0.955	0.723	0.515	0.275
	Other	184 (33.6)	0.562	0.439	0.804	0.342	**0.002**

p values ≤ 0.05 were presented in **boldface**.

Table 5 depicts the results of univariable and multivariable logistic regression analyses. Univariable analyses showed that the likelihood of practicing SM for individuals within the age group of 29–38 years was 1.72-fold (p-value = 0.047) compared to participants between 18–28 years of age. The chance of practicing SM for medical health professionals was 1.482-times higher (p-value = 0.046) than for non-medical health professionals. The likelihood of practicing SM for participants whose COVID-19 test was positive was 7.688-times (p-value < 0.001) more than for those who did not test for COVID-19. Individuals who were aware of the possible side effects of SM drugs were 2.266-times (p-value < 0.001) more likely to practice SM. Participants who received information regarding the possible side effects of the SM by the physician showed an almost 2 times (p-value = 0.045) higher chance of performing SM practices as compared to those who did not receive such information. As far as reasons are concerned, individuals who mentioned unavailability of the physician and difficulty in travelling/reaching healthcare professionals were found 2.062-times (p-value = 0.004) and 1.862-times (p-value =0.021) time more likely to perform SM, respectively.

The selection of variables for multivariable logistic regression analyses was based on the significance of the variables (p-values $\leq$ 0.05) in the univariable analysis. Furthermore, to confirm the best fitted model, different multivariable logistic models were run, for example, a multivariable model included all variables that were presented in univariable analysis, and another multivariable model included only those variables that were significant in univariable analysis. With the help of Akaike Information Criterion, AIC (the minimum values are better), it was found that the multivariable model presented in Table 5 was found to be better; the adjusted odds ratio and confidence interval are also reported in Table 5. Hence, after adjusting variables no. 1, 2, 3, 4, 5, 6, 8, 10, and 14 listed in Table 5, it was noted that variables 3 ("Tested for COVID") and 4 ("Were you aware of the possible side effects of the SM drugs?") showed significant (p-values $\leq$ 0.05) association as contributing factors for SM.

Table 5. Logistic regression analysis for identification of contributing factors for SM during COVID-19.

Variables	Categories	Practice SM No n (%)	Practice SM Yes n (%)	Univariable Logistic Regression C.O.R	Univariable Logistic Regression C.I	Univariable Logistic Regression p-Values	Multivariable Logistic Regression A.O.R	Multivariable Logistic Regression C.I	Multivariable Logistic Regression p-Values
1. Age	18–28	227 (67.0)	112 (33.0)	Ref		0.047 *	Ref		0.108
	29–38	33 (54.1)	28 (45.9)	1.72	0.990–2.987	0.054	1.446	0.778–2.687	0.244
	39–48	26 (81.3)	6 (18.8)	0.468	0.187–1.169	0.104	0.391	0.146–1.051	0.063
	49–58	16 (57.1)	12 (42.9)	1.52	0.695–3.322	0.294	1.438	0.597–3.461	0.418
2. Healthcare professional	Yes	131 (60.9)	84 (39.1)	1.482	1.007–2.181	0.046 *	1.163	0.740–1.828	0.513
	No	171 (69.8)	74 (30.2)	Ref			Ref		
3. Tested for COVID-19	Yes (the result was positive)	10 (29.4)	24 (70.6)	7.688	3.477–16.99	<0.001 *	5.258	2.261–12.229	<0.001 *
	Yes (the result was negative)	103 (57.9)	75 (42.1)	2.333	1.537–3.540	<0.001	1.884	1.189–2.987	<0.001 *
	No	189 (76.2)	59 (23.8)	Ref		<0.001	Ref		0.007
4. Were you aware of the possible side effects of the SM drugs?	Yes	181 (59.7)	122 (40.3)	2.266	1.463–3.508 *	<0.001 *	1.833	1.177–3.175	0.009 *
	No	121 (77.1)	36 (22.9)	Ref			Ref		
5. Does pharmacist demand for a prescription when you visit to buy medicines?	Yes	160 (61.8)	99 (38.2)	1.489	1.005–2.208 *	0.047 *	1.033	0.657–1.622	0.889
	No	142 (70.6)	59 (29.4)	Ref			Ref		
6. Did you receive information regarding the possible side effects of the SM drugs?	Yes, from a physician	67 (64.4)	37 (35.6)	Ref		0.005 *	Ref		0.125
	Yes, from a family member	29 (48.3)	31 (51.7)	1.963	1.014–3.694	0.045 *	1.46	0.710–3.003	0.304
	Yes, from a colleague	64 (64.0)	36 (36.0)	1.019	0.575–1.806	0.95	1.241	0.649–2.370	0.514
	Yes, from the Internet	15 (65.2)	8 (34.8)	1.068	0.556–2.056	0.844	1.235	0.583–2.641	0.581
	Yes, from other sources	39 (62.9)	23 (37.1)	0.966	0.374–2.491	0.943	1.1	0.383–3.159	0.859
		88 (79.3)	23 (20.7)	0.473	0.257–0.871	0.016 *	0.541	0.279–1.050	0.069
Reasons									
7. Already existing habits	Yes	26 (65.0)	14 (35.0)	1.032	0.523–2.038	0.928	-	-	-
	No	276 (65.7)	144 (34.3)	Ref			-	-	-
8. Unavailability of the physician	Yes	39 (51.3)	37 (48.7)	2.062	1.252–3.395	0.004 *	1.492	0.832–2.679	0.18
	No	263 (68.5)	121 (31.5)	Ref			Ref		
9. Financial issues	Yes	27 (69.2)	12 (30.8)	0.837	0.412–1.701	0.623	-	-	-
	No	275 (65.3)	146 (34.7)	Ref			-	-	-
10. Difficulty in travelling/reaching healthcare professionals	Yes	35 (53.0)	31 (47.0)	1.862	1.099–3.156	0.021 *	1.086	0.585–2.017	0.793
	No	267 (67.8)	121 (32.2)	Ref			Ref		

Table 5. Cont.

Variables	Categories	Practice SM		Univariable Logistic Regression			Multivariable Logistic Regression		
		No n (%)	Yes n (%)	C.O.R	CI	p-Values	A.O.R	CI	p-Values
11. Lack of effectiveness of medicines prescribed by physician	Yes	38 (65.5)	20 (34.5)	1.007	0.584–1.797	0.982	-	-	-
	No	264 (65.7)	138 (34.3)	Ref			-	-	-
12. Fear of contracting the virus	Yes	25 (61.0)	16 (39.0)	1.248	0.646–2.414	0.509	-	-	-
	No	277 (66.1)	142 (33.9)	Ref			-	-	-
13. Bad experience with physician	Yes	28 (63.6)	16 (36.4)	1.103	0.577–2.105	0.767	-	-	-
	No	274 (65.9)	142 (34.1)	Ref			-	-	-
14. Other	Yes	143 (77.7)	41 (22.3)	0.39	0.256–0.594	**<0.001 ***	0.639	0.380–1.074	0.091
	No	159 (57.6)	117 (42.4)	Ref			Ref		

C.O.R: Crude odds ratio (unadjusted OR), A.O.R: Adjusted OR; *: significant at ≤0.05, which are presented in **boldface**; multivariable logistic regression: adjustments were made for variables listed in the table for variables 1, 2, 3, 4, 5, 6, 8, 10 and 14.

4. Discussion

The purpose of the present study was to assess the characteristics and practices of SM in Sargodha, Pakistan, during the COVID-19 pandemic and to shed some light on the potential factors contributing to the practices of SM. According to our results, around one-third of the selected population has practiced SM, meaning that the majority still preferred/tried to establish contact with a physician or a licensed healthcare professional before consuming any medicine. Hence, the drugs received and utilized via personal prescriptions were higher than the rate of SM. Our findings (34.3%) regarding the use of SM were similar to findings from other developing countries after the onset of the pandemic, such as studies conducted in Togo (34.2%) [32] and Nigeria [33,34]. The main sources of drugs for SM were leftover prescriptions procured from friends and family, receiving drugs directly from family, and requesting them directly OTC from a pharmacy; similar sources as easy access to medications and SM were documented in a recent study from Dhaka, Bangladesh [35], and from previous studies in Rio Grande, Brazil [36], and Kuwait [37].

In this study, SM practice showed that those working in medical fields might be more fearful about the adverse effects of taking drugs inappropriately [38]; the possible reason for this could be better accessibility to relevant and trustworthy COVID-related information (from their workplace or from the internet), both about the prevention and the treatment of the illness. These findings are in line with a study conducted in India [39], where greater drug-related knowledge has led to concerned attitudes towards SM. On the other hand, identical studies have also been published noting the opposite, i.e., with significant levels of comprehension of OTC and POM drugs, including their prescription and adverse reactions, healthcare professionals were more likely to self-medicate during the outbreak [40]. Among our respondents, over half had never had a COVID-19 test of any kind, while the majority of those who had tests were documented as negative. This finding could be due to having a good degree of self-awareness about their health among people with a higher educational status [41]. The reasons for SM reported in this study were the unavailability of physicians, fears or difficulties in getting in contact with them, or bad experiences/ineffective treatments associated with visiting them, which were noted in other reports as well [32,33,36,37]. Fears of contracting the virus and difficulties in travelling to healthcare facilities were similarly documented in a study conducted in Lahore, Pakistan [42], and Dhaka, Bangladesh [35].

Our study reports that azithromycin was the most commonly used POM during the COVID-19 pandemic, while other notable allopathic medicines were acetaminophen, being the most commonly used for SM, and cough syrups, which is consistent with other reports in the context of COVID and SM [42]. The reason for azithromycin SM could be due to its properties being effective against COVID in vitro in addition to its proposed property to alleviate inflammation of the respiratory epithelium [43]. Acetaminophen was also highly noted among participants as a preventive measure against COVID-19; this drug has a widespread use already in SM for various indications, however, its use has expanded remarkably during the viral outbreak, both for its classical and novel supposed indications [44,45]. Ivermectin was also used as a preventative measure during the pandemic, as some early reports suggested a more promising outcome associated with supplementing the drug [46]; nevertheless, no recent clinical study has been successful in reliably confirming the usefulness of this compound in the prevention of COVID-19 [47]. Hydroxychloroquine was also extensively used in the initial stages of the pandemic as a preventive measure against COVID-19; studies of a different nature and quality have described the productive use of hydroxychloroquine and azithromycin for hospitalized individuals [48]; however, the utilization of hydroxychloroquine alone or with azithromycin may lead to substantial cardiac toxicities—leading to lethal arrhythmias in hospitalized COVID-patients—and highlighting that the use of these drugs as SM is questionable at best [49]. When it comes to dietary supplements to prevent/treat COVID, Vitamin C was used by approximately one third of participants; some studies have noted the efficacy of Vitamin C in the management of COVID-19 [50]. Nevertheless, it is also important to note that in high doses and when taken for extended periods of time, this vitamin may cause unwanted and harmful effects, like kidney stones [51]. Similarly, there has been considerable interest in Vitamin D supplementation for the prevention of acute respiratory tract infections and, in turn, COVID-19 [52,53]; but being a lipid-soluble vitamin, one has to be mindful with dosage to prevent hypervitaminosis and its associated adverse outcomes. According to this study, the participants used herbal medicines, i.e., Senna Makhi Kehwa, for the treatment and anticipation of contracting COVID-19. This may be explained by the fact that traditional medicines are habitually utilized as a result of the accessibility and lower expenses associated with herbal products [54]. It is also worth mentioning that the WHO has invited development throughout the world, including medicines of natural origins and herbal products, to explore potential therapeutics for COVID-19 [55].

The practice of SM has been previously noted to be highly prevalent in association with several ailments, including for the treatment of chronic pain [56], toothache and other dental indications [57], gastro-intestinal issues [58], and mood disorders [59]; nonetheless, with the onset of the COVID-19 pandemic, an increase in the prevalence of SM drug use associated with respiratory tract infections was noted. The WHO has predicted that the COVID-19 pandemic may last for a number of years, resulting in serious socio-economic consequences and changes in individuals' psycho-physical lifestyles, leading to deteriorating mental and physical health, which occurs in the backdrop of the unavailability of primary healthcare and mental care services [60]. With this in mind, national surveys on SM awareness and campaigns must be put forward to help educate laypeople and protect them from the potential harmful effects of the practice of SM.

The limitations of the present study must be acknowledged: firstly, the cross-sectional nature of the study design; the study was conducted in selected areas of Sargodha, with participants who were willing to participate in the research, which may have introduced bias into the results. Young adults and healthcare professionals are represented in high numbers among the participants. In this study, the practice of SM was associated with demographical patterns, i.e., age, gender, marital status, area of residence, and type of profession, however, this may not reflect the genuine image of SM in the entirety of Pakistan. Regarding statistical analyses, a limitation of the χ^2-square test is its sensitivity to sample size. When a big enough sample is employed, even small associations may become statistically significant. When applying the χ^2-square test, "statistically significant" does not automatically imply "meaningful". To establish causality, a more thorough examination would be needed, which we aimed to amend with the introduction of univariate and multivariable logistic regression analyses. Finally, the main limitation in conducting the present research-based study was the limited time-frame available to complete the study.

5. Conclusions

Self-medication (SM) has become a significant issue of health and well-being in developing countries, which has been exacerbated by the presently occurring COVID-19 pandemic. This study has concluded that the practice of self-medication is undertaken by approximately one-third of the population in Sargodha. The major contributing factors towards SM during COVID-19 were the unavailability of physicians, the lack of effectiveness of medicines prescribed by the physicians, and the fear of contracting the virus. Based on our results, various allopathic and natural alternative medicines were used for the prevention and treatment of COVID-19: azithromycin, acetaminophen, Ivermectin, and vitamin C and D were the most frequently consumed medicines and supplements. Medical health professionals, having comprehensive knowledge about drugs, are mostly involved in practicing SM. To minimize SM, the public must consult with a physician before administering any type of drug to establish a reliable diagnosis and to get a prescription for POM with recommended dosages. One of the pertinent arms of intervention to minimize SM practice is to improve awareness against misinformation about illegal COVID-19 preventive products and aiming to improve psychological health in the pandemic crisis (thus reducing anxiety and the compulsion to perform SM). Consciousness and understanding about the possible adverse effects of SM must be established and validated on a continuous level; in addition, on a commercial level, collaboration from pharmacists not to sell products (especially POM) without a certified prescription must be developed and implemented.

Supplementary Materials: The following supporting information can be downloaded at: https://www.mdpi.com/article/10.3390/tropicalmed7110330/s1. Supplementary Material S1: Instrument for data collection.

Author Contributions: S.A. and S.J. conceptualized and designed the study; J.A., M.G. and A.R. guided data analysis and interpretation; B.C. wrote the initial draft of the manuscript; L.-u.-R.K., M.M., M.G. and Z.S. critically reviewed the manuscript; S.A., A.R. and S.J. also supervised and administered the whole process of this research. All authors have read and agreed to the published version of the manuscript.

Funding: M.G. was supported by the János Bolyai Research Scholarship (BO/00144/20/5) of the Hungarian Academy of Sciences. The research study was supported by the ÚNKP-22-5-SZTE-107 New National Excellence Program of the Ministry for Innovation and Technology from the source of the National Research, Development and Innovation Fund. M.G. would also like to acknowledge the support of ESCMID's "30 under 30" Award.

Institutional Review Board Statement: The study was approved by the Institutional Advanced Studies and Research Board, University of Sargodha, Punjab, Pakistan (Ref No. SU/Acad/1723; 22 November 2021). The research committee of the hospital provided us with the joining letter to start our data collection. This study did not require clearance by an ethics board because it did not include human or animal subject trial.

Informed Consent Statement: Written informed consent was obtained from the respondents before participating in this study. Consent form includes the protection of privacy rights and agreement of voluntarily participation.

Data Availability Statement: All data generated during the study are presented in this paper.

Conflicts of Interest: The authors declare no conflict of interest, monetary or otherwise. The authors alone are responsible for the content and writing of this article.

References

1. Hernandez-Juyol, M.; Job-Quesada, J. Dentistry and self-medication: A current challenge. *Med. Oral Organo Of. De La Soc. Esp. De Med. Oral Y De La Acad. Iberoam. De Patol. Y Med. Bucal* **2002**, *7*, 344–347.
2. Aslam, A.; Gajdács, M.; Zin, C.S.; Ab Rahman, N.S.; Ahmed, S.I.; Zafar, M.Z.; Jamshed, S. Evidence of the Practice of Self-Medication with Antibiotics among the Lay Public in Low- and Middle-Income Countries: A Scoping Review. *Antibiotics* **2020**, *9*, 597. [CrossRef] [PubMed]
3. Sajith, M.; Suresh, S.M.; Roy, N.T.; Pawar, A. Self-Medication Practices Among Health Care Professional Students in a Tertiary Care Hospital, Pune. *Open Public Health J.* **2017**, *10*, 63–68. [CrossRef]
4. Pereira, F.S.V.T.; Stephan, C.; Bucaretchi, F.; Cordeiro, R. Automedicação em crianças e adolescentes. *J. De Pediatr.* **2007**, *83*, 453–458. [CrossRef]
5. Hughes, C.M.; McElnay, J.C.; Fleming, G.F. Benefits and Risks of Self Medication. *Drug Saf.* **2001**, *24*, 1027–1037. [CrossRef]
6. Abay, S.; Amelo, W. Assessment of Self-medication practices among medical, pharmacy, health science students in Gondar University. *Ethiopia* **2010**, *2*, 306–310. [CrossRef]
7. Burak, L.J.; Damico, A. College students' use of widely advertised medications. *J. Am. Coll. Health* **2000**, *49*, 118–121. [CrossRef]
8. Zafar, S.N.; Syed, R.; Waqar, S.; Zubairi, A.; Vaqar, T.; Shaikh, M.; Yousaf, W.; Shahid, S.; Saleem, S. Self-medication amongst university students of Karachi: Prevalence, knowledge and attitudes. *J. Pak. Med. Assoc.* **2008**, *58*, 214.
9. Sarahroodi, S.; Maleki-Jamshid, A.; Sawalha, A.F.; Mikaili, P.; Safaeian, L. Pattern of self-medication with analgesics among Iranian University students in central Iran. *J. Fam. Community Med.* **2012**, *19*, 125–129. [CrossRef]
10. Ehigiator, O.; Azodo, C.C.; Ehizele, A.O.; Ezeja, E.B.; Ehigiator, L.; Madukwe, I.U. Self-medication practices among dental, midwifery and nursing students. *Eur. J. Gen. Dent.* **2013**, *2*, 54–57. [CrossRef]
11. Klemenc-Ketis, Z.; Hladnik, Z.; Kersnik, J. A cross sectional study of sex differences in self-medication practices among university students in Slovenia. *Coll. Antropol.* **2011**, *35*, 329–334. [PubMed]
12. Helal, R.; Abou-ElWafa, H.S. Self-medication in university students from the city of Mansoura, Egypt. *J. Environ. Public Health* **2017**, *2017*, 9145193. [CrossRef] [PubMed]
13. Hussain, A.; Khanum, A. Self medication among university students of Islamabad, Pakistan-a preliminary study. *South. Med. Rev.* **2008**, *1*, 14–16.

14. Klemenc-Ketis, Z.; Hladnik, Z.; Kersnik, J. Self-Medication among Healthcare and Non-Healthcare Students at University of Ljubljana, Slovenia. *Med. Princ. Pr.* **2010**, *19*, 395–401. [CrossRef] [PubMed]
15. World Health Organization. *Guidelines for Developing National Drug Policies*; World Health Organization: Geneva, Switzerland, 1988.
16. Oyediran, O.O.; Ayandiran, E.O.; Olatubi, M.I.; Olabode, O. Awareness of risks associated with Self-medication among Patients attending General Out-patient Department of a Tertiary Hospital in South Western Nigeria. *Int. J. Afr. Nurs. Sci.* **2019**, *10*, 110–115. [CrossRef]
17. Uddin, T.M.; Chakraborty, A.J.; Khusro, A.; Zidan, B.R.M.; Mitra, S.; Bin Emran, T.; Dhama, K.; Ripon, K.H.; Gajdács, M.; Sahibzada, M.U.K.; et al. Antibiotic resistance in microbes: History, mechanisms, therapeutic strategies and future prospects. *J. Infect. Public Health* **2021**, *14*, 1750–1766. [CrossRef]
18. Arain, M.I.; Shahnaz, S.; Anwar, R.; Anwar, K. Assessment of Self-medication Practices During COVID-19 Pandemic in Hyderabad and Karachi, Pakistan. *Sudan J. Med. Sci.* **2021**, *16*, 347–354. [CrossRef]
19. Al-Mandhari, A.; WHO Regional Office for the Eastern Mediterranean; Samhouri, D.; Abubakar, A.; Brennan, R. Coronavirus Disease 2019 outbreak: Preparedness and readiness of countries in the Eastern Mediterranean Region. *East. Mediterr. Health J.* **2020**, *26*, 136–137. [CrossRef]
20. Al-Shammari, A.A.; Ali, H.; Alahmad, B.; Al-Refaei, F.H.; Al-Sabah, S.; Jamal, M.H.; Alshukry, A.; Al-Duwairi, Q.; Al-Mulla, F. The Impact of Strict Public Health Measures on COVID-19 Transmission in Developing Countries: The Case of Kuwait. *Front. Public Health* **2021**, *9*, 2395. [CrossRef]
21. James, H.; Handu, S.; Al Khaja, K.; Sequeira, R. Influence of medical training on self-medication by students. *Int. J. Clin. Pharmacol. Ther.* **2008**, *46*, 23–29. [CrossRef]
22. Onchonga, D. A Google Trends study on the interest in self-medication during the 2019 novel coronavirus (COVID-19) disease pandemic. *Saudi Pharm. J.* **2020**, *28*, 903–904. [CrossRef] [PubMed]
23. Lei, X.; Jiang, H.; Liu, C.; Ferrier, A.; Mugavin, J. Self-Medication Practice and Associated Factors among Residents in Wuhan, China. *Int. J. Environ. Res. Public Health* **2018**, *15*, 68. [CrossRef] [PubMed]
24. Kretchy, I.A.; Asiedu-Danso, M.; Kretchy, J.-P. Medication management and adherence during the COVID-19 pandemic: Perspectives and experiences from low-and middle-income countries. *Res. Soc. Adm. Pharm.* **2020**, *17*, 2023–2026. [CrossRef] [PubMed]
25. Xu, J.; Cao, B. Lessons learnt from hydroxychloroquine/azithromycin in treatment of COVID-19. *Eur. Respir. J.* **2021**, *59*, 2102002. [CrossRef]
26. Chauhan, V.; Galwankar, S.; Raina, S.; Krishnan, V. Proctoring hydroxychloroquine consumption for health-care workers in india as per the revised national guidelines. *J. Emerg. Trauma Shock* **2020**, *13*, 172–173. [CrossRef]
27. Suda, K.J.; Kim, K.C.; Hernandez, I.; Gellad, W.F.; Rothenberger, S.; Campbell, A.; Malliart, L.; Tadrous, M. The global impact of COVID-19 on drug purchases: A cross-sectional time series analysis. *J. Am. Pharm. Assoc.* **2021**, *62*, 766–774.e6. [CrossRef]
28. Geovan Menezes de Sousa, J.; de Oliveira Tavares, V.D.; de Meiroz Grilo, M.L.P.; Coelho, M.L.G.; de Lima-Araújo, G.L.; Schuch, F.B.; Galvão-Coelho, N.L. Mental health in COVID-19 pandemic: A meta-review of prevalence meta-analyses. *Front. Psychol.* **2021**, *12*, 703838. [CrossRef]
29. Raosoft Inc.: Sample Size Calculator. Available online: http://www.raosoft.com/samplesize.html (accessed on 13 August 2022).
30. Shakeel, S.; Iffat, W.; Qamar, A.; Rehman, H.; Ghuman, F.; Butt, F.; Rehman, A.U.; Madléna, M.; Paulik, E.; Gajdács, M.; et al. Healthcare Professionals' Compliance with the Standard Management Guidelines towards the Use of Biological Disease-Modifying Anti-Rheumatic Drugs in Rheumatoid Arthritis Patients. *Int. J. Environ. Res. Public Health* **2022**, *19*, 4699. [CrossRef]
31. Beaton, D.E.; Bombardier, C.; Guillemin, F.; Ferraz, M.B. Guidelines for the Process of Cross-Cultural Adaptation of Self-Report Measures. *Spine* **2000**, *25*, 3186–3191. [CrossRef]
32. Sadio, A.J.; Gbeasor-Komlanvi, F.A.; Konu, R.Y.; Bakoubayi, A.W.; Tchankoni, M.K.; Bitty-Anderson, A.M.; Gomez, I.M.; Denadou, C.P.; Anani, J.; Kouanfack, H.R.; et al. Assessment of self-medication practices in the context of the COVID-19 outbreak in Togo. *BMC Public Health* **2021**, *21*, 58. [CrossRef]
33. Wegbom, A.I.; Edet, C.K.; Raimi, O.; Fagbamigbe, A.F.; Kiri, V.A. Self-Medication Practices and Associated Factors in the Prevention and/or Treatment of COVID-19 Virus: A Population-Based Survey in Nigeria. *Front. Public Health* **2021**, *9*, 606801. [CrossRef] [PubMed]
34. Osemene, K.; Lamikanra, A. A Study of the Prevalence of Self-Medication Practice among University Students in Southwestern Nigeria. *Trop. J. Pharm. Res.* **2012**, *11*, 683–689. [CrossRef]
35. Nasir, M.; Chowdhury, S.; Zahan, T. Self-medication during COVID-19 outbreak: A cross sectional online survey in Dhaka city. *Int. J. Basic Clin. Pharmacol.* **2020**, *9*, 1325. [CrossRef]
36. Da Silva, M.G.C.; Soares, M.C.F.; Muccillo-Baisch, A.L. Self-medication in university students from the city of Rio Grande, Brazil. *BMC Public Health* **2012**, *12*, 339.
37. Abahussain, E.; Matowe, L.K.; Nicholls, P. Self-Reported Medication Use among Adolescents in Kuwait. *Med. Princ. Pr.* **2005**, *14*, 161–164. [CrossRef]
38. Jember, E.; Feleke, A.; Debie, A.; Asrade, G. Self-medication practices and associated factors among households at Gondar town, Northwest Ethiopia: A cross-sectional study. *BMC Res. Notes* **2019**, *12*, 153. [CrossRef]

39. Badiger, A.B.; Kundapur, R.; Jain, A.; Kumar, A.; Pattanshetty, S.; Thakolkaran, N.; Bhat, N.; Ullal, N. Self-medication patterns among medical students in south india. *Australas. Med. J.* **2012**, *5*, 217. [CrossRef]
40. López, J.J.; Dennis, R.; Moscoso, M. A study of self-medication in a neighborhood in Bogotá. *Rev. Salud Pública* **2009**, *11*, 432–442. [CrossRef]
41. Roberts, T.; Esponda, G.M.; Krupchanka, D.; Shidhaye, R.; Patel, V.; Rathod, S. Factors associated with health service utilisation for common mental disorders: A systematic review. *BMC Psychiatry* **2018**, *18*, 262. [CrossRef]
42. Azhar, H.; Tauseef, A.; Usman, T.; Azhar, Y.; Ahmed, M.; Umer, K.; Shoaib, M. Prevalence, Attitude and Knowledge of Self Medication during Covid-19 Disease Pandemic. *Pak. J. Med. Health Sci.* **2021**, 902–905. [CrossRef]
43. Gyselinck, I.; Janssens, W.; Verhamme, P.; Vos, R. Rationale for azithromycin in COVID-19: An overview of existing evidence. *BMJ Open Respir. Res.* **2021**, *8*, e000806. [CrossRef] [PubMed]
44. Shafie, M.; Eyasu, M.; Muzeyin, K.; Worku, Y.; Martín-Aragón, S. Prevalence and determinants of self-medication practice among selected households in Addis Ababa community. *PLoS ONE* **2018**, *13*, e0194122. [CrossRef] [PubMed]
45. Romano, S.; Galante, H.; Figueira, D.; Mendes, Z.; Rodrigues, A.T. Time-trend analysis of medicine sales and shortages during COVID-19 outbreak: Data from community pharmacies. *Res. Soc. Adm. Pharm.* **2020**, *17*, 1876–1881. [CrossRef] [PubMed]
46. Ford, N.; Vitoria, M.; Rangaraj, A.; Norris, S.L.; Calmy, A.; Doherty, M. Systematic review of the efficacy and safety of antiretroviral drugs against SARS, MERS or COVID-19: Initial assessment. *J. Int. AIDS Soc.* **2020**, *23*, e25489. [CrossRef] [PubMed]
47. Dong, L.; Hu, S.; Gao, J. Discovering drugs to treat coronavirus disease 2019 (COVID-19). *Drug Discov. Ther.* **2020**, *14*, 58–60. [CrossRef]
48. Arshad, S.; Kilgore, P.; Chaudhry, Z.S.; Jacobsen, G.; Wang, D.D.; Huitsing, K.; Brar, I.; Alangaden, G.J.; Ramesh, M.S.; McKinnon, J.E.; et al. Treatment with hydroxychloroquine, azithromycin, and combination in patients hospitalized with COVID-19. *Int. J. Infect. Dis.* **2020**, *97*, 396–403. [CrossRef]
49. Mercuro, N.J.; Yen, C.F.; Shim, D.J.; Maher, T.R.; McCoy, C.M.; Zimetbaum, P.J.; Gold, H.S. Risk of QT Interval Prolongation Associated With Use of Hydroxychloroquine With or Without Concomitant Azithromycin Among Hospitalized Patients Testing Positive for Coronavirus Disease 2019 (COVID-19). *JAMA Cardiol.* **2020**, *5*, 1036–1041. [CrossRef]
50. Hoang, B.X.; Shaw, G.; Fang, W.; Han, B. Possible application of high-dose vitamin C in the prevention and therapy of coronavirus infection. *J. Glob. Antimicrob. Resist.* **2020**, *23*, 256–262. [CrossRef]
51. Ferraro, P.M.; Curhan, G.C.; Gambaro, G.; Taylor, E.N. Total, Dietary, and Supplemental Vitamin C Intake and Risk of Incident Kidney Stones. *Am. J. Kidney Dis.* **2016**, *67*, 400–407. [CrossRef]
52. Martineau, A.R.; Jolliffe, D.A.; Hooper, R.L.; Greenberg, L.; Aloia, J.F.; Bergman, P.; Dubnov-Raz, G.; Esposito, S.; Ganmaa, D.; Ginde, A.A.; et al. Vitamin D supplementation to prevent acute respiratory tract infections: Systematic review and meta-analysis of individual participant data. *BMJ* **2017**, *356*, i6583. [CrossRef]
53. Margarucci, L.M.; Montanari, E.; Gianfranceschi, G.; Caprara, C.; Valeriani, F.; Piccolella, A.; Lombardi, V.; Scaramucci, E.; Spica, V. The role of vitamin D in prevention of COVID-19 and its severity: An umbrella review. *Acta Bio Med. Atenei Parm.* **2021**, *92*, e2021451.
54. Oreagba, I.A.; Oshikoya, K.A.; Amachree, M. Herbal medicine use among urban residents in Lagos, Nigeria. *BMC Complement. Altern. Med.* **2011**, *11*, 117. [CrossRef] [PubMed]
55. Chali, B.U.; Melaku, T.; Berhanu, N.; Mengistu, B.; Milkessa, G.; Mamo, G.; Alemu, S.; Mulugeta, T. Traditional Medicine Practice in the Context of COVID-19 Pandemic: Community Claim in Jimma Zone, Oromia, Ethiopia. *Infect. Drug Resist.* **2021**, *14*, 3773–3783. [CrossRef] [PubMed]
56. Alford, D.P.; German, J.S.; Samet, J.; Cheng, D.M.; Lloyd-Travaglini, C.A.; Saitz, R. Primary Care Patients with Drug Use Report Chronic Pain and Self-Medicate with Alcohol and Other Drugs. *J. Gen. Intern. Med.* **2016**, *31*, 486–491. [CrossRef] [PubMed]
57. Demeter, T.; Houman, A.B.; Gótai, L.; Károlyházy, K.; Kovács, A.; Márton, K.J. Effect of a gel-type denture adhesive on unstimulated whole saliva and minor salivary gland flow rates and on subjective orofacial sicca symptoms. *Orvosi Hetilap* **2018**, *159*, 1637–1644. [CrossRef]
58. Mehuys, E.; Verrue, C.; Van Borte, L.; De Bolle, L.; Van Tongelen, I.; Remon, J.P.; De Looze, D. Self-medication of upper gastrointestinal symptoms: A community pharmacy study. *J. De Pharm. De Belg.* **2009**, *43*, 890–898. [CrossRef]
59. Crum, R.M.; Mojtabai, R.; Lazareck, S.; Bolton, J.M.; Robinson, J.; Sareen, J.; Green, K.M.; Stuart, E.A.; La Flair, L.; Alvanzo, A.A.H.; et al. A Prospective Assessment of Reports of Drinking to Self-medicate Mood Symptoms With the Incidence and Persistence of Alcohol Dependence. *JAMA Psychiatry* **2013**, *70*, 718–726. [CrossRef]
60. Javed, B.; Sarwer, A.; Soto, E.B.; Mashwani, Z.U.R. The coronavirus (COVID-19) pandemic's impact on mental health. *Int. J. Health Plan. Manag.* **2020**, *35*, 993–996. [CrossRef]

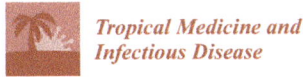

Article

Infectious Disease Modeling with Socio-Viral Behavioral Aspects—Lessons Learned from the Spread of SARS-CoV-2 in a University

Nuning Nuraini [1,*], Kamal Khairudin Sukandar [1], Maria Yulita Trida Tahu [1], Ernawati Arifin Giri-Rachman [2], Anggraini Barlian [2], Sri Harjati Suhardi [2], Udjianna Sekteria Pasaribu [1], Sonny Yuliar [3], Diky Mudhakir [4], Herto Dwi Ariesyady [5], Dian Rosleine [2], Iyan Sofyan [6] and Widjaja Martokusumo [7]

[1] Department of Mathematics, Faculty of Mathematics and Natural Sciences, Institut Teknologi Bandung, Bandung 40132, Indonesia
[2] School of Life Science and Technology, Institut Teknologi Bandung, Bandung 40132, Indonesia
[3] Center of Public Policy and Governance, Institut Teknologi Bandung, Bandung 40132, Indonesia
[4] School of Pharmacy, Institut Teknologi Bandung, Bandung 40132, Indonesia
[5] Faculty of Civil and Environmental Engineering, Institut Teknologi Bandung, Bandung 40132, Indonesia
[6] General Administration and Information Bureau, Institut Teknologi Bandung, Bandung 40132, Indonesia
[7] School of Architecture, Planning and Policy Development, Institut Teknologi Bandung, Bandung 40132, Indonesia
* Correspondence: nuning@math.itb.ac.id

Abstract: When it comes to understanding the spread of COVID-19, recent studies have shown that pathogens can be transmitted in two ways: direct contact and airborne pathogens. While the former is strongly related to the distancing behavior of people in society, the latter are associated with the length of the period in which the airborne pathogens remain active. Considering those facts, we constructed a compartmental model with a time-dependent transmission rate that incorporates the two sources of infection. This paper provides an analytical and numerical study of the model that validates trivial insights related to disease spread in a responsive society. As a case study, we applied the model to the COVID-19 spread data from a university environment, namely, the Institut Teknologi Bandung, Indonesia, during its early reopening stage, with a constant number of students. The results show a significant fit between the rendered model and the recorded cases of infections. The extrapolated trajectories indicate the resurgence of cases as students' interaction distance approaches its natural level. The assessment of several strategies is undertaken in this study in order to assist with the school reopening process.

Keywords: SIR model; socio-behavioral aspects; interaction distance; school reopening strategy

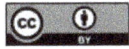

1. Introduction

In epidemiology, compartmental models are general modeling techniques used to understand the spread of disease, and they commonly consider three variables: S for those who are susceptible, I for those who are infected, and R for individuals who have recovered. Variations of the generic SIR model are available: the SIS model accommodates temporal immunity [1], the $SEIR$ model best represents the spread of disease with a significant latency period [2], and there are even combinations of the two [3]. The convenience of compartmental models in respect of adding more variables has resulted in their being widely used in infectious disease modeling [4]. Besides providing each state's estimated figure, this approach can also provide the reproductive ratio, which represents the expected number of secondary cases generated by one primary case [5–7]. In most of the constructed models, the reproductive ratio acts as a crucial threshold; above one indicates endemic, while below one indicates disease-free [8]. This is crucial for policymakers when regulating whether or not to ease restrictions amid disease spread.

However, generic compartmental models are sometimes based on assumptions that are not necessarily relevant; the population is considered closed in SIR models, whereas complete isolation was not followed in most regions, making them vulnerable to changes in the neighboring communities [9]. Another assumption that is commonly used in a generic model is that transmission and recovery rates are assumed to remain constant over time. Such a scenario will best represent disease that spreads in a population with no response to current disease prevalence, meaning that a high or low number of recorded cases will not affect the average socio-behavior of the population. The simplest case to consider is a disease spread within a closed population of sheep in a field [10]. When it comes to a human population, people's psychological behavior causes them to reduce their interaction intensity as the declared number of cases increases, which ought to vary the viral transmissibility [11]. Moreover, setting constant rates of transmission and recovery results in a high number of projected infected cases once the model is applied to a vast and highly populated community; this could be at the scale of entire nations [12]. According to recent studies, SIR-based predictions using early data for COVID-19 cases have shown an enormous figure for predicted cases, with the peak reaching up to 15–30% of the total population [13,14]. Nevertheless, an absence of the psychological behavior of the population could overestimate the prediction figure [15].

According to recent studies, there are so many studies that discuss the spread of the COVID-19 disease. Researchers developed various models and approaches from all over the world [16,17]. However, in this paper, we will discuss two major sources of transmission in some infectious diseases: direct contact and airborne transmission. In respect of the former, it is quite obvious that human-to-human transmission is mainly caused by direct contact such as talking at a close distance. The smaller the average interaction distance of people within a population, the greater the chance for pathogens to spread. By incorporating the effect of human psychological behaviors, it is natural to expect an increase in the average interaction distance given a high disease prevalence in a specific population, which will lead to a reduction in viral transmissibility. However, the latter source of transmission opens up possibilities for infections induced by the presence of airborne pathogens. This method of transmission is found in the spread of TB [18] and SARS-CoV-2 [19]. Although airborne pathogens can infect susceptible individuals, some studies have shown that most airborne pathogens can only last for a certain period. *Mycobacterium tuberculosis*, which attacks lungs and causes TB, can stay in the air for several hours depending on the environment [20], and SARS-CoV-2 can only last for hours in the air but can survive for up to a week on plastic [21]. In disease modeling, taking airborne pathogens into account is crucial, especially for those that have a significant period of viral survivability in the air.

The incorporation of the psychological behavior of society into responses to disease prevalence has been introduced in several works, such as Hua-Li et al. [11] and Oluyori et al. [22]. In practice, the authors define saturated transmission rates that are dependent on the figure of disease prevalence. The transmission rate is expected to increase for a low disease prevalence and start decreasing once the prevalence exceeds its critical point [11]. In 2021, Cabrera et al. [23] introduced a compartmental model that incorporates a socio-behavioral aspect in a slightly different way; they introduced the interaction distance to measure societal behaviors in response to disease prevalence. Hence, the nonlinear transmission rate integrates the interaction distances. However, the effect of airborne pathogens is rarely incorporated. One study conducted by Bazant and Bush in 2021 [24] demonstrates the significant effect of airborne transmissions on society regarding activities. Although airborne pathogens, especially SARS-CoV-2, can only last for hours, indoor transmission is crucial for infectious disease modeling, especially for school or office environments involving many indoor activities.

In this study, we constructed an SIR-based mathematical system that accommodates the two major causes of infection: direct contact and airborne transmission. The former source of infection, representing the socio-behavioral aspect, is based on the measure of the interaction distance of people in society. In 2021, Cabrera et al. [23] proposed adding a new variable that determines the interaction distance over time. The closer the interaction distance, the higher the chance of disease spread. The latter cause of infection, which represents viral characteristics, is incorporated by defining another variable that solely represents the concentration of pathogens in the air over time. We expect that the longer the pathogens can last in the air, the higher the concentrations over time, which leads to a higher chance of disease spread. Hence, the newly added variables will govern the transmission rate that eventually depends on the socio-viral behavioral aspects. In the analysis of the constructed model, we provide numerical results in respect of infections under different socio-viral behavioral aspects. The model performs well in depicting the spread of disease in societies under different rates of response, different rates of resistance to adopting new habits, and under different characteristics of the concerned diseases. As a case study, we applied the constructed models to the SARS-CoV-2 spread data that were collected in a university environment (Institut Teknologi Bandung College) in January 2022. The choice to use data from a university was made to ensure homogeneous socio-behavioral aspects for the whole society; no demographic is taken into account due to the homogeneity assumption [25–27]. The small scale of a university environment also ensures the involvement of pathogens in the air; the larger the scale of the observation, the smaller the effect of pathogens in the air. Lastly, we utilized the extrapolated figures to assess some strategic action plans related to SARS-CoV-2 infections in educational environments; school reopening schemes and vaccination implementation [28].

2. Context

Humans are mobile creatures who move in their part of an environment; they may meet an acquaintance or not. When the former scenario happens, they will likely move closer to reaching out to that acquaintance [29]. This phenomenon exemplifies the importance of interpersonal space (IPS) and peripersonal space (PPS) in which humans can perform body–environment interactions [30]. Although the dimensions of IPS and PPS include all directions, previous studies have only focused on a specific distance, i.e., the distance from the front of the person [31]. When it comes to understanding infectious diseases, the front-directed PPS is essential since most diseases, including SARS-CoV-2, are transmitted via the front parts of the human body. One unit that measures the intensity of PPS contact is the interaction distance, in which the closer the distance, the more intense the contact, which leads to an increase in the risk of disease transmission [32]. According to Sorokowska et al. [33], the preferred interpersonal distance of humans differs between different types of social relations (strangers, acquaintances, and partners). Table 1 provides a global comparison in respect of interaction distance.

Other than the interaction distance that causes direct transmissions, airborne transmission of some diseases is now widely recognized, especially for the spread of COVID-19 [34,35]. This approach accounts for the plausibility of infections caused by pathogen-bearing aerosols that are fine enough to be continuously mixed through an indoor space. Every infected individual present will contribute to the production of droplets containing the virus. Bazant and Bush [24], in their COVID-19 study, estimated the concentration of pathogens produced by a single infected individual in a well-mixed room for every breath, and for whispering and talking indoors.

However, other studies have shown that pathogens can remain active on other media, such as copper, cardboard, and plastic [21], for a certain period. Hence, other than significant airborne transmission indoors, pathogens that are attached to other media can also infect susceptible individuals. A study by Doremalen et al. provides the estimated critical periods of SARS-CoV (1 and 2) before they become inactive; these are given in Table 2. The estimations show that SARS-CoV can last up to 12 h in the air but can last longer on other media. This fact should indicate the importance of airborne pathogens and their attachment to other media in respect of understanding viral transmission. In this study we construct a mathematical model that incorporates both socio-behavioral and airborne pathogen effects.

Table 1. Average preferred interpersonal distance (in meters) for different types of social relations: strangers, acquaintances, and partners/close relations across all nations. The figure estimations were conducted by Sorokowska et al. [33].

Countries	Social Distance	Personal Distance	Intimate Distance
Romania, Hungary, Saudi Arabia, Turkey, Uganda	1.20–1.40 m	0.90–1.20 m	0.45–0.90 m
Pakistan, Estonia, Colombia, Hong Kong, China, Iran, Malaysia, Czech Republic, Portugal, Kenya, Switzerland, India, Indonesia, Croatia, Ghana, South Korea	1.05–1.20 m	0.75–1.05 m	0.40–0.75 m
Norway, Canada, Nigeria, Brazil, England, Mexico, Poland, Germany, USA, Kazakhstan, Italy, Serbia, Greece, Spain	0.90–1.05 m	0.60–0.75 m	0.40–0.60 m
Russia, Slovakia, Austria, Ukraine, Bulgaria, Peru, Argentina	0.70–0.90 m	0.60–0.70 m	0.30–0.50 m

Table 2. Estimated critical periods for SARS-CoV to remain active on several media.

Media	SARS-CoV-2	SARS-CoV-1
Aerosol	10.00 ± 2.00 h	8.00 ± 2.00 h
Copper	11.00 ± 6.00 h	19.00 ± 7.50 h
Cardboard	39.00 ± 9.00 h	8.00 ± 5.00 h
Stainless steel	72.00 ± 15.00 h	50.00 ± 10.00 h
Plastic	90.00 ± 10.00 h	90.00 ± 10.00 h

3. Proposed Model

In this study we used a generic model, but we separated those who had and had not received vaccines. This modification was based on the fact that the presence of immune titer in the human body can significantly prevent people from becoming infected, offering up to 90% protection [36]. Hence, there are three main state variables: susceptible (S), currently infected individuals (I), and removed individuals (R), with the total of six state variables created by adding subscripts v and u to each of the main states, representing the categories of being vaccinated and not, respectively. As shown in Figure 1, new infected individuals are generated from both S_u and S_v, caused by a direct interaction between susceptible and infectious individuals. After a specific period of infections, infected individuals will enter R, which represents being immune or deceased. We assume that there is no demographic change, which implies a constant population size: $N_u = S_u(t) + I(t) + R_u(t)$ and $N_v = S_v(t) + I_v(t) + R_v(t)$, for $t \geq 0$, and $N = N_u + N_v$ with a constant proportion of vaccinated and unvaccinated individuals. The model also assumes no significant difference in the recovery rates of vaccinated and unvaccinated individuals.

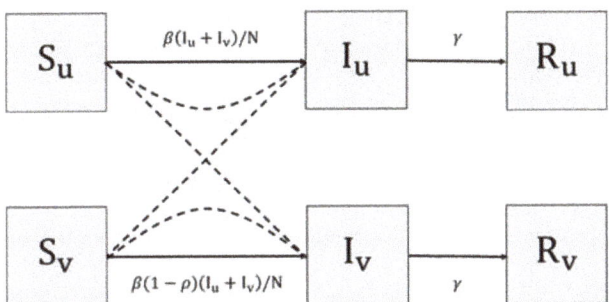

Figure 1. State-flow diagram of $\{SIR\}_{uv}$. Solid lines represent direct flow, while dashed lines represent interactions of states.

As shown in Figure 1, there are three parameters involved: transmission rate (β), recovery rate (γ), and vaccine effectiveness (ρ). The last two parameters are observable, i.e., their values can be measured and estimated using relevant information. Vaccine effectiveness, which ranges from 0 to 1, represents the protection induced by the vaccine. The higher this value, the lower the chance of people becoming infected once they interact with infectious individuals. Limited to the COVID-19 vaccine, the vaccine efficacy should vary depending on the manufacturer and COVID-19 variants [36]. The value of γ represents the rate of recovery, which governs the speed of transition from I to R. To make this realistic, γ^{-1} can be considered as the average infection period. In contrast, the rate of transmission β is unclear in terms of its physical representation; it summarizes all factors that produce infections. Hence, the value of β is considered unobservable. To incorporate the two major causes of infection as mentioned in Section 2, we added two additional lines to the system that represent the dynamics of the interaction distance D and the pathogen concentrations V. The final two variables dictate the dynamics of β resulting in the transmission rate that depends on the socio-viral behavioral aspect. A mathematical representation of the constructed model is given in the following form:

$$\begin{cases} S'_u = -\beta(I_u + I_v)S_u/N \\ I'_u = \beta(I_u + I_v)S_u/N - \gamma I_u \\ R'_u = \gamma I_u \\ S'_v = -\beta(1-\rho)(I_u + I_v)S_u/N \\ I'_v = \beta(1-\rho)(I_u + I_v)S_u/N - \gamma I_v \\ R'_v = \gamma I_u \end{cases} \quad (1)$$

with a constant population size N. The other two additional variables are D (in meters) and V (in quanta/m^3), representing the average interaction distance and viral loads over time. The formulation of D was first introduced by Cabrera et al. [23] along with the definition of the natural distancing habit D^* that could differ from one society to others—symbol D^* denotes the average of natural distancing behavior of society. The complete additional lines are given in the following systems:

$$\begin{cases} D' = -\lambda_1(D - D^*) + \lambda_2(I_u + I_v)/N \\ V' = \lambda_3(I_u + I_v) - \lambda_4 V \end{cases} \quad (2)$$

with non-negative initial conditions $\{S_u^0, I_u^0, R_u^0, S_v^0, I_v^0, R_v^0, D^0, V^0\}$ that are evaluated at the initial point $t = 0$. It is natural to assume that $I_u^0 = (1-\alpha)I^0$ and $I_v^0 = \alpha I^0$, for $I^0 = I_u^0 + I_v^0$, with α (in percent relative to the population size) representing the vaccine coverage. The addition of the two variables involves another four parameters. On one hand, the value of λ_2 (distance/time) represents how quickly people react to the current disease prevalence, i.e., the so-called rate of social response. By neglecting the first term, there are two scenarios that increase the interaction distance D: high values of the rate of response λ_2 or the disease prevalence I. Interestingly, setting λ_2 equals zero will lead to a situation where a society pays no attention to the current disease spread. Such a scenario drives the society to resort to their natural interaction distance D for $\lambda_1 \neq 0$. On the other hand, the rate λ_1 (1/time) measures the rate of resistance in society, per distance unit, to changing distancing behavior. It represents how quickly individuals return to their natural interaction distance D^* or their natural distancing habits. This rate is strongly related to the distancing culture. When we set a high value of λ_1, this results in a situation in which the society has a strong culture embedded, making it resistant to changes in behavior amid the current pandemic. In this study, we restrict the plausibility of $\lambda_1 = 0$ since we assume that every society has its own resistance in changing habits. When the disease prevalence approaches zero, then D' approaches $-\lambda_1(D - D^*)$, which leads to the convergence of D to D^* regardless of the initial condition D^0. More detailed formal analysis of System (1) and (2) are given in Appendix A.

While the first equation of System (2) portrays the socio-behavioral aspects, the second equation portrays the concentration of the pathogens. The rate λ_3 (quanta/(time m^3·person)) denotes the average concentration of viral/pathogens emitted by one infected individual per unit time. Face coverings and the practice of other social and respiratory etiquette will likely reduce the value of λ_3 and hence reduce the number of pathogens emitted into the air. The discharged microbes will remain suspended in the air in dust particles, respiratory particles, and water droplets [37]. However, pathogens will not last forever in the air (or other media); they will decay due to natural and human intervention. On the other hand, parameter λ_4 (1/time) denotes the removal rate of viral quanta in the air. A higher intervention of humans in the community, including through air filtering and periodical sanitation, can increase λ_4 and hence allow more microbes to decay or be inactive [38]. However, in most cases, λ_4 will only account for the natural effect of pathogen removal (subject to ambient temperature, humidity [21,39], and sunlight [40]), while human intervention can be represented by another functional term added to the dynamic of V [41]. Eventually, λ_1, λ_2, and λ_3 represent the socio-behavioral aspects in society while λ_4 represents the characteristics of the pathogens.

$$D(t) = D^* + \left(D^0 - D^*\right)e^{-\lambda_1 t} + \frac{\lambda_2}{N}\int_0^t I(s)e^{-\lambda_1(t-s)}ds \quad (3)$$

$$V(t) = V^0 e^{-\lambda_4 t} + \lambda_3 \int_0^t I(s)e^{-\lambda_4(t-s)}ds \quad (4)$$

Since the model adopts a uni-flow, then there exists τ such as $I(t) < \varepsilon, t > \tau$, for every $\varepsilon > 0$. In terms of epidemiology, the virus will always be eradicated to zero for large values of t since people will accumulate in the removed compartments. For the dynamics of D, the second and third terms approach zero as t approaches infinity, leaving only the first term that converges to D^*. However, the presence of V is strongly related to the presence of infectious individuals, who will vanish once the disease vanishes, no matter how large the initial condition. It should be noted that the proposed models do not consider reinfection or susceptible newborns. Hence, multiple disease outbreaks (if any) are expected to be driven by the change in interaction distance in society.

3.1. Observability of Socio-Behavioral Parameters

As discussed in the previous section, the model has 3 parameters that are related to the socio-behavioral aspects of society: λ_1, λ_2, and λ_3. It is clear from its definition that λ_3 is observable and that its value follows the estimations of the pathogen concentration per person per m^3. Bazant and Bush [24] and Miller et al. [42] provided estimated concentrations for several expiratory activities. Calibrated normal speaking activity is estimated to produce 72 infections quanta/m^3 while superspreading activity can contribute up to 970 infections quanta/m$_3$. However, the first two socio-behavioral parameters are not observable, i.e., the rate of social resistance λ_1 is not something that we can determine from the field. It combines all aspects that inhibit society in the change of behaviors.

The rate of social response, denoted by λ_2, has a dimension of meters per unit of time. In the absence of λ_1, the formula of D' reduces to only $D' = \lambda_2(I/N)$, with $I = I_u + I_v$. When $I = N$, then $D' = \lambda_2$, which is interpreted as the interaction distance increasing at the rate of λ_2 meters per unit time when the whole population is infected. Taking another scenario, $I = 1$ person results in $D' = \lambda_2/N$, which is considered as the λ_2/N increment of the interaction distance per unit of time when the society contains 1 infected individual. Henceforth, λ_2 is related to the quantity of the change in D for a certain disease prevalence. To understand this parameter more, let us take the solution of $D' = \lambda_2(I/N)$; $D(t) - D^0 = \lambda_2 \int_0^t (I(s)/N)ds$. By taking $D^0 = D^*$, then $\lambda_2 = (D(t) - D^*)/\int_0^t (I(s)/N)ds$. Expecting the presence of an average prevalence of $\bar{I}$ in the length of time T_2 will drive people in society to interact at the distance of $\bar{D}$, then λ_2 can be estimated using the following formula:

$$\lambda_2 = \frac{(\bar{D} - D^*)}{T_2\left(\frac{\bar{I}}{N}\right)} \quad (5)$$

Note that $\bar{I}/N$ represents the percentage of infections in society, i.e., the so-called point prevalence, denoted by $a\%$. Therefore, by knowing that the society is practicing distancing habits of $D = \bar{D}$ once the point prevalence is roughly $a\%$, we can estimate the expected value of λ_2 as the rate of social response amid the disease spread. Henceforth, $\lambda_2 = (\bar{D} - D^*)/(aT_2)$.

We can also consider the dynamics of D in the given system. When $(I_u + I_v)/N$ tends to zero, the effect of λ_2 is no longer significant; the whole second term will tend to zero, leaving $D' = -\lambda_1(\bar{D} - D^*)$. This simple ODE has a unique solution of $D(t) = D^* + D^0 e^{-\lambda_1 t}$. The higher the value of λ_1, the faster the dynamics of D to approach D^*. It is easy to prove that $\lim_{t\to\infty} D(t) = D^*$, regardless of the value of D^0. Hence, for an arbitrary small value $\varepsilon > 0$, there exists a value of T_1 that satisfies the following condition.

$$|D(t) - D^*| < \varepsilon \text{ for } t > T_1 \leftrightarrow \frac{|D(t) - D^*|}{D^0} < \frac{\varepsilon}{D^0} = \bar{\varepsilon} \text{ for } t > T_1 \quad (6)$$

We can manipulate the solution of $D(t)$ to reach $D^* + \bar{\varepsilon}$ in $t = T_1$ by adjusting the value of λ_1 as given by:

$$D^* + \varepsilon = D^* + D^0 e^{-\lambda_1 t} \to \lambda_1 = \frac{-\ln\left(\frac{\varepsilon}{D^0}\right)}{T_1} = -\frac{\ln(\bar{\varepsilon})}{T_1} \quad (7)$$

Henceforth, the rate of social resistance λ_1 can be evaluated using the estimated time for society to return to their natural interaction distance in the absence of disease spread, denoted by T_1; see Figure 2 for illustration. It should be noted that $\bar{\varepsilon}$ is an arbitrary small number $\varepsilon > 0$ divided by D^0. According to Equation (7), λ_1 takes the log value of $\bar{\varepsilon}$, which will be sensitive to the choice of $\bar{\varepsilon}$. Hence, it is natural to assume the relative deviation from D^* as $\bar{\varepsilon} = 1\%$, although the formula of λ_1 should clearly confirm that the value of λ_1 is dependent on the assumption.

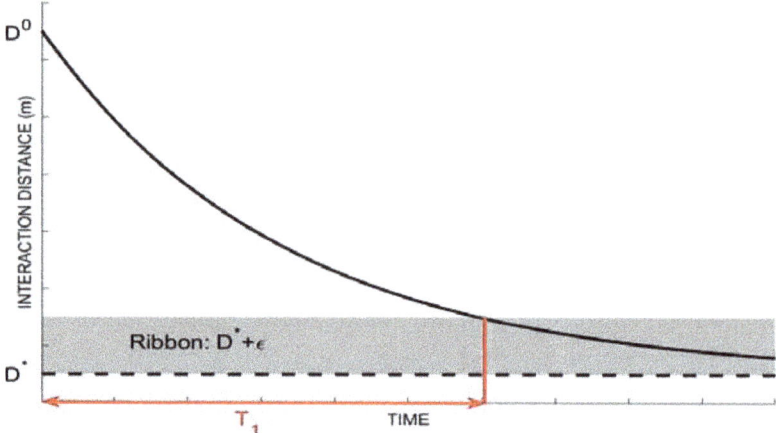

Figure 2. Illustration of rate of social resistance λ_1 by the given data for T_1.

3.2. Contact and Airborne-Based Transmission Rate

The rate of transmission is defined to be related to the interaction distance (D) and concentration of pathogens (V). In this study we accommodate two methods of transmission: contact-based and airborne-based transmission. Contact-based transmission is affected by the average interaction distance; the transmission rate decreases as the average interaction-distance increases, as people practice social-distancing. However, a high concentration of airborne pathogens contributes to an increase in the transmission rate.

$$\beta(D, V) = \beta^* \left(\frac{2D^*}{D^* + D} \right)^v \left(\frac{V + V^*}{V^*} \right)^w \qquad (8)$$

The definition of the contact-related transmission rate is adopted from [23], but we have added the effect of the current concentration of pathogens. The basic transmission rate β^* (1/time) is defined as constant, representing the basic probability of transmission per unit time. The second term (dimensionless) represents the effect of the average interaction-distance, which will decrease the overall β as D increases. The third term, however, represents how the concentration of pathogens affects the overall β value at which the risk of infection will rise as V increases. To keep the effect of V dimensionless, we divide V by the standard number of quanta exhaled by infectors per individual per m^3 per unit time. The adjuster levels of v and w are added to be fitted to the data, representing the strength of each source of infection in society.

3.3. Recovery Rate

Recovery rates (1/time) denote the quantity representing how fast infected individuals recover from the disease and, hence, build their immunity [43]. For some infectious diseases, the absence of healthcare might cause a longer infection period [27,44,45], specifically for COVID-19. Not limited to this disease, we define the implicitly time-dependent recovery rate as follows:

$$\gamma(I, K) = \gamma_0 + (\gamma_1 - \gamma_0) \frac{K}{I + K} \qquad (9)$$

where I denotes the state variable for infectious individuals and K denotes the constant healthcare capacity (beds). In addition, γ_1 and γ_0 are both recovery rates but represent different situations: excessive beds and collapsing health systems. On one hand, when the number of beds is excessive, then each of the infected individuals receives proper treatment and this leads to a shorter period of infections [45]. In other words, $\gamma(I, K)$ will achieve its maximum rate of recovery as K approaches infinity. Otherwise, $\gamma(I, K)$ will converge to γ_0 as the number of burdens is higher relative to the healthcare services [11]. Hence, the former denotes the maximum recovery rate given the proper treatment, while the latter denotes the lowest recovery rate achieved by patients treating themselves in order to recover. Figure 3 depicts the functional parameters and their dependent variables. Figure 3 (left) illustrates the effect of the average interaction distance that results in higher values of $\beta(D, V)$ as D approaches D^*. On the other hand, the rate of recovery follows Equation (9), which lessens the rate of the increase in the burden of cases down to γ_0. For the case with excessive healthcare capacities, the rate of recovery can be maximized up to γ_1, as shown in Figure 3 (right).

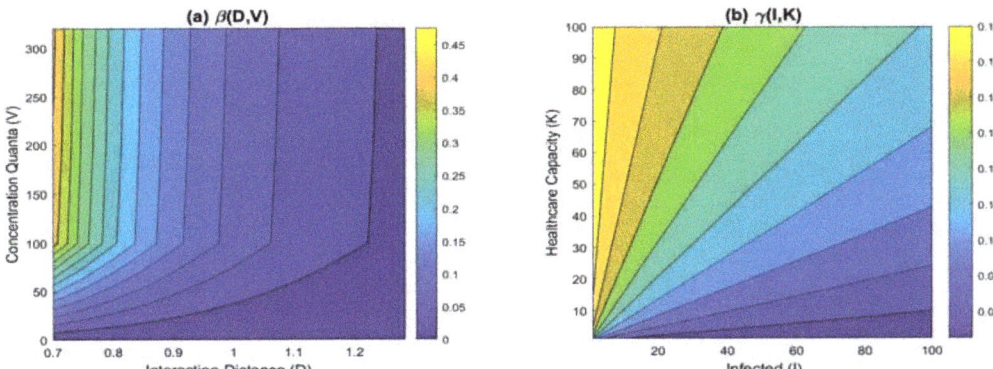

Figure 3. (a) Dependency of transmission rate β to D and V, by taking $\beta^* = 0.444$, $v = 7.680$, $w = 0.051$ and $D^* = 0.7$ m; (b) Effect of K and I to the rate of transmission by taking $\gamma_1 = 1/6$ (infection period of 6 days) and $\gamma_0 = 1/14$ (infection period of 14 days).

4. Numerical Results

In this study, the behavior of society that is being accommodated by the model is the rate of social resistance and social response. Socio-resistance rate, denoted by λ_1, represents the resistance of society to distancing their interactions due to the prevalence of people when I is not significantly zero. When the prevalence of people is close to zero, the resistance rate represents how fast the society moves back towards their natural interaction-distance D^*. In contrast, the rate of societal response represents the increase in interaction distancing per increase in point prevalence, which inhibits the disease spread when this value is high. In this section, we provide the number of infected individuals (per one thousand members of the population) for several values of λ_1 and λ_2.

4.1. Variations under Different Society Behaviors

The rate of social response is given in three scenarios (low, moderate, and high response), by taking values of $\lambda_2 = 0.20, 0.53$, and 0.87, respectively. These are based on the physical distancing campaign: (i) low social response drives people to physical distancing limited to $\overline{D} = 1$ m only, (ii) moderate can reach $\overline{D} = 1.5$ m, and (iii) high social response can reach up to 2 m. Table 3 shows the diverse approaches of countries in campaigning for physical distancing. We also set the rates of social resistance to $\lambda_1 = 0.15, 0.07$, and 0.05, which are based on $T_1 = 30, 60$, and 90 days, respectively. The ranges of λ_1 and λ_2 produced by Formulas (5) and (7) conform to those used in Cabrera et al. [23].

Table 3. Physical distancing campaigns among countries [46,47].

Countries	Physical Distancing (m)
Singapore, United Kingdom, Denmark, France, Hong Kong, China and France	1 m
Australia, Belgium, Greece, Germany, Italy, Spain, Portugal, Switzerland	1.5 m
Canada, United States	2 m

Figure 4 provides the numerical simulations for $I_u + I_v$ and D for the different pairwise scenarios of λ_1 and λ_2. As expected, the value of $D(t)$ will vary over time—increases as the disease prevalence increases. In all sub-figures, all dynamics for $D(t)$ always start from D^* as its natural distancing behavior when disease prevalence is around zero (no new cases recorded). However, as the disease prevalence rises, people in society build awareness to practice physical distancing which then increases the average distancing behavior D. As the new cases decrease to zero, it is natural that people in society return to their natural distancing D^*.

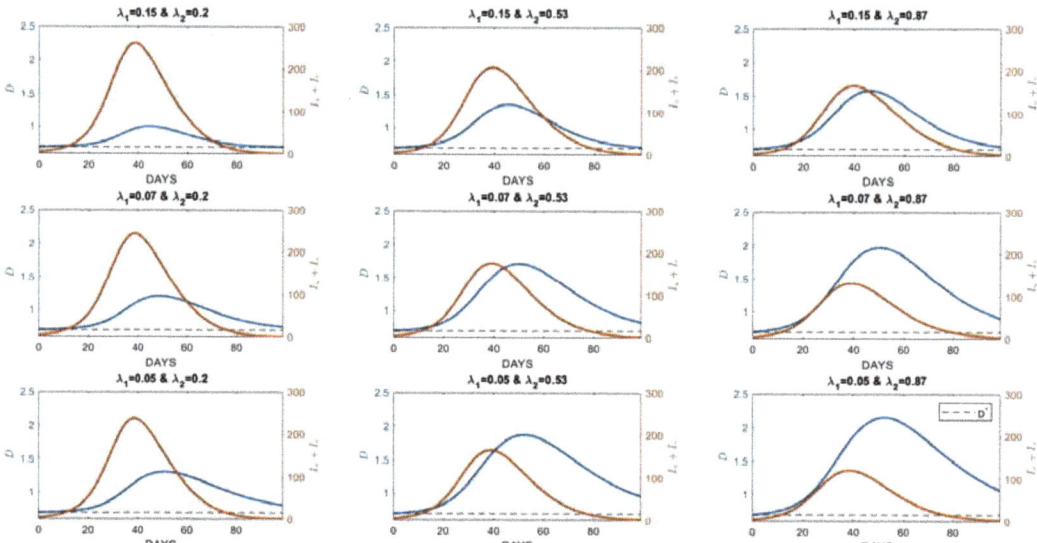

Figure 4. Numerical simulations for different values of the rate of resistance λ_1 and response to disease prevalence λ_2. Blue lines represent the average interaction distance, while the orange lines represent the burden of cases. The values of λ_1 and λ_2 are provided for three different values (low, moderate, high); $\lambda_2 = 0.20, 0.53, 0.87$ and $\lambda_1 = 0.05, 0.07, 0.15$. All figures were generated by choosing $N = 1000$ and $D^* = 0.7$ m and other parameters that evaluate the values of R_0 to exceed 1; $\rho = 0.5$, $\gamma_0 = 1/14$, $\lambda_1 = 1/6$.

The sub-figure in the left upper corner depicts the simulation results for a society with a lower response yet a higher resistance rate. Such a scenario results in a higher peak of the burden of cases relative to other scenarios. This result shows that if the society does not have enough awareness about the disease's prevalence, and has a strong resistance that inhibits the practice of physical distancing, the dynamics of D will be likely in around D^*, which results in a higher number of cases. Societies that campaign for close physical distancing (e.g., 1 m only), and have tendencies to always practice their natural habits, are likely represented by the left upper corner sub-figure. The figure situated at the center of the nine depicts simulations that apply to a society that has a considerably moderate level of resistance and response rate. The right lower corner depicts shows societies with a higher rate of response but a lower rate of resistance. Due to higher values of λ_2, every individual in the society moves further away relative to other scenarios and this results in a significant change in D relative to the value of D^*. When it comes to the figure of the burden of cases, this scenario estimates the lowest number of cases relative to other scenarios. Societies that practice physical distancing and have a tendency to keep practicing it in a longer period, even after the disease is no longer present, are best represented by this scenario, resulting in a lower burden of cases relative to other scenarios.

4.2. Variations under Different Pathogen Characteristics

Different pathogens lead to different survivability periods in the air or other media. The longer the pathogens are active as airborne pathogens, the more they accumulate, which increases the risk of infections. Characteristics of the observed pathogens are governed by parameter λ_4. In System (2), the term $-\lambda_4 V$ represents the concentration of pathogens per unit of time to become inactive. Figure 5 shows the dynamics of the disease prevalence $I_u + I_v$ under different periods of pathogens lasting in the air for the same parameters as used in Figure 4. In the lower-right picture, it is shown that pathogens that can last up to 48 h (red) can accumulate up to 300,000 quanta pathogens per m^3 and drive infections to as high as 23%. Figure 5a demonstrates how the dynamics of $I_u + I_v$ precede V on reaching a peak for exactly 2 days (48 h). It is natural to accept that the longer the period, the wider the gap between the occurrences of the two peaks. By setting a smaller period (higher λ_4), the dynamics of V decrease and so does $I_u + I_v$. Moreover, the peak of $I_u + I_v$ shifts to the right (see Figure 5b,c). More results on the model's sensitivity analysis are provided in Appendices B and C.

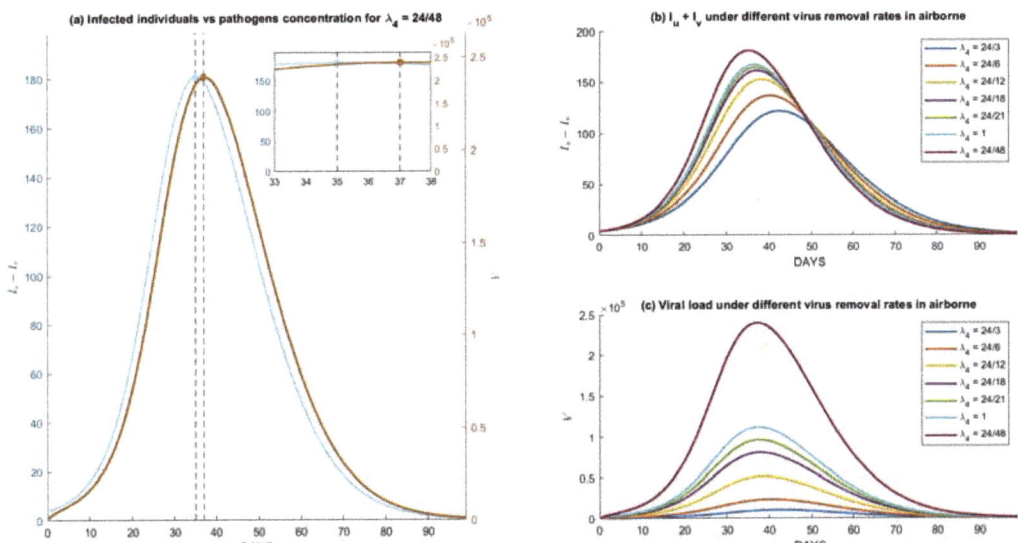

Figure 5. Numerical simulations of System (1) and (2) under different removal rates of airborne pathogens, that is implicated in the critical period of pathogens to remain active airborne: (a) comparison between the dynamics for infected individuals and viral load for a critical period of 48 h, which shows an exact lag of 48 h between the peak of infections and its viral loads, (b,c) dynamics for $I_u + I_v$ and its viral load under different critical periods of the airborne pathogen.

5. Case Study: SARS-CoV-2 Spread in School

As mentioned in the previous section, the proposed model incorporates the socio-behavioral aspects of people in the society combined with the effect of airborne transmission. When it comes to socio-behavioral aspects, we included social resistance and social response amid the disease spread, which limit the scope of the implementation. At the scale of nations, people in society comprise all levels of education, culture, habits, or even wealth [48], which leads to a variety in perceptions when dealing with disease spread; some may have higher awareness but some may not. This fact challenges the modeler regarding how to estimate λ_1 and λ_2 that will accurately portray the society. Hence, we designed the model to be applied to the scale of an educational or office environment. It is natural to expect the homogeneity of socio-behaviors, even homogeneity in age, in schools or offices. These limitations also support the involvement of airborne transmission due to the indoor activity in schools or offices [24]. Henceforth, this section provides the applications of the proposed model to understand the disease spread in a university environment.

5.1. Dataset and Parameters' Estimation

We collected the data in respect of the SARS-CoV-2 spread in a college environment, namely the Institut Teknologi Bandung (ITB), and data range from early January until late April 2022. The data comprise record daily cases, current active cases, and the total number of recovered individuals out of all enrolled students, lecturers, and college staff. Although students and staff do not stay at the college 24/7, it is reasonable to assume that they spend most of the time in the college environment. Here, we exclude the enrolled students that were infected in other cities due to the hybrid (online-offline) learning practice. The data are privately available at https://covidtrak.itb.ac.id/ (accessed on 1 April 2022), which is only accessible by ITB COVID-19 task-force members.

In terms of the parameter estimation, we only used data for the daily new cases from early January 2022 until late April 2022, which will be later denoted as D_a. Given in Table 4, System 204 and 210 involve 11 parameters, with only three of them being estimated by the integration of data D_a, namely β^*, v, and w, while other assumptions are as follows: the population size N equals 4000 (according to the report of the initial school reopening), the average vaccine efficacy $\rho = 0.37$ for SinoVac [36], $\gamma_0 = 1/14$, and $\gamma_1 = 1/6$, which represent the rate of recovery under lack of and excessive healthcare, respectively. In order to obtain the estimations of β^*, v, and w, we used a Markov Chain Monte Carlo (MCMC) method to estimate the whole distribution. The complete Bayesian hierarchy for the MCMC method is provided in Appendix D. Figure 6 shows the estimated posterior distribution of β^*, v, and w that was implemented to the data that resemble the recorded daily new cases.

Table 4. List of parameters used in evaluating the numerical simulation of System (1) and (2).

Notation	Description	Values
$\gamma_0(\gamma_1)$	COVID-19 recovery rate in the case of a lack of healthcare capacity (in the case of excessive healthcare). This parameter governs the time-dependent recovery rate	1/14 (1/6) 1/day
D^*	Natural interaction distance	1.2 m
β^*, v, and w	Intrinsic transmission rate and the contact and airborne transmission adjuster	Calibrated
ρ	Current vaccine efficacy, using SinoVac [29]	0.35
λ_1	The rate of social resistance in the observed community	0.07 1/day
λ_2	The rate of social response in the observed community	0.53 m/day

Table 4. *Cont.*

Notation	Description	Values
λ_3	Average concentration of airborne pathogens emitted by one infected individual per day	24 quanta/(day person·m^3) [24]
λ_4	Removal rate of airborne pathogens	2 1/day [21]

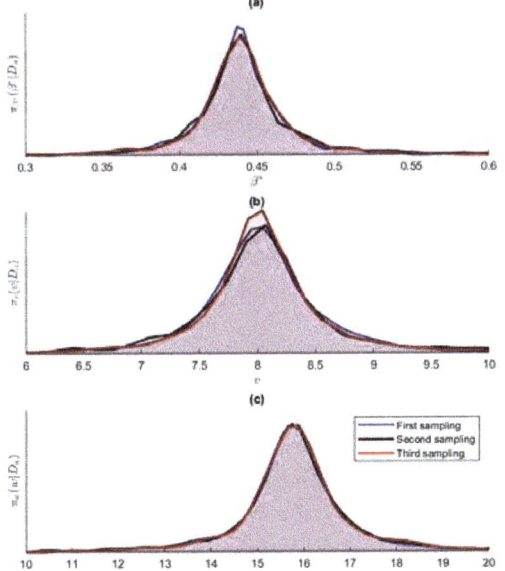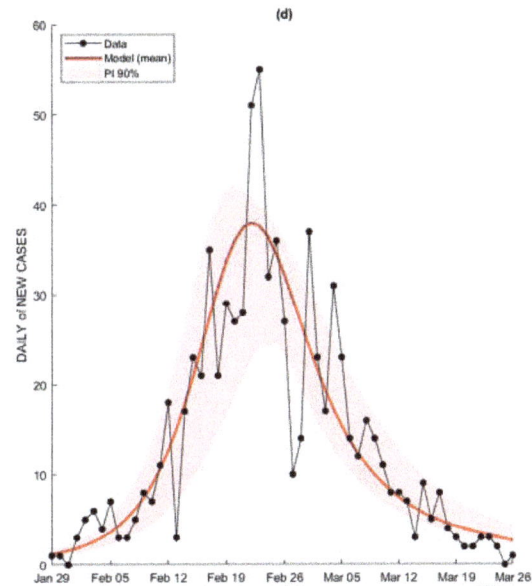

Figure 6. (a–c) Posterior distribution for β^*, v and w, estimated using MCMC method with prior of normal distributions: $\mathcal{N}(\mu, \sigma)$, with μ being the estimated single point and σ being a higher value to acquire the possibility of achieving the global minima. We generated three independent samples to portray the posterior density to ensure its consistency. (d) The comparison between the data (daily new cases) and the model with its 90% prediction interval.

5.2. Projected Number of Cases

Assuming no further changes in all parameters, the estimated posterior distribution of β^*, v, and w can be used to sample their values and generate the extrapolated trajectories for all states of the proposed model. Figure 7a and b show the projections of the disease prevalence in the university from early 2022 until mid-2023. Both consistently predict a significant decrease in the number of cases from May 2022, which implies a decrease in the average interaction distance D, approaching the social natural distancing D^*. Figure 7a–c clearly show that the figures are estimated with a relatively narrow prediction interval, which leads to high confidence in the results under the hold assumptions. As the average interaction distance D is around D^*, or, in other words, people in society behave as if there is no disease, the expected number of cases shown in Figure 7a,b increases in August 2022 and peaks in around October 2022, though the prediction interval is relatively wider compared to the previous period. These simulations show that the number of cases is expected to increase as D approaches D^*, without even considering reinfection due to immunity waning.

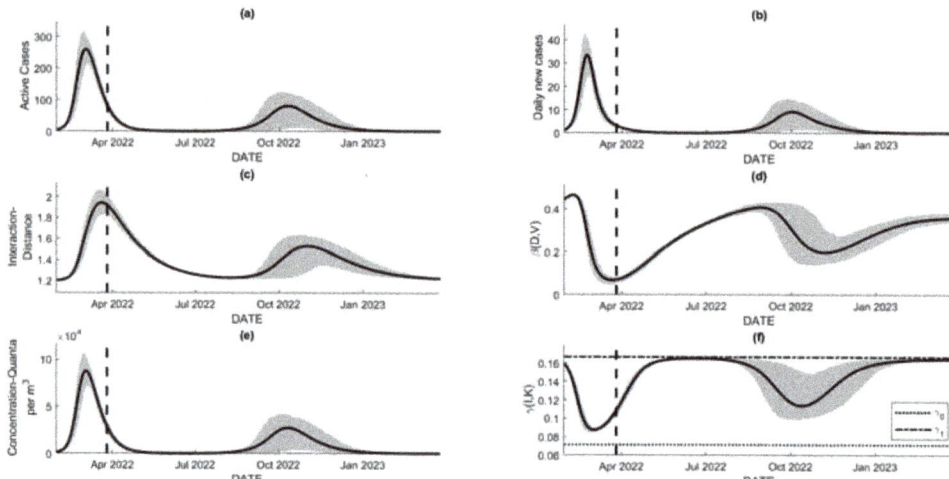

Figure 7. The extrapolated figures with the dashed line initiate the prediction window. The figures were evaluated using the estimated parameters obtained in the previous section, with the assumption of no significant change in parameters for the 365-day prediction intervals: (**a**,**b**) extrapolated number of active cases and daily new cases that levels off in around May to July 2022, but starts to increase on August and peaks on October 2022, (**c**) average interaction distance of society that will approach its natural distancing of $D^* = 1.2$ m as the number of cases decreases, but increases when the case resurgence is identified, (**d**) time-dependent transmission rate that gradually increasing as D approaches D^*, (**e**) dynamic for viral load over time that resembles that for active cases, and (**f**) time-dependent recovery rate that its values are bounded by γ_0 and γ_1.

Figure 7e depicts the dynamics of the pathogen concentrations in the observed area per m^3, which resembles the dynamics of the active cases over time. As stated in the previous section, the longer the pathogens can last in the air (or other media), the further the shift to the right relative to the dynamics of the active cases. In other words, the presence of $I_u + I_v$ contributes to the presence of pathogens that govern the rate of transmissibility. Figure 7d and f show the dynamics of $\beta = \beta(D, V)$ and $\gamma = \gamma(I, K)$. Although they are not directly dependent on time, they are time-dependent due to the dependency of D, V, and I to the unit of time. During the training time (initial time until the dashed lines), the rate of transmission β decreases due to the significant deviation of the average interaction distance relative to D^*. It is expected that the trajectories of β will increase during the prediction interval due to the decreasing values of D. For the rate of transmission, its value is always bounded within the $\gamma_0 - \gamma_1$ ribbon. The rate is expected to approach the maximum value of γ as the burden of cases approaches zero; otherwise, it approaches the minimum γ. For Figure 7f, we set $K = 100$, which represents the ability of the university hospital to accommodate only 100 patients at one time. This assumption causes a significant decrease in γ as the expected $I_u + I_v$ exceeds the value of K, depicting the ineffective health service as the burden exceeds its capacity.

5.3. Prospective Action Plans

Other than providing the extrapolated trajectories for all states, we are also interested in supplying numerical simulations related to prospective action plans for preventing the expected surge of COVID-19 in schools. This section provides the numerical assessment of three action plans: school reopening management, disinfection, and vaccine-related improvement.

5.3.1. School Reopening Management

Although technologies support students in attending online classes, the practice of in-person classes is still preferable. This fact should be the main reason for the massive reopening of most Indonesian schools, regardless of the level of education. However, this should challenge the previous simulations due to a significant change in the number of individuals in a school as it is reopened. Henceforth, we provide numerical simulations of all states, more concerned with $I_u + I_v$, as the number of individuals in a school varies due to the school reopening. In practice, we assume that all individuals (students, lecturers, and staff) can be considered vulnerable to the disease. The higher the number of susceptible individuals, the more individuals can be infected. Hence, it is natural to analyze the effect of the increase in N on the dynamics of $I_u + I_v$.

Mathematically speaking, $N = S_u + I_u + R_u + S_v + I_v + R_v$, which implies that $N' = S'_u + I'_u + R'_u + S'_v + I'_v + R'_v$. Substituting the derivatives of all states as stated in System (1), we have $N' = 0$, meaning that the population size remains unchanged. However, we modified the model to accommodate the change in the population size due to the school reopening. Since we assume that all new individuals enter compartments S_u and S_v (with the proportion governed by the vaccine coverage), we add recruitment terms f and g for S_u and S_v as given by Equation (10).

$$\begin{cases} S'_u = f - \beta(I_u + I_v)S_u/N \\ S'_v = g - \beta(1-\rho)(I_u + I_v)S_v/N \end{cases} \quad (10)$$

This gives us $N' = f + g$, for $f = f(t)$ and $g = g(t)$. Integrating both sides gives us $N(t) = \int_0^t (f(s) + g(s))ds$. If we choose $f(t) = (1-\alpha)N'_{obj}(t)$ and $f(t) = \alpha N'_{obj}(t)$, for a continuous and differentiable function $N_{obj}(t)$, then $f(t) + g(t) = N'_{obj}(t)$ and we expect that $N(t) = N_{obj}$. The simulation is conducted numerically, which includes the discretization of the time domain, and hence the condition of the differentiability of N_{obj} is no longer relevant. The subscript objwhich stands for 'objective', denotes the preferred dynamics of $N(t)$ that represent a certain school opening scheme. Hence, we can assess the effect of a specific school reopening scheme by choosing the appropriate function N_{obj} that depicts the expected dynamics of the total individuals at any time t. Then, we choose three different $N_{obj}(t)$ values that represent three interesting school reopening schemes:

1. **No school reopening (benchmark)** We preserve the size of the population as it was used to generate simulations in the previous section. We set $N = 4000$ for all $t > 0$, which leads to the constant population size for all time. This scenario is a benchmark for the other two scenarios.

2. **Gradual school reopening** A gradual school reopening is a scheme that admits students and academical staff gradually until, at some point, the total number of students and staff is reached. In the Institut Teknologi Bandung (ITB), there are approximately 20,000 students and academical staff at any time for a non-pandemic era, which starts with only 4000 individuals in a pandemic era (January until April 2022). Hence, we choose a simple-bounded linearly increasing function N_{obj} as given by:

$$N_{obj}(t) = \begin{cases} 4000 \ for \ t < 58 \\ 4000 + 114(t-59) \ for \ t \in [59, 200] \\ 20,000 \ for \ t > 201 \end{cases}$$

$t \in \mathbb{Z}^+$, with $t \in [0, 58]$, is the training data interval, which uses $N = 4000$. However, $t \in [200, end]$ represents the total school reopening that starts in September 1, 2022, with $N = 20,000$. The middle period of $t \in [59, 200]$ represents a linearly gradual reopening from 4000 to 20,000. In practice, it is easy to add that $f = 114(1-\alpha)$ and $g = 114\alpha$ during the period of reopening $t \in [59, 200]$, and $f = g = 0$ otherwise.

3. **Prevalence-tuned school opening** The last scenario accommodates the response of the school officials to reduce the school capacity as the disease prevalence level

increases. Hence, we assume that the number of N should be related to the number of I. We chose a negative exponential to represent the relation between N and I as follows:

$$N_{obj}(t) = (20,000 - 4000)e^{-kI(t)} + 4000.$$

This formulation suggests that as I is around zero, then the school officials are about to totally open the school, and $N = 20,000$. The opposite condition with a large number of I forces the school restriction and allows only 4000 individuals. This formulation of N_{obj} is not explicitly time-dependent; instead, it depends on the varying values of $I(t)$. In practice, we can set $f = (1-\alpha)(20,000 - 4000)ke^{-kt}I'(t)$ and $g = \alpha(20,000 - 4000)ke^{-kt}I'(t)$.

Figure 8 shows the numerical assessment of the three school reopening schemes. The simulations in red are the results that act as a benchmark for the other scenarios. This benchmark scenario gives the constant population size that drives the resurgence of the active cases around October as the average interaction distance increases. However, adding more people into the school through the gradual reopening scheme leads to more infections recorded, which reach a peak around July–August 2022. The surge is expected to happen since we add more people as N increases from 4000 to 20,000 in early September 2022. However, the infection-tuned scheme allows more people to enter the school relative to the other two schemes, yet results in lower cases compared to the second scenario. This is caused by the response of the school officials to reducing the school participants as the cases start to increase. This is the reason why cases increase in the same period as the second scheme but are significantly lower. By this simulation, all scenarios of reopening drive more people to enter the school, leading to more infections. The next section shows how the vaccine-related improvement can solve the problem of reopening without expecting any surge in infections.

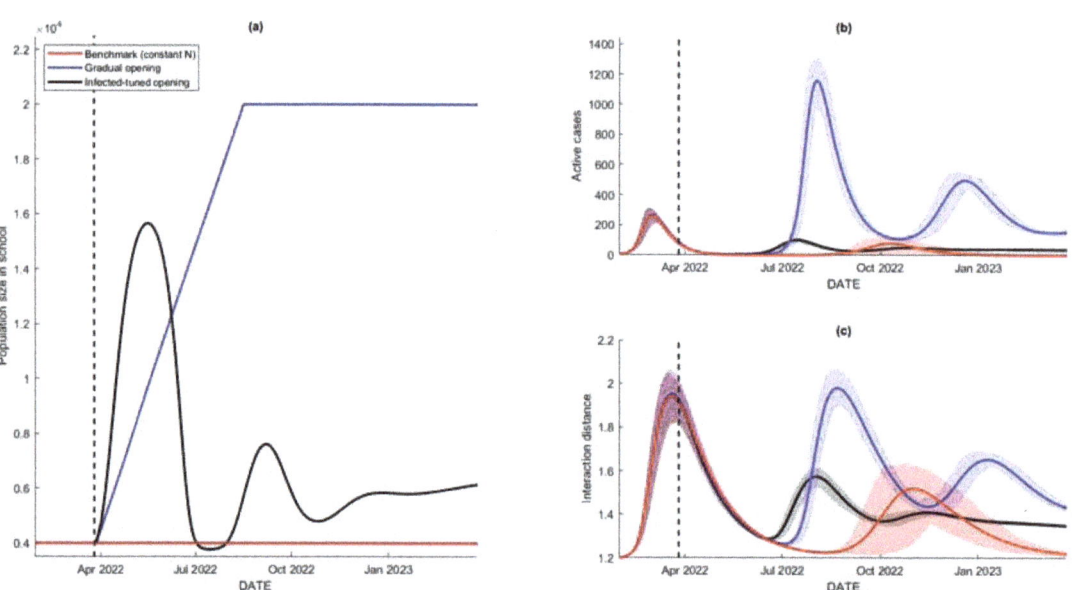

Figure 8. Numerical results of school reopening schemes: no reopening (benchmark) in red, gradual reopening in blue, and case-based reopening in black; (**a**) population sizes for the three scenarios during the school reopening, (**b**,**c**) simulations of the disease prevalence $I = I_u + I_v$ and the interaction distance D for different reopening schemes.

5.3.2. Vaccine Coverage and Effectiveness Improvement

Other than the physical distancing campaign, vaccination is one of the control measures in the spread of COVID-19, especially in a school environment. It has been shown that any school reopening leads to more infections recorded within the society. This section provides a simulation of the three reopening schemes whilst also varying the vaccine efficacy. By April 2022, the current average of vaccine efficacy is around 37%, as most Indonesians have been inoculated twice with SinoVac, which has 37% effectiveness in response to the Omicron variant. The improvement of the vaccine efficacy can be achieved by campaigning for a third vaccine dose with higher efficacy, such as Moderna, Pfizer, or Oxford AstraZeneca. Figure 9 shows the numerical simulations for different values of vaccine efficacy: $\rho = 37\%$, 50%, 65%, and 80%.

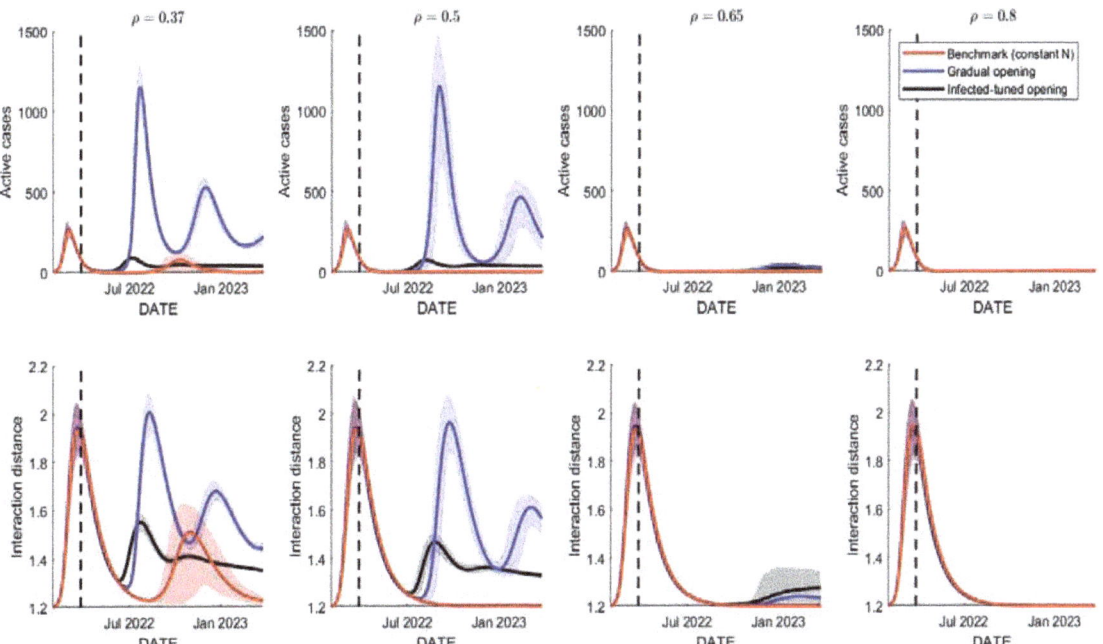

Figure 9. Simulations of the three school reopening schemes under different vaccine efficacies. Improving the vaccine efficacy should reduce the expected numbers of cases. The highest vaccine efficacy in response to the Omicron variant is about 71% [36].

The figure illustrates the effect of the improvement of the vaccine efficacy, by assuming that 80% of school attendees have received a full-dose vaccine with such efficacy. When the efficacy is improved from 37% to 50%, this affects the first scenario that has only 4000 and cases that are expected to occur in October 2022 vanish. However, $\rho = 50\%$ is not enough to reduce the other two scenarios (blue and black) significantly as the expected cases remain high for such scenarios. For $\rho = 65\%$, most of the expected cases are reduced significantly. Lastly, $\rho = 80\%$ or higher is expected to reduce a whole surge of cases, at least for the 365-day prediction interval. It can be seen that as the number of cases reduces to zero, the average interaction distance of people approaches its natural level, yet there is no trigger for more infections due to the acquisition of vaccine-induced immunity. These results suggest that any reopening scheme, up to a maximal school capacity of 20,000 individuals, will not lead to any surge in COVID-19 cases as long as 80% of the population has received a vaccine with a minimum 80% efficacy.

6. Conclusions

In this study, we provided a modified SIR-type model that incorporates socio-viral behavioral aspects. The first aspect (socio-behavioral) was added to the model by integrating the average interaction distance in society, while the other was added by integrating the critical period in which airborne pathogens remain active. In a general case, a society with a higher resistance rate λ_1 but a lower response rate λ_2 will record more total cases compared to other plausible scenarios. In other words, the mentioned scenario applies to society with people that are hardly accepting new distancing habits and that do not have the awareness of disease prevalence. In contrast, a society with people that easily adapt to new distancing behaviors due to disease transmission, representing a society with a higher λ_2 but a lower λ_1, will result in the least total cases compared to other scenarios. Furthermore, varying the critical period for active airborne pathogens also influence the model behaviors. The higher the critical period, the longer the airborne pathogens actively contribute to the increase in transmission rate.

As a case study, we implemented the proposed data on the spread of COVID-19 in a school environment to preserve the assumption of homogeneity in the population. Using the data on infections, we inferred the unknown parameters using the Bayesian approach. We have shown that the rendered model is well-depicting the training data. Using the inferred parameters, we extrapolated the model and came up with the evidence for a resurgence of cases in around August 2022. The resurgence of the case is purely implied by the return of society to its natural distancing behavior D^* when no new COVID-19 cases are recorded. The dynamics of airborne pathogens load V seem not to influence that significantly due to the short critical period of SARS-CoV-2 to remain active in the air.

In response to the resurgence of cases, we used the model to numerically assess some strategic actions, applicable to the school context, to prevent the resurgence. First, we define some reasonable school reopening schemes that influence the population size: no reopening, gradual reopening, and infection-tuned reopening. While the first has a constant population size N, the second is gradually increasing the population size until it reaches the maximum capacity. Different from the other two, the infection-tuned reopening is a scheme that increases N to its maximum capacity when no diseases are identified, but also allows for decreasing N as the number of cases increases. Though the third scheme seems not practical, an infection-tuned scheme is proven to be the most effective strategy to reopen the school and minimize the risk of the rerise of COVID-19. Second, since we have demonstrated that all school reopening schemes lead to the resurgence of COVID-19 cases, we provide a numerical simulation that justifies the importance of vaccine quality; coverage, and efficacy. With constant vaccination coverage, increasing the vaccine efficacy will reduce the risk of COVID-19 resurgence—a vaccine with an efficacy of more than 80% has been proven to effectively prevent the COVID-19 resurgence, regardless of how society behaves towards the disease spread.

Author Contributions: Conceptualization, N.N.; methodology, K.K.S. and N.N.; software, K.K.S.; validation, N.N., U.S.P., A.B., S.H.S., D.R., E.A.G.-R., S.Y., H.D.A., D.M., I.S. and W.M.; formal analysis, N.N., M.Y.T.T. and K.K.S.; investigation, N.N. and K.K.S.; resources, A.B., S.H.S., D.R., E.A.G.-R., S.Y., H.D.A., D.M., I.S. and W.M.; data curation, N.N., U.S.P., A.B., S.H.S., D.R., E.A.G.-R., S.Y., H.D.A., D.M., I.S. and W.M.; writing—original draft preparation, N.N. and K.K.S.; writing—review and editing, M.Y.T.T., A.B., S.H.S., D.R., E.A.G.-R., S.Y., H.D.A., D.M., I.S. and W.M.; visualization, K.K.S.; supervision, N.N.; project administration, N.N.; funding acquisition, E.A.G.-R. All authors have read and agreed to the published version of the manuscript.

Funding: This research is funded by Riset Unggulan 2022 with research grant number of 1V/IT1.C02/TA.00/2022 and ITB.

Institutional Review Board Statement: Not applicable.

Informed Consent Statement: Not applicable.

Acknowledgments: Authors would like to deliver a big appreciation for the ITB team for covidtrak that has voluntarily collecting data that was used for this research. We also should appreciate Yayasan ITB for funding this research. This research is funded by Riset Unggulan 2022 with research grant number of 1V/IT1.C02/TA.00/2022 and ITB.

Conflicts of Interest: The authors have no conflicts of interest to declare. All co-authors have seen and agree with the contents of the manuscript and there is no financial interest to report. We certify that the submission is original work and is not under review at any other publication.

Appendix A. Model Analysis and Threshold Number

For the sake of simplicity, we drop the vaccination effect and hence merge all compartments having indices u and v together. To generate both the disease-free and endemic equilibria, we added the natural disease in all state compartment (SIR), with μ represents the natural death rate. By substituting $\beta(D, V)$ and $\gamma(I, K)$ with those given by Equations (3) and (4), we have our system be rewritten as follows.

$$\begin{cases} S' = -\beta^* \left(\frac{2D^*}{D^*+D}\right)^v \left(\frac{V+V^*}{V^*}\right)^w \frac{SI}{N} \\ I' = \beta^* \left(\frac{2D^*}{D^*+D}\right)^v \left(\frac{V+V^*}{V^*}\right)^w \frac{SI}{N} - \left(\gamma_0 + (\gamma_1 - \gamma_0)\frac{K}{I+K}\right)I \\ R' = \left(\gamma_0 + (\gamma_1 - \gamma_0)\frac{K}{I+K}\right)I \\ D' = -\lambda_1(D - D^*) + \lambda_2(I/N) \\ V' = \lambda_3 I - \lambda_4 V \end{cases}$$

All plausible equilibria of System (5) are obtained by solving this nonlinear system, that is modified by adding the recruitment and natural death rate in order to get the Endemic Equilibrium.

$$0 = A - \beta^* \left(\frac{2D^*}{D^*+D}\right)^v \left(\frac{V+V^*}{V^*}\right)^w \frac{SI}{N} - \mu S$$

$$0 = \beta^* \left(\frac{2D^*}{D^*+D}\right)^v \left(\frac{V+V^*}{V^*}\right)^w \frac{SI}{N} - \left(\gamma_0 + (\gamma_1 - \gamma_0)\frac{K}{I+K}\right)I - \mu I$$

$$0 = \left(\gamma_0 + (\gamma_1 - \gamma_0)\frac{K}{I+K}\right)I$$

$$0 = -\lambda_1(D - D^*) + \lambda_2(I/N)$$

$$0 = \lambda_3 I - \lambda_4 V$$

The disease-free equilibrium (DFE) can be obtained by plugging $\hat{I} = 0$ to the system, which leads to $DFE = \{S^*, 0, R^*, D^*, 0\}$. Using the next generation matrix method, the formula of the basic reproductive ratio is given by

$$R_0 = \frac{\beta^*}{\gamma + \mu}$$

with the term of $\left(\frac{2D^*}{D^*+D}\right)^v \left(\frac{V+V^*}{V^*}\right)^w$ vanishes to 1 as all states approach the DFE. This quantity will determine whether the state will approach the DFE (when $R_0 < 1$) or otherwise approach the other equilibrium point, namely the EE.

Appendix B. Numerical Sensitivity Analysis of the Socio-Behavioral Parameters

In this study, the behaviors of society that being accommodated by the model is the rate of social resistance and social response. Socio-resistance rate, denoted with λ_1, represents the resistance of society for distancing their interaction due to the figure prevalence when I is not significantly zero. When the figure prevalence is close to zero, the resistance rate depicts how fast the society to live back with their natural interaction-distance D^*. In contrast, the rate of society response depicts the increase in interaction distancing per increase in point prevalence, which inhibits the disease spread when this value is set high. In this section, we provide the figure of infected individuals (per one thousand of population) as λ_1 and λ_2 is set varied.

Given in Figure A1, the setting of $\lambda_1 = 0$ while $\lambda_2 = 0.5$ depicts the situation that people in society tend to response to the figure prevalence by distancing interaction but have no intention to return on their previous interaction habit. The blue line in the bottom-left corner represents the average interaction-distance in the mentioned scenario that levels off in $D = 4.2$ without approaching the natural interaction-distance. By fixing $\lambda_2 = 0.5$, the increment of λ_1 will lower the average interaction-distance and fasten the dynamics of D to approach D^*. Poor society in certain regions tend to hasten on returning back on their previous habits (to work, study, etc) once the decrease in the point prevalence are declared, which in this model is considered to have relatively higher λ_1. In contrast, some regions in developed countries may have lower value of λ_1. Hence, the model requires the homogeneity of society; the smaller the society, the easier to assume, such as: students and academic staff in closed school, workers.

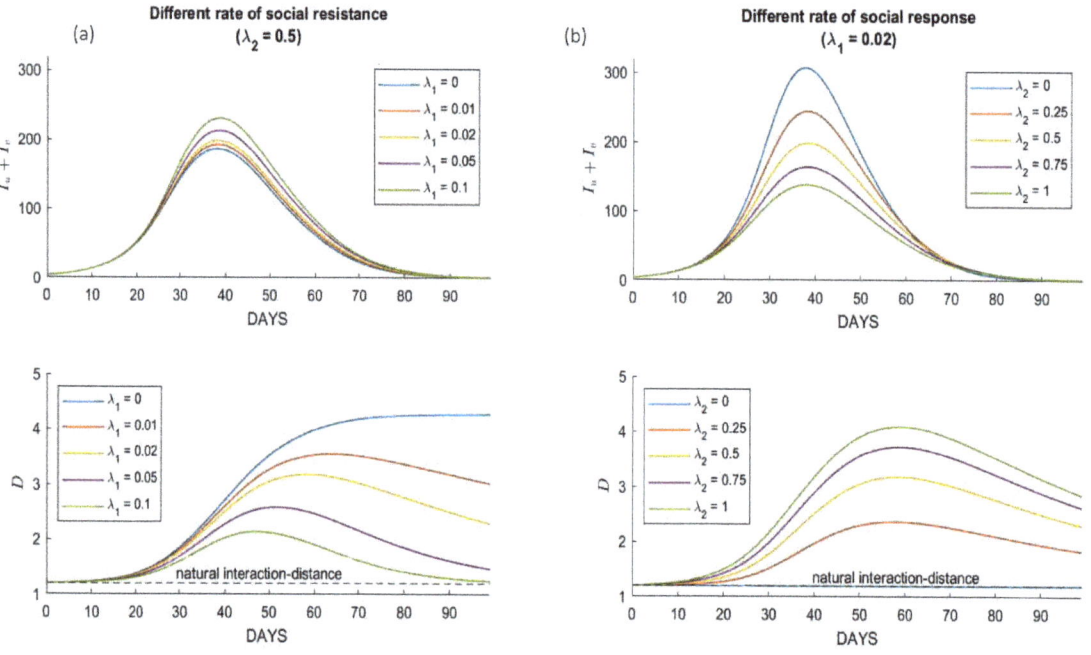

Figure A1. Number of infected individuals in society of population 1000 individuals under different values of socio-resistance and social response rates. (**a**) five different values of socio-resistance by setting $\lambda_2 = 0.5$. Each scenario has $\mathcal{R}_0 =$, for ascending order of λ_1. (**b**) Five different values of social response by setting $\lambda_1 = 0.02$.

Right-hand side figures in Figure A1 depicts how social response to point prevalence affects the dynamics of both infected individuals and interaction-distance. The scenario setting $\lambda_1 = 0$ portrays the society with no attention to current disease spread, implying to a steady interaction-distance to its natural habit. The higher the setting of λ_2, the more responsive the people in society to the current point prevalence.

Appendix C. Numerical Simulations under Different Healthcare Capacity

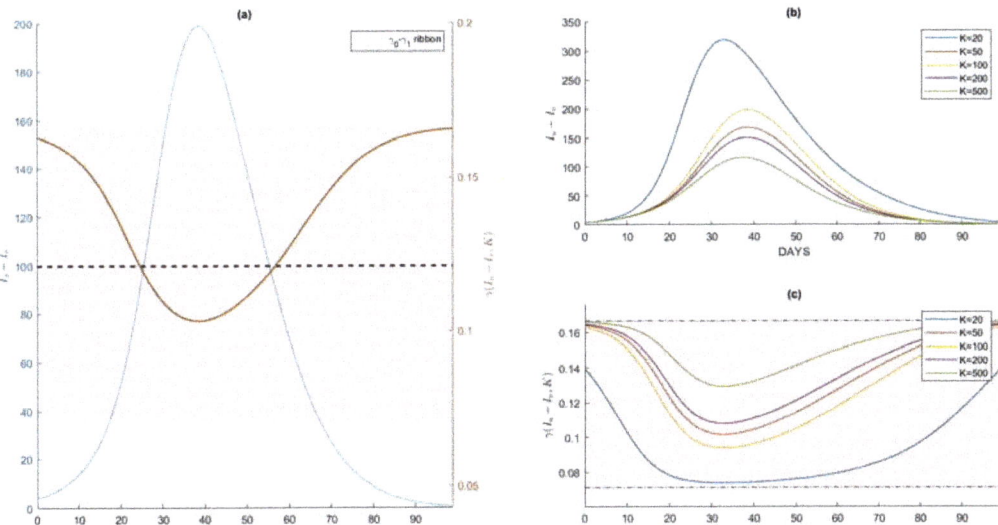

Figure A2. Numerical simulations under different values of healthcare capacities: (a) comparison between the dynamics of active cases and the rate of recovery using the same parameters as used in Figure A1, (b,c) sensitivity analysis of $I_u + I_v$ and the rate of recovery γ under different value of healthcare capacity K.

Appendix D. Bayesian Hierarchical for Parameters' Estimation

There are three parameters that are estimated by the integration of the provided data D_α. We assume that those three parameters are each a realization of a complete posterior distribution. Let us assume that $D_\alpha(i), i = 1, 2, \ldots, n$ denotes the daily cases of COVID-19 at day i, while $f(i; \hat{\theta})$ represents the dynamics of the daily cases evaluated from the proposed model given that $\hat{\theta} = [\beta^*, v, w]^T$. We expect that observation $D_\alpha(i)$ (experimental data or observed data) to be equal as the model response $f(i, \hat{\theta})$ plus the independent and identically distributed error ε_i, with mean zero and variance σ^2. Hence, we can write:

$$D_\alpha(i) = f(i; \hat{\theta}) + \varepsilon_i$$

with $\varepsilon_i \, N(0, \sigma^2)$. The goal is to estimate the posteriod distribution of $\pi(\hat{\theta}|D_\alpha(i))$, which quantify the probability of parameter $\hat{\theta}$ given the set of observational data.

$$\pi(\hat{\theta}|D_\alpha(i)) = \frac{\mathcal{L}(D_\alpha(i)|\hat{\theta})\pi_0(\hat{\theta})}{\mathcal{NL}}$$

with $\mathcal{L}(D_\alpha(i)|(\hat{\theta}))$ represent the likelihood and $\pi_0(\hat{\theta})$ is the prior knowledge of the estimated parameters. In terms of the data fitting, it is common to define the likelihood function as given in the following formula:

$$(D_\alpha(i)|(\hat{\theta})) = exp\left(-\frac{SS_q}{Var}\right)$$

with $SS_s = \sum_i^n (D_\alpha(i) - f(i; \hat{\theta}))^2$. We will use the MCMC method (with a Metropolis-Hastings Algorithm) to get samples from the posterior distributions given in 860. Since we have no prior knowledge for each of the estimated parameters, we choose the prior of normal distribution with zero mean, but high in variance. In MATLAB, we used the built-in function provided by Grinsted, A. available in https://www.mathworks.com/matlabcentral/fileexchange/49820-ensemble-mcmc-sampler (accessed on 17 June 2022).

References

1. Nakamura, G.M.; Martinez, A.S. Hamiltonian dynamics of the SIS epidemic model with stochastic fluctuations. *Sci. Rep.* **2019**, *9*, 15841. [CrossRef] [PubMed]
2. Carcione, J.M.; Santos, J.E.; Bagaini, C.; Ba, J. A Simulation of a COVID-19 Epidemic Based on a Deterministic SEIR Model. *Front. Public Health* **2020**, *8*, 230. [CrossRef] [PubMed]
3. Bjørnstad, O.N.; Shea, K.; Krzywinski, M.; Altman, N. The SEIRS model for infectious disease dynamics. *Nat. Methods* **2020**, *17*, 557–558. [CrossRef]
4. Tolles, J.; Luong, T. Modeling Epidemics with Compartmental Models. *JAMA* **2020**, *323*, 2515. [CrossRef] [PubMed]
5. Milligan, G. *Vaccinology: An Essential Guide*; Wiley Blackwell: Sussex, UK, 2015.
6. Susanto, H.; Tjahjono, V.; Hasan, A.; Kasim, M.; Nuraini, N.; Putri, E.; Kusdiantara, R.; Kurniawan, H. How Many Can You Infect? Simple (and Naive) Methods of Estimating the Reproduction Number. *Commun. Biomath. Sci.* **2020**, *3*, 28–36. [CrossRef]
7. Hasan, A.; Nasution, Y.; Susanto, H.; Putri, E.; Tjahjono, V.; Puspita, D.; Sukandar, K.; Nuraini, N.; Widyastuti, W. Modeling COVID-19 Transmissions and Evaluation of Large-Scale Social Restriction in Jakarta, Indonesia. *Commun. Biomath. Sci.* **2022**, *5*, 90–100. [CrossRef]
8. Katul, G.G.; Mrad, A.; Bonetti, S.; Manoli, G.; Parolari, A.J. Global convergence of COVID-19 basic reproduction number and estimation from early-time SIR dynamics. *PLoS ONE* **2020**, *15*, e0239800. [CrossRef]
9. Moein, S.; Nickaeen, N.; Roointan, A.; Borhani, N.; Heidary, Z.; Javanmard, S.H.; Ghaisari, J.; Gheisari, Y. Inefficiency of SIR models in forecasting COVID-19 epidemic: A case study of Isfahan. *Sci. Rep.* **2021**, *11*, 4725. [CrossRef]
10. Allen, L.J.S.; Brown, V.; Jonsson, C.; Klein, S.L.; Laverty, S.M.; Magwedere, K.; Owen, J.C.; Driessche, P.V.D. Mathematical modeling of viral zoonoses in wildlife. *Nat. Resour. Model.* **2011**, *25*, 5–51. [CrossRef]
11. Li, G.-H.; Zhang, Y.-X. Dynamic behaviors of a modified SIR model in epidemic diseases using nonlinear incidence and recovery rates. *PLoS ONE* **2017**, *12*, e0175789. [CrossRef]
12. Okabe, Y.; Shudo, A. A mathematical model of epidemics-a tutorial for students. *Mathematics* **2020**, *8*, 1174. [CrossRef]
13. Bertozzi, A.L.; Franco, E.; Mohler, G.; Short, M.B.; Sledge, D. The challenges of modeling and forecasting the spread of COVID-19. *Proc. Natl. Acad. Sci. USA* **2020**, *117*, 16732–16738. [CrossRef] [PubMed]
14. Wahyudi, B.A.; Palupi, I. Prediction of the peak COVID-19 pandemic in Indonesia using SIR model. *J. Teknol. Sist. Komput.* **2020**, *9*, 49–55. [CrossRef]
15. Weston, D.; Hauck, K.; Amlôt, R. Infection prevention behaviour and infectious disease modelling: A review of the literature and recommendations for the future. *BMC Public Health* **2018**, *18*, 336. [CrossRef]
16. Hufsky, F.; Lamkiewicz, K.; Almeida, A.; Aouacheria, A.; Arighi, C.; Bateman, A.; Baumbach, J.; Beerenwinkel, N.; Brandt, C.; Cacciabue, M.; et al. Computational strategies to combat COVID-19: Useful tools to accelerate SARS-CoV-2 and coronavirus research. *Brief. Bioinform.* **2021**, *22*, 642–663. [CrossRef]
17. Peter, S.; Dittrich, P.; Ibrahim, B. Structure and Hierarchy of SARS-CoV-2 Infection Dynamics Models Revealed by Reaction Network Analysis. *Viruses* **2020**, *13*, 14. [CrossRef]
18. Wisconsin, D. Infection Control and Prevention—Tuberculosis (tb). 2022. Available online: https://www.dhs.wisconsin.gov/ic/tb.htm (accessed on 1 April 2022).
19. CDC. Scientific Brief: Sars-cov-2 Transmission. 2022. Available online: https://www.cdc.gov/coronavirus/2019-ncov/science/science-briefs/sars-cov-2-transmission.html (accessed on 1 April 2022).
20. CDC. Tuberculosis: General Information. 2022. Available online: https://www.cdc.gov/tb/publications/factsheets/general/tb.htm (accessed on 31 May 2022).
21. Van Doremalen, N.; Bushmaker, T.; Morris, D.H.; Holbrook, M.G.; Gamble, A.; Williamson, B.N.; Tamin, A.; Harcourt, J.L.; Thornburg, N.J.; Gerber, S.I.; et al. Aerosol and Surface Stability of SARS-CoV-2 as Compared with SARS-CoV-1. *N. Engl. J. Med.* **2020**, *382*, 1564–1567. [CrossRef]
22. Oluyori, D.A.; Perez, A.C.; Okhuese, V.A.; Akram, M. Backward and hopf bifurcation analysis of an seirs COVID-19 epidemic model with saturated incidence and saturated treatment response (preprint work). *MedRxiv* 2020. [CrossRef]
23. Cabrera, M.; Córdova-Lepe, F.; Gutiérrez-Jara, J.P.; Vogt-Geisse, K. An SIR-type epidemiological model that integrates social distancing as a dynamic law based on point prevalence and socio-behavioral factors. *Sci. Rep.* **2021**, *11*, 10170. [CrossRef]
24. Bazant, M.Z.; Bush, J.W.M. A guideline to limit indoor airborne transmission of COVID-19. *Proc. Natl. Acad. Sci. USA* **2021**, *118*, e2018995118. [CrossRef]
25. Nuraini, N.; Sukandar, K.; Hadisoemarto, P.; Susanto, H.; Hasan, A.; Sumarti, N. Mathematical models for assessing vaccination scenarios in several provinces in Indonesia. *Infect. Dis. Model.* **2021**, *6*, 1236–1258. [CrossRef] [PubMed]
26. Aini, W.; Sukandar, K.K.; Nuraini, N.; Handayani, D. The Impact of Mass Exodus on the Resurgence of COVID-19 Cases: Case Study of Regions in Indonesia. *Front. Appl. Math. Stat.* **2022**, *8*, 912150. [CrossRef]
27. Sukandar, K.K.; Louismono, A.L.; Volisa, M.; Kusdiantara, R.; Fakhruddin, M.; Nuraini, N.; Soewono, E. A Prospective Method for Generating COVID-19 Dynamics. *Computation* **2022**, *10*, 107. [CrossRef]

28. Fuady, A.; Nuraini, N.; Sukandar, K.; Lestari, B. Targeted Vaccine Allocation Could Increase the COVID-19 Vaccine Benefits Amidst Its Lack of Availability. *Vaccines* **2021**, *9*, 462. [CrossRef]
29. Iachini, T.; Coello, Y.; Frassinetti, F.; Ruggiero, G. Body Space in Social Interactions: A Comparison of Reaching and Comfort Distance in Immersive Virtual Reality. *PLoS ONE* **2014**, *9*, e111511. [CrossRef]
30. Iachini, T.; Coello, Y.; Frassinetti, F.; Senese, V.P.; Galante, F.; Ruggiero, G. Peripersonal and interpersonal space in virtual and real environments: Effects of gender and age. *J. Environ. Psychol.* **2016**, *45*, 154–164. [CrossRef]
31. Matsuda, Y.; Sugimoto, M.; Inami, M.; Kitazaki, M. Peripersonal space in the front, rear, left and right directions for audio-tactile multisensory integration. *Sci. Rep.* **2021**, *11*, 11303. [CrossRef]
32. Salathé, M.; Kazandjieva, M.; Lee, J.W.; Levis, P.; Feldman, M.W.; Jones, J.H. A high-resolution human contact network for infectious disease transmission. *Proc. Natl. Acad. Sci. USA* **2010**, *107*, 22020–22025. [CrossRef]
33. Sorokowska, A.; Sorokowski, P.; Hilpert, P.; Cantarero, K.; Frackowiak, T.; Ahmadi, K.; Alghraibeh, A.M.; Aryeetey, R.; Bertoni, A.; Bettache, K.; et al. Preferred Interpersonal Distances: A Global Comparison. *J. Cross-Cultural Psychol.* **2017**, *48*, 577–592. [CrossRef]
34. Tang, J.W.; Bahnfleth, W.P.; Bluyssen, P.M. Dismantling myths on the airborne transmission of severe acute respiratory syndrome coronavirus-2 (SARS-coV-2). *J. Hosp. Infect.* **2021**, *110*, 89–596. [CrossRef] [PubMed]
35. Escombe, A.R.; Oeser, C.; Gilman, R.H.; Ñavincopa, M.; Ticona, E.; Martínez, C.; Caviedes, L.; Sheen, P.; Gonzalez, A.; Noakes, C.; et al. The Detection of Airborne Transmission of Tuberculosis from HIV-Infected Patients, Using an In Vivo Air Sampling Model. *Clin. Infect. Dis.* **2007**, *44*, 1349–1357. [CrossRef] [PubMed]
36. IHME. COVID-19 Vaccine Efficacy Summary. Available online: https://www.healthdata.org/covid/COVID-19-vaccine-efficacy-summary (accessed on 2 April 2022).
37. DDS. Airborne and Direct Contact Diseases. Available online: https://www.maine.gov/dhhs/mecdc/infectious-disease/epi/airborne/index.shtml (accessed on 16 March 2022).
38. Hammond, A.; Khalid, T.; Thornton, H.V.; Woodall, C.A.; Hay, A.D. Should homes and workplaces purchase portable air filters to reduce the transmission of SARS-CoV-2 and other respiratory infections? A systematic review. *PLoS ONE* **2021**, *16*, e0251049. [CrossRef] [PubMed]
39. Pyankov, O.V.; Bodnev, S.A.; Pyankova, O.G.; Agranovski, I.E. Survival of aerosolized coronavirus in the ambient air. *J. Aerosol Sci.* **2017**, *115*, 158–163. [CrossRef] [PubMed]
40. Ratnesar-Shumate, S.; Williams, G.; Green, B.; Krause, M.; Holland, B.; Wood, S.; Bohannon, J.; Boydston, J.; Freeburger, D.; Hooper, I.; et al. Simulated Sunlight Rapidly Inactivates SARS-CoV-2 on Surfaces. *J. Infect. Dis.* **2020**, *222*, 214–222. [CrossRef] [PubMed]
41. Riley, E.C.; Murphy, G.; Riley, R.L. Airborne spread of measles in a suburban elementary school. *Am. J. Epidemiol.* **1978**, *107*, 421–432. [CrossRef]
42. Miller, S.L.; Nazaroff, W.W.; Jimenez, J.L.; Boerstra, A.; Buonanno, G.; Dancer, S.J.; Kurnitski, J.; Marr, L.C.; Morawska, L.; Noakes, C. Transmission of SARS-CoV-2 by inhalation of respiratory aerosol in the Skagit Valley Chorale superspreading event. *Indoor Air* **2020**, *31*, 314–323. [CrossRef]
43. Gou, W.; Jin, Z. How heterogeneous susceptibility and recovery rates affect the spread of epidemics on networks. *Infect. Dis. Model.* **2017**, *2*, 353–367. [CrossRef]
44. Lee, B.Y.; Bartsch, S.M.; Ferguson, M.C.; Wedlock, P.T.; O'Shea, K.J.; Siegmund, S.S.; Cox, S.N.; McKinnell, J.A. The value of decreasing the duration of the infectious period of severe acute respiratory syndrome coronavirus 2 (SARS-CoV-2) infection. *PLOS Comput. Biol.* **2021**, *17*, e1008470. [CrossRef]
45. Ramatillah, D.L.; Isnaini, S. Treatment profiles and clinical outcomes of COVID-19 patients at private hospital in Jakarta. *PLoS ONE* **2021**, *16*, e0250147. [CrossRef]
46. Kelland, K. One Meter or Two? How Social Distancing Affects COVID-19 Risk. Available online: https://www.reuters.com/article/us-health-coronavirus-distance-explainer-idUSKBN23U22W (accessed on 23 June 2020).
47. CBCNews. Some Countries Reconsider 2-Metre Rule for Physical Distancing, But Not Here. 2020. Available online: https://www.cbc.ca/news/health/2-metres-coronavirus-covid-distancing-1.5624439 (accessed on 23 December 2021).
48. Henchoz, C.; Coste, T.; Wernli, B. Culture, money attitudes and economic outcomes. *Swiss J. Econ. Stat.* **2019**, *155*, 2. [CrossRef]

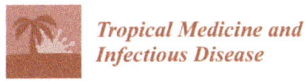

Article

A Risk Prediction Model and Risk Score of SARS-CoV-2 Infection Following Healthcare-Related Exposure

Kantarida Sripanidkulchai [1], Pinyo Rattanaumpawan [2], Winai Ratanasuwan [1], Nasikarn Angkasekwinai [2], Susan Assanasen [2], Peerawong Werarak [1], Oranich Navanukroh [1], Phatharajit Phatharodom [1] and Teerapong Tocharoenchok [3,*]

[1] Department of Preventive and Social Medicine, Faculty of Medicine Siriraj Hospital, Mahidol University, Bangkok 10700, Thailand
[2] Division of Infectious Diseases and Tropical Medicine, Department of Medicine, Faculty of Medicine Siriraj Hospital, Mahidol University, Bangkok 10700, Thailand
[3] Division of Cardiothoracic Surgery, Department of Surgery, Faculty of Medicine Siriraj Hospital, Mahidol University, Bangkok 10700, Thailand
* Correspondence: teerapong.toc@mahidol.ac.th; Tel.: +66-8-9688-0179

Abstract: Hospital workers are at high risk of contact with COVID-19 patients. Currently, there is no evidence-based, comprehensive risk assessment tool for healthcare-related exposure; so, we aimed to identify independent factors related to COVID-19 infection in hospital workers following workplace exposure(s) and construct a risk prediction model. We analyzed the COVID-19 contact tracing dataset from 15 July to 31 December 2021 using multiple logistic regression analysis, considering exposure details, demographics, and vaccination history. Of 7146 included exposures to confirmed COVID-19 patients, 229 (4.2%) had subsequently tested positive via RT-PCR. Independent risk factors for a positive test were having symptoms (adjusted odds ratio 4.94, 95%CI 3.83–6.39), participating in an unprotected aerosol-generating procedure (aOR 2.87, 1.66–4.96), duration of exposure >15 min (aOR 2.52, 1.82–3.49), personnel who did not wear a mask (aOR 2.49, 1.75–3.54), exposure to aerodigestive secretion (aOR 1.5, 1.03–2.17), index patient not wearing a mask (aOR 1.44, 1.01–2.07), and exposure distance <1 m without eye protection (aOR 1.39, 1.02–1.89). High-potency vaccines and high levels of education protected against infection. A risk model and scoring system with good discrimination power were built. Having symptoms, unprotected exposure, lower education level, and receiving low potency vaccines increased the risk of laboratory-confirmed COVID-19 following healthcare-related exposure events.

Keywords: COVID-19; SARS-CoV-2; occupational exposure; risk factors; personal protective equipment

1. Introduction

Healthcare workers are at high risk for exposure to COVID-19, both in the community and in the workplace when caring for patients [1]. Infection prevention and control practices are recommended for all hospital workers and include the use of personal protective equipment, physical distancing, source control measures, immunization, and post-exposure management [2]. The early assessment of risk and prompt management are important to protect the health and safety of personnel to prevent in-hospital transmission [3]. On the other hand, the isolation and quarantine associated with COVID-19 that are required of health workers place additional strain on healthcare services during periods of high demand. The individualized estimation of the infection risk of certain exposure of health workers is needed to guide optimal prevention and response strategies.

The exposure risk assessment and management system is currently mainly based on expert opinion, because only a few studies have addressed this problem, and there is the significant heterogeneity of operational definitions for variables that influence exposure risk, such as the measurement of contact duration, distance, the use of a face mask versus a respirator with eye protection, and differing vaccine regimens and efficacies [4–9]. Further, most COVID-19 healthcare exposure studies categorized exposure risk using multiple measures in combination (without complete details of individual exposure) and were conducted during periods when less contagious variants were circulating and different vaccine products and regimens were employed [9–11].

In the third quarter of 2021, Siriraj Hospital, a 2300-bed referral center in Bangkok with more than 16,000 employees, conducted more than 200 SARS-CoV-2 genetic tests per day for its personnel. Adapted from USCDC, WHO, European and Thailand public health interim guidelines, the hospital risk assessment and management system classified the risk of exposure and recommended appropriate testing times, work restrictions, and quarantine for those who were exposed to confirmed patients with COVID-19 [12–16]. Independent factors associated with COVID-19 infection could be identified using the large and detailed exposure dataset, demographic data, vaccination history, and complete entry and exit test status.

The objectives of this study are to identify independent factors associated with SARS-CoV-2 infection detected via RT-PCR in hospital workers following exposure(s) to confirmed positive patients and to build an evidence-based quantitative risk model and risk score for healthcare-related exposure.

2. Materials and Methods

2.1. Study Design, Setting, and Protocol

This study is a retrospective cohort analysis. From July 2021 to January 2022, during the increase in the number of cases of COVID-19 caused by the Delta variant, the hospital implemented a contact tracing and risk evaluation system based on exposure characteristics and immunization status to guide risk-specific SARS-CoV-2 tests, work restriction, and quarantine recommendations (Supplementary Tables S1–S3). Hospital workers who had been exposed to a confirmed case within the contagious period or had any symptoms related to SARS-CoV-2 (Appendix A) were evaluated as per hospital guidelines.

2.2. Data Collection and Preparation

Data collection was completed by exposed hospital workers or their representatives directly into a computer spreadsheet (infected person, worker identification, event details, symptoms, and immunization record). Completeness and accuracy were validated using mandatory field entry, data validation, and logic checks with feedback confirmation by responsible infection control officers. If personnel had multiple exposures to the same index person, the risk would be assigned to the highest risk event, and recommendations would be arranged according to the latest significant exposure. The classification of exposure risk (high, moderate, low or insignificant—based on the characteristics of exposure and the use of personal protective equipment (PPE) according to the consensus of the experts of the hospital detailed in Supplementary Table S1) and the recommendation were assigned by infectious disease specialists with the aid of software developed by the hospital. This exposure risk category was not introduced directly to the logistic regression model as all individual exposure criteria had already been included.

The variables of interest that were not included in the initial dataset (age, gender, education, and SARS-CoV-2 test results) and those subject to recall errors (immunization record) were provided by the hospital informatics and data innovation center. Missing and conflicting data were manually imputed based on available electronic hospital records.

2.3. Study Definition

2.3.1. Vaccine Formula and Potency Grouping

COVID-19 vaccination at least 14 days before exposure was considered to exert a full protective effect and was defined as the completion of the last dose. Due to the wide variety of vaccine combinations among Thai health workers [17], we classified all combination states into three distinct potency groups according to criteria adapted from Thai COVID-19 vaccination guidelines for a booster shot from the Ministry of Public Health in December 2021 (Supplementary Table S4) [18,19]. Low-potency combinations included any number of doses of an inactivated vaccine product, or a single dose of any other product (viral vector or mRNA). Moderate-potency combinations included two or more doses of an inactivated vaccine and at least one dose of either a viral vector product or an mRNA product. High-potency combinations included any dose of an inactivated product with at least one dose of viral vector product plus one dose of mRNA platform, or at least two doses of mRNA platform.

2.3.2. Laboratory Analysis and Case Definition

COVID-19 was diagnosed via SARS-CoV-2 genetic detection from respiratory samples using a real-time RT-PCR test, Allplex™ 2019-nCoV Assay (Seegene®, Seoul, Korea). The cycle threshold of <40 for the E and N gene and <42 for the RdRp gene was considered positive. To resolve the discrepancies between different genes tested, infectious disease specialists would define the status of the case based on their history and subsequent test(s).

2.4. Statistical Analysis

Continuous variables were reported as means with standard deviation and medians with interquartile range, while categorical data were reported using frequencies and percentages. The variables between groups were compared using the independent sample T test or Pearson's chi-square test (or nonparametric equivalents where appropriate), with statistical significance defined as a p value less than 0.05. Using multiple logistic regression, all variables with a p value less than 0.25 from univariate pre-screening entered the model provided they were present in at least 1% of the sample. Using the stepwise multivariate analysis, the variables that did not contribute to the model were eliminated either by exclusion or collapse to another category, whichever yielded maximal discrimination power from the ROC curve analysis. An additive risk score of predicted probability of COVID-19 infection was developed with coefficients from the final model (Appendix B). Model fit was accessed using the Hosmer and Lemeshow test. The logistic exposure risk calculator was built and is available at https://bit.ly/3uEi4W2 (accessed on 15 May 2022). All analyses were performed using SPSS™ software version 26.0 (IBM Corporation, Armonk, NY, USA) and Microsoft Excel™ software version 2203 (Microsoft Corporation, Redmond, WA, USA).

3. Results

The study flow diagram is illustrated in Figure 1. From 15 July to 31 December 2021, more than 19,000 hospital workers exposed to confirmed SARS-CoV-2 patients or who had symptoms related to COVID-19 were reported to infectious disease specialists. A total of 8557 entries were arranged for the RT-PCR test(s). After the exclusion of entries outside the scope of the study (uncertain contact history with various reasons for the RT-PCR test), duplicate entries and those without sufficient data for analysis, 7146 exposures were retained in the final dataset.

3.1. Baseline Characteristics

Of the 7146 exposures of 5449 hospital workers, 299 (4.2%) cases of COVID-19 infection were confirmed. The incidence of included events and COVID-19 detection gradually decreased during the study period (Supplementary Figure S1). The baseline characteristics of the included entries are listed in Table 1. The median age (range) of exposed hospital workers was 32 years (18–88), with women (73.8%) and healthcare personnel (Appendix A, 85.6%) being predominant. Among the hospital workers, the most common occupations were nurses and nurse/physician assistants (41.1%) followed by physicians/dentists and dentist assistants (12.6%), janitorial staff (12.3%), and administrative staff (12.3%). Less than 1% of the entries came from hospital workers with previous COVID-19 disease, and no hospital worker experienced repeated infection during the study period. In general, SARS-CoV-2 detections were more prevalent in exposures of workers with lower education (primary or secondary school; 7.7%), exposures without proper personal protective equipment or hygiene (i.e., high-risk exposure; 8.1%), exposures accompanied by fever or other symptoms related to COVID-19 (Appendix A, 14.3%), and exposures of hospital workers who had received vaccine combinations of lower potency (low potency; 14%).

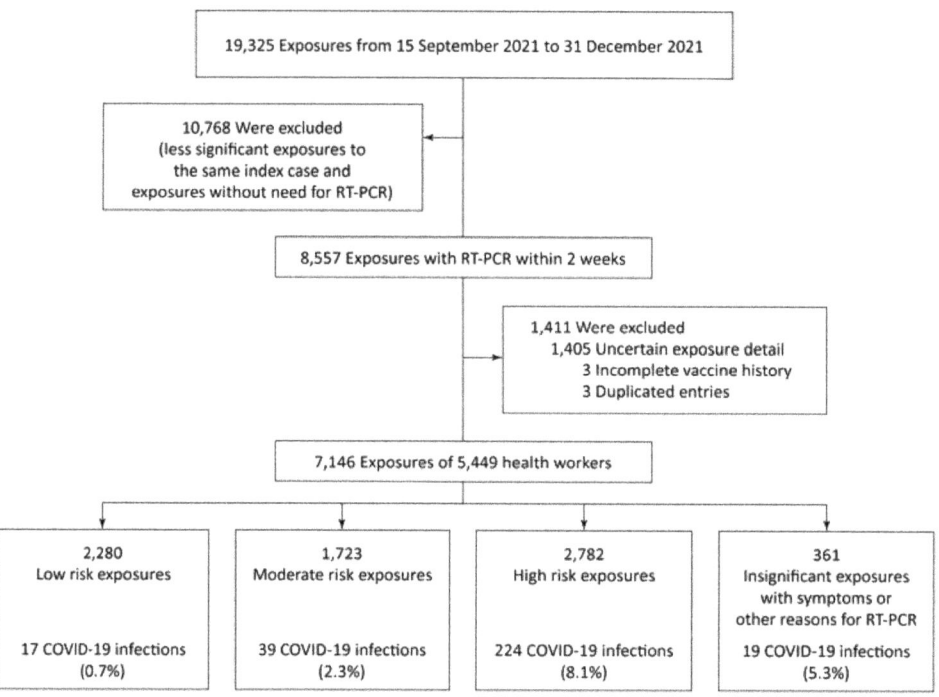

Figure 1. Consort type study flow diagram.

Table 1. Characteristics of occupational exposures to COVID-19 of hospital workers.

Characteristics	Subsequent COVID-19 Infection within 14 Days after Last Exposure			Total		p Value
	No	Yes				
	n = 6847	n = 299	Event Rate	n = 7146	% of Total	
Demographic						
Age at exposure, year						
Mean, standard deviation	34.95, 10.49	35.72, 10.64		34.98, 10.50		0.216
Median (interquartile range)	32 (27–42)	35 (26–44)		32 (27–42)		0.186
Gender						0.067
Male	1781	92	4.9%	1873	26.2%	
Female	5066	207	3.9%	5273	73.8%	
The highest education attainment						<0.001 §
Primary or secondary school	1599	133	7.7%	1732	24.2%	
Associate's degree	1296	69	5.1%	1365	19.1%	
Bachelor's degree	2846	80	2.7%	2926	40.9%	
Master's degree	762	12	1.6%	774	10.8%	
Doctoral degree	344	5	1.4%	349	4.9%	

Table 1. Cont.

Characteristics	Subsequent COVID-19 Infection within 14 Days after Last Exposure			Total		p Value
	No	Yes				
	n = 6847	n = 299	Event Rate	n = 7146	% of Total	
Role of hospital worker						0.620
Healthcare personnel	5864	253	4.1%	6117	86.6%	
Non-healthcare personnel	983	46	4.5%	1029	14.4%	
COVID-19 vaccination status						
Vaccines						<0.001
CoronaVac–CoronaVac	3684	190	4.9%	3874	54.2%	
CoronaVac–CoronaVac–ChAdOx-1	1203	47	3.8%	1250	17.5%	
CoronaVac–CoronaVac–BNT162b2	1070	18	1.7%	1088	15.2%	
ChAdOx-1	284	10	3.4%	294	4.1%	
ChAdOx-1–ChAdOx-1	219	9	3.9%	228	3.2%	
None	117	19	14.0%	136	1.9%	
ChAdOx-1–BNT162b2	116	1	0.9%	117	1.6%	
Others	154	5	3.1%	159	2.2%	
Potency of COVID-19 Vaccines *						<0.001 §
None	117	19	14.0%	136	1.9%	
Low-potency vaccines	4025	202	4.8%	4227	59.2%	
Moderate-potency vaccines	2537	77	2.9%	2614	37.6%	
High-potency vaccines	168	1	0.6%	169	2.4%	
The interval between the last dose of COVID-19 vaccines and exposure, day						
Mean, standard deviation	72.07, 33.36	73.78, 29.68		72.14, 33.22		0.351
Median (interquartile range)	72 (47–93)	75 (57–95)		72 (48–93)		0.302
Missing data	207	21		228	3.2%	
Previous COVID-19 infection						0.755 #
Absence	6564	290	4.2%	6854	99.1%	
Presence	62	3	4.6%	65	0.9%	
Exposure characteristics						
Infected person was wearing a mask/N95 respirator during exposure						<0.001
Yes	2897	61	2.1%	2958	41.4%	
No	3950	238	5.7%	4188	58.6%	
Distance of contact						<0.001
More than 1 m	1510	40	2.6%	1550	21.7%	
Less than 1 m	5337	259	4.6%	5596	78.3%	
Duration of exposure						<0.001
Less than 15 min	3380	53	1.5%	3433	48.0%	
More than 15 min	3467	246	6.6%	3713	52.0%	
Exposed hospital worker was wearing a mask/N95 respirator during exposure						<0.001
Yes	4535	91	2.0%	4626	64.7%	
No	2312	208	8.3%	2520	35.3%	
Exposed hospital worker was wearing a face shield during exposure						<0.001
Yes	1941	38	1.9%	1979	27.7%	
No	4906	261	5.1%	5167	72.3%	
Infected person was undergoing aerosol-generating procedures						0.186
No	6465	277	4.1%	6742	94.3%	
Yes; exposed hospital worker was wearing N95 respirator/PAPR and face shield	77	2	2.5%	79	1.1%	
Yes; exposed hospital worker was not wearing N95 respirator/PAPR and face shield	305	20	6.2%	325	4.5%	
Exposed hospital worker had direct contact with the aerodigestive secretion of the infected person						<0.001
No	6549	249	3.7%	6798	95.1%	
Yes	298	50	14%	348	4.9%	

Table 1. Cont.

Characteristics	Subsequent COVID-19 Infection within 14 Days after Last Exposure			Total		p Value
	No	Yes				
	n = 6847	n = 299	Event Rate	n = 7146	% of Total	
Exposure risk category by infectious disease physicians						<0.001
Low risk	2263	17	0.7%	2280	31.9%	
Moderate risk	1684	39	2.3%	1723	24.1%	
High risk	2558	224	8.1%	2782	38.9%	
Insignificant exposure with symptom(s) or reason(s) for RT-PCR	342	19	5.3%	361	5.1%	
Symptom of exposed hospital worker						
Fever or other COVID-19-related symptoms						<0.001
Absence	5073	103	2.0%	5176	79.1%	
Presence	1174	196	14.3%	1370	20.9%	

RT-PCR; reverse transcriptase–polymerase chain reaction, § linear-by-linear association, # Fisher's Exact test, other p value from independent samples T-test, Pearson Chi-Square test, or independent-samples Mann–Whitney U test, * adapted from Thai COVID-19 Vaccination Guidelines for a Booster Shot, Ministry of Public Health, December 2021.

All events were classified into four exposure risk categories: low (31.9%), moderate (24.1%), high (38.9%), and insignificant risk (but being tested due to COVID-19-related symptoms) (5.1%). This risk classification was highly correlated with the SARS-CoV-2 detection rate (0.7%, 2.3%, 8.1%, and 5.3%; $p < 0.001$). Most exposures (98.1%) came from personnel who had received at least one dose of the vaccine. The median interval from the last vaccination to the day of exposure was 72 days (range 14 to 236). More than half of the hospital workers (54.2%) received two doses of CoronaVac (SINOVAC Biotech, Beijing, China), 17.5% received an additional ChAdOx-1 (AstraZeneca, Oxford, UK; Cambridge, UK), 15.2% received an additional BNT162b2 (Pfizer-BioNTech, New York, USA; Mainz, Germany) vaccination as a booster, and 11.2% had other vaccine combinations. The remaining 136 exposures came from hospital workers who were not vaccinated at the time of exposure (1.9%).

Among the events with subsequent COVID-19 infection, the median time to detection after the last exposure was four days (interquartile range 1 to 7), with 90% of all detections occurring within 11 days from the last exposure (Supplementary Figure S2). No mortality was observed during the study period.

3.2. Factors Associated with SARS-CoV-2 Infection

After prescreening with univariate logistic regression, twelve factors entered the preliminary main effect model (Table 2), and nine remained in the final logistic model. There were two baseline characteristics and seven exposure-related factors that contributed to the risk of SARS-CoV-2 infection. All independent factors and weights associated with them are shown in Table 3. To calculate the predicted probability for SARS-CoV-2 genetic detection using an additive risk score, the points for factors present in a particular exposure are added to give an approximate percentage, as outlined in Table 4.

Table 2. Logistic regression analysis of variables associated with occupational SARS-CoV-2 infection among hospital workers.

Variable	Univariable Analysis			Multivariable Analysis		
	Crude OR	(95% CI)	p Value	Adjusted OR	(95% CI)	p Value
Demographic						
Age (year)	1.01	(1–1.02)	0.216	1.01	(1–1.02)	0.053
Male gender	1.26	(0.98–1.63)	0.068	1.11	(0.83–1.48)	0.480
The highest education attainment			<0.001			<0.001
Primary or secondary school (reference)						
Associate's	0.64	(0.47–0.86)	0.004	0.76	(0.54–1.06)	0.106
Bachelor's	0.34	(0.25–0.45)	<0.001	0.44	(0.32–0.61)	<0.001
Master's	0.19	(0.1–0.34)	<0.001	0.31	(0.17–0.58)	<0.001
Doctoral	0.18	(0.07–0.43)	<0.001	0.36	(0.14–0.92)	0.033
Role of worker: Healthcare personnel	0.92	(0.67–1.27)	0.620			
Exposure characteristics						
Infected person was not wearing a mask/N95 respirator during exposure	2.86	(2.15–3.81)	<0.001	1.45	(1–2.1)	0.048
Distance of exposure less than 1 m	1.83	(1.31–2.57)	<0.001	1.4	(0.97–2)	0.069
Duration of exposure more than 15 min	4.53	(3.35–6.11)	<0.001	2.51	(1.81–3.48)	<0.001
Exposed hospital worker not wearing a mask/N95 respirator during exposure	4.48	(3.49–5.77)	<0.001	2.54	(1.72–3.76)	<0.001
Exposed hospital worker not wearing face shield or goggles during exposure	2.72	(1.93–3.83)	<0.001	1.25	(0.78–1.98)	0.353
Infected person was undergoing aerosol-generating procedures			0.156			0.001
No (reference)						
Yes; exposed HCP was wearing N95 respirator/PAPR and face shield	0.61	(0.15–2.48)	0.486	1.28	(0.29–5.66)	0.748
Yes; exposed HCP was <u>not</u> wearing N95 respirator/PAPR and face shield	1.53	(0.96–2.44)	0.075	2.86	(1.64–5)	<0.001
Exposed hospital worker had direct contact with aerodigestive secretion of the infected person	4.41	(3.19–6.11)	<0.001	1.48	(1.02–2.15)	0.038
Symptoms of exposed hospital worker						
Fever or other COVID-19-related symptoms	5.44	(4.26–6.95)	<0.001	4.9	(3.78–6.34)	<0.001
COVID-19 vaccination status						
Potency of COVID-19 vaccines *			<0.001			<0.001
None (reference)						
Low-potency vaccines	0.31	(0.19–0.51)	<0.001	0.31	(0.18–0.54)	<0.001
Moderate-potency vaccines	0.19	(0.11–0.32)	<0.001	0.16	(0.09–0.3)	<0.001
High-potency vaccines	0.04	(0.01–0.28)	0.001	0.05	(0.01–0.41)	0.005
The interval between the last dose of COVID-19 vaccines and exposure (day)		(1–1.01)	0.402			
Previous COVID-19 infection: Yes	1.1	(0.34–3.51)	0.878			

* Adapted from Thai COVID-19 Vaccination Guidelines for a Booster Shot, Ministry of Public Health, December 2021.

Table 3. Independent risk factors associated with subsequent SARS-CoV-2 infection after occupational exposure among hospital workers, coefficients from the final logistic model, and weight (point) for the risk score.

Risk Factor	β	Odds Ratio (95% CI)	p Value	Point
The highest education attainment			<0.001	
Primary or secondary school (reference)				3
Undergraduate (associate's or bachelor's)	−0.64	0.53 (0.4–0.68)	<0.001	1
Postgraduate (master's or doctoral)	−1.13	0.32 (0.19–0.55)	<0.001	0
Infected person was not wearing a mask/N95 respirator during exposure	0.37	1.44 (1.01–2.07)	0.046	1
Distance of exposure less than 1 m without a face shield	0.33	1.39 (1.02–1.89)	0.038	1
Duration of exposure more than 15 min	0.93	2.52 (1.82–3.49)	<0.001	3
Exposed hospital worker was not wearing a mask/N95 respirator during exposure	0.91	2.49 (1.75–3.54)	<0.001	3
Exposed hospital worker was not wearing an N95 respirator and face shield/goggles while the infected person was undergoing aerosol-generating procedure	1.05	2.87 (1.66–4.96)	<0.001	3
Exposed hospital worker had direct contact with the aerodigestive secretion of the infected person	0.40	1.5 (1.03–2.17)	0.033	1
Fever or other COVID-19-related symptoms	1.60	4.94 (3.83–6.39)	<0.001	5
Potency of COVID-19 vaccines *			<0.001	
None (reference)				9
Low-potency vaccines	−1.19	0.3 (0.17–0.53)	<0.001	5
Moderate-potency vaccines	−1.79	0.17 (0.09–0.3)	<0.001	4
High-potency vaccines	−2.98	0.05 (0.01–0.4)	0.004	0
Constant	−3.69		<0.001	

* Adapted from Thai COVID-19 Vaccination Guidelines for a Booster Shot, Ministry of Public Health, December 2021.

Table 4. The predictive score for SARS-CoV-2 infection after occupational exposure among hospital workers.

Total Point	Predicted Probability of COVID-19 Infection (%)
0–9	0.05–0.93
10–14	1.28–4.60
15–16	6.28–8.51
17–19	11.44–19.94
20–23	25.70–48.09
24–29	56.27–86.92

Having a fever or other COVID-19-related symptoms was the strongest risk factor for SARS-CoV-2 genetic detection (adjusted OR 4.94, 95% CI 3.83–6.39). Other strong risk factors included performing an aerosol-generating procedure without full protection (aOR 2.87, 1.66–4.96), prolonged duration of contact (aOR 2.52, 1.82–3.49), and personnel not wearing a mask (aOR 2.49, 1.75–3.54). Direct contact with aerodigestive secretion, the infected person not wearing a mask, and close contact without proper eye protection carried smaller risks. Vaccination was protective against infection: aOR 0.05 (high-potency combinations), aOR 0.17 (moderate-potency combinations), and 0.3 (low-potency combination). Hospital workers with higher levels of education level were less likely to be infected.

The model fit was confirmed using the Hosmer and Lemeshow test (Chi-square 8.960, p 0.346). The discrimination power of the final logistic model and the risk scoring system accessed via ROC curves are depicted in Figure 2, which confirms the model's performance. The exposure risk categories also demonstrated good predictive power in the parallel analysis (adjusted OR 2.58 for moderate-risk and 8.53 for high-risk contact; Supplementary Table S5), but with a smaller area under the ROC curve at 0.827 (95% CI 0.804–0.849).

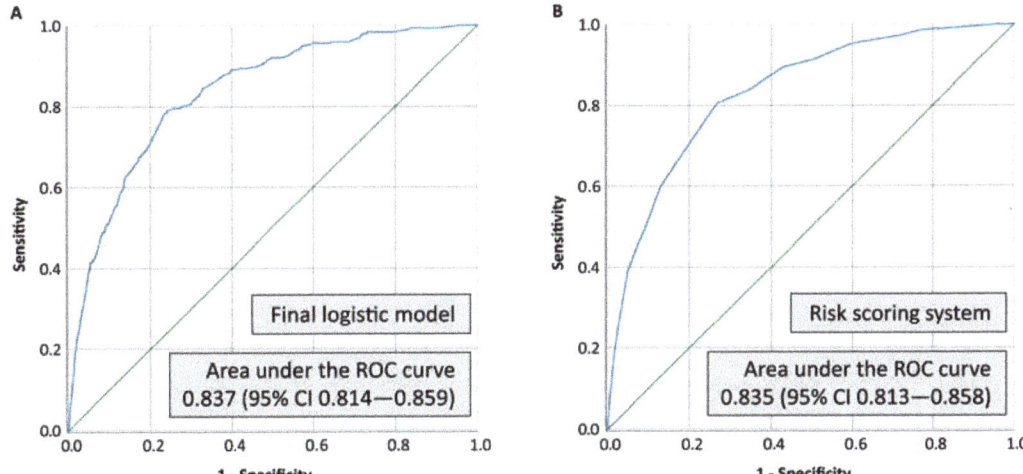

Figure 2. Areas under the ROC curve for the final logistic model (**A**) and the risk scoring system (**B**).

4. Discussion

Using information acquired from contact tracing during the Delta peak at 86–99% in the community [20–22], we developed a risk prediction model to estimate the risk of infection for hospital workers with different vaccination regimens following exposure to confirmed COVID-19 cases. Exposure type, the presence of symptoms, the appropriate use of PPE, education level, vaccination regimen, and time since the last dose each contributed important information regarding the risk of infection.

Having a fever or other COVID-19-related symptoms within two weeks was strongly predictive of a positive test. Similar to the previous report by Pienthong et al. [8], failure to comply with protective measures increased the risk of infection. For example, commencing an aerosol-generating procedure (Appendix A) without proper protective equipment (including an N95 respirator and eye protection) was the highest procedural risk in this study, followed closely by a prolonged duration of exposure and the worker not wearing a mask. Other violations of standard precautions and the improper use of PPE recommended by the WHO [23] also increased the risk of infection. One interesting finding to be noted is that an exposure distance of <1 m and not using an eye protection device failed to reach statistical significance in the preliminary effect model but showed significance when considering both factors together (i.e., a face shield is only beneficial when in close contact). This supports the adequacy of the universal droplet precautions despite recent evidence in favor of airborne precautions [24,25] given that no aerosol-generating procedure is being performed.

The most common vaccine regimen in this study, two doses of inactivated vaccines (low potency), provided the least protection against infection, while the second most common regimen, heterologous boosted inactivated vaccines (moderate potency), provided slightly better protection but much less when compared with the viral vector-mRNA combination (high potency). This is consistent with the previous report from Sritipsukho et al. [17] which underlined the importance of vaccine type over the number of doses. Our findings also validated our COVID-19 exposure risk category approach which was used to determine the need for RT-PCR testing and isolation during a period of manpower and resource limitation.

Although symptoms related to COVID-19 should be considered as a consequence of infection rather than a risk factor for infection, our data support that all symptomatic health workers with an exposure history during the epidemic should be tested, regardless of contact risk and immunologic status, provided that this policy does not overwhelm laboratory testing capacity. A significant portion of infected hospital workers tested positive before the initial recommended test date(s), which implied the benefit of the early test (and early detection) triggered by symptoms. This contrasts with other studies on symptomatic patients presenting at health services which demonstrated poor diagnostic accuracy of signs and symptoms [26,27]. An explanation might be that, in addition to being symptomatic, all of our included subjects must have certain exposure to an infected person.

Consistent with a 2020 study by Chadeau-Hyam et al., the level of education of the hospital workers was inversely correlated with the risk of testing positive [28]. This could be explained by better health literacy, self-awareness, and hygiene discipline. Educational achievement is also correlated with occupations that pose different risks of COVID-19 infection [29]. Improved educational interventions are additionally needed to increase awareness among workers with lower levels of education.

Most of the COVID-19 risk calculators available provide a very crude risk estimate based primarily on location, the nature of the activity, and the safety measures being taken [30]. Our risk calculator and score, on the contrary, provide an individualized risk assessment based on detailed exposure characteristics adjusted for vaccination status and socioeconomic background through educational attainment. To a certain extent, this tool has the utility to triage exposed individuals to prevent further infections in healthcare settings.

This study has several limitations. We did not include the severity of cases that got infected (i.e., CT value or hospitalization). Due to the retrospective nature of the observational study, some demographic information may have been missed. Furthermore, most of the data were entered by various staff with different levels of health knowledge. Therefore, misclassification may be an issue. The external validation of the risk model was also difficult to perform due to the rapid shift in the variants of concern and vaccine-induced immunity over time.

5. Conclusions

Having symptoms of COVID-19, inadequate personal protection, low education level, and not receiving a vaccine or receiving a low-potency vaccine regimen were found to be the main risks for COVID-19 infection among all healthcare-related exposures. Our quantitative exposure risk model and risk score have good predictive value and could help combat further spread among hospital workers according to their actual probability of infection.

Supplementary Materials: The following supporting information can be downloaded at: https://www.mdpi.com/article/10.3390/tropicalmed7090248/s1, Figure S1: Daily number and cumulative percentage of occupational exposures among healthcare personnel in the study, 15 September to 31 December 2021; Figure S2: Distribution of SARS-CoV-2 PCR assay detection day after last known exposure; Table S1: Exposure-characteristics-based risk classification; Table S2: Management of contact hospital workers in terms of guided testing and quarantine duration based on contact risk and vaccination history; Table S3: Definition of immunization during the study period; Table S4: Vaccine regimen potency grouping, adapted from Thai COVID-19 vaccination guidelines for a booster shot from the Ministry of Public Health as of December 2021; Table S5: Parallel analysis of variables associated with SARS-CoV-2 infection using exposure risk category, the final logistic model.

Author Contributions: Conceptualization, P.R. and T.T.; methodology, P.R. and T.T.; software, T.T.; formal analysis, P.R. and T.T.; investigation, K.S. and T.T.; data curation, K.S., P.R., W.R., N.A., P.W., S.A., P.P. and O.N.; writing—original draft preparation, K.S.; writing—review and editing, T.T., P.R., N.A. and S.A.; visualization, T.T.; supervision, P.R. project administration, K.S. and T.T. All authors have read and agreed to the published version of the manuscript.

Funding: This research received no external funding.

Institutional Review Board Statement: This study was approved by the Siriraj Institutional Review Board on 5 November 2021, which was in full compliance with international guidelines for human research protection such as the Declaration of Helsinki (Study Code 838/2564(IRB4)).

Informed Consent Statement: The patient consent was waived as it contained minimal risk to the subject.

Data Availability Statement: The datasets generated during and/or analyzed during the current study are available from the corresponding author upon reasonable request.

Acknowledgments: We thank the members of Infection Control Nurses, infectious disease specialists, Siriraj Informatics and Data Innovation Center, staff from the Department of Microbiology, Department of Immunology, and chiefs or representatives of each Division from the Faculty of Medicine Siriraj Hospital, Mahidol university who made the data reliable and available. We express our gratitude to Mark Simmerman for his insightful comments on manuscript and language editing. We also acknowledge the contributions of Chulaluk Komoltri from the clinical epidemiology unit for advice in the statistical analysis of this study.

Conflicts of Interest: The authors declare no conflict of interest.

Appendix A. Definition

- Healthcare workers or healthcare personnel include but are not limited to emergency medical service personnel, nurses, nursing assistants, physicians, technicians, therapists, phlebotomists, pharmacists, students and trainees, contractual staff not employed by the healthcare facility, and persons not directly involved in patient care, but who could be exposed to infectious agents that can be transmitted in the healthcare setting (e.g., clerical, dietary, environmental services, laundry, security, engineering and facilities management, administrative, billing, and volunteer personnel).
- Aerosol-generating procedure: a procedure that could generate more infectious aerosols than coughing, sneezing, talking, or breathing:
    - Open suctioning of airways;
    - Sputum induction;
    - Cardiopulmonary resuscitation;
    - Endotracheal intubation and extubation;
    - Non-invasive ventilation (e.g., BiPAP or CPAP);
    - Bronchoscopy;
    - Manual ventilation;
    - Nebulizer administration and high-flow oxygen delivery.
- Symptoms related to SARS-CoV-2 infection:
    - Fever or chill;
    - Fatigue;
    - Muscle ache;
    - Headache;
    - Cough;
    - Runny nose;
    - Sore throat;
    - Loss in the sense of smell or taste;
    - Shortness of breath;
    - Nausea;
    - Vomiting;
    - Diarrhea.

Appendix B. Mathematical Component of Risk Score

- For each independent risk factor:

$$\text{Weight (point)} := \lfloor \frac{\beta_i}{\beta_{min}} + \frac{1}{2} \rfloor, \text{ where } \beta_{min} = 0.328344912 \qquad (A1)$$

- For protective factor: education:

$$\text{Weight (point)} := \lfloor \frac{\beta_i}{\beta_{min}} + \frac{1}{2} \rfloor + 3, \text{ where } \beta_{min} = 0.328344912 \qquad (A2)$$

○ For protective factor: vaccination:

$$\text{Weight (point)} := \lfloor \frac{\beta_i}{\beta_{min}} + \frac{1}{2} \rfloor + 9, \text{ where } \beta_{min} = 0.328344912 \quad \text{(A3)}$$

References

1. Wang, D.; Hu, B.; Hu, C.; Zhu, F.; Liu, X.; Zhang, J.; Wang, B.; Xiang, H.; Cheng, Z.; Xiong, Y.; et al. Clinical Characteristics of 138 Hospitalized Patients With 2019 Novel Coronavirus-Infected Pneumonia in Wuhan, China. *JAMA* **2020**, *323*, 1061–1069. [CrossRef]
2. Branch-Elliman, W.; Savor Price, C.; McGeer, A.; Perl, T.M. Protecting the frontline: Designing an infection prevention platform for preventing emerging respiratory viral illnesses in healthcare personnel. *Infect. Control Hosp. Epidemiol.* **2015**, *36*, 336–345. [CrossRef] [PubMed]
3. COVID-19: Occupational Health and Safety for Health Workers: Interim Guidance. Available online: https://www.who.int/publications/i/item/WHO-2019-nCoV-HCW_advice-2021-1 (accessed on 29 May 2022).
4. Ashinyo, M.E.; Dubik, S.D.; Duti, V.; Amegah, K.E.; Ashinyo, A.; Larsen-Reindorf, R.; Kaba Akoriyea, S.; Kuma-Aboagye, P. Healthcare Workers Exposure Risk Assessment: A Survey among Frontline Workers in Designated COVID-19 Treatment Centers in Ghana. *J. Prim. Care Community Health* **2020**, *11*, 2150132720969483. [CrossRef] [PubMed]
5. Maltezou, H.C.; Dedoukou, X.; Tseroni, M.; Tsonou, P.; Raftopoulos, V.; Papadima, K.; Mouratidou, E.; Poufta, S.; Panagiotakopoulos, G.; Hatzigeorgiou, D.; et al. SARS-CoV-2 Infection in Healthcare Personnel with High-risk Occupational Exposure: Evaluation of 7-Day Exclusion From Work Policy. *Clin. Infect. Dis.* **2020**, *71*, 3182–3187. [CrossRef] [PubMed]
6. Wang, Y.; Wang, L.; Zhao, X.; Zhang, J.; Ma, W.; Zhao, H.; Han, X. A Semi-Quantitative Risk Assessment and Management Strategies on COVID-19 Infection to Outpatient Health Care Workers in the Post-Pandemic Period. *Risk Manag. Healthc. Policy* **2021**, *14*, 815–825. [CrossRef] [PubMed]
7. Cook, T.M. Personal protective equipment during the coronavirus disease (COVID) 2019 pandemic—A narrative review. *Anaesthesia* **2020**, *75*, 920–927. [CrossRef] [PubMed]
8. Pienthong, T.; Khawcharoenporn, T.; Apisarnthanarak, P.; Weber, D.J.; Apisarnthanarak, A. Factors Associated with COVID-19 Infection Among Thai Health Care Personnel with High Risk Exposures: The Important Roles of Double Masking and Physical Distancing while Eating. *Infect. Control Hosp. Epidemiol.* **2022**, 1–9. [CrossRef]
9. Gragnani, C.M.; Fernandes, P.; Waxman, D.A. Validation of Centers for Disease Control and Prevention level 3 risk classification for healthcare workers exposed to severe acute respiratory coronavirus virus 2 (SARS-CoV-2). *Infect. Control Hosp. Epidemiol.* **2021**, *42*, 483–485. [CrossRef] [PubMed]
10. Vargese, S.S.; Dev, S.S.; Soman, A.S.; Kurian, N.; Varghese, V.A.; Mathew, E. Exposure risk and COVID-19 infection among frontline health-care workers: A single tertiary care centre experience. *Clin. Epidemiol. Glob. Health* **2022**, *13*, 100933. [CrossRef] [PubMed]
11. Wan, K.S.; Tok, P.S.K.; Yoga Ratnam, K.K.; Aziz, N.; Isahak, M.; Ahmad Zaki, R.; Nik Farid, N.D.; Hairi, N.N.; Rampal, S.; Ng, C.W.; et al. Implementation of a COVID-19 surveillance programme for healthcare workers in a teaching hospital in an upper-middle-income country. *PLoS ONE* **2021**, *16*, e0249394. [CrossRef] [PubMed]
12. Interim Guidance for Managing Healthcare Personnel with SARS-CoV-2 Infection or Exposure to SARS-CoV-2. Available online: https://www.cdc.gov/coronavirus/2019-ncov/hcp/guidance-risk-assesment-hcp.html (accessed on 13 May 2022).
13. Interim Infection Prevention and Control Recommendations for Healthcare Personnel during the Coronavirus Disease 2019 (COVID-19) Pandemic. Available online: https://www.cdc.gov/coronavirus/2019-ncov/hcp/infection-control-recommendations.html (accessed on 13 May 2022).
14. Contact Tracing in the European Union: Public Health Management of Persons, Including Healthcare Workers, Who Have Had Contact with COVID-19 Cases—Fourth Update. Available online: https://www.ecdc.europa.eu/en/covid-19-contact-tracing-public-health-management (accessed on 13 May 2022).
15. Risk Assessment and Management of Exposure of Health Care Workers in the Context of COVID-19: Interim Guidance. Available online: https://www.who.int/publications/i/item/risk-assessment-and-management-of-exposure-of-health-care-workers-in-the-context-of-covid-19-interim-guidance (accessed on 15 May 2022).
16. Guidelines for Surveillance and Investigation of Coronavirus Disease 2019 (COVID-19). Available online: https://ddc.moph.go.th/viralpneumonia/eng/file/guidelines/g_GSI_22Dec21.pdf (accessed on 15 May 2022).
17. Sritipsukho, P.; Khawcharoenporn, T.; Siribumrungwong, B.; Damronglerd, P.; Suwantarat, N.; Satdhabudha, A.; Chaiyakulsil, C.; Sinlapamongkolkul, P.; Tangsathapornpong, A.; Bunjoungmanee, P.; et al. Comparing real-life effectiveness of various COVID-19 vaccine regimens during the delta variant-dominant pandemic: A test-negative case-control study. *Emerg. Microbes Infect.* **2022**, *11*, 585–592. [CrossRef] [PubMed]
18. Ministry of Public Health's Guidelines for Vaccination against COVID-19. Available online: https://ddc.moph.go.th/vaccine-covid19/getFiles/14/1639630757714.pdf (accessed on 21 May 2022).
19. Ministry of Public Health's Guidelines for COVID-19 Vaccination as a Booster Shot. Available online: https://ddc.moph.go.th/vaccine-covid19/getFiles/14/1640232499139.pdf (accessed on 21 May 2022).

20. Report on the Results of Surveillance for COVID-19 Strains during 24–30 July 2021. Available online: https://www3.dmsc.moph.go.th/post-view/1234 (accessed on 20 May 2022).
21. Report on the Results of Surveillance for COVID-19 Strains during 2–8 October 2021. Available online: https://www3.dmsc.moph.go.th/post-view/1328 (accessed on 20 May 2022).
22. Report on the Results of Surveillance for COVID-19 Strains during 1 November–11 February 2022. Available online: https://www3.dmsc.moph.go.th/post-view/1481 (accessed on 20 May 2022).
23. Infection Prevention and Control during Health Care When Coronavirus Disease (COVID-19) Is Suspected or Confirmed: Interim Guidance. Available online: https://apps.who.int/iris/handle/10665/332879 (accessed on 20 May 2022).
24. Bahl, P.; Doolan, C.; de Silva, C.; Chughtai, A.A.; Bourouiba, L.; MacIntyre, C.R. Airborne or Droplet Precautions for Health Workers Treating Coronavirus Disease 2019? *J. Infect. Dis.* **2022**, *225*, 1561–1568. [CrossRef] [PubMed]
25. Lewis, D. Why the WHO took two years to say COVID is airborne. *Nature* **2022**, *604*, 26–31. [CrossRef] [PubMed]
26. French, N.; Jones, G.; Heuer, C.; Hope, V.; Jefferies, S.; Muellner, P.; McNeill, A.; Haslett, S.; Priest, P. Creating symptom-based criteria for diagnostic testing: A case study based on a multivariate analysis of data collected during the first wave of the COVID-19 pandemic in New Zealand. *BMC Infect. Dis.* **2021**, *21*, 1119. [CrossRef] [PubMed]
27. Struyf, T.; Deeks, J.J.; Dinnes, J.; Takwoingi, Y.; Davenport, C.; Leeflang, M.M.; Spijker, R.; Hooft, L.; Emperador, D.; Domen, J.; et al. Signs and symptoms to determine if a patient presenting in primary care or hospital outpatient settings has COVID-19. *Cochrane Database Syst. Rev.* **2021**, *2*, CD013665. [CrossRef] [PubMed]
28. Chadeau-Hyam, M.; Bodinier, B.; Elliott, J.; Whitaker, M.D.; Tzoulaki, I.; Vermeulen, R.; Kelly-Irving, M.; Delpierre, C.; Elliott, P. Risk factors for positive and negative COVID-19 tests: A cautious and in-depth analysis of UK biobank data. *Int. J. Epidemiol.* **2020**, *49*, 1454–1467. [CrossRef] [PubMed]
29. Lu, M. The Front Line: Visualizing the Occupations with the Highest COVID-19 Risk. Available online: https://www.visualcapitalist.com/the-front-line-visualizing-the-occupations-with-the-highest-covid-19-risk/ (accessed on 20 May 2022).
30. Eisenstein, M. What's your risk of catching COVID? *Nature* **2020**, *589*, 158–159. [CrossRef]

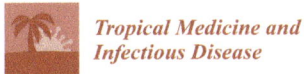

Article

Mortality in Four Waves of COVID-19 Is Differently Associated with Healthcare Capacities Affected by Economic Disparities

Lan Yao [1], J. Carolyn Graff [2], Lotfi Aleya [3], Jiamin Ma [1,4], Yanhong Cao [5], Wei Wei [5], Shuqiu Sun [5], Congyi Wang [6], Yan Jiao [1], Weikuan Gu [1,7,*], Gang Wang [4] and Dianjun Sun [5,*]

1. Department of Orthopedic Surgery and BME-Campbell Clinic, University of Tennessee Health Science Center, Memphis, TN 38163, USA
2. College of Nursing, University of Tennessee Health Science Center, Memphis, TN 38105, USA
3. Chrono-Environnement Laboratory, UMR CNRS 6249, Bourgogne Franche-Comté Université, CEDEX 21010, F-25030 Besançon, France
4. The First Affiliated Hospital of Harbin Medical University, 23 Youzheng Street, Nangang District, Harbin 150001, China
5. Center for Endemic Disease Control, Chinese Center for Disease Control and Prevention, Harbin Medical University, 157 Baojian Road, Harbin 150081, China
6. The Center for Biomedical Research, Department of Respiratory and Critical Care Medicine, NHC Key Laboratory of Respiratory Diseases, Tongji Hospital, Tongji Medical College, Huazhong University of Science and Technology, Wuhan 430030, China
7. Research Service, Memphis VA Medical Center, 1030 Jefferson Avenue, Memphis, TN 38104, USA
* Correspondence: wgu@uthsc.edu (W.G.); hrbmusdj@163.com (D.S.); Tel.: +1-901-448-2259 (W.G.); +86-451-86612695 (D.S.)

Abstract: Background: The greatest challenges are imposed on the overall capacity of disease management when the cases reach the maximum in each wave of the pandemic. Methods: The cases and deaths for the four waves of COVID-19 in 119 countries and regions (CRs) were collected. We compared the mortality across CRs where populations experience different economic and healthcare disparities. Findings: Among 119 CRs, 117, 112, 111, and 55 have experienced 1, 2, 3, and 4 waves of COVID-19 disease, respectively. The average mortality rates at the disease turning point were 0.036, 0.019. 0.017, and 0.015 for the waves 1, 2, 3, and 4, respectively. Among 49 potential factors, income level, gross national income (GNI) per capita, and school enrollment are positively correlated with the mortality rates in the first wave, but negatively correlated with the rates of the rest of the waves. Their values for the first wave are 0.253, 0.346 and 0.385, respectively. The r value for waves 2, 3, and 4 are −0.310, −0.293, −0.234; −0.263, −0.284, −0.282; and −0.330, −0.394, −0.048, respectively. In high-income CRs, the mortality rates in waves 2 and 3 were 29% and 28% of that in wave 1; while in upper-middle-income CRs, the rates for waves 2 and 3 were 76% and 79% of that in wave 1. The rates in waves 2 and 3 for lower-middle-income countries were 88% and 89% of that in wave 1, and for low-income countries were 135% and 135%. Furthermore, comparison among the largest case numbers through all waves indicated that the mortalities in upper- and lower-middle-income countries is 65% more than that of the high-income countries. Interpretation: Conclusions from the first wave of the COVID-19 pandemic do not apply to the following waves. The clinical outcomes in developing countries become worse along with the expansion of the pandemic.

Keywords: COVID-19; economy; income levels; mortality; waves; policy; turning points

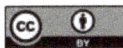

1. Introduction

A considerable amount of research has been conducted to better understand factors influencing mortality caused by the pandemic of COVID-19 [1–7]. Most data are based on the first wave, while some are based on the combination of the first and second waves of the pandemic [1–7]. None of these studies revealed the impact of income levels, with other factors, such as transportation and population density, regarded as the major predictive factors in the pandemic [6–8]. A report based on the second wave of the COVID-19 pandemic indicated that COVID-19 was more severe on the African continent than the first wave [1]. The question remains as to whether economic levels affect the mitigation of COVID-19 in stages such as in waves 2, 3, and 4.

Based on reports from Worldometers (https://www.worldometers.info/coronavirus/ (accessed on 14 January 2022)) [9] and the World Health Organization (WHO) Coronavirus (COVID-19) Dashboard (https://covid19.who.int/ (accessed on 14 January 2022)) [2], accessed in early 2022, more than 100 countries and regions (CRs) have experienced more than three waves of the disease. These data provide a chance to compare the influential factors in fighting COVID-19 in up to four waves of the disease among CRs at different economic levels.

In order to measure the overall capacity of CRs in fighting COVID-19, this study focuses on the time points of the mortality rate derived from two intrinsic turning points, the maximum of case and death numbers, during each wave of the pandemic. For each CR, we measure its capacity in the management of the disease by the mortality rate at the turning point of the disease.

Income level in a country or region reflects the level of resources and medical facilities that determine the overall capacity of fighting a pandemic. Because the COVID-19 disease became pandemic, the income level in a country or regional level was essential for fighting the disease. In particular, when the disease reaches a maximum level, it challenges the biomedical capability of a country or region. The mortality rate at the time of the disease peak days indicates whether the medical resource is good enough to deal with the hospitalized patients. This study examines the relationship between income level and mortality at the peak of the disease, and determines how different countries at different income levels fight COVID-19 pandemics.

2. Methods

2.1. Data Sources

We conducted correlation analyses between mortality rates at peak points in different waves and a total of 49 potential influential factors: comparisons of mortality rates at peak points among different levels of incomes, the mortality rates at the maximum case numbers among all waves in different income levels, and time- and case-adjusted mortality rates among different income levels. The average numbers of cases and deaths of seven days in the peak days of different waves of COVID-19 were collected from Worldometers, and confirmed with the WHO Coronavirus (COVID-19) Dashboard. Population statistics were collected from Worldometers (https://www.worldometers.info/world-population/population-by-country/ (accessed on 14 January 2022)). Data collection started on 21 January 2022 and ended on 2 February 2022.

2.2. Influential Factors

The information of potential factors from each CR was collected from the World Bank. A total of 49 potential influential factors were collected. These factors include→Forest area (% of land area), →Rural population (% of total population)→Surface area (sq. km), →Mortality rate, under-5 (per 1000 live births), →Incidence of tuberculosis (per 100,000 people), →Access to electricity (% of population), →CO_2 emissions (metric tons per capita), →Urban population, →Energy use (kg of oil equivalent per capita), →Urban population (% of total population), →Adjusted net savings, including particulate emission damage (% of GNI), →Expense (% of GDP), →Foreign direct investment, net inflows (BoP, current USD), →Gross savings (% of GDP), →Exports of goods and services (% of GDP), →Imports of goods and services (% of GDP), →Government expenditure on education, total (% of GDP), →Literacy rate, youth total (% of people ages 15–24), →Unemployment, total (% of total labor force), →Population living in slums (% of urban population), →Cause of death, by communicable diseases and maternal, prenatal and nutrition conditions (% of total), →Refugee population by country or territory of origin, →Hospital beds (per 1000 people),

→Prevalence of overweight, weight for height (% of children under 5), →Specialist surgical workforce (per 100,000 population), →Air transport, registered carrier departures worldwide, →Annual freshwater withdrawals, total (billion cubic meters), →Fixed telephone subscriptions (per 100 people), →Fixed broadband subscriptions (per 100 people), →Secure Internet servers (per 1 million people), International tourism, receipts (% of total exports),→Researchers in R&D (per million people), →PM2.5 air pollution, population exposed to levels exceeding WHO guideline value (% of total), →Population in the largest city (% of urban population), →Top countries in number of air passengers carried in 2019, →Ownership of passenger cars (units per thousand persons). Income levels of CRs were obtained from the World Bank's Atlas method, which relies on the gross national income (GDP) per capita in 2019 at nominal values as an indicator of income.

2.3. Criteria of Data Collection

Inclusion criteria: (1) For the first three waves of the pandemic, data were collected from CRs with at least 100,000 reported total cases; (2) for wave 4, additional data were collected from CRs with a reported total case number of more than 50,000; and (3) at least one visible turning point was reported in at least one wave in both of the cases and deaths, judged by two authors. Exclusion criteria: (1) no obvious turning point in the data in either cases or deaths; (2) the number of deaths on the turning point was less than 3; and (3) the days of turning points between cases and death were more than 2 months.

2.4. Definition of Waves and Turning Points

A disease wave is defined as the cases and deaths that had turning points (peak days) and were flanked on both sides by days with a smaller number of cases or deaths (Figure S1). The average number of seven days was used to define the turning point (or peak) of a wave [2]. The cases turning point was defined as the day with the largest number of average cases in seven days (the seven-day average). Case numbers on each side of the peak must decrease at least 10%, in comparison with the number on a peak day. The same criteria were also used to determine the peak of deaths.

2.5. Definition of Mortality at the Day of the Turning Point

The mortality of each wave is defined as the average number of seven days at the death turning point divided by the average number of seven days at the case turning point in the same wave. When the number of days between a case turning point and a death turning point is the smallest, then these case and death points are considered to be in the same wave. If the days between these two turning points are more than two months, they are not regarded as the same wave, even when there is not any wave during the pandemic.

2.6. Data Uniformity and Bias Checking

Data collection was conducted by two investigators and double-checked by a third researcher. Outliers identified by individual authors were discussed by at least two authors. Peak days and data on peak days were double-checked by two additional authors. Statistical analyses were conducted by two authors to ensure accuracy. Wave numbers were adjusted based on timeline and case numbers to evaluate the accuracy of the data analysis.

3. Statistical Analysis

Data analysis was conducted in the following ten steps. (1) CRs names, days of case peak in a wave, number of cases of a wave, days of death peaks, and number of deaths on the peak days were collected and stored in an Excel file. A total of 49 influence factors of CRs were collected in a separate Excel file. (2) Mortality at the peak of each wave was calculated by dividing the seven-day average number of the day of the death peak with the seven-day average number of cases on the day of the cases peak. (3) The correlation coefficient (r) between these mortality and influential parameters were calculated with the formula function of Excel. Student *t*-tests were conducted with paired comparison and two tailed distributions. (4) Influential factors with positive or negative impacts were selected for evaluation. (5) Mortalities in three waves in different income levels of CRs were analyzed and compared with each other. (6) The numbers of waves were adjusted according to the time of the waves and compared among different income levels. (7) Case-number-weighted mortalities among three waves were compared among CRs in different income levels. (8) Mortalities in the largest waves among CRs were compared to investigate the capability of fighting COVID-19 when facing the greatest challenge in CRs at different income levels. (9) Case-number-based normalization was done with the following formula: W(eight) = D * Ci/Ct. Where W = the case-number-weighted death rate, D = death number in a specific wave; Ci = the case number of the same individual CRs, and Ct = the total number of cases in a disease wave. (10) Figures for mortality were visualized using the Chart function in Excel, including those of the Australian Bureau of Statistics, GeoNames, Microsoft, Navinfo, and TomTom.

4. Results

4.1. Mortality Turning Points in the First Wave of COVID-19 Compared to Other Waves

As of 21 January 2022, more than 100,000 cases were reported from each of the 119 CRs. Among them, only two CRs did not exhibit any distinctive wave (Table S1). Among the remaining CRs, 55 experienced four waves, 102 showed three waves, 112 had at least two waves and 117 had at least one wave (Figure 1A–D). The average mortalities for the waves 1, 2, 3, and 4 were 0.0359, 0.0194, 0.0168, and 0.0145, respectively. There were no correlations between the first wave and the rest of three waves, with r values of 0.20, 0.06, and −0.04 for waves 2, 3, and 4 (Figure 1E–G). However, there were correlations among the remaining three waves, with r values of 0.57, 0.48, and 0.49 for wave 2 vs. 3, 2 vs. 4, and 3 vs. 4, respectively (Figure 1H–J). The distribution among CRs on mortality rates at the peak points among four waves varies significantly (Figure 1). In the first wave, the high mortality rates were mainly identified in European and North American CRs; conversely, in the other waves, the high mortality rates occurred among developing countries, mainly among African, Southeastern Asian, and South American CRs.

Table S1 shows the days, and the number of cases and deaths at the turning points of different waves. There are great variations in cases and number of deaths among different countries. It is astonishing to see the extremely high death rate among developed countries. For example, the death rates in France, the UK, Italy, the Netherlands, and Belgium were 21.5%, 18.9%, 14.5%, 13.5%, and 19.7%. These data hinted at a high death rate in the developed countries in the first wave. However, the death rate of the same countries in wave 2 are 1.2%, 1.9%, 2.1%, 0.8%, and 1.2%. These vast changes indicated that better biomedical resources were effectively utilized when the developed countries were ready for the pandemic of COVID-19. In contrast, there is no such a significant change in mortality between wave 1 and wave 2 among developing countries (Figure 1). Therefore, our follow-up analysis focused on the differences among countries at different income levels.

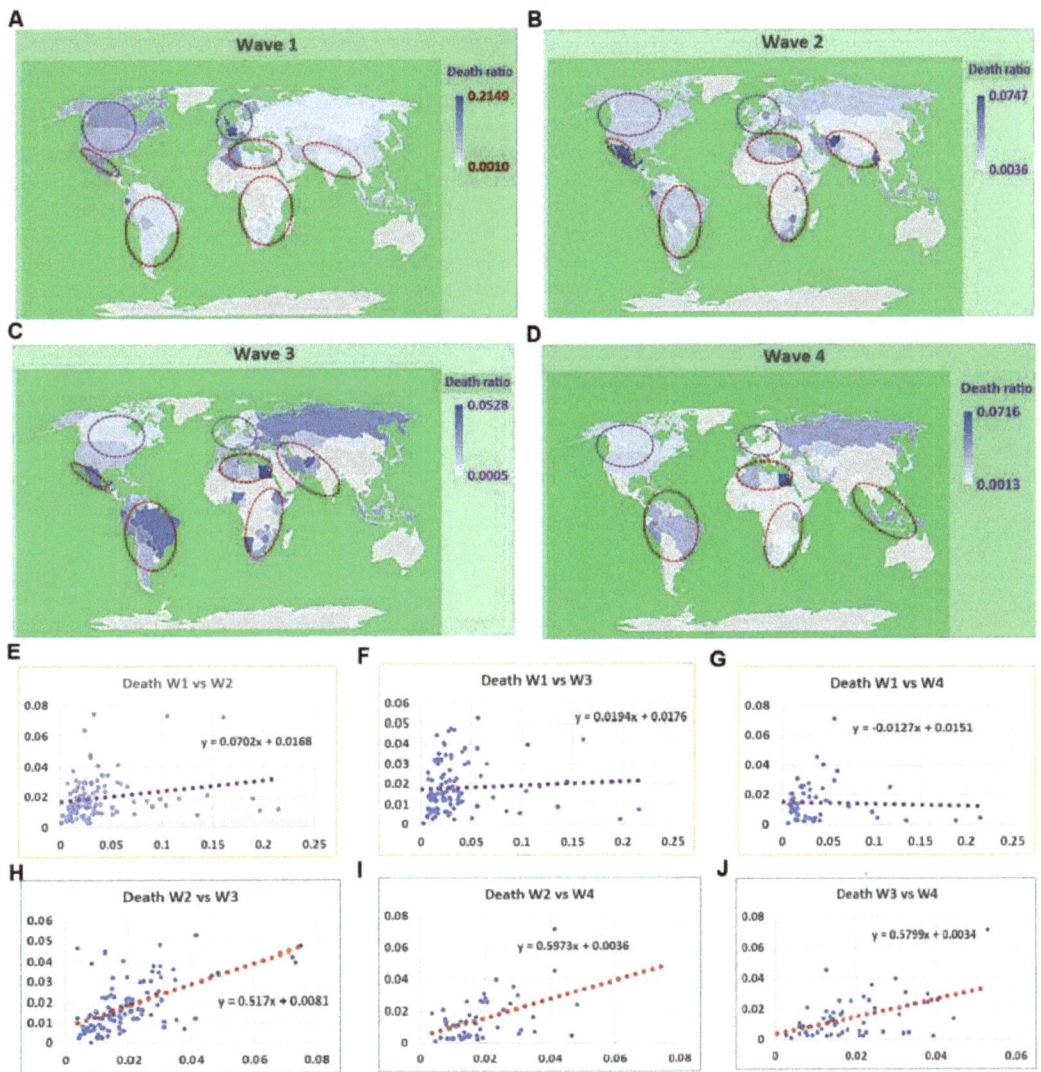

Figure 1. Mortality at the case turning point of the COVID-19 pandemic for 119 countries and regions (CRs). Blue circles indicate the developed CRs, and red circles indicate developing CRs. (**A–D**) The mortalities in CRs for waves 1, 2, 3, and 4. In wave 1, the mortalities in developed CRs were higher than other CRs while the mortalities in the waves 2, 3, and 4 in the developing CRs were higher than that in developed CRs. (**E–G**) The correlation of mortality between wave 1 and the other three waves, 2, 3, and 4. (**H–J**) The correlation among waves 2, 3, and 4.

4.2. Influential Factors for the Mortalities among CRs

Among 49 potential influencing factors, 9 showed at least one r with an absolute value more than 0.3 (Figure S2, Tables S2 and S3). The correlation between the mortality rate and these nine factors showed an opposite direction between the first wave and the subsequent three waves (Figure 2A). In the first wave, factors of categories including economic levels (income, GNI per capita, researchers in R&D, broadband subscriptions, school enrollment), aging population (aged 65 and older and life expectancy), and transportation (owners of passenger cars) are all positively correlated to the mortality rate. These results are consistent with the previous literature findings that economy and transportation boosted the transmission, which caused the high mortalities, particularly within the aged population at the early stage of the COVID-19 pandemic [10,11]. However, in the remaining waves, these factors are either negatively or not correlated to the mortality rate. In particular, the income level, GNI per capita, and researchers in R&D (per million people) (Figure S2) were all negatively correlated to the death rate for waves 2, 3, and 4 (Figure 2B–D). The r values for income for waves 1, 2, 3, and 4 were 0.26, −0.31, −0.26, and −0.33, respectively. The r values for GNI for the waves 1, 2, 3, and 4 were 0.35, −0.29, −0.28, and −0.39, respectively. The values for researchers in R&D for the waves 1, 2, 3, and 4 were 0.37, −0.14, −0.31, and −0.42, respectively. As shown above, these 49 factors are collected from the World Bank, and the data range from 2017 to 2019. Through analysis of all 49 potential factors, we found that only 9 factors show a possible influence on the COVID-19 disease pandemic. Among these nine factors, income level was our focus in this study. Other factors may have their effects and may be analyzed in future studies. For example, passenger cars are closely related to the traveling capacity; as traveling is an important factor for COVID-19 transmission, future studies on this aspect are necessary.

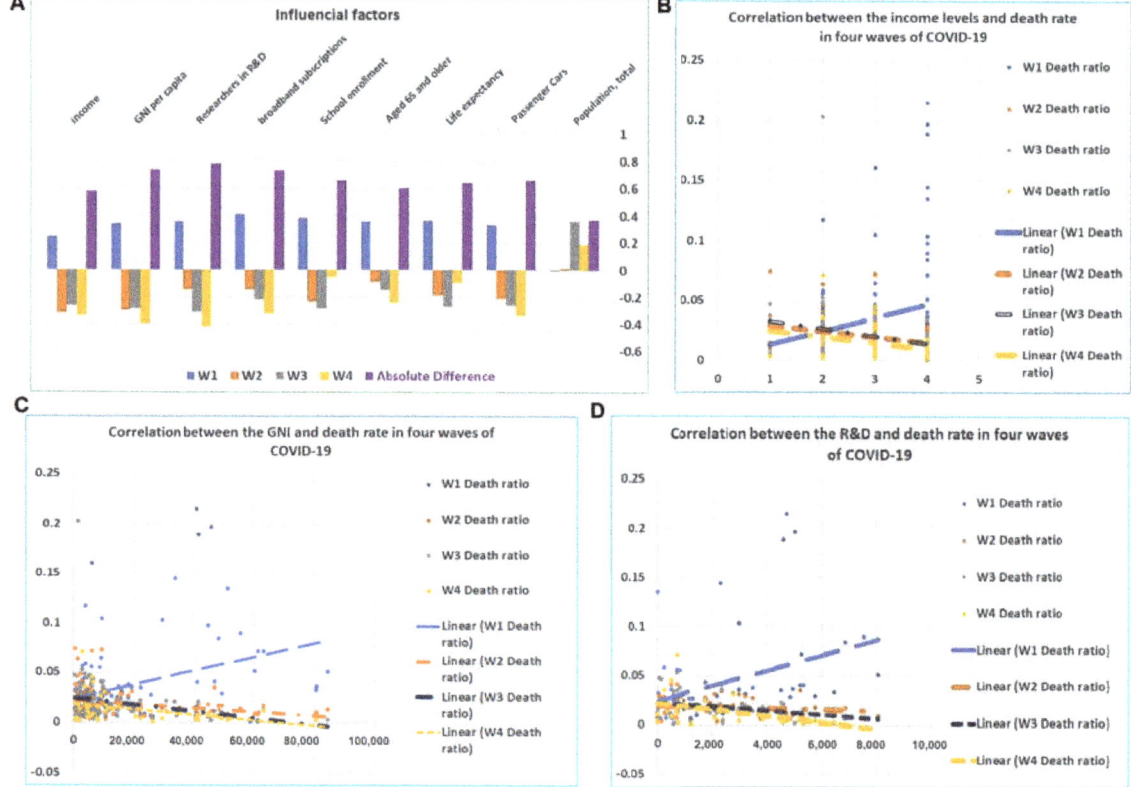

Figure 2. Influential factors on the mortality of COVID-19 during four waves of pandemics. (**A**) Total of nine factors showed r values of more than 3 in at least one wave. The correlations between these nine factors and mortality in wave 1 are in an opposite direction when comparing these correlations with that of waves 2, 3, and 4. (**B**–**D**) The correlations between the mortality in the four waves and income levels (2B), GNI (2C), and R&D (2D). In each case, wave 1 showed positive correlations, while the other waves showed none or negative correlations.

4.3. Mortality of COVID-19 at Peak Point Varied across CRs with Different Income Levels

The patterns of mortality rates at the turning points among different income levels were further assessed in the first three waves which contain an adequate number CRs for analysis in groups at different income levels. Compared to the mortalities in wave 1, the reduction rate of the mortalities in waves 2 and 3 were significantly different among CRs at different income levels (Figure 3A). Among CRs at a high-income level, the mortalities in waves 2 and 3 were equal to 29% and 28% of that in wave 1, while in the upper-middle-income CRs, the rate was 76% and 79% for wave 2 and 3. The lower-middle-level CRs had rates of 88% and 90%, while among low-income levels, the rates were 135% and 135% (Figure 3B–E). Thus, the lower the income level, the slower the reduction rate in the mortalities in the later waves of the disease.

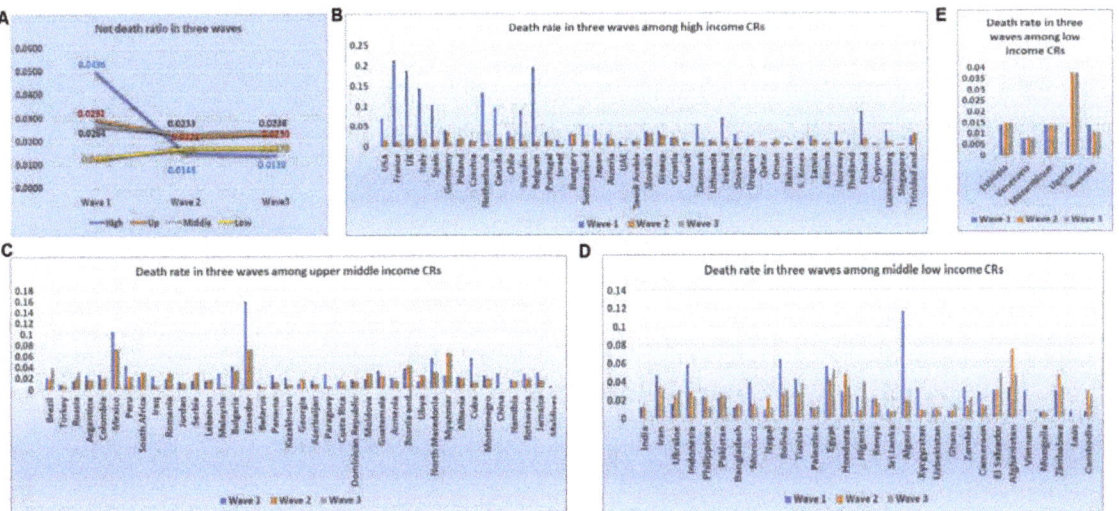

Figure 3. Turning point mortalities during the first three waves of COVID-19 disease in countries according to income levels. (**A**) The average mortalities for waves 1, 2, and 3 in countries of high-, upper-middle-, and lower-middle-incomes, respectively. (**B**) The mortality in three waves in CRs of high-income levels. (**C**) The mortality in three waves in CRs of upper-middle-income levels. (**D**) The mortality in three waves in CRs of lower-middle-income levels. (**E**) The mortality in three waves in CRs of low-income levels.

4.4. Developing Countries' Challenges when COVID-19 Reaches the Largest Scale

In order to examine the capacity for fighting COVID-19 when facing the largest challenge, we compared the mortalities among the largest waves in CRs at different income levels. Such a comparison revealed a significant difference between developed and developing CRs (Table S4). The average mortality in high-income CRs was 0.013, while the average mortalities among upper- and lower-middle-income CRs were 0.021. P values from *t*-tests between high-income CRs and upper- and lower-middle-income CRs were 0.001 and 0.002, while the *p* value between upper- and lower-middle-income CRs was 0.999. The mortality rates among these three categories were different, while the mortality rates within each category were similar (Figure 4A). The mortality rates in the majority of high-income CRs are below 0.02 (Figure 4A), while in the upper- and lower-middle-income CRs, the rates in about 50% of CRs are between 0.02 and 0.04 (Figure 4C,D).

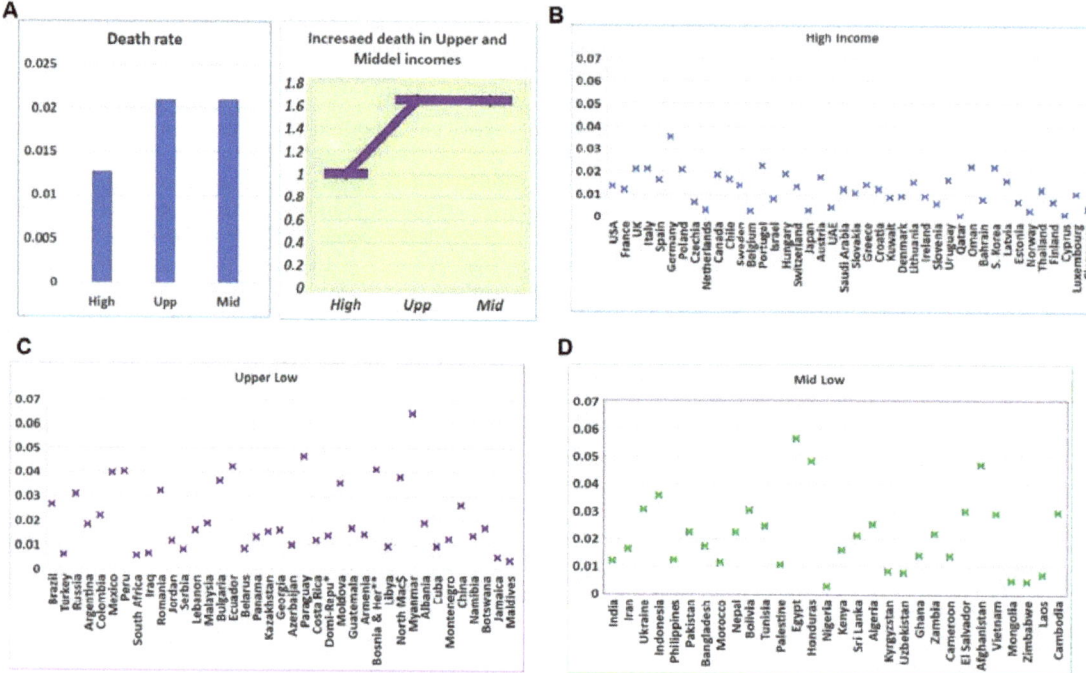

Figure 4. Mortalities in CRs of different income levels at the largest scale of the pandemic. (**A**) Left panel shows the mortality rate in CRs according to income level when COVID-19 reaches the largest scale. Right panel shows the percentages of upper- and lower-middle-income levels in comparison with CRs at a high-income level. (**B**) Distributions of mortalities of CRs at the high-income level. (**C**) Distributions of mortalities of CRs at the upper-middle-income level. (**D**) Distributions of mortalities of CRs at the lower-middle-income level.

4.5. Timeline-Adjusted Comparisons among Different Waves

Due to the variations in the spreading of the disease across the world, the time of the same wave among different CRs differed. Comparison was further conducted on the timeline base for different waves. The waves are re-divided based on the timeline of approximately before July of 2020, between July and November 2020, between November 2020 and March/April 2021, and after, for waves 1, 2, 3, and 4, respectively. The disease patterns among different income levels are compared among these four waves. Data for such a comparison showed similar patterns to the non-time adjusted mortalities among different income levels among the first three waves (Figure 5A). Patterns in different waves indicated that in the high-income CRs, the mortality in the first wave was higher than that in subsequent waves (Figure 5B), while in the CRs with other income levels, the mortalities were higher in the later waves than that in the first wave (Figure 5C,D).

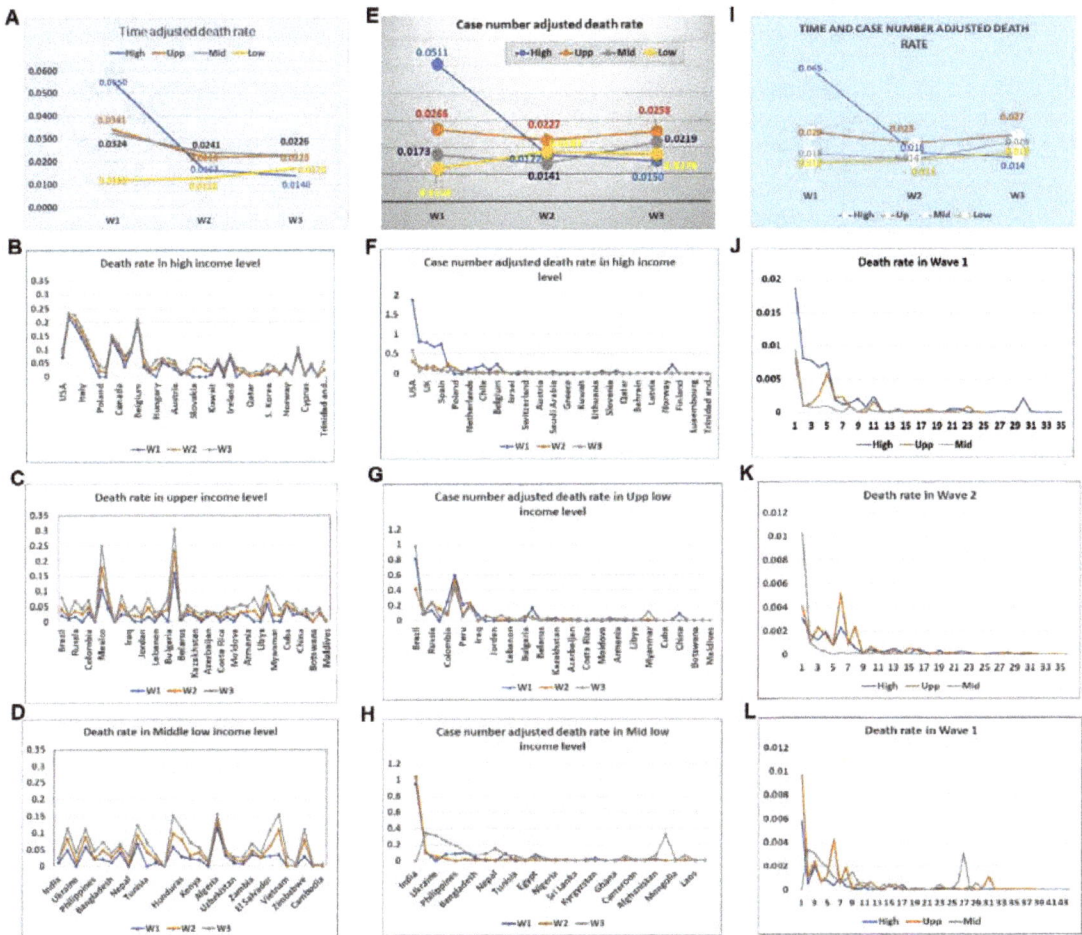

Figure 5. Mortalities based on timeline and case-number-adjusted data. (**A–D**) Mortalities based on timeline-adjusted data. (**A**) The average number of deaths in CRs at different income levels in three waves of disease based on the timeline. (**B**) Distributions of mortalities in high-income level CRs by timeline. (**C**) Distributions of mortalities in upper-middle-income level CRs by timeline. (**D**) Distributions of mortalities in lower-middle-income level CRs by timeline. (**E–H**) Mortalities based on case-number-adjusted data. (**E**) The average number of deaths in CRs at different income levels in three waves of disease by cases. (**F**) Distributions of mortalities in high-income level CRs by cases. (**G**) Distributions of mortalities in upper-middle-income level CRs by cases. (**H**) Distributions of mortalities in lower-middle-income level CRs by cases. (**I–L**) Mortalities based on timeline- and case-number-adjusted data. (**I**) The average number of deaths in CRs at a different income level in three waves of disease by timeline and cases. (**J**) Distributions of mortalities in high-income level CRs by timeline and cases. (**K**) Distributions of mortalities in upper-middle-income level CRs by timeline and cases. (**L**) Distributions of mortalities in lower-middle-income level CRs by timeline and cases.

4.6. Comparison of Normalized Data Based on Case Number among Different Waves

In order to confirm the impact of income levels, we examined the patterns of disease waves using normalized mortality rates based on the case numbers. The normalized data showed that the disease patterns in three waves are similar to that of non-normalized data.

The wave 1 mortality rate in high-income CRs was higher than the wave 1 rates in CRs with other income levels, while in waves 2 and 3, the mortality rates in CRs with other income levels were higher than that of the high-income CRs (Figure 5E). Comparing the mortalities of three waves in the CRs indicated that in the high-income level, the rate of the first wave was higher than that of the other waves. On the contrary, the mortality rates in CRs with middle- and low-income levels increased in waves 2 and 3 (Figures 5F and 6).

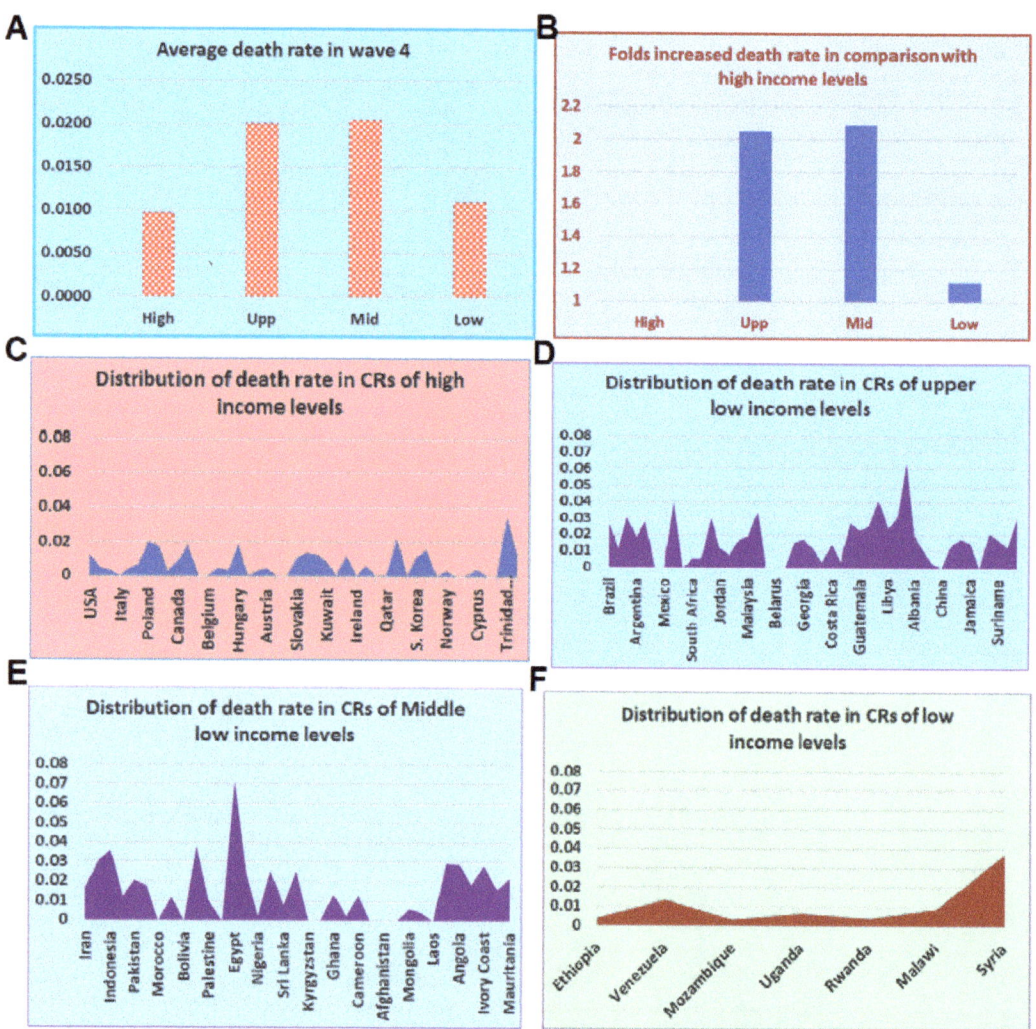

Figure 6. Mortality rates at the turning points during wave 4 of COVID-19 disease in CRs with different income levels. (**A**) Average mortality rates in CRs by income level. (**B**) Fold increase in the upper- and lower-middle, and low income CRs compared to high-income CRs. (**C**) Distributions of mortality rates of CRs at the high-income level. (**D**) Distributions of mortality rates of CRs at the upper-middle-income level. (**E**) Distributions of mortality rate of CRs at the lower-middle-income level. (**F**) Distributions of mortality rate of CRs at the low-income level.

4.7. Comparison Based on Timeline and Case Normalized Data among Different Waves

When data were normalized based on both the timeline and case numbers, the patterns of three waves of the pandemics were similar to the non-modified original data. The mortality rate in the first wave in the high-income CRs was much higher than that of the other income categories, while in the third wave, its mortality became the lowest among all income levels (Figure 5I). The distributions of mortality rates of CRs among waves 1, 2, and 3 showed the same patterns (Figure 5J–L).

4.8. Wave 4 Preliminary Data and Increasing Lags Based on Income

In our initial evaluation among different income levels, we omitted wave 4 data because there was a significantly smaller number of CRs in the fourth wave compared to the other waves. Instead, we included 19 additional CRs with more than 50,000 cases for a preliminary analysis for wave 4. The majority of these additional CRs are from the African region (Tables S5 and S6). Among these 19 CRs, 11 had a visible wave 4 based on our team's judgment. By adding data from these 11 CRs, we were able to compare the mortality rates among all CRs at four levels of income. Results suggest that the mortality rate in high-income CRs was less than 1% (Figure 6A), while in the upper- and lower-middle-income CRs, the mortalities were as high as 2%. The increased mortality rates in CRs of upper- and lower-middle-incomes reached 100% (Figure 6B). In the low-income CRs, the mortality was higher than 1% with a small number of cases (Figure 6B), which may increase in the future. The distribution of the mortality rates among CRs of these four income levels showed a difference between the CRs of high-income and CRs at the other income levels (Figure 6C–F).

5. Discussion

Our data indicate that conclusions from previous considerable research on the factors influencing COVID-19 rates and deaths were not applicable to the overall COVID-19 pandemic because these results are based on data from the first wave. The occurrence of the first wave has its special characteristics because COVID-19 originated from a metropolis and spread at an unprecedented fast speed through travelling and close contact. Thus, the economic powered convenience of traveling and population density were the major factors [8–10] for the disease spreading. It first reached the developed countries and caused high mortality under an urgent and unprepared situation. In comparison, the first wave of the developing CRs happened later than the high-income CRs. It would have caused many more mortalities if the early phase of the pandemic had reached low-income CRs.

One of the most important findings from this study is that economic disparities affect the capabilities of low-income CRs in fighting the COVID-19 pandemic [10]. The data from waves 2 and 3 confirmed that, in the same situation, developing CRs suffer more than developed countries. There are significant differences in the mortality among different waves of the pandemic in CRs at different income levels. Among high-income CRs, the mortality rates ranged from as high as 5% in wave 1 to approximately 1.4% in wave 3, a 3-fold decrease. Conversely, in the upper- and lower-middle-income CRs, the mortality rates did not decrease during waves 2 and 3. The mortality rates of the CRs with upper- and lower-middle-incomes were approximately 180% of that in high-income countries. Preliminary data from wave 4 support the findings from the previous three waves on the influence of economic disparities in fighting COVID-19.

The influence of income inequalities on the COVID-19 pandemic in waves 2 and 3 was confirmed by multiple types of analyses due to the complexity of the COVID-19 pandemics across different regions of the world. The data were first shown based on the data from waves of original sequential numbers. This analysis was entirely based on the numbers of waves of the pandemic when comparing among CRs at different income levels. The second comparison was conducted based on the time-sequence of the waves. The third comparison was based on the adjusted data by the number of cases of the peak in the waves. Finally, the data were compared with both timeline- and case-number-adjusted data. All analyses showed the same pattern of negative effects on mortalities by the income levels during waves 2 and 3. Even in wave 4, when the omicron was less severe in symptoms and the world was better prepared with a variety of approaches, the mortalities in the high-income CRs were below 1% and the CRs of upper- and lower-middle-incomes were still as high as 2%. Although data from low-income CRs were missing and incomplete, the mortality was still higher than that of CRs of high-income levels.

One important comparison in our study is the mortality levels when the pandemic reached the highest case numbers among different waves in CRs of different income levels. Case numbers reaching the maximum number was most challenging to CRs' capability to fight the COVID-19 pandemic. This comparison clearly demonstrated that the high-income CRs have advantages in the prevention of deaths among their infected population. Different waves happened at different time points. It is important to analyze these different waves at different time points. For example, wave 1 in most of the world occurred before the middle of 2020, while wave 2 occurred during the period between the latter half of 2020 and early 2021, and wave 3 occurred between early 2021 to the middle-to-late of 2021. The importance of time point is not only for the time sequential of the different waves, but also for reflecting the stages of disease variations and virus mutations. The same wave represents the same disease nature and pandemic pattern at a defined period of time. We used average mortality data from each country and conducted a two samples t-test to compare the mean of different mortalities. In this way, we could tell the variations of mortality over time.

Two distinguishing features of this study are the analysis of data by waves and the focus on the peaks of the waves. As our data has shown, different waves of the COVID-19 pandemic occurred at different times, and in different regions, environments, and situations. Examining different waves individually reveals various features of these waves. Examining the mortality rate during the peaks of the waves allows us to obtain the data showing the real capability of CRs in fighting the pandemic. This analysis enables us to examine the mortality at the same point from different CRs. In this case, the collected data are comparable.

The positive association between mortality and three other factors in wave 1, ownership of passenger cars (units per thousand persons), percent of population aged 65 and older, and life expectancy at birth, and the non- or negative correlations in other waves of the pandemics provide support that the influential factors for wave 1 do not have the same effect for the rest of the COVID-19 pandemic. In fact, the negative correlations between the car owners and mortality rates in other waves suggest that access to hospitals enhances the chance of survival of patients in the high-income CRs. The consistency of negative correlations between the mortality rates and economic factors such as income level, GNI per capita, and car ownership, indicate that economic levels play essential roles in CRs' capability to fight COVID-19.

Due to the limited availability of data, our initial analyses did not include the low-income countries as a separate category when analyzing the influence of income levels in the first three waves. However, based on our preliminary data from seven low-income CRs and a total of more than 12,000 cases, the mortality rate in the low-income CRs was higher than that of the high-income CRs. In considering the data from waves 2 and 3, it is anticipated that the situation in the low-income CRs will worsen when the pandemic reaches the same scale as that of high-income CRs. The longer the pandemic period is, the worse the mortality rates will be in the low-income countries.

Our study has some limitations. The days of turning point and the waves were arbitrarily determined by our authors, mainly based on the data provided by the Worldometers. The data from Worldometers are not always consistent with that from WHO websites. There were subtle differences in numbers, although these differences did not affect the results. We decided to use the data from Worldometers because of the data convenience as it provides daily numbers of cases and deaths with figures and seven-day averages. It is possible that the data from low-income CRs may not be as complete as that of CRs at other income levels, most likely due to the problems in disease surveillance or data collection.

Many factors have been reported as influential factors on the mortality of COVID-19. However, our analysis indicated that only a few factors affect mortality. Surprisingly, cases per million and population density did not show an overall significant impact on the mortality rate. The most likely reason is that influential factors in one or more places or countries may not be included in our analysis of 119 CRs.

As the vaccination and medical treatment develop, the economic advantage of high-income CRs will become more evident. If medical resources cannot be supplied in low- or lower-middle-income CRs, the mortalities in these CRs will increase before they begin decreasing. Because different waves of COVID-19 have different characterizations, the relation between income level and the latest waves of the COVID-19 pandemic may be different from these four waves in our analysis. In particular, omicron has become the dominant virus variant over the world. How the income level affects the pandemic of omicron will be an important question to ask. Furthermore, new variants with new infection characterization and disease features may appear in the future. Therefore, it is essential to monitor the dynamic changes of pandemic pattern with updated information for future studies.

6. Conclusions

Our analysis indicated that there are significant differences in disease mortality rates and influential factors between wave 1 and the subsequent waves up to January 2022. Economic disadvantages of developing CRs contributed to more suffering from the COVID-19 pandemic. As time goes on, the vaccination coverage and medical treatment in developed CRs has enabled low mortality rates. The prolonged COVID-19 pandemic causes an increase of mortalities in the developing CRs due to the lack of fighting resources, which are economically dependent.

7. Research in Context

Evidence Before This Study. The majority reported influential factors on the pandemic COVID-19 are based on the data from the early stage, i.e., the first wave of the pandemic. The few studies on individual waves did not conduct comparison of either multiple waves of the disease or on the disease turning points of the different waves worldwide.

Added Value of this Study. In this study, analysis based on the data from turning points and different waves of the COVID-19 enabled a detailed examination of the relationship between the influential factors and mortalities across CRs around the world. The use of data from the largest wave and the use of time- and case-adjusted data strengthened the finding that economic inequality affects the capacity of lower income CRs to fight the COVID-19 pandemic.

Implications of the Available Evidence. This comprehensive analysis of the mortalities in multiple waves of the COVID-19 pandemic in CRs at different income levels provides a deeper understanding about the influential factors among different waves and the significant role of economic levels in fighting the pandemic. The results suggest that developing CRs may continue to suffer more, while the developed CRs have greatly reduced the death rate from COVID-19 with economic driven research and development on vaccination and treatment. Our data also serves as a warning that serious outcomes in low-income countries may occur in the absence of intervention from the developed CRs.

Supplementary Materials: The following supporting information can be downloaded at: https://www.mdpi.com/article/10.3390/tropicalmed7090241/s1. Figure S1: Example of visible and non-visible turning points; Figure S2: Correlations of potential influential factors and death rates in four waves; Table S1: Days, number of cases and deaths at turning point of different waves; Table S2: Correlations between influential factors and death rate at turning pints of four waves; Table S3: Relationship of income, GNI and R and D to death rates at four waves; Table S4: The death rates at turning points in the largest wave of CRs of different income levels; Table S5: Time and case number adjusted mortality rate in CRs of different income levels; Table S6: Additional data for wave 4 from CRs with 50,000 case or more.

Author Contributions: L.Y. and W.G. collected and analyzed data and drafted the manuscript; L.Y., Y.C., J.C.G. and W.G. participated in the data collection and confirmation; L.Y., J.M., W.G. and L.A. participated in the data analysis and manuscript draft; Y.C., J.M., W.W., S.S., C.W., Y.J., G.W., D.S. and W.G. interpreted the results and edited the manuscript; W.G. and D.S. designed the project. All authors have read and agreed to the published version of the manuscript.

Funding: This work was partially supported by funding from the University of Tennessee Health Science Center (R073290109) to W.G. in Memphis, TN, USA, and grant 90DDUC0058 to J.C.G. from the U.S. Department of Health and Human Services, Administration for Community Living.

Institutional Review Board Statement: Not applicable.

Informed Consent Statement: Not applicable.

Data Availability Statement: All COVID-19 cases, deaths, and dates collected are either presented in the article and supplymentary materials or available online at https://www.worldometers.info/coronavirus (accessed on 14 January 2022).

Acknowledgments: The authors alone are responsible for the views expressed in this article, which do not necessarily represent the decisions, policy, or views of any institution or organization represented by the authors.

Conflicts of Interest: We declare no competing interest.

References

1. Salyer, S.J.; Maeda, J.; Sembuche, S.; Kebede, Y.; Tshangela, A.; Moussif, M.; Ihekweazu, C.; Mayet, N.; Abate, E.; Ouma, A.O.; et al. The first and second waves of the COVID-19 pandemic in Africa: A cross-sectional study. *Lancet* **2021**, *397*, 1265–1275. [CrossRef]
2. Wang, L.; Li, J.; Guo, S.; Xie, N.; Yao, L.; Cao, Y.; Day, S.W.; Howard, S.C.; Graff, J.C.; Gu, T.; et al. Real-time estimation and prediction of mortality caused by COVID-19 with patient information based algorithm. *Sci. Total Environ.* **2020**, *727*, 138394. [CrossRef] [PubMed]
3. Carbonell, R.; Urgelés, S.; Rodríguez, A.; Bodí, M.; Martín-Loeches, I.; Solé-Violán, J.; Díaz, E.; Gómez, J.; Trefler, S.; Vallverdú, M.; et al. Mortality comparison between the first and second/third waves among 3795 critical COVID-19 patients with pneumonia admitted to the ICU: A multicentre retrospective cohort study. *Lancet Reg. Health Eur.* **2021**, *11*, 100243. [CrossRef] [PubMed]
4. Jassat, W.; Mudara, C.; Ozougwu, L.; Tempia, S.; Blumberg, L.; Davies, M.-A.; Pillay, Y.; Carter, T.; Morewane, R.; Wolmarans, M.; et al. Difference in mortality among individuals admitted to hospital with COVID-19 during the first and second waves in South Africa: A cohort study. *Lancet Glob. Health* **2021**, *9*, e1216–e1225. [CrossRef]
5. Zeiser, F.A.; Donida, B.; da Costa, C.A.; Ramos, G.D.O.; Scherer, J.N.; Barcellos, N.T.; Alegretti, A.P.; Ikeda, M.L.R.; Müller, A.P.W.C.; Bohn, H.C.; et al. First and second COVID-19 waves in Brazil: A cross-sectional study of patients' characteristics related to hospitalization and in-hospital mortality. *Lancet Reg. Health Am.* **2022**, *6*, 100107. [CrossRef] [PubMed]
6. Yao, L.; Li, M.; Wan, J.Y.; Howard, S.C.; Bailey, J.E.; Graff, J.C. Democracy and case fatality rate of COVID-19 at early stage of pandemic: A multicountry study. *Environ. Sci. Pollut. Res. Int.* **2022**, *29*, 8694–8704. [CrossRef] [PubMed]
7. Karmakar, M.; Lantz, P.M.; Tipirneni, R. Association of Social and Demographic Factors with COVID-19 Incidence and Death Rates in the US. *JAMA Netw. Open* **2021**, *4*, e2036462. [CrossRef] [PubMed]
8. Yin, H.; Sun, T.; Yao, L.; Jiao, Y.; Ma, L.; Lin, L.; Graff, J.C.; Aleya, L.; Postlethwaite, A.; Gu, W.; et al. Association between population density and infection rate suggests the importance of social distancing and travel restriction in reducing the COVID-19 pandemic. *Environ. Sci. Pollut. Res. Int.* **2021**, *28*, 40424–40430. [CrossRef] [PubMed]
9. Worldometers. COVID-19 Coronavirus Pandemic. Available online: https://www.worldometers.info/coronavirus/ (accessed on 14 January 2022).
10. Ma, L.; Yu, Z.; Jiao, Y.; Lin, L.; Zhong, W.; Day, S.W.; Postlethwaite, A.; Chen, H.; Li, Q.; Yin, H.; et al. Capacity of transportation and spread of COVID-19-an ironical fact for developed countries. *Environ. Sci. Pollut. Res. Int.* **2021**, *28*, 37498–37505. [CrossRef] [PubMed]
11. Kim, S.Y.; Yoo, D.M.; Min, C.; Choi, H.G. The Effects of Income Level on Susceptibility to COVID-19 and COVID-19 Morbidity/Mortality: A Nationwide Cohort Study in South Korea. *J. Clin. Med.* **2021**, *10*, 4733. [CrossRef] [PubMed]

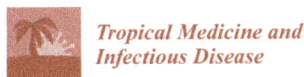 *Tropical Medicine and Infectious Disease*

Article

Comparison of Four Real-Time Polymerase Chain Reaction Assays for the Detection of SARS-CoV-2 in Respiratory Samples from Tunja, Boyacá, Colombia

Lorenzo H. Salamanca-Neita [1,2,*], Óscar Carvajal [1], Juan Pablo Carvajal [1], Maribel Forero-Castro [2] and Nidya Alexandra Segura [2,*]

1 Laboratorio Carvajal IPS, SAS, Tunja 150003, Colombia
2 Facultad de Ciencias, Grupo de Investigación en Ciencias Biomédicas, Universidad Pedagógica y Tecnológica de Colombia, Tunja 150003, Colombia
* Correspondence: lhsalamanca@uniboyaca.edu.co (L.H.S.-N.); nidya.segura@uptc.edu.co (N.A.S.)

Citation: Salamanca-Neita, L.H.; Carvajal, Ó.; Carvajal, J.P.; Forero-Castro, M.; Segura, N.A. Comparison of Four Real-Time Polymerase Chain Reaction Assays for the Detection of SARS-CoV-2 in Respiratory Samples from Tunja, Boyacá, Colombia. *Trop. Med. Infect. Dis.* **2022**, *7*, 240. https://doi.org/10.3390/tropicalmed7090240

Academic Editors: John Frean, Peter A. Leggat and Lucille Blumberg

Received: 19 July 2022
Accepted: 2 September 2022
Published: 10 September 2022

Publisher's Note: MDPI stays neutral with regard to jurisdictional claims in published maps and institutional affiliations.

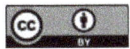

Copyright: © 2022 by the authors. Licensee MDPI, Basel, Switzerland. This article is an open access article distributed under the terms and conditions of the Creative Commons Attribution (CC BY) license (https://creativecommons.org/licenses/by/4.0/).

Abstract: Coronavirus disease (COVID-19) is an infectious disease caused by SARS-CoV-2. In Colombia, many commercial methods are now available to perform the RT-qPCR assays, and laboratories must evaluate their diagnostic accuracy to ensure reliable results for patients suspected of being positive for COVID-19. The purpose of this study was to compare four commercial RT-qPCR assays with respect to their ability to detect the SARS-CoV2 virus from nasopharyngeal swab samples referred to Laboratorio Carvajal IPS, SAS in Tunja, Boyacá, Colombia. We utilized 152 respiratory tract samples (Nasopharyngeal Swabs) from patients suspected of having SARS-CoV-2. The diagnostic accuracy of GeneFinder[TM] COVID-19 Plus RealAmp (In Vitro Diagnostics) (GF-TM), One-Step Real-Time RT-PCR (Vitro Master Diagnostica) (O-S RT-qPCR), and the Berlin modified protocol (BM) were assessed using the gold-standard Berlin protocol (Berlin Charité Probe One-Step RT-qPCR Kit, New England Biolabs) (BR) as a reference. Operational characteristics were estimated in terms of sensitivity, specificity, agreement, and predictive values. Using the gold-standard BR as a reference, the sensitivity/specificity of the diagnostic tests was found to be 100%/92.7% for GF-TM, 92.75%/67.47% for O-S RT-qPCR, and 100%/96.39% for the BM protocol. Using BR as a reference, the sensitivity/specificity for the diagnostic tests were found to be 100%/92.7% for the GF-TM assay, 92.72%/67.47% for the O-S RT-qPCR, and 100%/96.39% for BM. Relative to the BR reference protocol, the GF-TM and BM RT-PCR assays obtained similar results (k = 0.92 and k = 0.96, respectively), whereas the results obtained by O-S-RT-qPCR were only moderately similar. We conclude that the GF-TM and BM protocols offer the best sensitivity and specificity, with similar results in comparison to the gold-standard BR protocol. We recommend evaluating the diagnostic accuracy of the OS-RT-qPCR protocol in future studies with a larger number of samples.

Keywords: severe acute respiratory syndrome coronavirus 2 (SARS-CoV2); COVID-19; molecular diagnostics; real-time polymerase chain reaction (RT-qPCR)

1. Introduction

The outbreak of the coronavirus disease in 2019, also known as COVID-19, the causative agent of which is novel severe acute respiratory syndrome coronavirus 2 (SARS-CoV-2), was first detected in China on 31 December 2019 [1]. It was quickly (30 January 2020) declared a pandemic by the World Health Organization (WHO), becoming the first global public health emergency of the 21st century [2]. COVID-19 is becoming increasingly common in the population. Likewise, fear is generated due to the appearance of new variants, which is why vaccine-mediated immunity is needed to avoid the possible appearance of new variants capable of escaping the immune system [3]. Given the high speed of spread and the high cost of health services associated with this viral disease, as well as the lack of effective treatment, diagnosis is essential with continuous evaluation of the kits offered on the market, as well as strategies to generate safe and effective vaccines for vulnerable and susceptible populations and improve response and coverage strategies in health systems [4].

Since the pandemic was declared, the National Institute of Health reports that at least 525,609,637 people have been infected, with 6,277,241 deaths reported globally as of June 2022. In Colombia, 6,099,111 million cases have been reported, with 4214 active cases and 139,833 deaths. In the Department of Boyacá, Colombia, where the study population is located, 125,328 cases were reported during the same period, with a total of 2785 patient deaths (National Institute of Health, 2021, https://www.ins.gov.co/Noticias/Paginas/Coronavirus.aspx accessed on 18 August 2022). The viral genome of SARS-CoV-2 was sequenced on 3 February 2020 by the Shanghai Public Health Clinical Center, Fudan University, Shanghai, China. Thanks to the complete genomic sequencing of this new virus, the development of several vaccines and treatments against this viral disease have been developed. Similarly, the complete sequence allowed for the advancement of various diagnostic protocols for the identification of specific sequences of the viral genome. Specificity was improved using molecular techniques, such as PCR and the implementation of duplex PCR. The latter helped to decrease the time necessary to obtain test results and increase the processing capacity of laboratories worldwide [5].

Given that new variants of SARS-CoV-2 present with specific mutations, PCR assays could fail to detect some viral genes. In general, molecular kits should target conserved sites (e.g., genomic sequences that are the least likely to accumulate mutations over time). In this stage of the SARS-CoV-2 pandemic, an unprecedented number of genomes are available that can readily identify suitable candidates within conserved sites for diagnosis. These molecular assays involve protocols and procedures that allow SARS-CoV-2 to be identified using specific genes, such as E, RdRp, S, and N, among others. Although the virus has undergone multiple mutations, several studies have shown that most of the mutations occur in the region that encodes the spike protein in specific sites of its genome. As a result, the development of tests against other viral proteins has been recommended because the use of S might decrease specificity and cause false-negative test results [6].

To address the diagnosis of this viral disease in Colombia, the head of the National Institute of Health had to face the challenge of implementing diagnostic techniques based on World Health Organization (WHO) recommendations and the national guidelines for the laboratory surveillance of respiratory viruses. Therefore the diagnosis of SARS-CoV-2 is based on the regulations stipulated by the WHO, which recommended the Charité Berlin protocol as the gold standard in diagnostic laboratories, which was implemented in Colombia under the supervision of the Colombian National Institute of Health in collaborating laboratories (https://www.ins.gov.co/Pruebas_Rapidas/2.%20Protocolo%20Est%C3%A1ndar%20para%20validaci%C3%B3n%20de%20PR%20en%20Colombia.pdf accessed on 18 August 2022). Currently, several commercial kits are offered for the molecular diagnosis and identification of SARS-CoV-2 in Colombia, and laboratories must evaluate the diagnostic accuracy of these kits to ensure reliable results with respect to suspected COVID-19 patients.

The objective of this study was to compare four commercial RT-qPCR assays for the detection of the SARS-CoV2 virus using nasopharyngeal swab samples referred to Laboratorio Carvajal IPS, SAS in Tunja, Boyacá, Colombia. This research was approved by the research ethics committee of the Universidad Pedagógica y Tecnológica de Colombia, which was provided in the city of Tunja on 18 November 2021.

2. Materials and Methods

2.1. Study Design

A single-center prospective study was performed on 152 samples from female (70) and male (82) patients suspected of SARS-CoV2 infection in the department of Boyacá, Colombia. Samples with evidence of inadequate storage; presence of microbial, fungal, or chemical contamination in solvents or reagents; or a volume less than 250 µL, as well as alterations or modifications in labeling, were excluded.

2.2. Sample Collection and Preservation

A total of 152 samples from suspected COVID-19 patients were collected from the upper respiratory tract using nasopharyngeal swabs [7]. Samples were immediately placed into sterile tubes containing 3 mL of viral transport medium (VTM) [8]. The samples were stored at a temperature between 2 °C and 8 °C and sent to the molecular biology laboratory of Carvajal Laboratorio IPS SAS to confirm the presence or absence of viral RNA.

We followed the guidelines established by the National Institute of Health of Colombia (INS) (https://www.ins.gov.co/buscador-eventos/Informacindelaboratorio/Lineamientosparalavigilanciaporlaboratoriodevirusrespiratorios.pdf accessed on 18 August 2022), the Ministry of Health and Social Protection of Colombia (Minsalud) (https://www.minsalud.gov.co/sites/rid/Lists/BibliotecaDigital/RIDE/VS/ED/VSP/psps03-lineamiento-bioseguridad-red-nal-lab.pdf accessed on 18 August 2022), and the provisional biosecurity guidelines of "Laboratory for the handling and transport of samples associated with the new coronavirus 2019 (2019-nCoV)" (https://www.minsalud.gov.co/sites/rid/Lists/BibliotecaDigital/RIDE/VS/ED/VSP/psps02-lineamientos-gmuestras-pandemia-sars-cov-2-col.pdf accessed on 18 August 2022) for the reception of samples suspected of SARS-CoV-2 positivity.

The samples were received along with a referral form, "INS Basic Data Report Sheet 346", which included names and surnames of each patient, date of first symptoms of the disease, date of sampling, type of sample (nasopharyngeal aspirate, bronchoalveolar lavage, necropsy, etc.), and any additional epidemiological or clinical data (https://www.ins.gov.co/buscador-eventos/Lineamientos/345_ESI_Irag_2022.pdf accessed on 18 August 2022). All samples met the criteria listed in the Guidelines for Laboratory Surveillance of Respiratory Viruses and the Manual of Sampling for Microbiological Analysis of the Ministry of Health of Bogotá [9].

2.3. RNA Extraction

Samples were processed at the same as the kits, so it was not necessary to thaw and freeze them again, thus avoiding RNA damage. RNA was extracted from the virus was with a Nextractor® NX-48S automated nucleic acid extraction system (Genolutium, Gangseo-gu, Seoul, Korea) using an AN NX-48s viral RNA extraction kit (Genolutium, Gangseo-gu, Seoul, Korea) as a reagent, which is compatible with the automation system, following the protocol established by the manufacturer. This system is automated, which favors a reduction in handling errors, prevents cross contamination, and significantly reduces processing times. Viral RNAs were stored at −80 °C for further analysis by RT-qPCR.

2.4. Real-Time Polymerase Chain Reaction (RT-qPCR)

In this study, the diagnostic accuracy of GeneFinder™ COVID-19 Plus RealAmp (In Vitro Diagnostics) (GF-TM), One-Step Real-Time RT-PCR (Vitro Master Diagnostica, Granada, España) (O-S RT-qPCR), and the Berlin modified protocol (BM) was assessed. The gold-standard Berlin protocol (Berlin Charité Probe One-Step RT-qPCR Kit, New England Biolabs, Ipswich, Massachusetts) (BR) was used as a reference. Table 1 shows the characteristics of each commercial kit evaluated during the study.

SARS-CoV-2 positivity was confirmed by RT-qPCR using the E, N, and RdRp genes in the GF-TM, O-S RT-qPCR, and BM protocols, respectively. In contrast, the BR reference protocol diagnoses SARS-CoV-2 by the amplification and detection of a region of the E gene, which is shared by various betacoronaviruses of the Sarbecovirus subgenus. In these samples, a positive PCR test was performed in order to detect a specific region of SARS-CoV-2 located in the RdRp gene. For the purpose of reducing these limitations, a duplex PCR test for the detection of the E and RNase P genes, designated the gold standard, was validated. A performance panel was performed with positive and negative samples for SARS-CoV-2 viral RNA. Additionally, the RNase P gene was included as a control to identify the viability of the samples, and to rule out the presence of PCR inhibitors or poor extraction of viral RNA, PCR-grade water was used as negative control for RT-PCR.

Table 1. Characteristics of the commercial kits assessed for the detection of SARS-CoV-2.

Feature	GF-TM	O-S RT-qPCR	BM	BR
Manufacturer	In Vitro Diagnostics	Vitro Master Diagnostica	Forest University	New England Biolabs
Sample types	Bronchoalveolar lavage fluid, nasopharyngeal swabs, oropharyngeal swabs, nasal swabs, mid-turbinate nasal swabs, or sputum specimens	Bronchoalveolar lavage fluid and nasopharyngeal swabs	Nasopharyngeal swabs and oropharyngeal swabs	Bronchoalveolar lavage fluid, nasopharyngeal swabs, and oropharyngeal swabs
Sample volume required	5 µL	8 µL	5 µL	5 µL
Extraction required	Yes	Yes	Yes	Yes
Target gene of SARS-CoV-2	E, N, and RdRp	E and N	E and N	And
Internal quality control	RNAse P	RNAse P	RNAse P	RNAse P
Analytical sensitivity	RdRp: 10 copies/test	Gen N: 10 copies/test	Gen N: 10 copies/test	Gen N: 10 copies/test
	N: 10 copies/test	Gen E: 10 copies/test	Gen E: 10 copies/test	Gen E: 10 copies/test
	E: 10 copies/test			
Analytical specificity	1	1	1	1
Maximum performance per kit	100 samples	100 samples	Not specified	100 samples
Test run time	1 h 35'	1 h 2'	1 h 5'	43'
Recommended platform	Biosystems® 7500 Real-Time PCR Instrument (ABI 7500). StepOneTM Real-Time PCR System (Applied Biosystems). CFX96TM Real-Time PCR Detection System (Bio-Rad).	QuantStudioTM 3 Real-Time PCR System (Applied Biosystems). QuantStudioTM 5 Real-Time PCR System (Applied Biosystems). Biosystems® 7500 Real-Time PCR Instrument (ABI 7500). StepOne PlusTM Real-Time PCR System (Applied Biosystems). StepOneTM Real-Time PCR System (Applied Biosystems). CFX96TM Real-Time PCR Detection System (Bio-Rad). Rotor—Gene—Q (Qiagen).	CFX96TM Real-Time PCR Detection System (Bio-Rad).	CFX96TM Real-Time PCR Detection System (Bio-Rad). QuantStudioTM 5 Real-Time PCR System (Applied Biosystems).

Abbreviations: GeneFinder™ COVID-19 Plus RealAmp (In Vitro Diagnostics): GF-TM; One-Step Real-Time RT-PCR (Vitro Master Diagnostica): O-S RT-qPCR; Berlin modified protocol: BM; and gold-standard Berlin protocol (Berlin Charité Probe One-Step RT-qPCR Kit, New England Biolabs): BR.

For each amplification event, a reaction was performed using a total volume of 25 µL containing 5 µL of RNA extracted in the previous step, 12.5 µL of 2× reaction buffer provided with the Superscript III one-step RT-PCR amplification system with Taq Platinum

Polymerase (Invitrogen; containing 0.4 mM of each dNTP and 3.2 mM of magnesium sulfate), 1 µL of reverse transcriptase, 0.4 µL of 50 mM of magnesium sulfate solution (not provided with the kit), 1 µg of non-acetylated bovine serum albumin, and 1.5 µL of each primer from a stock solution of 10 µM. RT-qPCR was performed using a CFX-96 for 10 min at 55 °C, 3 min at 95 °C, 45 cycles of 15 s at 95 °C, and 30 s at 58 °C [10]. The data were analyzed using Bio-Rad CFX Manager software (version 3.1.3090.1022; Applied Biosystems, Waltham, MA, USA). The primers and probe sequences of primers were established by each of the commercial firms based on "Diagnostic detection of 201-nCoV by real-time RT-PCR protocol—Berlin 2020" (https://www.who.int/docs/default-source/coronaviruse/protocol-v2-1.pdf accessed on 18 August 2022).

GF-TM and O-S RT-qPCR were performed according to the manufacturers' recommendations. The BM protocol was supplied by the Laboratory of Virology at the Universidad del Bosque and modified from the Charité Berlin protocol (https://www.who.int/docs/default-source/coronaviruse/protocol-v2-1.pdf accessed on 18 August 2022) by including a single multiplex PCR reaction for the identification of the E and N genes. All assays used RNA genomic SARS-CoV2, which was provided by the INS or reference laboratories as a positive control (Table 1).

2.5. Statistical Analysis

The distribution of the variables was assessed with Kolmogorov–Smirnov test. Categorical data were summarized as absolute frequencies and percentages, whereas categorical variables were summarized as relative and absolute frequencies.

Sensitivity and specificity were calculated in 2 × 2 tables at each level. The sensitivity (95% CI), specificity (95% CI), and positive and negative predictive values were calculated using BR as the gold standard. Matched pairs of recorded cycle threshold values (Ct values) were compared using the Spearman correlation coefficient. Indeterminate results were excluded from the data analysis.

Diagnostic similarities among GF-TM, O-S RT-qPCR, BM, and the gold-standard BR were calculated using accordance analysis with the Fleiss' Cohen's kappa (κ) test, in which $\kappa > 0.80$ signifies a high similarity between methods. A value of $p < 0.05$ was considered statistically significant. Obtained data were systematized in Microsoft Excel v15.0, and all statistical analyses were performed with IBM® SPSS® 22.0 software (IBM, Armonk, NY, USA).

To evaluate the amplification of genes E and RNase P, the fold change (FC) was calculated using R version 4.2.1 software; the obtained values indicate the number of times that the fluorescence emitted increases or decreases in relation to the reference gene.

3. Results

Comparison of the Results between the Four RT-qPCR Assays

A total of 152 samples from patients suspected of having COVID-19 ranging in age from 1 to 81 years were included in our analysis. A total of 82 samples from men, and 70 samples were from women. Most of the samples belonged were collected from adults between the ages of 25 and 64 years, corresponding to the working age population (57.9%), followed by adolescents between the ages of 15 and 24 years (21.1%), elderly aged 65 years old and older (14.5%), children between the ages of 5 and 14 years (5.3%), and children under 5 years of age (1.3%). Supplementary Table S1 details the primary data obtained from this study; data were analyzed using OpenEpi® software.

Table 2 shows the comparative results between the four investigated RT-qPCR assays. Using BR as reference, a total of 152 samples were tested (62 positive and 83 negative), and the sensitivity/specificity of the diagnostic tests was found to be 100%/92.7% for the GF-TM assay, 92.72%/67.47% for the O-S RT-qPCR assay, and 100%/96.39% for the BM assay. Relative the BR reference protocol, the GF-TM and BM RT-PCR assays achieved similar results (k = 0.92 and k = 0.96 respectively), whereas the results obtained with O-S-RT-qPCR were less similar (Table 2). Supplementary Table S2 details the concordant and discordant results in the 152 analyzed samples.

Table 2. Comparison of results between the four molecular assays for the detection of SARS-CoV-2 using the Berlin protocol (BR) as a reference (n = 152, of which 62 were positive and 83 were negative).

Assay		BR Positive	BR Negative	Kappa (k) (±95% cL)	Sensitivity	Specificity	PPV	PNV	GIVES
GF-TM	Positive	69	6	0.92	100%	92.70%	92%	100%	96.05%
	Negative	0	77						
O-S RT-qPCR	Positive	64	27	0.58	92.75%	67.47%	70.33%	91.48%	78.95%
	Negative	5	56						
BM	Positive	69	3	0.96	100%	96.39%	100%	95.87%	98.30%
	Negative	0	80						

Abbreviations: GeneFinder™ COVID-19 Plus RealAmp (In Vitro Diagnostics): GF-TM; One-Step Real-Time RT-PCR (Vitro Master Diagnostica): O-S RT-qPCR; Berlin modified protocol: BM; gold-standard Berlin protocol (Berlin Charité Probe One-Step RT-qPCR Kit, New England Biolabs): BR; predictive positive value: PPV; predictive negative value: PNV; diagnostic accuracy: DA.

Figure 1 shows the correlation of Ct cycle threshold values between the RT-qPCR assays for the detection of the SARS-CoV2 virus. We observed a statistically significant strong positive correlation between BM versus BR protocols ($r = 0.746$, $p < 0.0001$) and between the GF-TM and BR ($r = 0.622$, $p < 0.001$) protocols. Likewise, there was a significant moderately positive correlation between the O-S RT-qPCR and BR ($r = 0.482$, $p < 0.001$) protocols.

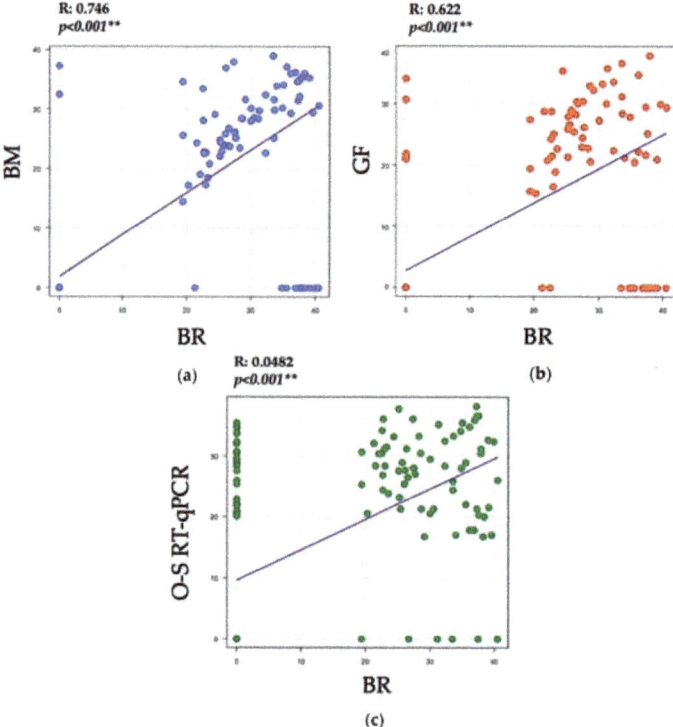

Figure 1. Correlation of Ct values between the RT-qPCR assays for the detection of the SARS-CoV2 virus. (**a**) Correlation of Ct values of E gene between the BM and BR protocols (**b**) Correlation of Ct values of E gene between the GF-TM and BR protocols (**c**) Correlation of Ct values of E gene between the O-S RT-qPCR and BR protocols. Abbreviations: GeneFinder™ COVID-19 Plus RealAmp (In Vitro Diagnostics): GF-TM; One-Step Real-Time RT-PCR (Vitro Master Diagnostica): O-S RT-qPCR; Berlin modified protocol: BM; gold-standard Berlin protocol (Berlin Charité Probe One-Step RT-qPCR Kit, New England Biolabs): BR. (p-value < 0.001 ** is highly significant).

ROC curve analysis indicated that the best diagnostic kit was the BM, with a predictive capacity of 93%; followed by the GF-TM kit, with a predictive capacity of 87%; and the O-S RT-qPCR kit, with a predictive capacity of 79.7% (Table 3).

Table 3. Comparative ROC curve analysis between the RT-qPCR assays for the detection of the SARS-CoV2 virus.

Test Result Variable	Area	Desv. Error [a]	Asymptotic Significance [b]	95% Asymptotic Confidence Interval	
				Lower Limit	Upper Limit
BM	93.0%	0.025	<0.001	88%	98%
GF-TM	87.0%	0.033	<0.002	81%	93%
O-S RT-qPCR	79.7%	0.037	<0.003	72%	87%

Abbreviations: GeneFinder™ COVID-19 Plus RealAmp (In Vitro Diagnostics): GF-TM; One-Step Real-Time RT-PCR (Vitro Master Diagnostica): O-S RT-qPCR; Berlin modified protocol: BM; gold-standard Berlin protocol (Berlin Charité Probe One-Step RT-qPCR Kit, New England Biolabs): BR. (Desv. Error [a]: quantifies the oscillations of the sample mean around the population mean, Asymptotic significance [b]: degree of compatibility between the proposed population value and the available sample information).

In terms of the optimal cycle threshold point evaluated using the Youden index, the BM and GF-TM kits had an excellent specificity and good sensitivity, whereas the O-S RT-qPCR Kit had a good sensitivity but a poor specificity. For the BM Kit, a value greater than 7.2 is considered positive for COVID-19, with a sensitivity of 89.9% and a specificity of 97.6%. Similarly, GF-TM kit values higher than 7.7 are considered positive for COVID-19, with a sensitivity of 79.7% and a specificity of 94%. The O-S RT-qPCR assay is relatively unreliable for the detection of COVID-19, given its optimal cutoff point of 8.4, although it achieves 92.8% sensitivity, whereas its specificity is only 68.7%, meaning that it has a false-positive rate of more than 30%.

To assess the efficiency of the diagnostic kits according to the levels of fluorescence emitted during the amplification process of the E and RNase P genes compared to the gold-standard BR, comparative groups were formed. For group 1, the E gene of BR was taken as a reference; compared to the E gene of GF-TM and the E gene of BM, the efficiency of BR was better than that of BM and GF-TM, as the level of BR fluorescence was 1.4-fold higher than that emitted by the E gene of BM and GF-TM. Similarly, a comparison of the RNase P established that the BR kit fluorescence was 1.3-fold higher than that of GF-TM and BM kits. In group 2, the E gene of the BR was taken as a reference again; however, this time, it was compared with the E gene of GF-TM and the E gene of O-S RT-qPCR, revealing that the efficiency of the E gene of BR was better than that of GF-TM and O-S RT-qPCR, as the BR fluorescence level was 1.3-fold greater than that emitted by the E genes of GF-TM and O-S RT-qPCR. However, for RNase P, the BR kit emitted 0.5-fold more fluorescence than both GF-TM and O-S RT-qPCR. Finally, regarding group 3, the E gene of the BR was evaluated as a reference and compared with the E gene of BM and O-S RT-qPCR; in this case, the behavior of the three kits was similar, as the level of fluorescence of the two compared kits was 0.1-fold higher in relation to that of the BR. In contrast, for RNase P, the BM and O-S RT-qPCR kits presented a 0.7-fold higher level of fluorescence than that of the BR (Table 4).

Table 4. Fold change of fluorescence levels for genes E and N in three kits assessed in comparison to BR.

Gen/Reference Kit	Gen	Group/Kit	Normalized	Fold Change	Relative Expression	Error
E-BR	E	GF-TM	2.75	0.00	1.00	8.26
		BM	1.30	−1.45	2.73	8.36
	E	GF-TM	2.75	0.00	1.00	8.26
		O-S RT-qPCR	1.43	−1.32	2.49	8.33
	E	BM	1.30	0.00	1.00	8.36
		O-S RT-qPCR	1.43	0.13	0.91	8.33
RNAse P-BR	RNAse P	GF-TM	1.93	0.00	1.00	3.75
		BM	0.61	−1.32	2.50	2.75
	RNAse P	GF-TM	1.93	0.00	1.00	3.75
		O-S RT-qPCR	1.40	−0.53	1.44	6.54
	RNAse P	BM	0.61	0.00	1.00	2.75
		O-S RT-qPCR	1.40	0.79	0.58	6.54

Abbreviations: GeneFinder™ COVID-19 Plus RealAmp (In Vitro Diagnostics): GF-TM; One-Step Real-Time RT-PCR (Vitro Master Diagnostica): O-S RT-qPCR; Berlin modified protocol: BM; gold-standard Berlin protocol (Berlin Charité Probe One-Step RT-qPCR Kit, New England Biolabs): BR.

Table 5 describes the basic advantages and disadvantages of the RT-qPCR assays used to screen for of severe acute respiratory syndrome coronavirus 2 (SARS-CoV-2) with respect to the number of genes detected by the kit, processing time, sample volume, and reagent volume.

Table 5. Summary of the basic advantages and disadvantages of the real-time polymerase chain reaction assays used to screen for severe acute respiratory syndrome coronavirus 2 (SARS-CoV-2).

RT-qPCR Assay	Advantages	Disadvantages
GF-TM	Identification of three target genes: genes E, N, and RdRp and their reagents	Dependency on commercial company
	Easy-to-handle preparation of the reagents	Kit for 100 tests High cost of market availability
O-S RT-qPCR	Short amplification time compared to the other kits: 1 h 2′	Dependence on commercial company
	Identification of two gene targets: E and N	Kit for 100 tests
BM	Identification of two target genes: E and N Easy preparation of reagents for large volumes	Kit for 100 tests High cost of market availability
BR	Reference protocol for molecular detection developed by the Charité Virology Institute Recommended by PAHO for the universal monitoring of SARS-CoV-2 Kit for more than 1000 reactions	Personnel required to prepare reagents Manufacturer outside the country

Abbreviations: GeneFinder™ COVID-19 Plus RealAmp (In Vitro Diagnostics): GF-TM; One-Step Real-Time RT-PCR (Vitro Master Diagnostica): O-S RT-qPCR; Berlin modified protocol: BM; gold-standard Berlin protocol (Berlin Charité Probe One-Step RT-qPCR Kit, New England Biolabs): BR.

4. Discussion

Molecular tests based on the identification of specific genes of SARS-CoV-2 that are currently offered on the market and that are used in both symptomatic and asymptomatic patients are characterized by high specificity and low sensitivity, sometimes generating false-negative results [11]. Although the qRT-PCR technique is highly efficient, some studies have shown that it can generate false negatives [11], which could cause a risk to the patient, their family, the community, and the health system, as an infected person could, as a result of an erroneous result, spread the infection. On the other hand, in the clinical setting, it should be clear that the accuracy of diagnostic tests can be influenced by the stage of the patient's disease and the quality of the samples [12]. In addition, several authors have shown that false negatives can be determined by multiple factors, including poorly trained personnel, incorrectly collected samples, possible errors in the batches of primers and other reagents used for analysis, lack of information from manufacturers, and traceability of the reference materials. Furthermore, it should be emphasized that the RT-PCR technique is not 100% sensitive and specific for other pathogens of importance in the clinical setting, as indicated by data obtained for the diagnosis of SARS-CoV-2 [13,14].

In clinical samples, a positive sample is defined as a Ct value of any specific gene for SARS-CoV-2 of less than or equal to 43; on the contrary, an amplification value greater than 43 is considered a negative result. As an internal control, RNAse P must be present in each sample, and its Ct value must be less than 35 to validate the test. If this gene does not amplify, the test must be invalidated, and the extraction must be repeated (https://www.aidian.eu/uploads/NO-Dokumenter-og-materiell/ES-Products/ELITech/GeneFinder-COVID-19-RealAmp-Plus-Kit_Full-manual_V1_IVD.PDF accessed on 18 August 2022). According to our results, discordant samples were observed in 37 of the 152 samples analyzed. This discrepancy could be associated with the design of the primers by the manufacturers and the fact that the target genes to be identified vary between the diagnostic kits, which might cause changes om the Ct values owing to the amount of RNA assessed; likewise, the viral load of the patient can affect the results. Furthermore, to date, there is no standard methodology, such as calibrators or reference material, among others, that allows for standardization of values between kits offered on the market.

The design of real-time multiplex PCR kits, which identify several target genes in a single reaction, offers lower efficiency in terms of fluorescence levels, in addition to longer amplification times compared to a monoplex PCR, which recognizes a target gene in a single reaction. The most common cause of this effect is the competition for components of the master mix, such as dNTPs and MgCl2, among others, i.e., the more genes of interest identified, as in the case of kits for the diagnosis of SARS-CoV-2 investigated in the present study (BM, GF-TM, and O-S RT-q-PCR, which identify the RdRp, N, E, and RNAse P genes in a single reaction) the lower the levels of fluorescence and the longer the amplification time compared to the kit BR, which identifies only the E and RNAse P genes, which can explain, at least in part, the calculated FC data [15,16].

We evaluated the diagnostic accuracy of four commercially available RT-qPCR methods for the detection of SARS-CoV2 from respiratory samples referred to the Laboratorio Carvajal IPS, SAS in Tunja, Boyacá, Colombia. Our results can help to ensure that tests offered for the screening of SARS-CoV-2 in Colombian patients who are suspected of having COVID-19 meet the criteria for optimal performance.

The current study provides a comprehensive and independent comparison of the analytical performance of primer–probe sets for SARS-CoV-2 testing in several parts of the world. Our findings show a high similarity with respect to the analytical sensitivities for SARS-CoV-2 detection, indicating that the outcomes of different assays are comparable. The primary exception to this is the One-Step Real-Time RT-PCR (Vitro Master Diagnostica, Spain) (O-S RT-qPCR), which had the lowest sensitivity of the investigated kits, consistent with the results of a previous study [17].

This study demonstrates that RT-qPCR significantly improves accuracy and reduces the false-negative rate in the diagnosis of SARS-CoV-2 in pharyngeal swab specimens, which represent a convenient and simple sampling method. Furthermore, qPCR is sensitive and suitable for low-viral-load specimens from patients under isolation and observation who may not be exhibiting clinical symptoms. Finally, RT-qPCR can be used to quantitatively monitor patients to evaluate disease progression [18].

We conclude that the GF-TM and BM protocols offer optimal sensitivity and specificity, as well as results to those of the gold-standard BR protocol, possibly due to the design of the primers. We recommend evaluating the diagnostic accuracy of the OS-RT-qPCR protocol in future studies with a larger number of samples. We recommend that laboratories evaluate the diagnostic accuracy of RT-qPCR assays used for the detection of the SARS-CoV2 virus to ensure reliable results for patients who are suspected of being COVID-19-positive.

Supplementary Materials: The following are available online at https://www.mdpi.com/article/10.3390/tropicalmed7090240/s1, Table S1: Primary data obtained from four real-time polymerase chain reaction assays for the detection of SARS-CoV-2 in respiratory samples from Tunja, Boyacá, Colombia, Table S2. Description of the concordant and discordant results found in 152 analyzed samples. A. Concordant results of positive samples between the investigated kits and their amplification Ct, B. Concordant results of negative samples between the investigated different kits, C. Discordant results between the investigated kits.

Author Contributions: Conceptualization, L.H.S.-N., M.F.-C. and N.A.S.; methodology, L.H.S.-N., M.F.-C. and N.A.S.; software, L.H.S.-N., Ó.C. and J.P.C.; validation, L.H.S.-N., Ó.C. and J.P.C.; formal analysis, L.H.S.-N., M.F.-C. and N.A.S.; investigation, L.H.S.-N., Ó.C., J.P.C., M.F.-C. and N.A.S.; resources, L.H.S.-N., Ó.C., J.P.C., M.F.-C. and N.A.S.; data curation, L.H.S.-N.; writing—original draft preparation, L.H.S.-N., M.F.-C. and N.A.S.; writing—review and editing, L.H.S.-N., M.F.-C. and N.A.S.; visualization, L.H.S.-N., M.F.-C. and N.A.S.; supervision, Ó.C., J.P.C., M.F.-C. and N.A.S.; project administration, L.H.S.-N., Ó.C. and J.P.C.; funding acquisition, L.H.S.-N., Ó.C. and J.P.C. All authors have read and agreed to the published version of the manuscript.

Funding: This study was derived from the research study entitled: "Fortalecimiento de capacidades instaladas de Ciencia y Tecnología de Carvajal Laboratorios IPS SAS para atender problemáticas asociadas con agentes biológicos de alto riesgo para la salud humana en el Departamento de Boyacá", funded by the Ministerio de Ciencia Tecnología e Innovación (Minciencias) (SIGP CODE: 78326; BPIN: 2020000100102).

Institutional Review Board Statement: The study was conducted according to the guidelines of the Declaration of Helsinki, and the protocol was approved by the Ethics Review Committee of the Universidad Pedagógica y Tecnológica de Colombia on 18 November 2021.

Informed Consent Statement: No informed consent was given for the research because previously characterized RNAs from the biobank of the molecular biology area of Carvajal, IPS laboratory were used.

Acknowledgments: The authors from Laboratorio Carvajal IPS, SAS acknowledge the hard work of their research and laboratory team members. This manuscript was developed within the framework of an institutional agreement between the Research Group in Biomedical Sciences of the UPTC (GICBUPTC) of Universidad Pedagógica y Tecnológica de Colombia, Tunja, Boyacá, Colombia, and the Laboratorio Carvajal IPS, SAS.

Conflicts of Interest: The authors declare no conflict of interest.

References

1. Wang, M.-Y.; Zhao, R.; Gao, L.-J.; Gao, X.-F.; Wang, D.-P.; Cao, J.-M. SARS-CoV-2: Structure, Biology, and Structure-Based Therapeutics Development. *Front. Cell. Infect. Microbiol.* **2020**, *10*, 587269. [CrossRef] [PubMed]
2. Kumar, A.; Prasoon, P.; Kumari, C.; Pareek, V.; Faiq, M.A.; Narayan, R.K.; Kulandhasamy, M.; Kant, K. SARS-CoV-2-specific virulence factors in COVID-19. *J. Med. Virol.* **2021**, *93*, 1343–1350. [CrossRef] [PubMed]
3. Liu, Q.; Qin, C.; Liu, M.; Liu, J. Effectiveness and safety of SARS-CoV-2 vaccine in real-world studies: A systematic review and meta-analysis. *Infect. Dis. Poverty* **2021**, *10*, 132. [CrossRef] [PubMed]
4. Ling, Y.; Zhong, J.; Luo, J. Safety and effectiveness of SARS-CoV-2 vaccines: A systematic review and meta-analysis. *J. Med. Virol.* **2021**, *93*, 6486–6495. [CrossRef] [PubMed]
5. Wu, F.; Zhao, S.; Yu, B.; Chen, Y.-M.; Wang, W.; Song, Z.-G.; Hu, Y.; Tao, Z.-W.; Tian, J.-H.; Pei, Y.-Y.; et al. A new coronavirus associated with human respiratory disease in China. *Nature* **2020**, *579*, 265–269. [CrossRef] [PubMed]
6. Wang, H.; Jean, S.; Eltringham, R.; Madison, J.; Snyder, P.; Tu, H.; Jones, D.M.; Leber, A.L. Mutation-Specific SARS-CoV-2 PCR Screen: Rapid and Accurate Detection of Variants of Concern and the Identification of a Newly Emerging Variant with Spike L452R Mutation. *J. Clin. Microbiol.* **2021**, *59*, e00926-21. [CrossRef]
7. Liu, M.; Li, Q.; Zhou, J.; Ai, W.; Zheng, X.; Zeng, J.; Liu, Y.; Xiang, X.; Guo, R.; Li, X.; et al. Value of swab types and collection time on SARS-CoV-2 detection using RT-PCR assay. *J. Virol. Methods* **2020**, *286*, 113974. [CrossRef] [PubMed]
8. McAuley, J.; Fraser, C.; Paraskeva, E.; Trajcevska, E.; Sait, M.; Wang, N.; Bert, E.; Purcell, D.; Strugnell, R. Optimal preparation of SARS-CoV-2 viral transport medium for culture. *Virol. J.* **2021**, *18*, 53. [CrossRef] [PubMed]

9. Castro, A.L.L.; Rodríguez, R.B.; Mojica, F.I.L.; Andrade, J.L.C. *Manual de Toma de Muestras para Análisis Microbiologico*, 1st ed.; Saludcapital: Bogota, Colombia, 2015; Volume 2015.
10. Corman, V.M.; Landt, O.; Kaiser, M.; Molenkamp, R.; Meijer, A.; Chu, D.K.W.; Bleicker, T.; Brünink, S.; Schneider, J.; Schmidt, M.L.; et al. Detection of 2019 novel coronavirus (2019-nCoV) by real-time RT-PCR. *Eurosurveillance* **2020**, *25*, 2000045. [CrossRef]
11. Pecoraro, V.; Negro, A.; Pirotti, T.; Trenti, T. Estimate false-negative RT-PCR rates for SARS-CoV-2. A systematic review and meta-analysis. *Eur. J. Clin. Investig.* **2022**, *52*, e13706. [CrossRef] [PubMed]
12. Guo, W.; Zhou, Q.; Xu, J. Negative results in nucleic acid test of COVID-19 patients: Assessment from the perspective of clinical laboratories. *Ann. Palliat. Med.* **2020**, *9*, 4246–4251. [CrossRef] [PubMed]
13. Eguchi, H.; Horita, N.; Ushio, R.; Kato, I.; Nakajima, Y.; Ota, E.; Kaneko, T. Diagnostic test accuracy of antigenaemia assay for PCR-proven cytomegalovirus infection—systematic review and meta-analysis. *Clin. Microbiol. Infect.* **2017**, *23*, 907–915. [CrossRef] [PubMed]
14. Wei, Z.; Zhang, X.; Wei, C.; Yao, L.; Li, Y.; Xu, H.; Jia, Y.; Guo, R.; Wu, Y.; Yang, K.; et al. Diagnostic accuracy of in-house real-time PCR assay for Mycobacterium tuberculosis: A systematic review and meta-analysis. *BMC Infect. Dis.* **2019**, *19*, 701. [CrossRef] [PubMed]
15. Kim, H.-K.; Oh, S.-H.; Yun, K.A.; Sung, H.; Kim, M.-N. Comparison of Anyplex II RV16 with the xTAG Respiratory Viral Panel and Seeplex RV15 for Detection of Respiratory Viruses. *J. Clin. Microbiol.* **2013**, *51*, 1137–1141. [CrossRef] [PubMed]
16. Gwyn, S.; Abubakar, A.; Akinmulero, O.; Bergeron, E.; Blessing, U.N.; Chaitram, J.; Coughlin, M.M.; Dawurung, A.B.; Dickson, F.N.; Esiekpe, M.; et al. Performance of SARS-CoV-2 Antigens in a Multiplex Bead Assay for Integrated Serological Surveillance of Neglected Tropical and Other Diseases. *Am. J. Trop. Med. Hyg.* **2022**, *107*, 260–267. [CrossRef] [PubMed]
17. Vogels, C.B.F.; Brito, A.F.; Wyllie, A.L.; Fauver, J.R.; Ott, I.M.; Kalinich, C.C.; Petrone, M.E.; Casanovas-Massana, A.; Muenker, M.C.; Moore, A.J.; et al. Analytical Sensitivity and Efficiency Comparisons of SARS-CoV-2 qRT-PCR Primer-Probe Sets. *Nat. Microbiol.* **2020**, *5*, 1299–1305. [CrossRef] [PubMed]
18. Dong, L.; Zhou, J.; Niu, C.; Wang, Q.; Pan, Y.; Sheng, S.; Wang, X.; Zhang, Y.; Yang, J.; Liu, M.; et al. Highly accurate and sensitive diagnostic detection of SARS-CoV-2 by digital PCR. *Talanta* **2021**, *224*, 121726. [CrossRef] [PubMed]

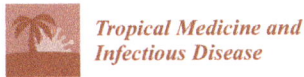 *Tropical Medicine and Infectious Disease*

Article

Transmission Dynamics and Genomic Epidemiology of Emerging Variants of SARS-CoV-2 in Bangladesh

Md. Abu Sayeed [1,2], Jinnat Ferdous [1,2], Otun Saha [3], Shariful Islam [1,2], Shusmita Dutta Choudhury [1,2], Josefina Abedin [1,2], Mohammad Mahmudul Hassan [4,5] and Ariful Islam [1,2,6,*]

1. EcoHealth Alliance New York, New York, NY 10018, USA
2. Institute of Epidemiology, Disease Control and Research (IEDCR), Dhaka 1212, Bangladesh
3. Department of Microbiology, Noakhali Science and Technology University, Noakhali 3814, Bangladesh
4. Faculty of Veterinary Medicine, Chattogram Veterinary and Animal Sciences University, Chattogram 4225, Bangladesh
5. Queensland Alliance for One Health Sciences, School of Veterinary Science, The University of Queensland, Gatton, QLD 4343, Australia
6. Centre for Integrative Ecology, School of Life and Environmental Science, Deakin University, Melbourne, VIC 3216, Australia
* Correspondence: arif@ecohealthalliance.org

Abstract: With the progression of the global SARS-CoV-2 pandemic, the new variants have become more infectious and continue spreading at a higher rate than pre-existing ones. Thus, we conducted a study to explore the epidemiology of emerging variants of SARS-CoV-2 that circulated in Bangladesh from December 2020 to September 2021, representing the 2nd and 3rd waves. We collected new cases and deaths per million daily data with the reproduction rate. We retrieved 928 SARS-CoV-2 sequences from GISAID and performed phylogenetic tree construction and mutation analysis. Case counts were lower initially at the end of 2020, during January–February and April–May 2021, whereas the death toll reached the highest value of 1.587 per million on the first week of August and then started to decline. All the variants (α, β, δ, η) were prevalent in the capital city, Dhaka, with dispersion to large cities, such as Sylhet and Chattogram. The B.1.1.25 lineage was prevalent during December 2020, but the B.1.617.2/δ variant was later followed by the B.1.351/β variant. The phylogeny revealed that the various strains found in Bangladesh could be from numerous countries. The intra-cluster and inter-cluster communication began in Bangladesh soon after the virus arrived. The prominent amino acid substitution was D614G from December 2020 to July 2021 (93.5 to 100%). From February–April, one of the VOC's important mutations, N501Y substitution, was also estimated at 51.8%, 76.1%, and 65.1% for the α, β and γ variants, respectively. The γ variant's unique mutation K417T was detected only at 1.8% in February. Another frequent mutation was P681R, a salient feature of the δ variant, detected in June (88.2%) and July (100%). Furthermore, only one γ variant was detected during the entire second and third wave, whereas no η variant was observed in this period. This rapid growth in the number of variants identified across Bangladesh shows virus adaptation and a lack of strict quarantine, prompting periodic genomic surveillance to foresee the spread of new variants, if any, and to take preventive measures as soon as possible.

Keywords: reproduction rate; phylogenetic analysis; clade GK; D614G; P681R

Citation: Sayeed, M.A.; Ferdous, J.; Saha, O.; Islam, S.; Choudhury, S.D.; Abedin, J.; Hassan, M.M.; Islam, A. Transmission Dynamics and Genomic Epidemiology of Emerging Variants of SARS-CoV-2 in Bangladesh. *Trop. Med. Infect. Dis.* 2022, 7, 197. https://doi.org/10.3390/tropicalmed7080197

Academic Editors: Peter A. Leggat, John Frean and Lucille Blumberg

Received: 3 July 2022
Accepted: 11 August 2022
Published: 20 August 2022

Publisher's Note: MDPI stays neutral with regard to jurisdictional claims in published maps and institutional affiliations.

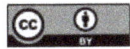

Copyright: © 2022 by the authors. Licensee MDPI, Basel, Switzerland. This article is an open access article distributed under the terms and conditions of the Creative Commons Attribution (CC BY) license (https://creativecommons.org/licenses/by/4.0/).

1. Introduction

The novel viral pneumonia cases, characterized by high fever, dry cough, and occasionally catastrophic hypoxia, reported for the first time in Wuhan, China, in December 2019 had an epidemiological link with the live animal market [1]. The etiological agent was named severe acute respiratory syndrome coronavirus 2 (SARS-CoV-2) by the International Committee on Taxonomy of Viruses (ICTV) [2]. The first sequence of SARS-CoV-2 grouped the virus under the Sarbecovirus subgenus of the Coronaviridae family, typically categorized as Beta coronavirus [3,4]. By May 2021, the virus spanned over 203 countries of the world, with around 170 million cases and 0.35 million deaths [5], with a case fatality rate of 10% [6], which is higher than the seasonal flu outbreak (0.1–0.2%) [7]. SARS-CoV-2 is a highly recombinogenic virus, with 29903 nucleotides. The single-strand RNA virus has six functional open reading frames (ORFs), including replicas (ORF1a/ORF1b), spike (S), envelope, membrane, and nucleocapsids organized from 5' to 3' directions [8].

Mutations of the virus arise in almost every cycle. Frequent mutations, which are estimated roughly at 1.17–1.36×10^{-3} base substitutions per site per year [9] of the genomic composition, make the virus prone to continuous evolution, ultimately leading to the formation of new variants (variant of concern (VOC): Alpha/α (lineage B.1.1.7), Beta/β (lineage B.1.351), Gamma/γ (lineage P.1), Delta/δ (lineage B.1.617.2); variant of interest (VOI): Lambda (lineage C.37), Mu (lineage B.1.621), Epsilon (lineages B.1.429, B.1.427, CAL.20C), Zeta (lineage P.2), Theta (lineage P.3), Eta (lineage B.1.525), Iota (lineage B.1.526), Kappa (lineage B.1.617.1)). Several variants of SARS-CoV-2 have raised public health awareness due to their infectious nature. Among them, the α variant under the Pango lineage B.1.1.7 and GISAID clade GRY was first documented in the United Kingdom in September 2020 (a.k.a. 20B/501Y.V1 variant of concern (VOC) 202012/01). The β variant under the Pango lineage B.1.351 and GISAID clade GH/501Y.V2 was first detected in South Africa in May 2020. On the other hand, the VOC under P.1 lineage and GR clade/501Y.V3 was designated as Gamma γ VOC, and was isolated in Brazil. Another important VOC is δ, which originated in India in October 2020 and belongs to the B.1.617.2 lineage and G/478K.V1 clade (https://www.who.int/en/activities/tracking-SARS-CoV-2-variants/, accessed on 25 January 2022) [10]. The current circulating virus differs from the Wuhan variant at around 20 points in their genomes [11]. The different variants, such as the Brazilian variant P.1 lineage, emerged from the B.1.1.28 lineage due to 10 unique mutations in the virus genome, including spike protein (D614G), receptor-binding domain (RBD) (K417T, E484K, and N501Y), N-terminal domain (NTD) (L18F, T20N, P26S, D138Y, and R190S) and furin cleavage site (H655Y) [12]. The lineage B.1.1.7 emerged due to the major change in the amino acid asparagine by tyrosine at the 501 position of the spike protein, along with other mutations, increasing the transmissibility of the virus. Many more variants of the mother SARS-CoV-2 virus strain have also been reported in different countries and regions such as California, Nigeria, and India [13,14].

Phylogenetic analysis of the GISAID sequences identified different clusters named clades, where O was the ancestral type detected from Wuhan [15,16]. In early January and February 2020, the viruses were classified into clades 19A and 19B (L and S) [17]. Around 70% prevalent clade was L-type detected in the early stages from Wuhan, where S-type was also the ancestral type whose frequency decreased over the next few months. Again, A2a or Clade G, the ancestor of clades 20A-C, were identified in February, characterized by a specific non-synonymous mutation (D614G) in the spike protein [11]. Bangladesh experienced the start of the pandemic in March 2020 [18]. Since then, the devastating spread at the community level has continued. In the earlier period, the virus spread following a typical exponential growth curve with a higher reproduction rate [19]. Initially, to curb the transmission, the Government of Bangladesh implemented a countrywide lockdown procedure, but some unusual activities maintained the upward trend of the curve. However, by the end of July 2020, the curve sloped down, and the reproduction rate started to decline [20]. Meanwhile, the world started facing the challenges of different new variants of SARS-CoV-2. By December 2020, the new UK and South African variants were detected in Bangladesh [21]. In addition, the neighboring country, India, faced the havoc of COVID-19. After the end of May 2021, around 28 million people were affected, with the death of around 0.32 million [22]. The sequencing of the virus isolated from affected patients in India revealed a shared set of four genetic variant mutations in the genome of the core virus, which enhanced the effectiveness and transmissibility at an unbound rate [23].

In Bangladesh, the first α variant B.1.1.7 was detected at the end of January 2021 (GISAID). Since then, the case count has started to increase dramatically. Finally, the Government imposed the countrywide second lockdown procedure. Meanwhile, the sequencing of the virus identified 84 α-VOCs, which were first detected in the UK, 28 β-VOCs, which were first detected in South Africa, 44 δ-VOCs, which were first detected in India, 1 γ-VOC, which was first detected in Brazil/Japan, and 14 variant under investigation (VUI) Epsilon variants, first detected in Nigeria (www.GISAID.org, accessed on 15 January 2022). However, after two months of the lockdown, the Government decided against resuming normal activities. Therefore, in this study, we presented the case and death rates per million and showed the epidemiological and genomic diversity of SARS-CoV-2 variant strains in the Bangladesh population.

2. Materials and Methods

2.1. Temporal and Spatial Epidemiology of COVID-19

The Government of Bangladesh has been reporting daily COVID-19 cases through media briefings since 8 March 2020. The database is open for everyone to learn about the existing situation. We collected daily new cases and new deaths per million from 1 December 2020 to 15 September 2021. The number of cases and deaths per day was extracted from an online web portal (https://ourworldindata.org/coronavirus, accessed on 25 March 2022) because the data are open-sourced and the author declared that all visualizations, data and code produced by the web are completely open under the Creative Commons BY license and anyone has the permission to use, distribute and reproduce the data in any medium [24]. As the WHO and Worldometer coronavirus databases are also being updated on a real-time basis for every parameter, we included data from these two websites also [22,25]. The number of new cases and new death per day per million were presented graphically. From these data, we calculated the reproduction rate (R_t) of COVID-19 for each day and presented them graphically [19]. We produced a geospatial map in ArcGIS 10.3, visualizing the spatial distribution of different VOCs according to the districts of Bangladesh [20].

2.2. Genomic Epidemiology

2.2.1. Retrieval of Genomic Sequences and Metadata

From the Global Initiative on Sharing All Influenza Data (GISAID), we retrieved SARS-CoV-2 genomic metadata of Bangladeshi strains from 1 December 2020 to 15 September 2021. A total of 928 variant sequences were deposited during this time frame and were used in this study. We considered the genome length of 29,000 nucleotides for substitution mutation and phylogenetic analysis. This study did not include partial genomes with exceptionally high variation counts, gaps, or genomes that lacked a complete history of the patients/sampling location/collection date. Furthermore, genomic sequences that contained legionary characters (N, R, X, and Y) other than A, T, G, and C were omitted from the study [26]. We carried out the selection process by using manual sorting in MEGA 7. After that, we used pyfasta (https://github.com/brentp/pyfasta, accessed on 25 March 2022) to segment the whole genome into 2 different files, each with approximately 450 sequences. We aligned each file using the MAFFT web server, employing access modifiers, as described by Katoh et al. [27]. We used the complete genome sequence of the SARS-CoV-2 Wuhan-Hu-1 strain (accession NC 045512, version NC 045512.2). To filter all the ambiguous and low-quality sequences, we used the Sequence Cleaner (https://github.com/metageni/Sequence-Cleaner, accessed on 25 March 2022), applying specified parameters of minimum length ($m = 3822$), percentage N ($mn = 0$), maintaining all duplicates, and remove any ambiguous sequences. To find the gap-containing strains for deletion analysis, we used the SeqKit toolbox [28]. To delete the internal stop codon-containing sequences, we used the SEquence DAtaset builder [29]. Reference genomes from various nations were chosen based on the BLAST hit of the selected genomes (Supplementary File S1). The genomic sequences of the SARS-CoV-2 strains were aligned using the online Virus Pathogen Resource (https://www.viprbrc.org/, accessed on 25 March 2022) database and the MEGA 7 tool. The MSA file was then loaded with Jalview visualization software to remove redundancies from the sequences under study [30].

2.2.2. Genome-Wide Analysis of Bangladeshi SARS-CoV-2 Variants

We initially analyzed the SARS-CoV-2 sequence by using "One Click Workflows" (https://ngphylogeny.fr/workflows/oneclick/, accessed on 4 October 2021), as described by Lemoine et al. [31]. We followed the standard process of phylogenetic tree building steps, including multiple alignments, alignment curation, tree formation, and visualization described by earlier researchers [32–35]. We used a web-based program, "Nextstrain" (https://clades.nextstrain.org, accessed on 25 March 2022), to generate the clade-designated tree. We used a subset of all the emerging virus sequences for making variant-specific phylogenetic trees using the neighbor-joining methods described by Islam et al. [19]. Furthermore, to identify the possible transmission routes of every reported variant in Bangladesh, all interactive phylogenetic reconstructions were carefully evaluated to discover the likely ancestral sources of the Bangladeshi SARS-CoV-2 variant genomes. Each branch tip bearing a Bangladeshi genome found in accessible Nextstrain clades was recognized in the original phylogeny. That branch was then examined backwards in the tree, until all the closely related exogenous strains and their countries of origin were discovered. We used the automated global map-based analysis in auspice version 0.5.0 (https://auspice.us, accessed on 25 March 2022) by Nextstrain [36] to visualize the transmission paths.

Finally, the aligned sequences were viewed for mutation analysis with MEGA 7 and the Virus Pathogen Resource (https://www.viprbrc.org/, accessed on 25 March 2022) to identify the deletions and insertions compared to the reference genome. Furthermore, mutations that result in amino acid substitutions were investigated using the Wuhan reference sequence and the GISAID platform, which included the CoVserver enabled by GISAID in the GIDAID EpiCoV database, as well as a blast (https://blast.ncbi.nlm.nih.gov/, accessed on 25 March 2022) of the entire genome and individual proteins [37].

3. Results

3.1. Epidemiology of COVID-19 in Bangladesh

3.1.1. Temporal Distribution of COVID-19 Cases and Deaths during 2nd and 3rd Wave

At the end of 2020, COVID-19 cases were 6.157 per million, and the death rate was 0.17 per million in Bangladesh. During March–April and June–July 2021, we witnessed the 2nd and 3rd waves of COVID-19, respectively. The cases started increasing on 2 March, and reached the highest on 7 April 2021. Then, the case counts declined gradually and reached the lowest count in the middle of May. After that, the case count suddenly increased from the middle of June and reached 53.5 cases per million at the end of the month. From 1 July, the cases per million increased and peaked at 97.5 on 28 July. From August onwards, the new cases reduced slowly and reached 11.7 cases per million on 15 September 2021 (Figure 1).

Similarly, the number of deaths increased from the end of March to the end of April. The death count reached the optimum level of around 0.680 death per million cases on 19 April. Then, there was a gradual declining trend with a zigzag pattern. However, after 13 June, the number of deaths increased again and reached 0.698 per million on 30 June. From the start of July, the deaths per million followed an upward trend to reach its highest at 1.551 on 27 July. Again, the death toll decreased to 1.275 per million on 30 July, then started floating and reached its highest at 1.587 per million on 10 August, then finally declined and reduced to 0.247 on 15 September 2021 (Figure 1).

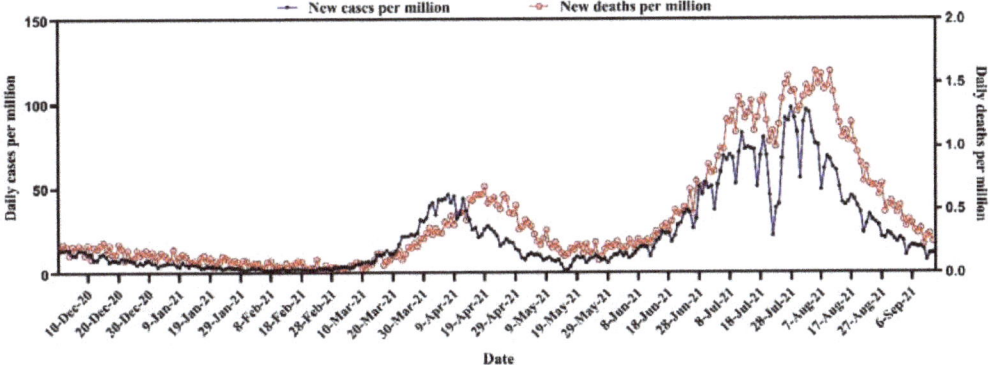

Figure 1. Temporal trend of COVID-19 cases and deaths in Bangladesh (per million).

3.1.2. Daily Reproduction Rate of COVID-19 Cases during 2nd and 3rd Wave

The overall R_t was just over one (1.02) on 1 December 2020. The R_t decreased to less than one and maintained a plateau until 22 February 2021. After that, the reproduction rate increased by over one and reached its highest at 1.67 on 23 March 2021. Then, the reproduction rate started declining and dropped below one again and reached its lowest value of 0.57 on 14 May 2021. However, from May 20, the reproduction rate started to increase and reached 1.45 on 28 June 2021. In the first half of July, the R_t was over one and decreased below one on 19 July. The R_t was less than one until 23 July and then again increased above one during the last few days of July, which persisted until 4 August. After that, the R_t decreased to less than one, and this trend persisted until 15 September 2021 (Figure 2).

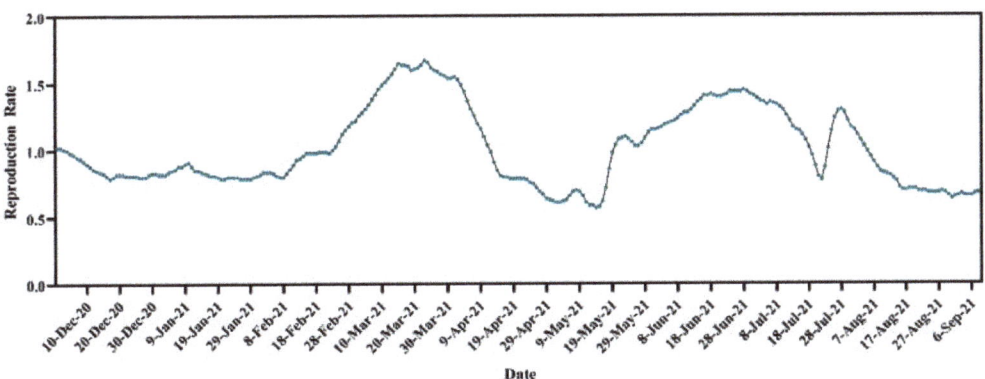

Figure 2. Temporal dynamics of reproduction rate of SARS-CoV-2 cases in Bangladesh (https://ourworldindata.org/coronavirus, accessed on 15 September 2021).

3.1.3. Spatial Distribution of Emerging Variants of COVID-19 in Bangladesh

The highest percentage of all the variants, α, β, γ, and δ, was found in the Dhaka district. In addition, the α variant was also prevalent in the Sylhet and Chattogram districts. The Chattogram district also had a higher frequency of the β variant. Another peripheral district, Nawabganj, had a higher number of cases due to the δ variant (Figure 3). The frequency of the area-specific VOCs is given in Supplementary File S2.

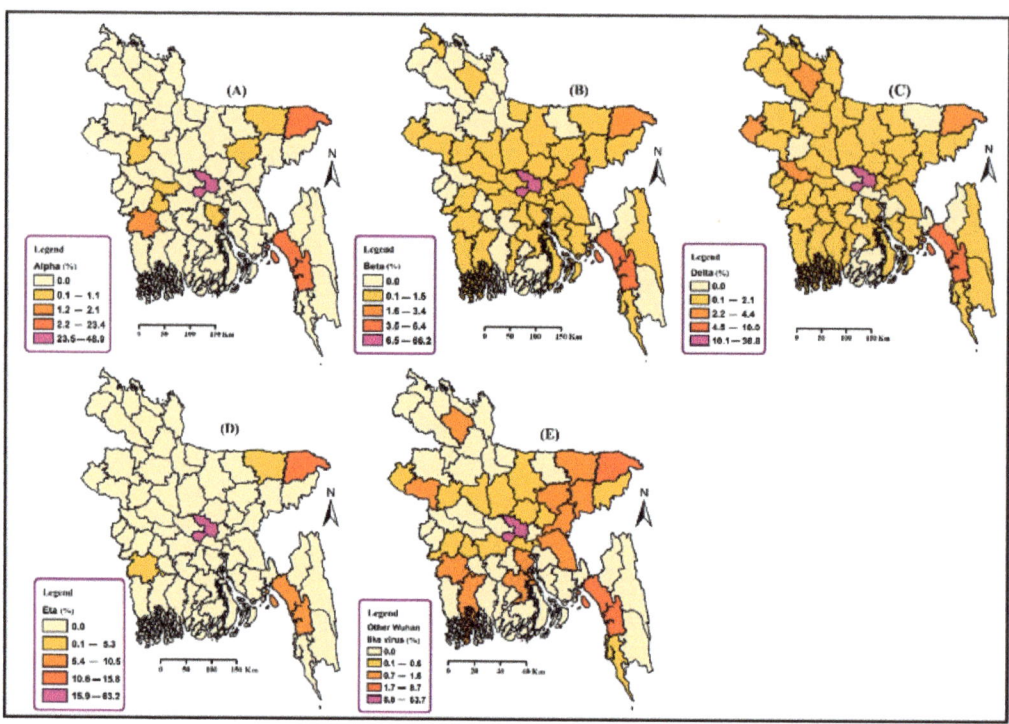

Figure 3. Spatial distribution of (**A**) Alpha variants (%); (**B**) Beta (%); (**C**) Delta (%); (**D**) Eta (%) variants of SARS-CoV-2; and (**E**) other Wuhan-like strains (%) in Bangladesh from December 2020 to 15 September 2021. We have omitted the Gamma variant as only one sequence has been reported in GISAID and visualization of a single virus might mislead the geographic distribution of the variant.

3.1.4. Clade and Lineage Diversity of SARS-CoV-2 in Bangladesh

We have studied 928 genome sequences of SARS-CoV-2 reported from Bangladesh from December 2020 to 15 September 2021. From December 2020 to February 2021, the GR clade was the most prevalent (87.04, 77.7, 65%, respectively) among all the clades. However, in March and April, GH was Bangladesh's most highly distributed clade. The scenario changed in May and June, when most cases were affected by strains under the clade GK. The GK clade prevailed in Bangladesh until July 2021 (Figure 4).

A variety of lineages have reigned in Bangladesh since December 2020. In December 2020, January, and February 2021, the most prevalent lineage was B.1.1.25 (83.3, 74.1, and 38.3%, respectively). However, along with B.1.1.25, another lineage, the α variant B.1.1.7, also increased in Bangladesh during February 2021. However, in March and April, the β variant B.1.351.3 was the most dominant (67.8% and 76.7%, respectively), whereas lineage B.1.617.2 (δ variant) was predominant in May, June and July 2021 (43.2, 87.6 and 100%, respectively) (Figure 5).

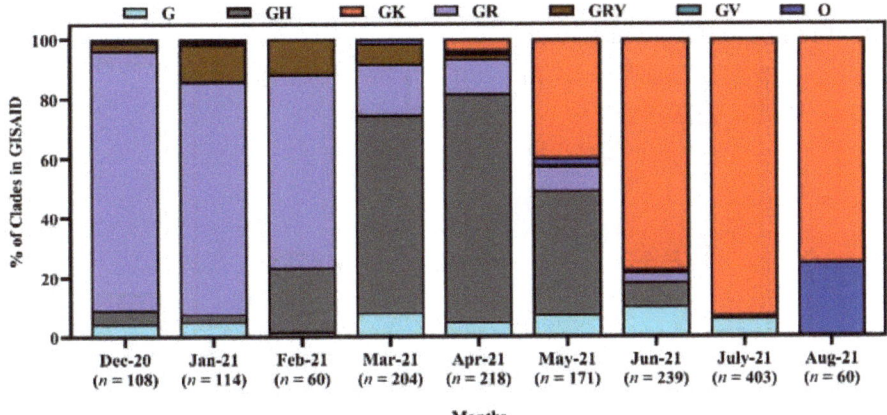

Figure 4. Clade diversity of SARS-CoV-2 in Bangladesh from December 2020 to September 15, 2021. Here, the clades are based on the marker variants **G**: C241T,C3037T,A23403G includes S-D614G; **GH**: C241T,C3037T,A23403G,G25563T includes S-D614G + NS3-Q57H; **GK**: C241T,C3037T,A23403G,C22995A S-D614G + S-T478K; **GR**: C241T,C3037T,A23403G,G28882A includes S-D614G + N-G204R; **GRY**: C241T,C3037T,21765-21770del,21991-21993del,A23063T,A23403G,G28882A includes S-H69del, S-V70del, S-Y144del, S-N501Y + S-D614G + N-G204R; **GV**: C241T,C3037T,A23403G,C22227T includes S-D614G + S-A222V; **O**: Includes S: C8782T,T28144C includes NS8-L84S + L: C241,C3037,A23403,C8782,G11083,G26144,T28144 + V: G11083T,G26144T NSP6-L37F + NS3-G251V [38].

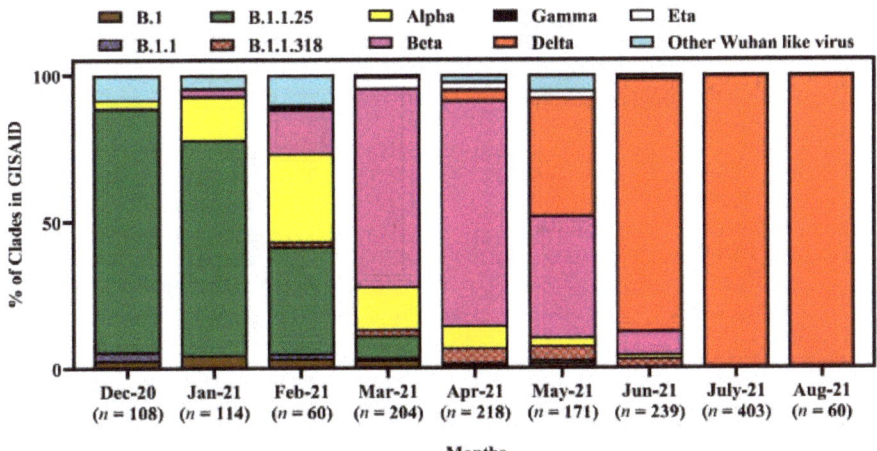

Figure 5. Lineage diversity of SARS-CoV-2 in Bangladesh from December 2020 to 15 September 2021.

3.2. Transmission Route of Emerging Variants in Bangladesh

Figure 6 shows the transmission pathways of the emerging variants from different countries to Bangladesh. The VOC B.1.1.7 was mainly introduced into Bangladesh from European countries, such as Germany, UAE, African countries, and the Philippines. The B.1.525 entered mainly from African countries to Bangladesh. In addition, the Delta (B.1.617.2) variant entered from India (Figure 6).

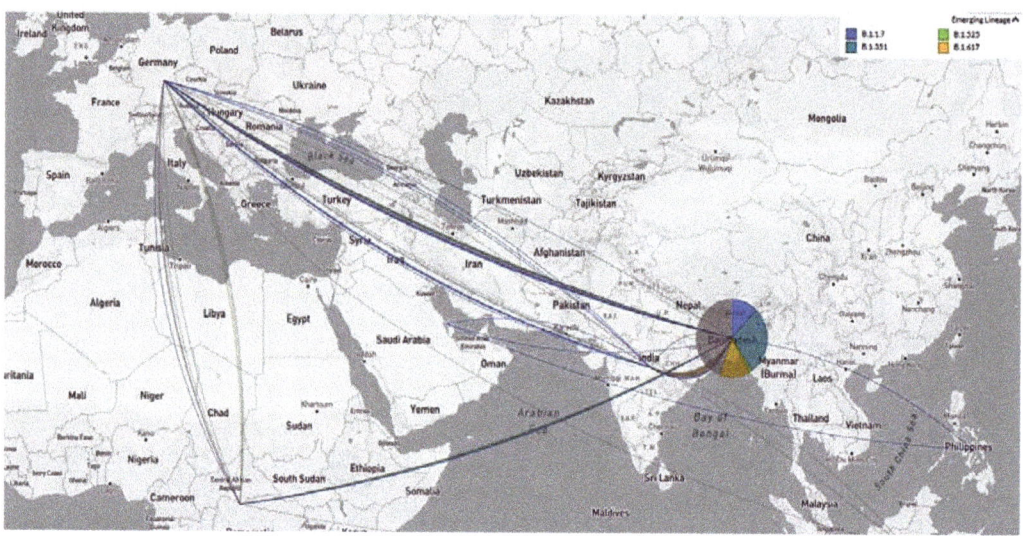

Figure 6. Emerging variant's geographic transmission lines to Bangladesh (live display at nextstrain.org/ncov, accessed on 15 September 2021).

3.3. Genomic Epidemiology of SARS-CoV-2 Variant of Concern (VOC) in Bangladesh

3.3.1. 20I/501Y.V1, Alpha Variants/B.1.1.7 in Bangladesh

The Alpha variants/B.1.1.7 of SARS-CoV-2 in Bangladesh showed fourteen different instances of clustering with sequences from around the world. Most of the Bangladeshi strains clustered with virus sequences from Singapore, France, Ireland, England, Norway, Bulgaria, Switzerland, South Korea, Netherlands, Austria, Hong Kong, India, and Romania. Some of the reported sequences clustered with sequences from the USA, Canada, Germany, and Sweden (Figure 7).

Figure 7 also suggests multiple viral introductions into Bangladesh from several countries. The sample EPI-ISL-1750957 from Bangladesh is closely related to the sample EPI-ISL-878860 isolated in England. Another Bangladeshi sample EPI-ISL-1750958 is highly similar to the sample EPI-ISL-1754743 from France. The two samples EPI-ISL-1750960 and EPI-ISL-1550506 are close to the EPI-ISL-1511507 sample from the USA, EPI-ISL-1742872 from Canada, and EPI-ISL-1743960 from the USA. The distinct Bangladeshi sample EPI-ISL-1669904 has also shown similarities with samples from France (EPI-ISL-1035928).

3.3.2. 20H/501Y.V2, Beta Variants in Bangladesh

All the three-pangolin lineages of Beta variants (B.1.351, B.1.351.2 and B.1.351.3) were observed in Bangladesh (Figures 8 and 9). The B.1.351 circulated in Dhaka, Chattogram, and Sirajgonj from March to May 2021. Later in June, it was found in the Brahmanbaria and Sylhet districts. The source of introduction of B.1.351 was likely South Africa, Canada, Spain, USA.

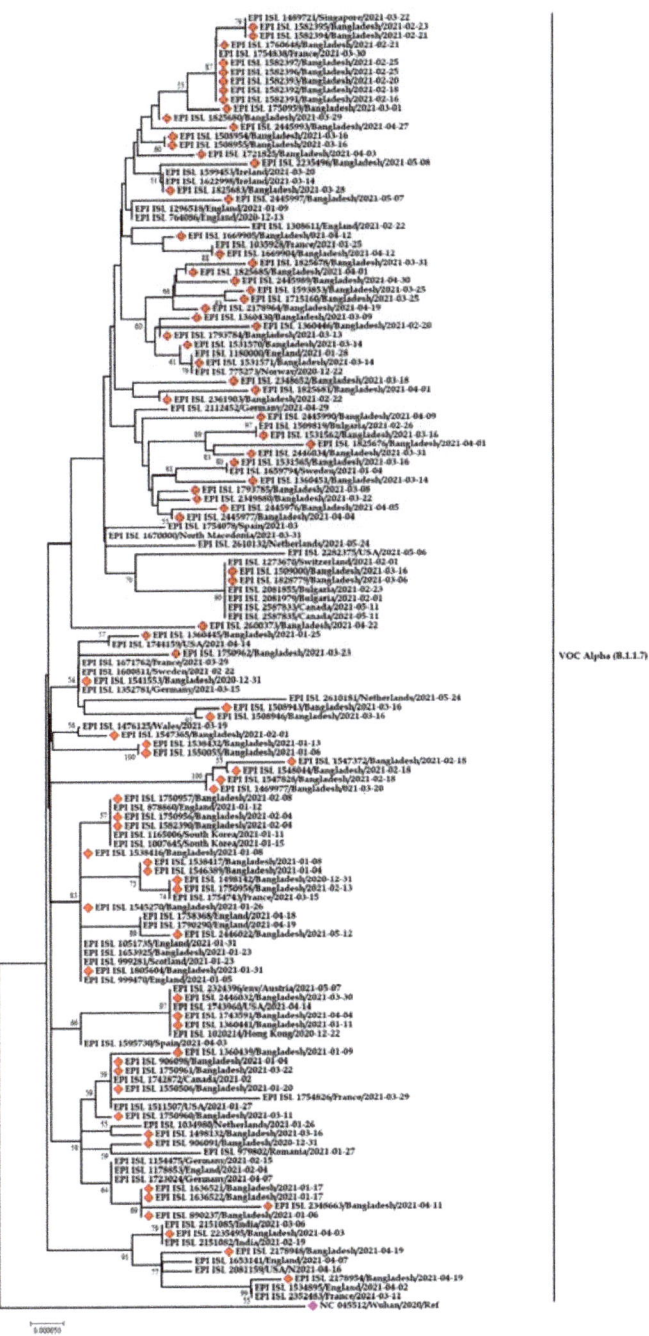

Figure 7. Phylogenetic analysis of emerging Alpha variants of SARS-CoV-2 in Bangladesh. Here, red diamond dots denote Bangladeshi Alpha variants SARS-CoV-2 viruses, and pink dots denote the Wuhan-Hu-1 viruses.

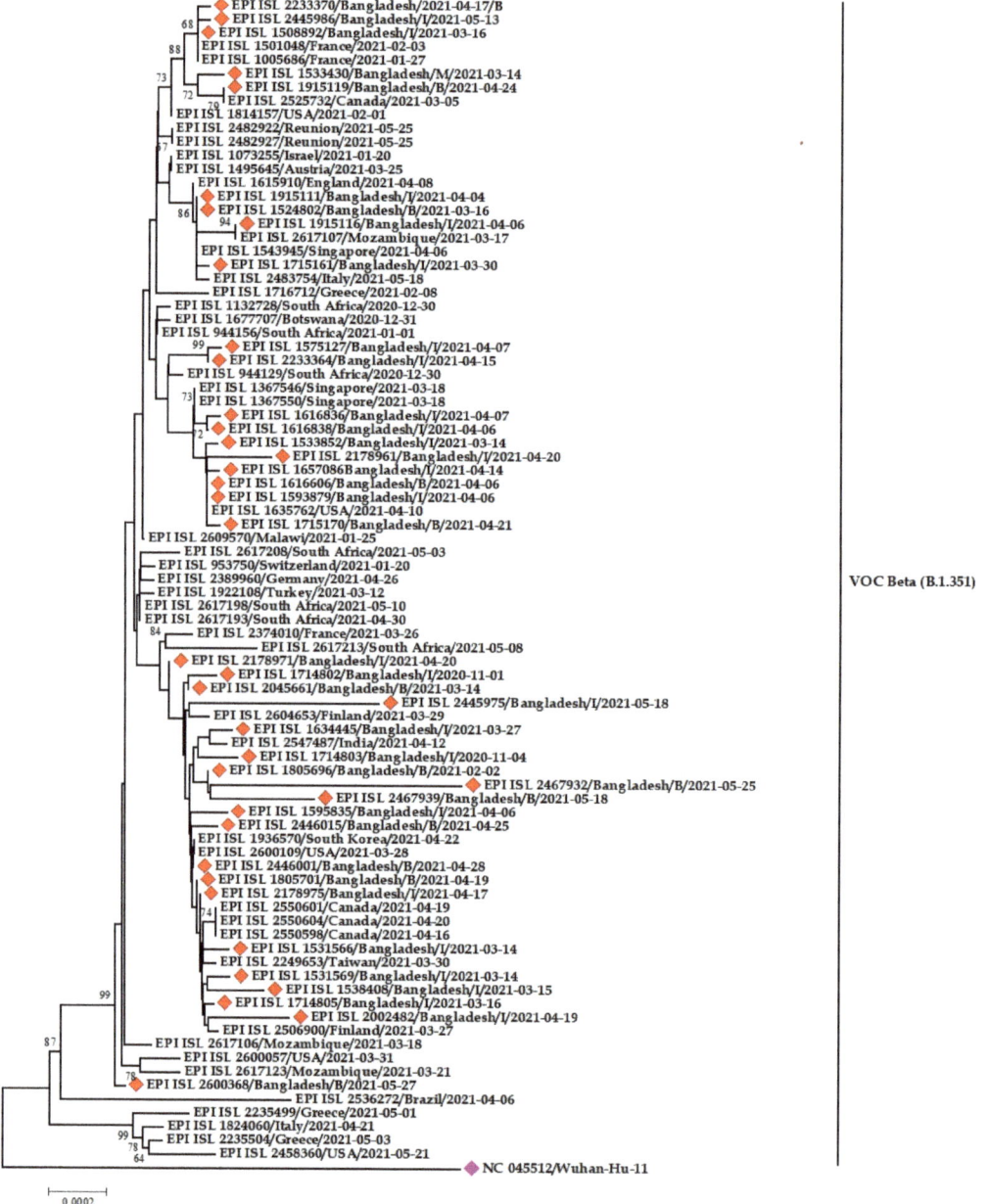

Figure 8. Phylogenetic analysis of emerging Beta variants of SARS-CoV-2 in Bangladesh. Here, red diamond dots denote Beta variant SARS-CoV-2 viruses, and pink dots denote Wuhan-Hu-1 viruses.

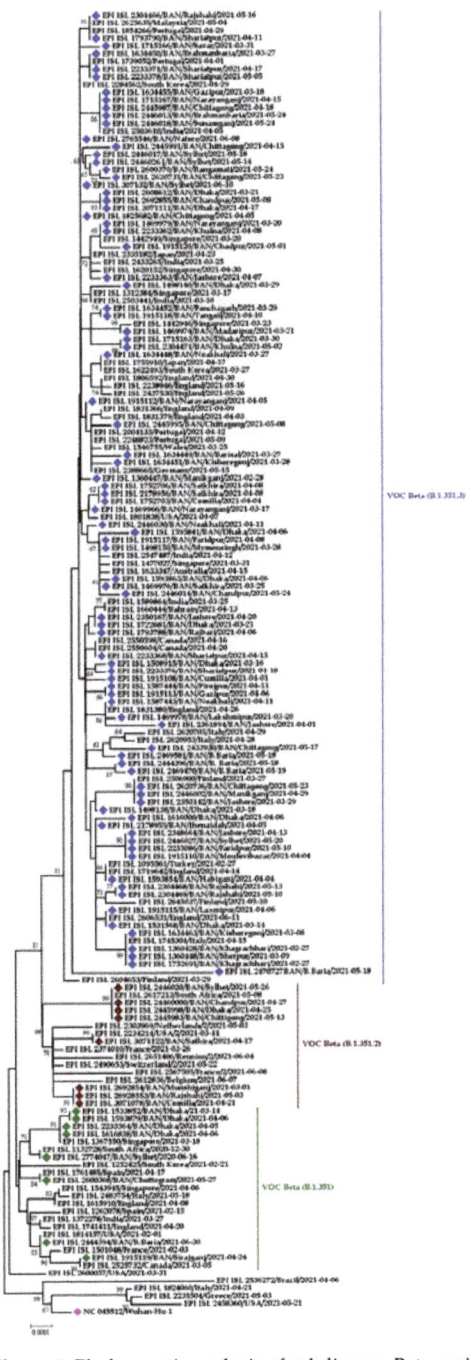

Figure 9. Phylogenetic analysis of sub-lineage Beta variant B.1.351.3 in Bangladesh. Here, blue dots denote Beta (B.1.351.1) SARS-CoV-2 viruses, and maroon, green and pink dotes denote B.1.351.2, B.1.351, and Wuhan-Hu-1 viruses, respectively.

The Bangladeshi strains clustered with virus sequences were reported from mainly European countries and the Middle east. The Bangladeshi Beta variants have a likeness to virus sequences reported from England, Germany, Switzerland, Scotland, Italy, Turkey, and Jordan (Figure 8).

B.1.351.2 was found in Munshigonj in March but in Dhaka, Chandpur, Sathira and Comilla in April 2021. Later in May, it was distributed to other districts, such as Rajshahi, Chattogram and Sylhet. On the other hand, the sub-lineage B.1.351.3 of Beta variants formed twelve different clusters. This lineage was circulating in Manikgonj and Khagrachhari during February 2021. The strain from Manikgonj stands alone in the phylogenetic tree without resembling other strains. However, the strain from Khagrachari later spread to Sherpur and Kishoregonj districts in March. The strain spread from Dhaka to other districts during March, April, and May (Figure 9).

3.3.3. VOC G/452R.V3 Delta Variant (B.1.617.2) in Bangladesh

Among the three three pangolin lineages of the Delta variant, only one (B.1.617.2) was detected in Bangladesh. This variant was thought to be introduced in April in Dinajpur, Jhenaida, Dhaka, or Khulna. The strains from Dhaka showed nucleotide similarity with a strain (EEPI ISL 2189738) from India. The phylogeny illustrates the direct relationship between strains from India and Dinajpur, Chapai-nawabgonj, Khulna, Dhaka, and Chattogram. After arriving in Bangladesh, the virus began to spread at a neighborhood level and expanded throughout the county quickly (Figure 10). In the phylogenetic tree (Delta V), it was discovered that when one virus was detected in Jashore, it was also reported in other parts of the country, including Noakhali, Laxmipur, Gopalganj, and Narshingdi, demonstrating community-level transmission of Indian-originated viruses. Another cluster supports community transmission of the Delta variant strain of SARS-CoV-2 virus from Jashore to other districts (Dhaka, Chattogram, Sylhet, Habigonj, Tangail, and Rangpur) (Figure 10).

3.3.4. VUI G/484K.V3 and VOC GR/501Y.V3 Variants in Bangladesh

The Eta variants of SARS-CoV-2 Bangladeshi strains clustered with virus sequences were reported from the USA, England, Togo, Ghana, Singapore, Nigeria, Germany, and France, whereas only one Gamma variant was reported from Bangladesh, which clustered with strains from Brazil, Canada, Japan, and Singapore (Figure 11).

3.3.5. Point Mutation Analysis of SARS-CoV-2 in Different Time Period in Bangladesh

The highest amino acid substitution was D614G from December 2020 to July 2021. This mutation was present in almost all the sequences from Bangladesh (ranging from 93.5 to 100%). The overall P681H mutation was detected at a low percentage (ranging from 4.8 to 35.7%) from Dec to July. E484K was found at the highest proportion during March (64.7%) and April (65.1%), 2021. At the same time, K417N was more prevalent in March (65.2%). N501Y is one of the critical mutations for the α, β and γ variants. During February, March, and April, the N501Y substitution was found at 51.8, 76.1, and 65.1%, respectively.

The K417T mutation was detected only at 1.8% in February. On the other hand, another frequent mutation was P681R in June (88.2%) and July (100%). Some other significant mutations, D950N and L452R. D950N, L452R, T478K, were frequently increased from May and detected in 82.4, 94.1, and 88.2% of sequences, respectively, in July (Figure 12).

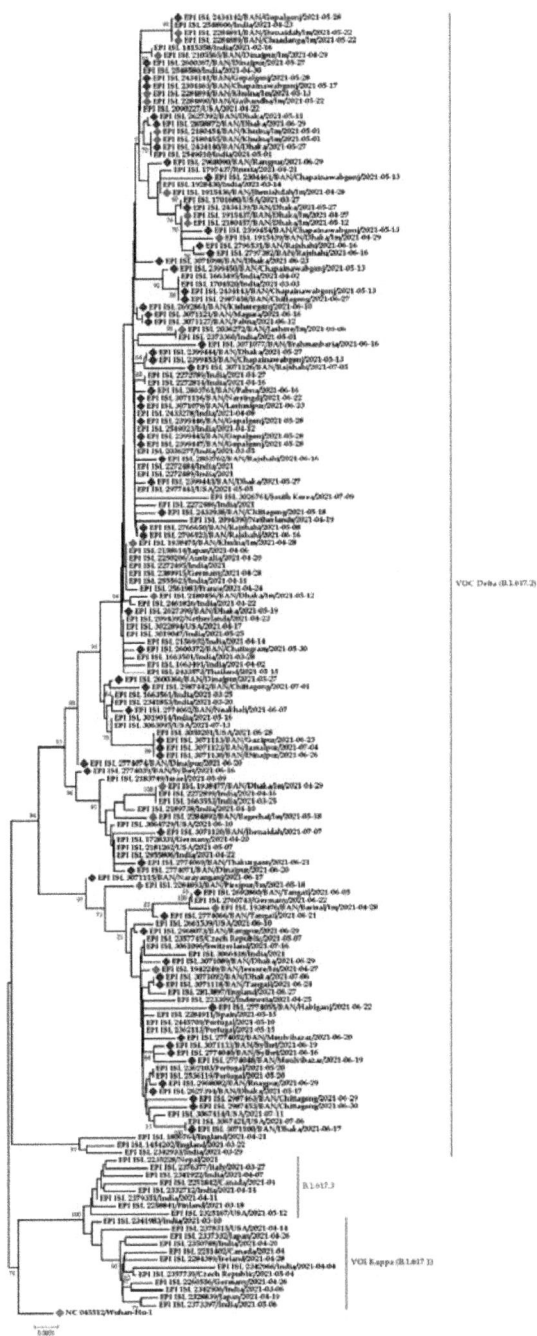

Figure 10. Phylogenetic analysis of sub-lineage of Delta variant (B.1.617.2) in Bangladesh. Here, maroon dots denote community transmission of Delta variant SARS-CoV-2 viruses; blue and pink dotes denote imported SARS-CoV-2 Delta variant and Wuhan-Hu-1 viruses, respectively. B.1.617.3 and B.1.617.1 were used as out group here.

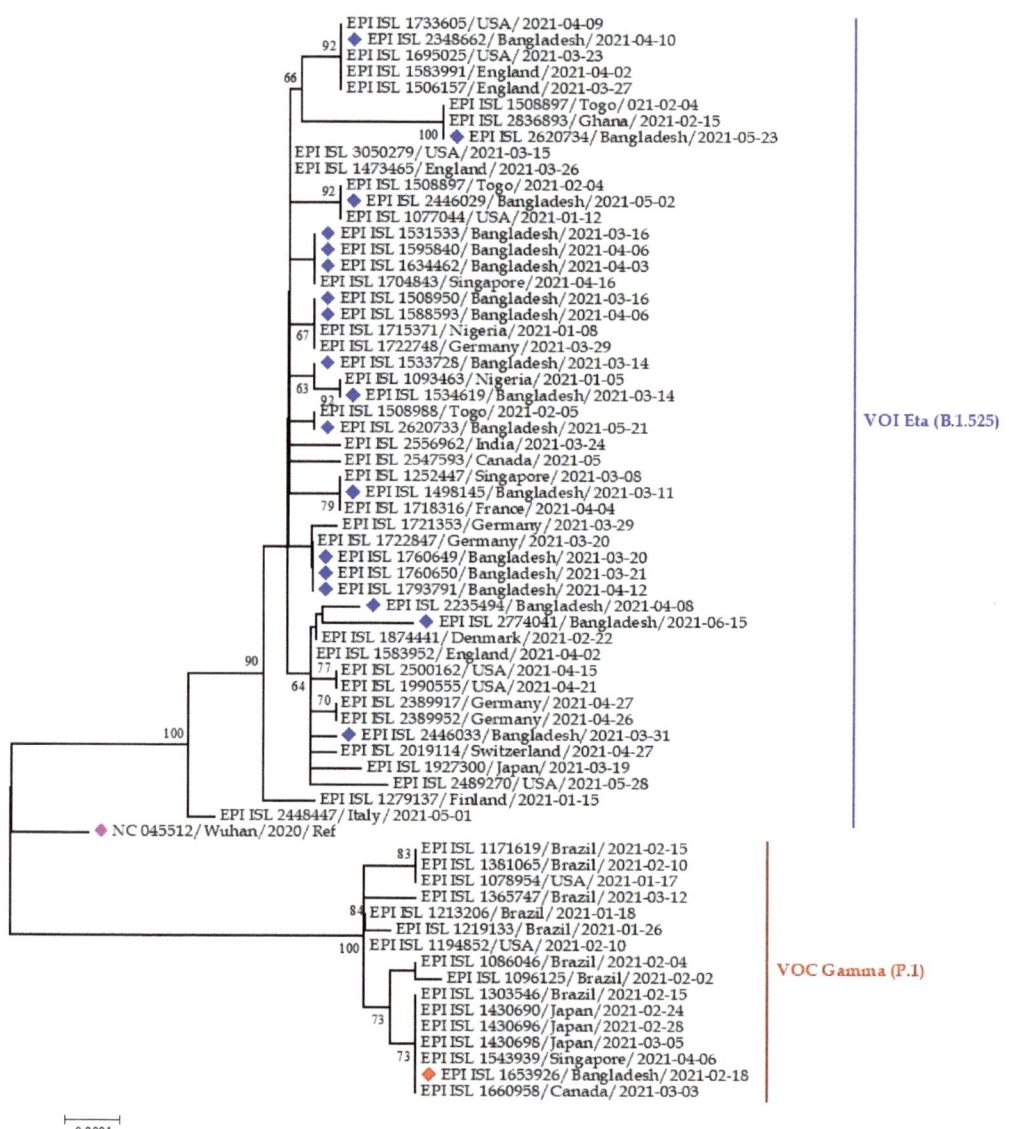

Figure 11. Phylogenetic analysis of emerging Eta and Gamma variants of SARS-CoV-2 Bangladeshi isolates. Here, blue dots denote Eta variant SARS-CoV-2 viruses; red and pink dotes denote Gamma variant and Wuhan-Hu-1 viruses, respectively.

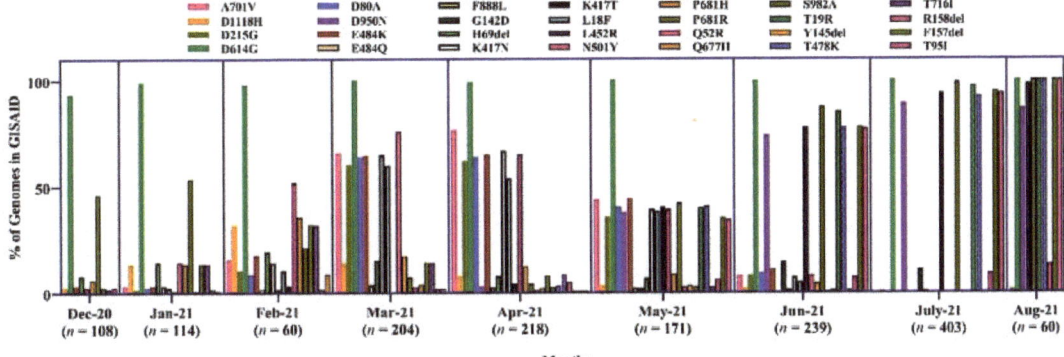

Figure 12. Proportion of amino acid mutations in the spike protein of SARS-CoV-2 sequences in Bangladesh.

3.3.6. Variant Specific Mutation Analysis of SARS-CoV-2 in Bangladesh

Again, we present the variant-specific substitution mutations in the spike protein in Figure 13. In the case of the Alpha variant (N = 94), the most frequent substitution mutation was observed at D1118H (n = 94), followed by S982A (n = 93) and P681H (n = 91). In the case of the Beta variant, the substitution mutation D614G (n = 408) was more commonly observed, followed by A701V (402) and K417N (371). In the Delta variant (N = 702), the highest substitution was D614G (n = 701), followed by some other unique mutation, including T19R (n = 688), R158del (n = 641) and D950N (n = 627). In the Eta variant (N = 19), the most frequent substitution was A67V (n = 19) (Figure 13). We detected only one Gamma variant, which has been omitted from this analysis.

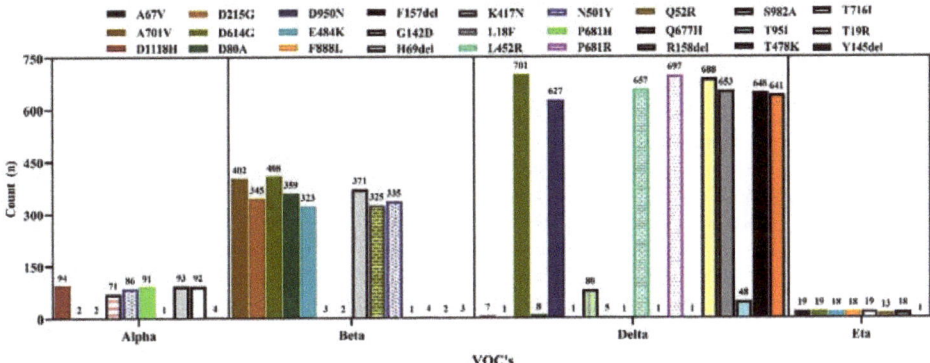

Figure 13. Frequency of substitution mutations in the spike protein of VOCs' sequences in Bangladesh.

4. Discussion

4.1. Spatial and Temporal Epidemiology of COVID-19 in Bangladesh

In 2020, Bangladesh was able to combat the initial SARS-CoV-2 outbreak wave successfully [39]. We observed that the second wave of COVID-19 cases gradually started to spreadin early March, with a notable spike in cases occurring around the middle of April. From February to March 2021, Bangladesh began to experience the severity of the second wave of COVID-19 cases and deaths related to the β variant (also known as the South African variant) [40]. A nationwide lockdown successfully reduced SARS-CoV-

2 transmission during this time (12 to 15 April 2021), from daily 3.15 to 2.35 cases per 100,000 population [41]. Although the Government started mass vaccination on 7 February 2021, ninety percent of all variants during April and May 2021 were Beta variants [42]. However, the double mutant Delta variant (B.1.617.2) was discovered for the first time in Bangladesh on May 8th, 2021; since then, the third wave of COVID-19 appeared with a sharp increase at the end of June 2021, with 68% prevalence [43]. Additionally, 20–55% of those who had previously recovered from COVID-19 caused by the other variant were infected by this strain [44]. The variant also exerted roughly eight-fold less sensitivity to Oxford-AstraZeneca and Pfizer-BioNTech vaccine-generated immunity compared to the Alpha variant, according to a number of epidemiological and in vitro findings [45]. Therefore, the protective effects of vaccination were not observed at that time; however, the mass vaccination program has proven to be successful, with the reduction in daily new cases and deaths in recent times. In our analysis, we found a peak at the third wave by the end of July when only 0.94% people of this country received their first shot of the vaccine, which was much lower that other countries across the world [24]. Moreover, the reproduction rate increased simultaneously, along with the progression of the 2nd and 3rd waves. The timeline of the 2nd and 3rd waves of COVID-19 in Bangladesh corresponds with the introduction of several variants of concern into the country [40].

Several studies reported that participants have more knowledge about the disease's risk; thus, they wear masks in public places [46,47]. However, Bangladesh still faced the second and third waves of COVID-19. Considering the vast population of Bangladesh, only a small number of test centers are available. Furthermore, a longer time is needed for the COVID-19 test results to return [48]. Almost 19% of patients were asymptomatic when they tested positive for COVID-19 during the second wave. In addition, a similar percentage of patients did not know how they became infected, and both urban and rural areas were affected equally [49]. So, people roam freely before testing positive for COVID-19 and spread the infection to other exposed humans. Additionally, if the residents practiced strict preventive measures, there would not be a surge of COVID-19 cases in Bangladesh. The 2nd and 3rd waves resulted from people not maintaining social distance, unwillingness to wear masks, and scarcity of vaccines for susceptible populations. All these factors collectively favor the rapid spread of the virus and the emergence of a higher number of cases in Bangladesh.

With the progression of the global SARS-CoV-2 pandemic, the new variants are becoming more infectious and continue spreading at a higher rate in contrast to pre-existing variants, due to changes in the virus genomic composition [50,51]. All the variants, α, β, γ, δ, and η, were most prevalent in the central districts, such as Dhaka. All the VOCs were more prevalent in Dhaka because it is the port of entry for millions of people every day. Dhaka is the capital city of Bangladesh. It connects other districts via rail, air, and waterways. Dhaka has an international airport, a few ferry ghats, and several rail stations. These ports of entry make Dhaka vulnerable to all the emerging variants. So, it is not surprising to observe the presence of all the variants in the capital district. The only exception was the δ variant, which was distributed to the peripheral districts along with Dhaka. This variant was responsible for Bangladesh's 3rd wave of COVID-19 [52]. The δ variant originated in the neighboring country India [53]. The peripheral districts, such as Comilla, Dinajpur, and Sylhet, have borders with India. People come and go through the border daily for various purposes. As a result, the Delta variant was dominant in those peripheral districts. In addition, dustbins are unavailable in rural areas, so people dump their wastes on roadside pits or drain water bodies, and vacant plots near houses [54]. These factors also contribute to viral spreading in peripheral districts.

There was a changing pattern in the clade prevalence in Bangladesh from December 2020 to September 2021. Although initially, the clade GR was predominant, later it reduced, and there was a rise in clade GK in Bangladesh. A similar changing pattern of lineages from B.1.1.25 to B.1.617.2 has been observed over the same period. The changing pattern in the lineage's distribution corresponds to the gradual spread of β and δ variants during the 2nd and 3rd waves of COVID-19 in Bangladesh [55].

4.2. Transmission Dynamics and Phylogeny of Emerging Variants in Bangladesh

The investigative genomic analysis of the emerging variants confers the high prevalence of α, β, and δ, the significant determining variants for Bangladesh's second and third wave [21]. We revealed the possible origin and transmission route of the emerging variants in Bangladesh through Nexstrain and phylogenetic analyses. The emerging variants' introduction to Bangladesh was through European and African countries. This fact was again re-confirmed based on the evidence presented in the phylogenetic trees. The variants circulating in Bangladesh are of European origin, mainly England, France, Germany, Ireland, Italy, and the USA. However, some viral sequences demonstrate similarities with other Asian countries, including Singapore, Japan, and South Korea, which has already been established by earlier studies [56,57]. All the clustering of the Bangladeshi sequences indicates the virus's transmission from expatriates to the community, which might be due to an improperly structured quarantine facility for travelers in Bangladesh. Multiple introductions have been recorded from Italy, India, and the UK [58]. The clustering of α and β variants of SARS-CoV-2 in Bangladesh illustrated that the virus reached the community transmission level, and only one Eta variant indicates the lack of community transmission of the emerging Eta variants.

We also conducted mutation analyses for all the Bangladeshi sequenced strains of SARS-CoV-2 deposited in the GISAID. D614G is the most dominant mutation in the Bangladeshi strains [19]. Similarly, the mutations that are important for several VOCs were recorded from the sequences of infected patients and environments in Bangladesh [19,59,60]. The Alpha, Beta and Gamma variants were common during March and April, but later in June–July, the Delta variant replaced other VOCs. Therefore, Delta variant-related mutations were increasing gradually [55,60].

The global SARS-CoV-2 vaccines are currently available for human immunization. Moreover, variant-proof COVID-19 vaccines and pan-Beta coronavirus vaccines are in the development stage that could, in the future, protect against multiple COVID-19 variants and other Beta coronaviruses, such as MERS and SARS [61,62]. Although there are around 115 vaccines that have been reported, among which some are available for immunization, about 53.1% of people have received at least one dose of any COVID-19 WHO-approved vaccine across the globe, whereas in Bangladesh, around 87 million people only received their vaccine in November 2021 [63]. However, the overall immunization rate depends on the people's acceptance of vaccines, which is still questionable [64]. In addition, a considerable level of people need to be vaccinated to attain herd immunity [65]. Therefore, the government, policy planners, and stakeholders should take action with regard to people's apprehensiveness towards immunization against SARS-CoV-2 to break the transmission dynamics.

5. Conclusions

COVID-19 started to impact human lives in Bangladesh in the first quarter of 2020. From the end of 2020, the case counts were lower. Nevertheless, during March–April and June–July 2021, we witnessed the 2nd and 3rd waves of COVID-19. Although initially, Bangladesh dealt with only COVID-19, from December 2020, several variants of concerns started to arise. The variants were prevalent in Dhaka, the capital city, with frequent dispersion to other large cities, such as Sylhet and Chattogram. Simultaneously, the Delta variants were prevalent in border districts, as they originated in India. Initially, the GR clade was higher, and then gradually, clade GK replaced it. Similarly, lineage B.1.1.25 was prevalent during December 2020; however, later, the Delta variant prevailed in Bangladesh. Detection of specific mutations related to specific variants further confirms the results. There are also phylogenetic relations between Bangladeshi strains and strains from other countries. Thus, we recommend frequent genomic surveillance to forecast the spreading of new variants, if any, and to take preventive steps as soon as possible.

Supplementary Materials: The following supporting information can be downloaded at: https://www.mdpi.com/article/10.3390/tropicalmed7080197/s1, File S1: SARS-CoV-2 genome sequence metadata; File S2: District wise frequency of VOC's.

Author Contributions: Conceptualization, A.I.; methodology, M.A.S. and A.I.; software, M.A.S., O.S. and A.I.; data curation, M.A.S., S.D.C. and J.A.; formal analysis, M.A.S., A.I. and O.S.; writing—original draft preparation, M.A.S., J.F. and A.I.; writing—review and editing, M.A.S., A.I., J.F., J.A., S.I., S.D.C. and M.M.H.; visualization, M.A.S., O.S. and A.I.; supervision, A.I. and M.M.H. All authors have read and agreed to the published version of the manuscript.

Funding: The authors did not receive any external funds to conduct this research. However, the research team was partially supported by NIH U01AI153420 through EcoHealth Alliance.

Institutional Review Board Statement: Not applicable.

Informed Consent Statement: Not applicable.

Data Availability Statement: All data generated or analyzed during this study are included in this published article (and its Supplementary Information files).

Acknowledgments: We thank the Directorate General of Health Services (DGHS) and Institute of Epidemiology Disease Control and Research (IEDCR) Bangladesh, for sharing COVID-19 outbreak data with the public. We gratefully acknowledge all of the scientists from the originating laboratories who collected the samples, and providing sequencing data to the GISAID database, which was used in the analyses presented in this paper. The authors appreciate the Institute of Epidemiology, Disease Control and Study (IEDCR) and EcoHealth Alliance's continuous support of our research team.

Conflicts of Interest: The authors declare that they have no conflict of interest.

References

1. Islam, A.; Ferdous, J.; Sayeed, M.A.; Islam, S.; Kaisar Rahman, M.; Abedin, J.; Saha, O.; Hassan, M.M.; Shirin, T. Spatial epidemiology and genetic diversity of SARS-CoV-2 and related coronaviruses in domestic and wild animals. *PLoS ONE* **2021**, *16*, e0260635. [CrossRef] [PubMed]
2. Bchetnia, M.; Girard, C.; Duchaine, C.; Laprise, C. The outbreak of the novel severe acute respiratory syndrome coronavirus 2 (SARS-CoV-2): A review of the current global status. *J. Infect. Public Health* **2020**, *13*, 1601–1610. [CrossRef] [PubMed]
3. Jin, Y.-H.; Cai, L.; Cheng, Z.-S.; Cheng, H.; Deng, T.; Fan, Y.-P.; Fang, C.; Huang, D.; Huang, L.-Q.; Huang, Q.J. A rapid advice guideline for the diagnosis and treatment of 2019 novel coronavirus (2019-nCoV) infected pneumonia (standard version). *Mil. Med. Res.* **2020**, *7*, 4. [CrossRef] [PubMed]
4. Islam, A.; Ferdous, J.; Islam, S.; Sayeed, M.A.; Dutta Choudhury, S.; Saha, O.; Hassan, M.M.; Shirin, T. Evolutionary dynamics and epidemiology of endemic and emerging coronaviruses in humans, domestic animals, and wildlife. *Viruses* **2021**, *13*, 1908. [CrossRef]
5. Goswami, D.; Kumar, M.; Ghosh, S.K.; Das, A. Natural product compounds in alpinia officinarum and ginger are potent SARS-CoV-2 papain-like protease inhibitors. *ChemRxiv* **2020**, 1–16. [CrossRef]
6. Munster, V.J.; Koopmans, M.; Van Doremalen, N.; Van Riel, D.; De Wit, E. A novel coronavirus emerging in China—key questions for impact assessment. *N. Engl. J. Med.* **2020**, *382*, 692–694. [CrossRef]
7. CDC. 2018–19 Influenza Illnesses, Medical Visits, Hospitalizations, and Deaths Averted by Vaccination. Available online: www.cdc.gov/flu (accessed on 1 June 2021).
8. Cella, E.; Benedetti, F.; Fabris, S.; Borsetti, A.; Pezzuto, A.; Ciotti, M.; Pascarella, S.; Ceccarelli, G.; Zella, D.; Ciccozzi, M.J.C.; et al. SARS-CoV-2 Lineages and Sub-Lineages Circulating Worldwide: A Dynamic Overview. *Chemotherapy* **2021**, *66*, 3–7. [CrossRef]
9. Ko, K.; Nagashima, S.; Bunthen, E.; Ouoba, S.; Akita, T.; Sugiyama, A.; Ohisa, M.; Sakaguchi, T.; Tahara, H.; Ohge, H.; et al. Molecular characterization and the mutation pattern of SARS-CoV-2 during first and second wave outbreaks in Hiroshima, Japan. *PLoS ONE* **2021**, *16*, e0246383. [CrossRef]
10. Yadav, P.D.; Nyayanit, D.A.; Sahay, R.R.; Sarkale, P.; Pethani, J.; Patil, S.; Baradkar, S.; Potdar, V.; Patil, D.Y. Isolation and characterization of the new SARS-CoV-2 variant in travellers from the United Kingdom to India: VUI-202012/01 of the B. 1.1. 7 lineage. *J. Travel Med.* **2021**, *28*, taab009. [CrossRef]
11. Srivastava, S.; Banu, S.; Singh, P.; Sowpati, D.T.; Mishra, R.K. SARS-CoV-2 genomics: An Indian perspective on sequencing viral variants. *J. Biosci.* **2021**, *46*, 22. [CrossRef]
12. Wang, P.; Casner, R.G.; Nair, M.S.; Wang, M.; Yu, J.; Cerutti, G.; Liu, L.; Kwong, P.D.; Huang, Y.; Shapiro, L.; et al. Increased resistance of SARS-CoV-2 variant P. 1 to antibody neutralization. *Cell Host Microbe* **2021**, *29*, 747–751.e744. [CrossRef] [PubMed]

13. Happi, A.N.; Ugwu, C.A.; Happi, C.T. Tracking the emergence of new SARS-CoV-2 variants in South Africa. *Nat. Med.* **2021**, *27*, 372–373. [CrossRef] [PubMed]
14. Zhang, W.; Davis, B.D.; Chen, S.S.; Martinez, J.M.S.; Plummer, J.T.; Vail, E. Emergence of a novel SARS-CoV-2 variant in Southern California. *JAMA* **2021**, *325*, 1324–1326. [CrossRef] [PubMed]
15. Wu, F.; Zhao, S.; Yu, B.; Chen, Y.-M.; Wang, W.; Song, Z.-G.; Hu, Y.; Tao, Z.-W.; Tian, J.-H.; Pei, Y.-Y.; et al. A new coronavirus associated with human respiratory disease in China. *Nature* **2020**, *579*, 265–269. [CrossRef] [PubMed]
16. Zhou, P.; Yang, X.-L.; Wang, X.-G.; Hu, B.; Zhang, L.; Zhang, W.; Si, H.-R.; Zhu, Y.; Li, B.; Huang, C.-L.; et al. A pneumonia outbreak associated with a new coronavirus of probable bat origin. *Nature* **2020**, *579*, 270–273. [CrossRef]
17. Tang, X.; Wu, C.; Li, X.; Song, Y.; Yao, X.; Wu, X.; Duan, Y.; Zhang, H.; Wang, Y.; Qian, Z.J.; et al. On the origin and continuing evolution of SARS-CoV-2. *Natl. Sci. Rev.* **2020**, *7*, 1012–1023. [CrossRef]
18. Islam, A.; Sayeed, M.A.; Rahman, M.K.; Ferdous, J.; Shano, S.; Choudhury, S.D.; Hassan, M.M. Spatiotemporal patterns and trends of community transmission of the pandemic COVID-19 in South Asia: Bangladesh as a case study. *Biosaf. Health* **2021**, *3*, 39–49. [CrossRef]
19. Islam, A.; Sayeed, M.A.; Rahman, M.K.; Zamil, S.; Abedin, J.; Saha, O.; Hassan, M.M. Assessment of basic reproduction number (R0), spatial and temporal epidemiological determinants, and genetic characterization of SARS-CoV-2 in Bangladesh. *Infect. Genet. Evol.* **2021**, *92*, 104884. [CrossRef]
20. Islam, A.; Sayeed, M.A.; Rahman, M.K.; Ferdous, J.; Islam, S.; Hassan, M.M. Geospatial dynamics of COVID-19 clusters and hotspots in Bangladesh. *Transbound. Emerg. Dis.* **2021**, *68*, 3643–3657. [CrossRef]
21. Saha, S.; Tanmoy, A.M.; Hooda, Y.; Tanni, A.A.; Goswami, S.; Al Sium, S.M.; Sajib, M.S.I.; Malaker, R.; Islam, S.; Rahman, H. COVID-19 rise in Bangladesh correlates with increasing detection of B. 1.351 variant. *BMJ Glob. Health* **2021**, *6*, e006012. [CrossRef]
22. Worldometers. COVID-19 Coronavirus Pandemic. 2021. Available online: https://www.worldometers.info/coronavirus/ (accessed on 17 September 2021).
23. Banu, S.; Jolly, B.; Mukherjee, P.; Singh, P.; Khan, S.; Zaveri, L.; Shambhavi, S.; Gaur, N.; Reddy, S.; Kaveri, K. A distinct phylogenetic cluster of Indian SARS-CoV-2 isolates. In Proceedings of the Open Forum Infectious Diseases, Hyderabad, Telangana, India, 18 September 2020.
24. Ritchie, H.; Mathieu, E.; Rodés-Guirao, L.; Appel, C.; Giattino, C.; Ortiz-Ospina, E.; Macdonald, J.H.B.; Beltekian, D.; Roser, M. Coronavirus Pandemic (COVID-19). Available online: https://ourworldindata.org/coronavirus (accessed on 22 March 2020).
25. WHO. Coronavirus Disease (COVID-19) Update. Available online: https://www.who.int/bangladesh/emergencies/coronavirus-disease-(covid-19)-update (accessed on 10 September 2021).
26. Saha, O.; Hossain, M.S.; Rahaman, M.M. Genomic exploration light on multiple origin with potential parsimony-informative sites of the severe acute respiratory syndrome coronavirus 2 in Bangladesh. *Gene Rep.* **2020**, *21*, 100951. [CrossRef] [PubMed]
27. Katoh, K.; Misawa, K.; Kuma, K.i.; Miyata, T. MAFFT: A novel method for rapid multiple sequence alignment based on fast Fourier transform. *Nucleic Acids Res.* **2002**, *30*, 3059–3066. [CrossRef]
28. Shen, W.; Le, S.; Li, Y.; Hu, F. SeqKit: A cross-platform and ultrafast toolkit for FASTA/Q file manipulation. *PLoS ONE* **2016**, *11*, e0163962. [CrossRef] [PubMed]
29. SEDA. The SEDA Manual. Available online: https://www.sing-group.org/seda/manual/index.html (accessed on 20 March 2022).
30. Waterhouse, A.M.; Procter, J.B.; Martin, D.M.; Clamp, M.; Barton, G.J. Jalview Version 2—A multiple sequence alignment editor and analysis workbench. *Bioinformatics* **2009**, *25*, 1189–1191. [CrossRef] [PubMed]
31. Lemoine, F.; Correia, D.; Lefort, V.; Doppelt-Azeroual, O.; Mareuil, F.; Cohen-Boulakia, S.; Gascuel, O. NGPhylogeny. fr: New generation phylogenetic services for non-specialists. *Nucleic Acids Res.* **2019**, *47*, W260–W265. [CrossRef]
32. Katoh, K.; Standley, D.M. MAFFT multiple sequence alignment software version 7: Improvements in performance and usability. *Mol. Biol. Evol.* **2013**, *30*, 772–780. [CrossRef]
33. Criscuolo, A.; Gribaldo, S. BMGE (Block Mapping and Gathering with Entropy): A new software for selection of phylogenetic informative regions from multiple sequence alignments. *BMC Evol. Biol.* **2010**, *10*, 210. [CrossRef]
34. Lefort, V.; Desper, R.; Gascuel, O. FastME 2.0: A comprehensive, accurate, and fast distance-based phylogeny inference program. *Mol. Biol. Evol.* **2015**, *32*, 2798–2800. [CrossRef]
35. Letunic, I.; Bork, P.J. Interactive Tree Of Life (iTOL) v4: Recent updates and new developments. *Nucleic Acids Res.* **2019**, *47*, W256–W259. [CrossRef]
36. Hadfield, J.; Megill, C.; Bell, S.M.; Huddleston, J.; Potter, B.; Callender, C.; Sagulenko, P.; Bedford, T.; Neher, R.A. Nextstrain: Real-time tracking of pathogen evolution. *Bioinformatics* **2018**, *34*, 4121–4123. [CrossRef]
37. Saha, O.; Islam, I.; Shatadru, R.N.; Rakhi, N.N.; Hossain, M.S.; Rahaman, M.M. Temporal landscape of mutational frequencies in SARS-CoV-2 genomes of Bangladesh: Possible implications from the ongoing outbreak in Bangladesh. *Virus Genes* **2021**, *57*, 413–425. [CrossRef] [PubMed]
38. GISAID. Clade and Lineage Nomenclature, 2 March 2021. Available online: https://www.gisaid.org/resources/statements-clarifications/clade-and-lineage-nomenclature-aids-in-genomic-epidemiology-of-active-hcov-19-viruses/ (accessed on 20 September 2021).
39. Bari, R.; Sultana, F. Second Wave of COVID-19 in Bangladesh: An integrated and coordinated set of actions is crucial to tackle current upsurge of cases and deaths. *Front. Public Health* **2021**, *9*, 699918. [CrossRef] [PubMed]

40. Imran, M.A.; Noor, I.U.; Ghosh, A. Impact of Lockdown Measures and Meteorological Parameters on the COVID-19 Incidence and Mortality Rate in Bangladesh. *Infect. Microbes Dis.* **2021**, *3*, 41. [CrossRef]
41. Welch, S.B.; Kulasekere, D.A. The Interplay Between Policy and COVID-19 Outbreaks in South Asia: Longitudinal Trend Analysis of Surveillance Data. *JMIR Public Health Surveill.* **2021**, *7*, e24251. [CrossRef] [PubMed]
42. Rahman, M.; Shirin, T.; Rahman, S.; Rahman, M.M.; Hossain, M.E.; Khan, M.H.; Rahman, M.Z.; Arifeen, S.E.; Ahmed, T. The emergence of SARS-CoV-2 variants in Dhaka city, Bangladesh. *Transbound. Emerg. Dis.* **2021**, *68*, 3000–3001. [CrossRef] [PubMed]
43. Bari, M.S.; Hossain, M.J.; Akhter, S.; Emran, T.B. Delta variant and black fungal invasion: A bidirectional assault might worsen the massive second/third stream of COVID-19 outbreak in South-Asia. *Ethics Med. Public Health* **2021**, *19*, 100722. [CrossRef]
44. Devnath, P.; Hossain, M.J.; Emran, T.B.; Mitra, S. Massive third-wave COVID-19 outbreak in Bangladesh: A co-epidemic of dengue might worsen the situation. *Future Virol.* **2022**, *17*, 347–350. [CrossRef]
45. Mlcochova, P.; Kemp, S.A.; Dhar, M.S.; Papa, G.; Meng, B.; Ferreira, I.A; Datir, R.; Collier, D.A.; Albecka, A.; Singh, S. SARS-CoV-2 B. 1.617. 2 Delta variant replication and immune evasion. *Nature* **2021**, *599*, 114–119. [CrossRef]
46. Hossain, M.A.; Jahid, M.I.K.; Hossain, K.M.A. Knowledge, attitudes, and fear of COVID-19 during the Rapid Rise Period in Bangladesh. *PLoS ONE* **2020**, *15*, e0239646. [CrossRef]
47. Ferdous, M.Z.; Islam, M.S. Knowledge, attitude, and practice regarding COVID-19 outbreak in Bangladesh: An online-based cross-sectional study. *PLoS ONE* **2020**, *15*, e0239254. [CrossRef]
48. Rahaman, K.R.; Mahmud, M.S.; Mallick, B. Challenges of Testing COVID-19 Cases in Bangladesh. *Int. J. Environ. Res. Public Health* **2020**, *17*, 6439. [CrossRef] [PubMed]
49. Ali, M.R.; Hasan, M.A.; Rahman, M.S.; Billah, M.; Karmakar, S.; Shimu, A.S.; Hossain, M.F.; Maruf, M.M.H.; Rahman, M.S.; Saju, M.S.R.; et al. Clinical manifestations and socio-demographic status of COVID-19 patients during the second-wave of pandemic: A Bangladeshi experience. *J. Infect. Public Health* **2021**, *14*, 1367–1374. [CrossRef]
50. Cacciapaglia, G.; Cot, C.; Sannino, F. Second wave COVID-19 pandemics in Europe: A temporal playbook. *Sci. Rep.* **2020**, *10*, 15514. [CrossRef] [PubMed]
51. Salyer, S.J.; Maeda, J.; Sembuche, S.; Kebede, Y.; Tshangela, A.; Moussif, M.; Ihekweazu, C.; Mayet, N.; Abate, E.; Ouma, A.O.; et al. The first and second waves of the COVID-19 pandemic in Africa: A cross-sectional study. *Lancet* **2021**, *397*, 1265–1275. [CrossRef]
52. Afrin, S.Z.; Islam, M.T.; Paul, S.K.; Kobayashi, N.; Parvin, R. Dynamics of SARS-CoV-2 variants of concern (VOC) in Bangladesh during the first half of 2021. *Virology* **2021**, *565*, 29–37. [CrossRef]
53. Kirola, L. Genetic emergence of B.1.617.2 in COVID-19. *New Microbes New Infect.* **2021**, *43*, 100929. [CrossRef] [PubMed]
54. Sheheli, S. Waste disposal and management system in rural areas of mymensingh. *Progress. Agric.* **2007**, *18*, 241–246. [CrossRef]
55. Afrad, M.H.; Khan, M.H.; Rahman, S.I.A.; Bin Manjur, O.H.; Hossain, M.; Alam, A.N.; Khan, F.I.; Afreen, N.; Haque, F.T.; Thomson, N.R.; et al. Genome Sequences of 15 SARS-CoV-2 Sublineage B.1.617.2 Strains in Bangladesh. *Microbiol. Resour. Announc.* **2021**, *10*, e0056021. [CrossRef]
56. Shishir, T.A.; Naser, I.B.; Faruque, S.M. In silico comparative genomics of SARS-CoV-2 to determine the source and diversity of the pathogen in Bangladesh. *PLoS ONE* **2021**, *16*, e0245584. [CrossRef]
57. Parvez, M.S.A.; Rahman, M.M.; Morshed, M.N.; Rahman, D.; Anwar, S.; Hosen, M.J. Genetic analysis of SARS-CoV-2 isolates collected from Bangladesh: Insights into the origin, mutational spectrum and possible pathomechanism. *Comput. Biol. Chem.* **2021**, *90*, 107413. [CrossRef]
58. Al Nahid, A.; Ghosh, A. Investigating the possible origin and transmission routes of SARS-CoV-2 genomes and variants of concern in Bangladesh. *Infect. Genet. Evol.* **2021**, *95*, 105057. [CrossRef] [PubMed]
59. Islam, A.; Sayeed, M.; Kalam, M.; Ferdous, J.; Rahman, M.; Abedin, J.; Islam, S.; Shano, S.; Saha, O.; Shirin, T. Molecular epidemiology of SARS-CoV-2 in diverse environmental samples globally. *Microorganisms* **2021**, *9*, 1696. [CrossRef] [PubMed]
60. Islam, A.; Sayeed, M.A.; Kalam, M.A.; Fedous, J.; Shano, S.; Abedin, J.; Islam, S.; Choudhury, S.D.; Saha, O.; Hassan, M.M. Transmission Pathways and Genomic Epidemiology of Emerging Variants of SARS-CoV-2 in the Environment. *COVID* **2022**, *2*, 916–939. [CrossRef]
61. Islam, A.; Ferdous, J.; Islam, S.; Sayeed, M.A.; Rahman, M.K.; Saha, O.; Hassan, M.M.; Shirin, T. Transmission dynamics and susceptibility patterns of SARS-CoV-2 in domestic, farmed, and wild animals: Sustainable One health surveillance for conservation and public health to prevent future epidemics and pandemics. *Transbound. Emerg. Dis.* **2021**, 1–21. [CrossRef] [PubMed]
62. Dolgin, E. Pan-coronavirus vaccine pipeline takes form. *Nat. Rev. Drug Discov.* **2022**, *21*, 324–326. [CrossRef]
63. Anon. Our World in Data, Coronavirus (COVID-19) Vaccinations. Available online: https://ourworldindata.org/covid-vaccinations (accessed on 10 November 2021).
64. Lazarus, J.V.; Ratzan, S.C.; Palayew, A.; Gostin, L.O.; Larson, H.J.; Rabin, K.; Kimball, S.; El-Mohandes, A. A global survey of potential acceptance of a COVID-19 vaccine. *Nat. Med.* **2021**, *27*, 225–228. [CrossRef]
65. Malik, A.A.; McFadden, S.M.; Elharake, J.; Omer, S.B. Determinants of COVID-19 vaccine acceptance in the US. *eClinicalMedicine* **2020**, *26*, 100495. [CrossRef]

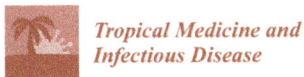 *Tropical Medicine and Infectious Disease*

Article

Coordination and Management of COVID-19 in Africa through Health Operations and Technical Expertise Pillar: A Case Study from WHO AFRO One Year into Response

Nsenga Ngoy [1], Ishata Nannie Conteh [1], Boniface Oyugi [1,2], Patrick Abok [1], Aminata Kobie [1], Peter Phori [1], Cephas Hamba [1], Nonso Ephraim Ejiofor [1], Kaizer Fitzwanga [1], John Appiah [1], Ama Edwin [1], Temidayo Fawole [1], Rashidatu Kamara [1], Landry Kabego Cihambanya [1], Tasiana Mzozo [3], Caroline Ryan [3], Fiona Braka [1], Zabulon Yoti [1], Francis Kasolo [1], Joseph C. Okeibunor [1,*] and Abdou Salam Gueye [1]

[1] World Health Organisation, Regional Office for Africa, Emergency Preparedness and Response Programme, Cité du Djoué, Brazzaville P.O. Box 06, Congo
[2] Centre for Health Services Studies (CHSS), University of Kent, George Allen Wing, Canterbury CT2 7NF, UK
[3] World Health Organisation, Regional Office for Africa, Emergency Preparedness and Response Programme, Nairobi Hub, United Nations Office in Nairobi UN Avenue Gigiri, Nairobi 00100, Kenya
* Correspondence: okeibunorj@who.int

Abstract: Background: following the importation of the first Coronavirus disease 2019 (COVID-19) case into Africa on 14 February 2020 in Egypt, the World Health Organisation (WHO) regional office for Africa (AFRO) activated a three-level incident management support team (IMST), with technical pillars, to coordinate planning, implementing, supervision, and monitoring of the situation and progress of implementation as well as response to the pandemic in the region. At WHO AFRO, one of the pillars was the health operations and technical expertise (HOTE) pillar with five sub-pillars: case management, infection prevention and control, risk communication and community engagement, laboratory, and emergency medical team (EMT). This paper documents the learnings (both positive and negative for consideration of change) from the activities of the HOTE pillar and recommends future actions for improving its coordination for future emergencies, especially for multi-country outbreaks or pandemic emergency responses. **Method:** we conducted a document review of the HOTE pillar coordination meetings' minutes, reports, policy and strategy documents of the activities, and outcomes and feedback on updates on the HOTE pillar given at regular intervals to the Regional IMST. In addition, key informant interviews were conducted with 14 members of the HOTE sub pillar. **Key Learnings:** the pandemic response revealed that shared decision making, collaborative coordination, and planning have been significant in the COVID-19 response in Africa. The HOTE pillar's response structure contributed to attaining the IMST objectives in the African region and translated to timely support for the WHO AFRO and the member states. However, while the coordination mechanism appeared robust, some challenges included duplication of coordination efforts, communication, documentation, and information management. **Recommendations:** we recommend streamlining the flow of information to better understand the challenges that countries face. There is a need to define the role and responsibilities of sub-pillar team members and provide new team members with information briefs to guide them on where and how to access internal information and work under the pillar. A unified documentation system is important and could help to strengthen intra-pillar collaboration and communication. Various indicators should be developed to constantly monitor the HOTE team's deliverables, performance and its members.

Keywords: coronavirus; coordination; health operations and technical expertise; AFRO

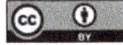

1. Introduction

The first human case of Coronavirus disease 2019 (COVID-19), caused by the SARS-CoV-2 virus, was identified in Wuhan in the People's Republic of China on 30 December

2019 [1]. Soon after, the World Health Organisation (WHO) declared the outbreak as a public health emergency of international concern (PHEIC) and as a pandemic on 30 January and 11 March 2020, respectively [2]. Following the first COVID-19 case importation into Egypt on 14 February 2020, the disease has spread to the whole continent. As of 25 February 2021, a total of 111,762,965 COVID-19 confirmed cases (distributed as per Figure 1) and 2,479,678 deaths had been recorded, with 2.5% (2,789,965) of the cumulative global cases and 2.9% (71,204) of cumulative global deaths coming from the WHO African Region.

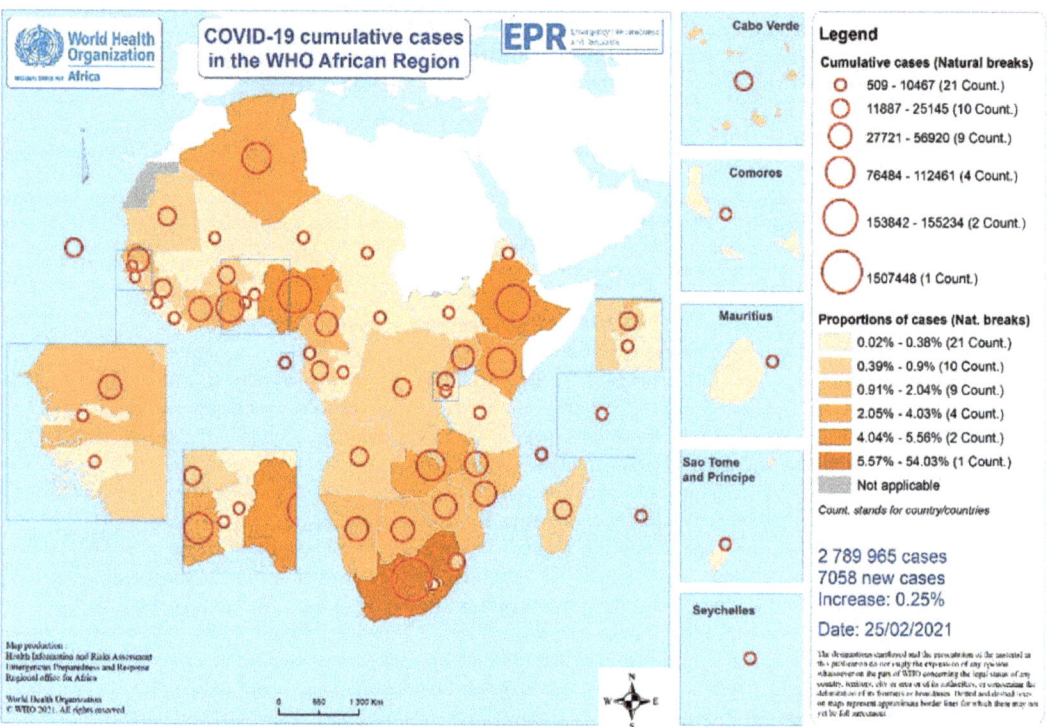

Figure 1. Geographic Distribution of Cumulative COVID-19 in the WHO African Region (Source: IMST presentations).

The number of cases and deaths recorded in Africa when writing this paper (March 2021) was much lower than predicted [3]. Several reasons have been advanced for these low numbers, including the role of aridity and temperature in transmission, demographic characteristics (distribution of age), the difference in identification of cases, and death detection capacity [4–9], and the possible contribution of pre-existing immunity from other viral infections [10]. Others have indicated that the numbers are due to the underestimation of the true magnitude of the pandemic resulting from weak surveillance systems [11,12] as postulated by the low rate of testing per population in the continent with ratios of as low as 1072 or 1441 tests per one million population in South Sudan and Niger, respectively [13].

However, the extent to which each (or a combination or interaction) of these factors has impacted the relatively low number of cases and deaths is yet to be fully explored. Nevertheless, what is clear is that the vast experience of responding to frequent outbreaks and emergencies has put the African Region in a comparatively better prepared position, and hence could mobilise the response capacity better than other regions. Besides the existing challenges of poverty and fragile health systems, the COVID-19 pandemic contributed to the disruption in its socio-economic activities in Africa, such as the breakdown in the delivery of health services [14]. The disruptions were largely from the measures put forward to curb the spread of the COVID-19 and included lockdowns, closure of borders and schools, restriction of travel, trade, and mass gatherings. These actions (such as border closures and lockdowns) taken by the countries in Africa helped slow the spread of COVID-19 on the continent.

In addition, most countries in the region rapidly instituted the incident management support team (IMST), a WHO system for coordinating and managing public health events in line with the WHO Emergency Response Framework [15]. The IMST is based on recognised best practices of emergency management included within the health sector. The critical functions for emergency response under the IMST are leadership, partner coordination, information and planning, health operations and technical expertise (HOTE), operations support and logistics, and finance and administration [16]. Prior to the first reported COVID-19 case in the WHO Africa region, a preparedness IMST was activated to assess, prepare, monitor, detect, and rapidly respond to the first case. Due to the nature of the emergency (involving all 47 countries in the region), an inter-cluster IMST structure that included repurposed staff from across the different clusters in the AFRO regional office was activated. The IMST is headed by the regional director with a designated incident manager (IM) that deals with the daily operations of the response. The IMST meets daily to share information and discuss strategic and operational issues to guide each country's pandemic support and follow up action points for the technical staff to act. Figure 2 shows the first IMST structures for the AFRO pandemic response, which was then revised in April 2020 to Figure 3 after a regional interaction review (IAR) was conducted, which was necessary due to the protracted nature of the pandemic (the revised structure is discussed in detail below).

This paper documents the learnings (both positive and negative for consideration of change) from the activities of the HOTE pillar and recommends future actions for improving its coordination for future emergencies, especially for multi-country outbreaks or pandemic emergency responses. The HOTE pillar comprises of five sub-pillars, namely case management (CM), infection prevention and control (IPC), laboratory support, risk communication and community engagements (RCCE), and emergency medical teams (EMTs), all of which involve specific technical expertise that focuses on building a country's capacity and providing technical and operational support in the response [17,18]. We focus on the HOTE because it is the core operational and interventional pillar, forming the driving force of response under the IMST and because its operation exceeded the usual country-level cooperation that the WHO country office (WCO) has with the member states [16]. While other IMST pillars are important, the HOTE pillar plays a significant role in linking the WHO with the Ministry of Health (MOH) and its partners to ensure optimal coverage and quality of health services in response to emergencies by promoting the implementation of the most effective, context-specific public health interventions and clinical services by operational partners. For instance, the pillar links directly with the member states' MOHs by providing SOPs, technical guidelines, the best practices and protocols that promote adequate responses and quality of health services in response to emergencies. Through the guidelines, HOTE fosters the implementation of the most effective and context-specific public health interventions. Adequately, the pillar assesses different interventions to provide a regional profile that guides the MOHs need to deploy experts on the subject matter and organise virtual and onsite training needs. HOTE also ensure optimal coverage and clinical services by linking with operational partners and providing essential supplies such as personal protective equipment, medical oxygen, etc. Further, unlike other pillars in the IMST, the focus on the HOTE pillar is to provide up-to-date, evidence-based field operations, policies, and guidance.

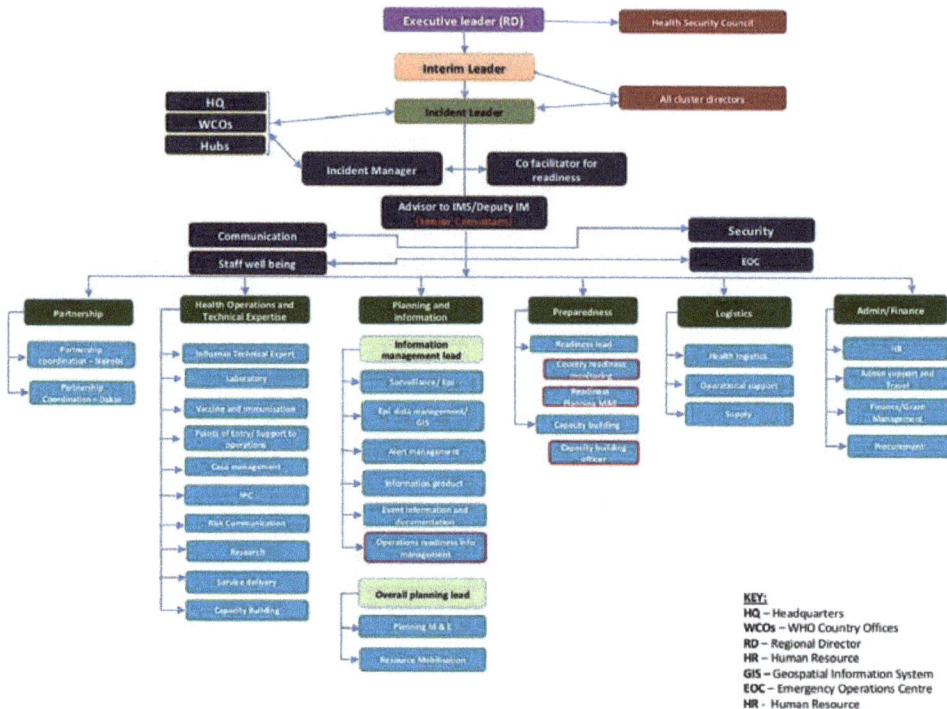

Figure 2. AFRO COVID-19 AFRO Incident Management Support Team (IMST) for preparedness and response (Note: four sub pillar teams have been highlighted by a red blank because their functions were often cross-cutting across the other pillars but also supported countries work).

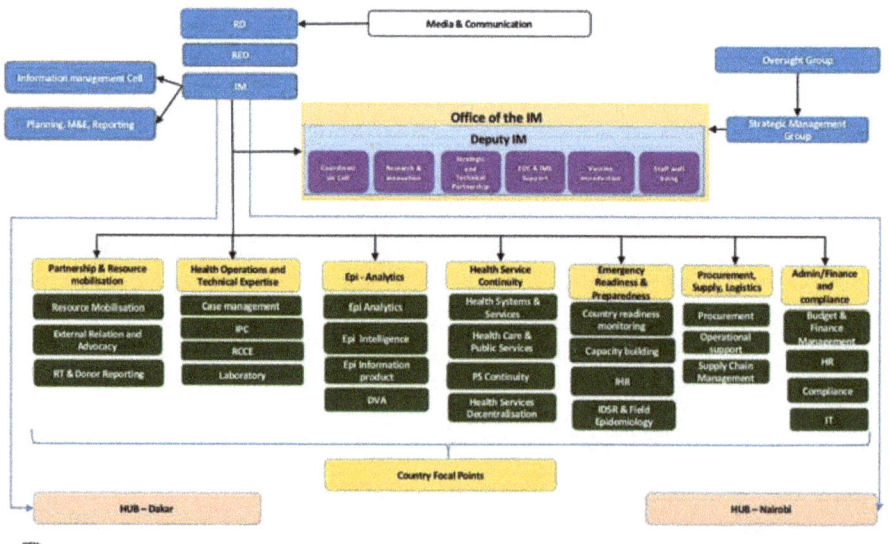

Figure 3. Revised AFRO IMST structure.

2. Methods

A mixed methods, case study methodology as defined by Yin [19] was utilized in this study. It focuses on the coordination and response to the COVID-19 pandemic from the HOTE pillar's perspective. The parameters studied included all activities implemented by the HOTE pillar one-year post activation of the IMST for the pandemic in the AFRO region as defined in the comprehensive Strategic Preparedness and Response Plan (SPRP) February-December 2020 updated (May 2020) [20]. The analysis was done using mixed methods to converge the findings to increase validity and to have individual components complementing each other, thus providing better explanations for the phenomenon under investigation [21].

Firstly, we retrieved the retrospective information on the activities and operations of the HOTE pillar, background information, historical insight into the pillar work, and a picture of how WHO AFRO or its emergency program fared over time [22]. The information was retrieved through a document review of available reports and surveys, periodicals, and monthly bulletins accessed through the WHO website. Those that were not publicly available such as HOTE minutes, confidential reports, and manuals, were gathered from the key informants who were part of the HOTE team from the onset of the pandemic. Additionally, the pandemic response staff from the two regional hubs of WHO (Dakar and Nairobi) and the planning, monitoring, and evaluation cell were requested to provide any other relevant documents and information on local policies, strategies and work plans that were deemed useful for the study.

Secondly, key informant interviews (n = 14) were conducted with purposively selected staff heading different sub-pillars in HOTE and the focal persons supporting individual countries who had been involved since the pandemic began and since the pillar was instituted. One researcher (BO) conducted the interviews using a semi-structured interview guide that was developed based on the content and gaps identified from the document review. The interviews were used to verify findings or corroborate evidence from the document reviews [22]. All the participants who agreed to undertake the interviews were invited to participate after being explained for the study purpose, and they gave verbal informed consent. The interviews were conducted in English and audio-recorded, and each lasted between 30–45 min. All the IDIs were transcribed verbatim in English and compared against their respective audio files by one researcher BO. All the validated transcripts were extracted in MS Excel for ease of management and transparency of the analysis process. All information/data provided from the document review and key informant interviews were synthesised using thematic analysis into thematic areas around learnings.

3. Findings

The pandemic response revealed that shared decision making, collaborative coordination, and planning have been significant in the COVID-19 response in Africa. The HOTE pillar's response structure contributed to attaining the IMST objectives in the African region and translated to timely support for the WHO AFRO and the member states.

The Changes in the Organisational Structure of Health Operations and Technical Expertise Pillar during the Pandemic and the Roles of the Sub Pillars

The HOTE is a critical pillar in the COVID-19 response and ensures that optimal and quality guidance of emergency response services are effectively communicated to African region countries. This pillar also provides updated evidence-based field operations, policies, guidance, and technical expertise during the response. In January 2020, during the preparedness phase and the initial stage of the outbreak, the HOTE pillar had ten sub pillars: influenza, CM, IPC, laboratory support, RCCE, vaccines and immunisation, POE/support to the operation, research, service delivery/health services continuity, and capacity building. Following the global pandemic declaration in March 2020, the AFRO region IMST structure was revised with the HOTE pillar reduced to six sub pillars: influenza, vaccines and immunisation, POE/support to the operation, research, and capacity building.

As the pandemic evolved, the HOTE pillar was further revised in August 2020 to five sub-pillars: CM, IPC, laboratory support, RCCE and emergency medical teams (EMT). Additionally, through the WHO AFRO emergency hubs in Dakar, Senegal and Nairobi, Kenya, the HOTE pillar working with the country focal persons provided/s daily strategic support to countries on the various operational and response activities. The country focal points (CFP) team was created when the size of the pandemic grew, requiring that the HOTE responds to a multiplicity of country requests. The CFPs were constituted to provide frequent engagement with the countries to monitor the evolution of the pandemic and flag issues of support. The criteria used for modification of the HOTE pillar was based on the findings of the Intra Action Review (IAR) carried out on the IMST, which provided lessons to situate better the pillars as part of the Incident Management System (IMS) as guided by the Emergency Response Framework (ERF) [16].

Currently, the HOTE pillar activities coordination is led by a pillar lead who coordinates the five sub pillars' operations (Figure 3). The pillar lead participates in the cross-pillar meetings at the IMST strategic meeting and is the pillar's voice to the management. Having a HOTE pillar team lead working with the sub pillar leads has been an effective way of outlining the pillar needs, making strategic guidance on the management of COVID-19 across the region, and identifying the gaps that need the attention of the administration. The pillar lead has also been able to link the team to other pillars and units (such as the CFPs) to update the regional management on the countries' ongoing preparedness and response activities (Table 1). Overall, the operations of the HOTE pillar have focused on the dissemination of strategic and technical guidance adapted to regional contexts; reinforcement of capacities, including the deployment of experts; further expansion of laboratory diagnostic capacities for COVID-19 in all countries; resource mobilisation at regional and country levels; and supporting the distribution of essential supplies such as personal protective equipment (PPE), laboratory equipment and reagents, and other medical devices to member states. HOTE pillar support to countries at regional, national, and sub-national levels was clearly defined in a comprehensive SPRP February-December 2020 updated (May 2020) [20].

Table 1. Interventions and activities of HOTE pillar lead, sub-pillars, and cross pillar coordination (from 25 February to 25 February 2021).

Pillar/Sub-Pillar	Interventions	Activities
Pillar Lead (1)	- Provide guidance and leadership of the pillar.	- Coordinate the operations of the five sub-pillars - Represents the pillar in the cross-pillar meetings at the IMST strategic meeting - The lead represents the voice of the pillar and communicates all their needs to the management.
IPC (7)	- Strengthen patients' treatment and prevent transmission to staff, all patients/visitors, and the community against COVID-19 infection by reviewing, updating, and disseminating existing and interim IPC protocols, including triage.	- Build capacity of health care workers on IPC for COVID-19 and SARIs (staff, training, supplies-PPEs, and equipment) for member states. - Provide strategic guidance to countries on all aspects of the pandemic response relating to the IPC component - Provide countries with the technical recommendations and tools necessary for their application - Strengthen the capacities of countries in the implementation of interventions, as well as in monitoring and evaluation - Strengthen the activities carried out by the other sub-pillars because of their transversal nature
RCCE (6)	- Strengthen public awareness through an integrated risk communication and community engagement approach on the COVID-19, including a psycho-social component in 47 Member States.	- Strengthen the identification of RCCE actions towards specific population groups and settings to address knowledge, rumours, and misinformation in 47 Member states.

Table 1. Cont.

Pillar/Sub-Pillar	Interventions	Activities
CM (5)	- Improve clinical care for COVID-19 patients through slowing and stopping transmission, finding, isolating, and testing every suspected case, and provide timely, appropriate care to affected patients.	- Support clinical CM for COVID-19 patients in Member States' treatment facilities through training, developing guidance and SOPs, assessments for screening/isolation capacity, ICU units, and related medical supplies access.
Laboratory (5)	- Strengthen and maintain regional and country surveillance systems to gather data on alerts, suspected cases and confirmed COVID-19 cases in collaboration with partners.	- Provide laboratory support at National and Sub-national levels, including reagents and other supplies to the Member States.
EMT (2)	- Strengthen and establish the regional training centre; and the national EMTs	- Enhance collaboration/coordination with Member states, Africa CDC, Regional Economic Communities, National and International NGOs and UN resident coordinators (RCs) to mobilise experts and safe deployment to support the response.

Note: () shows the number of staff.

4. Key Learnings

4.1. HOTE Intra and Extra Team Coordination

The HOTE pillar holds a weekly strategic meeting where the sub-pillars present updates on key activities undertaken and plans for the upcoming week. In addition, challenges and issues experienced by individual countries are also presented and discussed to provide solutions. In collaboration with the cross-pillar lead and using available data, deep-dive discussions are held to address cross-cutting issues in countries and outcomes of these discussions are presented at the main IMST meetings. At the pandemic's peak, cross pillar discussions were held every week, and were further relaxed to a biweekly basis as the country's epidemiological situation improved. Concerning the regional IMST meetings, daily meetings were held with all pillar leads and team members (including senior management representations) at the start of the pandemic. As the regional epidemiological situation improved, the frequency reduced to three times a week and two times a week as from March 2021.

Given that daily IMST meetings were a useful platform for information sharing and learning, the HOTE pillar lead or a designated pillar team member regularly presented to the IMST on the pillars ongoing activities with other team members providing additional information comments.

The cross-pillar discussion helped provide solutions to the ongoing challenges that countries faced, e.g., the surge response to South Africa. It allowed the staff better to understand the impact of the new disease- COVID-19. As shown in Figure 3, the CFPs are part of the AFRO IMST for COVID-19 and provide the overall country coordination, guidance, technical and operation support to WHO country offices (WCO) regarding emergency response management under the IMST. They link the WCO and IMST at the regional office and headquarters. Functionally, they report to the HOTE team lead as per the IMST. They perform information management roles (such as ensuring WCO sitrep and the dashboard of major events in countries are updated and shared regularly) and monitor and follow up on the countries' operational support. Otherwise they are involved in resource mobilisation in-country and externally, and follow up with the implementation of the response plan and utilisation of mobilised funds. Other roles include surge support for HR and supplies; planning, managing, and monitoring performance standards and key performance indicators during operations response; conducting the countries' needs, gaps, and capacity assessments/analyses; and leading capacity building roles.

Therefore, the collaboration between the CFPs and the HOTE was important as they brought the various challenges that countries were facing, the role or support that the AFRO IMST provided to the member states, and the country's best practices key upcoming events.

While the HOTE team members would also attend the country meeting to respond to questions and requests for the WHO AFRO management, the CFPs returned the key responsibility of leading discussions with countries. Equally significant was the lateral coordination and collaboration between HOTE and other pillars (such as epi-analytics (see Figure 3 for more sub pillars)). The pillars within the IMST are interlinked, and each contributed to the other's work, with the overall outcome being the achievement of the strategic objectives under the COVID-19 Strategic Preparedness and Response Plan (SPRP) 2020 [17,18].

For instance, the collaboration between epi-analytics and HOTE teams would generate cross pillar presentations that summarise a country's concerns or challenges, such as evidence of increasing healthcare workers infection or poor case management. This strategic information and solutions are subsequently shared with the AFR senior management for endorsement of proposed actions. As a result of the strategic role that the HOTE pillar played, it was noted that countries would get in touch directly with the HOTE team members to follow up on the envisaged/expected supports; thus demonstrating that countries appreciated the support they were getting from HOTE.

4.2. Internal and External Coordination Meetings

The internal and external coordination meeting of the HOTE pillar went through several changes as the pandemic evolved. At the start, sub-pillars under the HOTE pillar would meet during a weekly meeting at which the challenges and planned activities for the week would be discussed. From this sub-pillar collaboration, it was easy to learn what the other teams were doing, and it allowed pillars to request support help from others. Additionally, alternative discussions through communication by email normally brought about a significant response from different sub pillars whenever it was needed, as a result of the comradeship created through the weekly meetings. Furthermore, to enhance the coordination of various sub pillar components, the team worked closely with the emergency Hubs, whose roles were linked to the team. This coordination process effectively enabled policymakers to set forth actions that ensured best practices with the desired goal [23].

During the early phase of the pandemic, the general HOTE coordination meetings were poorly attended and unnecessarily long. The poor attendance may be attributed to the timing and conflicting meetings that the different pillar members attended, which subsequently led to the slow implementation and follow up of planned actions. Also, given that the various sub-pillar members were working virtually from different countries, a difference in the time zones may have been a factor in the poor attendance at the HOTE meetings. Thus, coordinating HOTE meetings was a major challenge and required cooperation from all involved to achieve the desired objective of the pillar.

4.3. HOTE Collaboration with Countries

Early in the pandemic, there was non-synchronised coordination between the HOTE pillar with the countries. The sub pillar team members would join in the different country's meetings and teleconferences (TCs) to understand the countries' challenges and, where possible, offer on-the-spot technical guidance. In some countries it yielded positive results, as some countries that reached out to HOTE pillar members received help with operational and technical needs requested.

With time, the HOTE meetings with member states focused on helping the countries meet their objectives/goals. Through this collaboration, countries developed trust in the support provided by the HOTE pillar team and would engage in unrelated areas surrounding their respective ministries of health. Requests whose solutions were not readily available were referred to the AFRO management support. A provision of the solution to the countries strengthened the WHO's credibility in the countries and provided an opportunity for countries to improve their health workforce and health systems.

However, the attendance of countries TCs by HOTE sub pillar members and the designated country focal points based at the hubs were met with resistance and were perceived negatively in some countries. Moreover, the WHO AFRO through HOTE or other region pillars would be demurred by some countries as making demands for information rather than supporting and offering solutions to the response. Working through the CFPs and the two hubs as the entry point to the countries was a more acceptable way of coordinating the support of member states. However, the CFPs assigned to respective countries would be overwhelmed with the meetings and follow-ups, given that they were concerned with coordinating other activities other than just the pandemic.

On several occasions, countries preferred to directly interact with the HOTE team members who were thought to have additional capacity to address their requests. Occasionally, this was also due to the fact that urgent information requested by countries sent through the CFPs by the HOTE team was not transmitted to the respective countries on time, thus causing delays.

In other cases, when the countries dealt directly with the CFPs—especially when following up on financial support—the CFPs would reach out to the HOTE team members directly and follow up the same work. On some occasions, when the CFPs would be on leave or have conflicting activities from other assignments, there would be gaps in the countries' meeting attendance and communication. There were also delays in sourcing information from teams in member states, which hampered much-needed interventions to curb the pandemic. The other pillars were equally affected, resulting in a resurgence of the cases in most countries and increased mortality. However, when the CFPs communication teams were more established and straightened, a collaborative approach was taken, which led to reduced delays.

4.4. Intra-Communication among HOTE Members

Clear, well-defined communication creates an effective team, although this is usually an insidious process [24]. At the onset of the pandemic, there was a lack of clarity about the different sub-pillar members' responsibilities and roles and the communication channels between the different sub-pillars to management. This was particularly evident with some sub-pillars not creating time for orientation/briefing of new team members who joined at different times during the pandemic, making it difficult for the team to be on the same page. There appeared to be some team members who did not understand their roles and responsibilities from the onset, and this made it difficult for them to fit in the HOTE pillar structure.

To address the above, sub-pillar team leaders defined the roles and responsibilities for each member. The new team members had difficulty finding their way around the organisation. For instance, it took a long time to have the members set up with email systems to ease coordination within the response structure, and when it was done, it was not very clear whom/where to access information. Consequently, failing to get the new members timely access to the organisation's email account hampered their coordination work with the countries, since some countries did not respond to HOTE members communicating with them through personal email accounts. Nonetheless, with some countries' ways of working (not responding to emails from personal mail addresses without the WHO domains and feeling bombarded), it remains a challenge to get a timely response from them.

It was not always easy to get information about internal coordination mechanisms and meetings within WHO. When some members participated in the discussions, it appeared as though they didn't understand what the meeting was all about and thus would not effectively implement session follow up actions. Because of the lack of introduction/induction of new HOTE and IMST members, not all team members within the sub pillars were receptive, as some could not respond to emails from the unknown (new) team members. The lack of adequate orientation of the members was most significant, especially for those who came mid-pandemic and did not know where to go or understand the organisation's processes. In some instances where orientation was provided, there would be a lack of guidance on accessing the technical reports, which may have resulted in duplication of efforts in producing some reports and briefs. It was, however, easier to get information from the management and incident management leadership than at the technical level.

4.5. Documentation and Information Management

We find that multiple information sharing channels under the HOTE pillar were conveying different information about the pillar. Potentially this may have fuelled different results among the sub pillars, causing poor utilisation of the available information to guide the ongoing pandemic support. There was a significantly large amount of information produced and collected by the different sub pillars that was not being utilised for strategic decision making, or that would require a unified way of constellating. The team members' strength was more geared towards providing technical guidance to the member states rather than synthesising the information. At the later pandemic stage, the emergency information management was set within the HOTE pillar to support information synthesis and consolidation between the different sub pillars to aid in strategic decision making and unified documentation. This helped strengthen the intra pillar information management. However, gathering information between some of the sub pillars was still not straightforward.

4.6. Monitoring Objectives

Based on the results, it was difficult to ascertain whether the HOTE pillar had achieved its intended objective. This was because the pillar did not have objectively verified indicators that they would use to track the pillar's performance during the year; however, the sub-pillars had indicators. At the HOTE pillar's operations level, it felt like the pillar was working without a strategy. When it came to writing the different reports for the pillar, each team was writing in an unfocused and uncoordinated way without really focusing on the indicators that the HOTE pillar wanted to achieve. Overall, this made it hard for HOTE to report achievement against indicators.

5. Discussion and Conclusions

The coordination and management of the COVID-19 pandemic is a complex undertaking that requires consolidated effort in synchronising actions and multilateral decisions. A well-coordinated response is the fastest way to transition out of a pandemic [25], and this entails skilled professionals being fully capacitated to respond to public health emergencies [26]. As previously shown by WHO [27], the early stages of an outbreak require various synergic components such as coordinating response, communication, ensuring health intervention, and managing information. Similarly, these components should have amenable objectives that will characterise the scope of activities [28]. The results under the HOTE pillar have shown that shared decision-making, collaborative coordination, and planning have been significant in the COVID-19 pandemic response from an African context.

The AFRO region IMST objectives are spelt out in the COVID-19 SPRP 2020 [17,18]. While the objectives of each of the sub pillars under the HOTE pillar's response structure are included in the SPRP, the findings on monitoring and evaluation have shown that it is difficult to ascertain whether the HOTE pillar had achieved its intended objective. Interestingly, the amalgamation of some sub pillars to HOTE came mid-response, and the SPRP 2020 outlined the sub pillar objectives while the SPRP 2021 was created to improve the objectives. However, through the response structure, the sub-pillar teams have been able to timely support the member states (particularly allowing countries to operationalise the in-country response's management structure as defined based on the country plans). Additionally, the structure has been useful in notifying the senior management at WHO AFRO on the needs (for the countries) and strategic directions.

However, the results have also shown that while coordination is critical in standardised situations, uncertainties and complex scenarios present challenges for coordination research practices [29]. For instance, the limitations on the coordination meetings' attendance, intrapillar interaction challenges, and even the countries' challenges all may have hampered the progress of the response from the onset. However, given the changes made progressively as the pandemic progressed, it was easy to support the countries. As observed in the management of the Ebola outbreak in West Africa, the separation of the technical and operational components of the response coordination under the IMST streamlined the coordination and enabled the experts to support their technical work [30]. The experience with the coordination of the HOTE pillar builds into the framework proposed by Hernantes et al. [31] and addresses the four specific challenges characterising crisis management, including the heterogeneity of the actors and stakeholders involved, multi-dimension effects, the diversity of activities to build resiliency, and the centrality of knowledge transfer and sharing mechanisms.

Nonetheless, we believe that sustaining the coordination approach could enhance IMST management of pandemic objectives of a similar magnitude in AFRO. We propose the following recommendations to strengthen the approach.

The main strength of this study was the triangulation of data/information from the document review and interviews, which provided a platform for gaining a deeper and broader understanding of the different coordination aspects of the HOTE pillar. The main limitation was capturing the learnings as both positive and negative aspects rather than using a framework. However, the analysis was adequately driven by data through thematic analysis.

6. Recommendations

As WHO AFRO continues to support the member states, we propose changes to the work approaches that could tackle the challenges that our review has revealed. For instance, we suggest that both internal and external meetings have agendas shared in advance and that the calendar invites are shared with all the members in advance. This would allow participants to prepare in advance and even adequately engage with the content of the meetings. Through this, it will also be possible to sufficiently capture the notes for the records of the meetings and share them with participants to track the meeting action points or requests from member states. Moreover, requested information could be streamlined to key questions from the countries, CFPs, and the two regional hubs. Once streamlined, there is a need to agree on how the information could flow through the country hubs or focal points and then to HOTE or even IMST. This could help define a unified flow of information and a better understanding of the countries' challenges and reduce the relayed responses from them. Also, we propose that we have a streamlined way of requesting information and come together as a pillar to submit our work.

Besides, the roles and responsibilities of each pillar member should be streamlined and identified. This would enhance better knowledge and performance of each member and even ease the justification of the roles to the senior management. It would also be imperative to have a HOTE introductory note indicating where and how to access new members' information, besides having an orientation to understand the organisations' way of working. The notes and the orientation would help set up the new members joining the team and share the visions and objectives of the different sub pillars. It would help the team remain strategic in achieving its key goals and expectations without delays and making the members who join mid emergency feel welcome. Also, at the onset of the teams, it is imperative to have key performance indicators (KPIs) for each member to achieve a common goal. This is essential to help to improve our strength in our systems and improve the quality of care. Besides, continued collaboration between different pillars—given that we are intricately woven together—would produce better performance outputs.

There is a need to continue working towards achieving a unified documentation component so that the pillar can speak from a unified position. This helps to strengthen what we do as a pillar, and it also allows the pillar to communicate to IMST on the activities that we do, and they can contribute directly to IMST objectives. Besides, it provides a unified way to guide the member states and gives us an opportunity and the sub pillars to focus our energies on providing technical guidance to countries.

The sub pillar indicators should be defined to the team to know whether the intended performance is being achieved or not. Additionally, it would be imperative to add coordination level indicators to examine the role of coordination in achieving the sub pillars' objectives. Constantly monitoring the deliverable indicators' performance would ensure that we are—as a team—discussing the problems (technical and financial) and identifying the solutions.

Author Contributions: Conceptualization, N.N. and B.O.; methodology, B.O. and I.N.C.; software, B.O.; validation, N.N, and P.A.; formal analysis, B.O.; investigation, B.O.; resources, I.N.C., P.A., N.E.E., A.K., P.P., C.H., N.E.E., K.F., J.A., A.E., T.F., R.K., L.K.C., T.M., C.R.; data curation, B.O.; writing—original draft preparation, B.O.; writing—review and editing, N.N., B.O., I.N.C., P.A., N.E.E., A.K., P.P., C.H., N.E.E., K.F., J.A., A.E., T.F., R.K., L.K.C., T.M., C.R.; visualization, B.O.; supervision, N.N., I.N.C., F.B., Z.Y., F.K.; project administration, J.C.O.; funding acquisition, F.B., Z.Y., F.K., A.S.G. All authors have read and agreed to the published version of the manuscript.

Funding: This research received no external funding.

Institutional Review Board Statement: The study was conducted according to the guidelines of the Declaration of Helsinki, and approved by the WHO Regional Office for Africa COVID-19 IMST and the regional office publication review committee.

Informed Consent Statement: Informed consent was obtained from all subjects involved in the study.

Data Availability Statement: All required data is present in the manuscript.

Conflicts of Interest: None declared.

References

1. World Health Organisation. *Novel Coronavirus (2019-nCoV)*; Situation Report—1; World Health Organisation: Geneva, Switzerland, 2020. Available online: https://www.who.int/docs/default-source/coronaviruse/situation-reports/20200121-sitrep-1-2019-ncov.pdf (accessed on 7 January 2020).
2. World Health Organisation. *Listings of WHO's Response to COVID-19*; World Health Organisation: Geneva, Switzerland, 2020. Available online: https://www.who.int/news/item/29-06-2020-covidtimeline (accessed on 7 January 2020).
3. Quaife, M.; van Zandvoort, K.; Gimma, A.; Shah, K.; McCreesh, N.; Prem, K.; Barasa, E.; Mwanga, D.; Kangwana, B.; Pinchoff, J.; et al. The impact of COVID-19 control measures on social contacts and transmission in Kenyan informal settlements. *BMC Med.* **2020**, *18*, 316. [CrossRef] [PubMed]
4. Diop, B.Z.; Ngom, M.; Biyong, C.P.; Biyong, J.N.P. The relatively young and rural population may limit the spread and severity of COVID-19 in Africa: A modelling study. *BMJ Glob. Health.* **2020**, *5*, e002699. [CrossRef] [PubMed]
5. Gilbert, M.; Pullano, G.; Pinotti, F.; Valdano, E.; Poletto, C.; Boëlle, P.-Y. Preparedness and vulnerability of African countries against importations of COVID-19: A modelling study. *Lancet* **2020**, *395*, 871–877. [CrossRef]
6. Nkengasong, J.N.; Mankoula, W. Looming threat of COVID-19 infection in Africa: Act collectively, and fast. *Lancet* **2020**, *395*, 841–842. [CrossRef]
7. Hopman, J.; Allegranzi, B.; Mehtar, S. Managing COVID-19 in low-and middle-income countries. *JAMA.* **2020**, *323*, 1549–1550. [CrossRef]
8. Martinez-Alvarez, M.; Jarde, A.; Usuf, E.; Brotherton, H.; Bittaye, M.; Sameteh, A.L.; Antonio, M.; Vives-Tomas, J.; D'Alessandro, U.; Roca, A. COVID-19 pandemic in west Africa. *Lancet Glob. Health* **2020**, *8*, e631–e632. [CrossRef]
9. Nguimkeu, P.; Tadadjeu, S. Why is the Number of COVID-19 Cases Lower Than Expected in Sub-Saharan Africa? A Cross-Sectional Analysis of the Role of Demographic and Geographic Factors. *World Dev.* **2021**, *138*, 105251. [CrossRef]
10. Doshi, P. COVID-19: Do many people have pre-existing immunity? *BMJ* **2020**, *370*, m3563. [CrossRef]
11. Haider, N.; Osman, A.Y.; Gadzekpo, A.; Akipede, G.O.; Asogun, D.; Ansumana, R.; Lessells, R.J.; Khan, P.; Hamid, M.M.A.; Yeboah-Manu, D.; et al. Lockdown measures in response to COVID-19 in nine sub-Saharan African countries. *BMJ Glob. Health* **2020**, *5*, e003319. [CrossRef]
12. Bankole, T.O.; Omoyeni, O.B.; Oyebode, A.O.; Akintunde, D.O. Low incidence of COVID-19 in the West African sub-region: Mitigating healthcare delivery system or a matter of time? *J. Public Health* **2020**, *30*, 1179–1188. [CrossRef]
13. Worldometer: Coronavirus Update (Live). Available online: https://www.worldometers.info/coronavirus/ (accessed on 26 October 2020).
14. Yaya, S.; Otu, A.; Labonté, R. Globalisation in the time of COVID-19: Repositioning Africa to meet the immediate and remote challenges. *Glob. Health* **2020**, *16*, 1–7. [CrossRef] [PubMed]

15. World Health Organisation. *Operational Review of the WHO AFRO IMST to COVID-19 Pandemic Response*; World Health Organisation: Brazaville, Congo, 2020.
16. World Health Organization. *Emergency Response Framework (ERF)*, 2nd ed.; World Health Organization: Geneva, Switzerland, 2017. Available online: https://apps.who.int/iris/bitstream/handle/10665/258604/9789241512299-eng.pdf (accessed on 2 June 2021).
17. World Health Organisation. *Report on the Strategic Response to COVID-19 in the WHO African Region: February–December 2020*; WHO Regional Office for Africa: Brazzavile, Congo, 2020.
18. World Health Organisation. *Strategic Response Plan for the WHO African Region: February–December 2020 (Update 4 May 2020)*; World Health Organisation: Brazzavile, Congo, 2020. Available online: https://www.afro.who.int/sites/default/files/2021-04/SPRP%20BUDGET%200520_01.pdf (accessed on 30 July 2021).
19. Yin, K.R. *Case Study Research and Applications: Design and Methods*, 6th ed.; SAGE Publications: Thousand Oaks, CA, USA, 2018.
20. World Health Organisation. *Health Operation and Technical Expertise*; Pillar Progressive Report for COVID-19; World Health Organisation: Geneva, Switzerland, 2020.
21. Heale, R.; Forbes, D. Understanding triangulation in research. *Evid. Based Nurs.* **2013**, *16*, 98. [CrossRef] [PubMed]
22. Bowen, G.A. Document analysis as a qualitative research method. *Qual. Res. J.* **2009**, *9*, 27–40. [CrossRef]
23. Uneke, C.J.; Langlois, E.V.; Uro-Chukwu, H.C.; Chukwu, J.; Ghaffar, A. Fostering access to and use of contextualised knowledge to support health policy-making: Lessons from the Policy Information Platform in Nigeria. *Health Res. Policy Syst.* **2019**, *17*, 1–12. [CrossRef] [PubMed]
24. Cohn, K.H. Developing effective communication skills. *J. Oncol. Pract.* **2007**, *3*, 314–317.
25. Forman, R.; Atun, R.; McKee, M.; Mossialos, E. 12 Lessons learned from the management of the coronavirus pandemic. *Health Policy* **2020**, *124*, 577–580. [CrossRef]
26. Savoia, E.; Massin-Short, S.B.; Rodday, A.M.; Aaron, L.A.; Higdon, M.A.; Stoto, M.A. Public health systems research in emergency preparedness: A review of the literature. *Am. J. Prev. Med.* **2009**, *37*, 150–156. [CrossRef]
27. World Health Organisation. *Managing Epidemics: Key Facts About Major Deadly Diseases*; World Health Organisation: Geneva, Switzerland, 2018. Available online: https://www.who.int/emergencies/diseases/managing-epidemics-interactive.pdf (accessed on 23 March 2021).
28. Hung, K.; Mashino, S.; Chan, E.; MacDermot, M.; Balsari, S.; Ciottone, G.; Della Corte, F.; Dell'Aringa, M.; Egawa, S.; Evio, B.; et al. Health Workforce Development in Health Emergency and Disaster Risk Management: The Need for Evidence-Based Recommendations. *Int. J. Environ. Res. Public Health* **2021**, *18*, 3382. [CrossRef]
29. Margherita, A.; Elia, G.; Klein, M. Managing the COVID-19 emergency: A coordination framework to enhance response practices and actions. *Technol. Forecast. Soc. Chang.* **2021**, *166*, 120656. [CrossRef]
30. Olu, O.O.; Lamunu, M.; Chimbaru, A.; Adegboyega, A.; Conteh, I.; Nsenga, N.; Sempiira, N.; Kamara, K.-B.; Dafae, F.M. Incident management systems are essential for effective coordination of large disease outbreaks: Perspectives from the coordination of the Ebola outbreak response in Sierra Leone. *Front. Public Health* **2016**, *4*, 254. [CrossRef]
31. Hernantes, J.; Rich, E.; Laugé, A.; Labaka, L.; Sarriegi, J.M. Learning before the storm: Modeling multiple stakeholder activities in support of crisis management, a practical case. *Technol. Forecast. Soc. Chang.* **2013**, *80*, 1742–1755. [CrossRef]

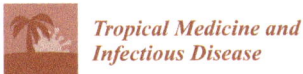 *Tropical Medicine and Infectious Disease*

Article

Dengue and COVID-19: Managing Undifferentiated Febrile Illness during a "Twindemic"

Liang En Wee [1,*], Edwin Philip Conceicao [2], Jean Xiang-Ying Sim [1,2], May Kyawt Aung [2], Aung Myat Oo [2], Yang Yong [2], Shalvi Arora [2] and Indumathi Venkatachalam [1,2]

1. Department of Infectious Diseases, Singapore General Hospital, Singapore 169608, Singapore; jean.sim.x.y@singhealth.com.sg (J.X.-Y.S.); indumathi.venkatachalam@singhealth.com.sg (I.V.)
2. Department of Infection Prevention and Epidemiology, Singapore General Hospital, Singapore 169608, Singapore; conceicao.edwin.philip@sgh.com.sg (E.P.C.); may.kyawt.aung@sgh.com.sg (M.K.A.); aung.myat.oo@sgh.com.sg (A.M.O.); yang.yong@sgh.com.sg (Y.Y.); shalvi.arora@sgh.com.sg (S.A.)
* Correspondence: ian.wee.l.e@singhealth.com.sg

Citation: Wee, L.E.; Conceicao, E.P.; Sim, J.X.-Y.; Aung, M.K.; Oo, A.M.; Yong, Y.; Arora, S.; Venkatachalam, I. Dengue and COVID-19: Managing Undifferentiated Febrile Illness during a "Twindemic". *Trop. Med. Infect. Dis.* **2022**, *7*, 68. https://doi.org/10.3390/tropicalmed7050068

Academic Editor: Richard J. Maude

Received: 2 April 2022
Accepted: 30 April 2022
Published: 7 May 2022

Publisher's Note: MDPI stays neutral with regard to jurisdictional claims in published maps and institutional affiliations.

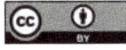

Copyright: © 2022 by the authors. Licensee MDPI, Basel, Switzerland. This article is an open access article distributed under the terms and conditions of the Creative Commons Attribution (CC BY) license (https:// creativecommons.org/licenses/by/ 4.0/).

Abstract: Background: During the COVID-19 pandemic, distinguishing dengue from COVID-19 in endemic areas can be difficult, as both may present as undifferentiated febrile illness. COVID-19 cases may also present with false-positive dengue serology. Hospitalisation protocols for managing undifferentiated febrile illness are essential in mitigating the risk from both COVID-19 and dengue. Methods: At a tertiary hospital contending with COVID-19 during a dengue epidemic, a triage strategy of routine COVID-19 testing for febrile patients with viral prodromes was used. All febrile patients with viral prodromes and no epidemiologic risk for COVID-19 were first admitted to a designated ward for COVID-19 testing, from January 2020 to December 2021. Results: A total of 6103 cases of COVID-19 and 1251 cases of dengue were managed at our institution, comprising a total of 3.9% (6103/155,452) and 0.8% (1251/155,452) of admissions, respectively. A surge in dengue hospitalisations in mid-2020 corresponded closely with the imposition of a community-wide lockdown. A total of 23 cases of PCR-proven COVID-19 infection with positive dengue serology were identified, of whom only two were true co-infections; both had been appropriately isolated upon admission. Average length-of-stay for dengue cases initially admitted to isolation during the pandemic was 8.35 days (S.D. = 6.53), compared with 6.91 days (S.D. = 8.61) for cases admitted outside isolation (1.44 days, 95%CI = 0.58–2.30, p = 0.001). Pre-pandemic, only 1.6% (9/580) of dengue cases were admitted initially to isolation-areas; in contrast, during the pandemic period, 66.6% (833/1251) of dengue cases were initially admitted to isolation-areas while awaiting the results of SARS-CoV-2 testing. Conclusions: During successive COVID-19 pandemic waves in a dengue-endemic country, coinfection with dengue and COVID-19 was uncommon. Routine COVID-19 testing for febrile patients with viral prodromes mitigated the potential infection-prevention risk from COVID-19 cases, albeit with an increased length-of-stay for dengue hospitalizations admitted initially to isolation.

Keywords: dengue; COVID-19; SARS-CoV-2; undifferentiated febrile illness; antigen testing

1. Introduction

During the COVID-19 pandemic, several dengue-endemic countries in Asia and South America have experienced concurrent outbreaks of dengue and COVID-19 [1–4]. In the early stages of illness, dengue and COVID-19 can be difficult to distinguish because clinical and laboratory features may potentially overlap, presenting as undifferentiated fever associated with nonspecific signs and symptoms [2]. Co-occurrence and potential co-infection of these two viral diseases introduces a significant burden on healthcare systems, particularly in tropical countries where arboviral diseases are endemic [3]. During overlapping "twin-demics" of dengue and COVID-19, all cases of undifferentiated febrile illness may need to be managed as COVID-19 until proved otherwise via diagnostic testing, with significant implications on healthcare resources. Misdiagnosis or delay in diagnosis of dengue is also conceivable because of the similarities in clinical manifestations of these two diseases [4,5]. Reliance on diagnostic testing to distinguish these two diseases further strains laboratory capacity, especially in resource-limited settings where molecular testing for SARS-CoV-2 and dengue may be unavailable [2]. Rapid serological tests can play a crucial role in dengue diagnostics, especially in low-resource settings where resource-intensive laboratory tests such as polymerase-chain-reaction (PCR) may not be routinely available [6]. Similarly, rapid-antigen-detection (RAD) testing for SARS-CoV-2 has been introduced as a useful component of hospital triage protocols to guide isolation measures and aid targeted admission [7]. However, RAD tests for SARS-CoV-2 may still yield false-negatives and need to be interpreted cautiously, especially in the context of significant contact history or clinical syndromes compatible with COVID-19 [8]. Similarly, there have been reports of false-positive dengue serology with rapid diagnostic tests (RDTs) in cases of COVID-19 [9], resulting in inadvertent exposure of other healthcare workers (HCWs) and patients [10,11]. The triage of patients presenting with undifferentiated febrile illness poses a potential challenge in tropical countries with co-circulating and nonspecific presentations of dengue infection and COVID-19.

In Singapore, a Southeast Asian tropical city-state, successive pandemic waves of COVID-19 were encountered during an ongoing dengue epidemic. In mid-2020, a surge in COVID-19 infections was reported, corresponding to ongoing outbreaks amongst migrant workers living in communal dormitories [12]. This coincided with the imposition of lockdown measures to reduce community transmission of SARS-CoV-2, shifting working patterns into residences, resulting in increased dengue transmission [13]. Dengue is endemic in tropical Singapore [14]. Early on in the COVID-19 pandemic, recognizing that COVID-19 could potentially manifest as undifferentiated viral fever with minimal respiratory symptoms [15], all patients hospitalized for undifferentiated fever were admitted to designated isolation areas where COVID-19 was first ruled out [16]. However, adopting such a broad approach for isolation triage posed its own difficulties in terms of practicality and costs, with 10% of hospital bed capacity set aside for isolation areas [17]. There were sustainability issues, especially due to strain from successive waves of COVID-19 caused by more infectious SARS-CoV-2 variants, including the SARS-CoV-2 delta variant (B.1.617.2) [18]. At our institution, the largest public hospital in Singapore, a triage strategy of routine SARS-CoV-2 testing at admission triage for all febrile patients was utilized, initially with PCR and subsequently supplemented by RAD testing. We evaluated the success of this strategy over a two-year period.

2. Materials and Methods

2.1. Institutional Setting and Study Period

The Singapore General Hospital is the largest public tertiary hospital in Singapore, with 1785 beds. The first case of COVID-19 in Singapore, in a traveller from Wuhan, was reported from our institution on 23 January 2020 [17]. Over a two-year study period (January 2020 to December 2021), our hospital's epidemiology team tracked the number of lab-confirmed cases of dengue and COVID-19 managed in our institution. Cases of dengue were diagnosed using a combination of serology, antigen or PCR for additional confirmatory testing; in our institution, dengue diagnostic tests were ordered at the discretion of the primary physician when a clinical syndrome suggestive of dengue was encountered. Cases of COVID-19 were diagnosed using PCR on various molecular platforms. Aggregated descriptive statistics, including length-of-stay (LoS), admission to isolation areas, and in-hospital mortality, were collected for all dengue inpatients during the COVID-19 pandemic and compared against a 2-year pre-pandemic period (January 2018–December 2019). Potential cases of co-infection with both SARS-CoV-2 and dengue were defined as testing positive for SARS-CoV-2 on PCR, as well as having a positive dengue serology result within 48 h of hospitalization; all potential cases were reviewed to exclude false-positive dengue serology.

2.2. Workflow for Patients Presenting with Undifferentiated Fever during the COVID-19 Pandemic

From the onset of the COVID-19 pandemic in January 2020, all patients with fever (defined as a single tympanic temperature of $\geq$37.8 °C) presenting to our institution were triaged in designated "fever areas" of the emergency department (ED), where HCWs used full personal protective equipment (PPE), comprising N95 respirators, gowns, gloves and eye protection, and infrastructural enhancements were introduced, such as partitions between patient cubicles and more frequent cleaning, to mitigate potential exposure to an unsuspected case of COVID-19 [19]. Basic investigations, including bloods and chest radiographs, were performed routinely for all patients presenting with fever in the ED, to aid in risk stratification. Dengue RDTs were also available in the ED. SARS-CoV-2 testing via PCR was available from the onset of the pandemic. While testing was initially ordered at the discretion of the primary physician based on case-definitions issued by the World Health Organisation (WHO) and our local Ministry of Health (MOH), from April 2020 onward, all admissions with fever were routinely screened for SARS-CoV-2 [16], and from June 2021, all admissions were universally screened for SARS-CoV-2 given large community outbreaks attributed to the SARS-CoV-2 delta variant (B.1.617.2 [18]. This degree of enhanced surveillance for SARS-CoV-2 allowed us to determine with certainty the extent of co-infection with both SARS-CoV-2 and dengue amongst all inpatients in the pandemic period, and detect cases of COVID-19 with false-positive dengue serology on RDTs. Given the significant turnaround time required for SARS-CoV-2 testing via PCR, initially patients with undifferentiated fever and no epidemiological risk for COVID-19 were preferentially admitted to designated isolation areas where patients were nursed either in single rooms or cohort rooms with 2–3 patients to a room (modified from usual norm of 5–6 bedded open-plan cohorted cubicles) [17]. HCWs in these wards used full PPE, comprising N95 respirators, gowns, gloves and eye protection when caring for these patients, until the results of SARS-CoV-2 testing returned [17]. From June 2021 onward, in addition to PCR, RAD testing for SARS-CoV-2 was also carried out in the ED for all admissions, with a turnaround time of 15 min [8]. Patients with a positive RAD result were admitted to negative-pressure single rooms in the isolation ward (IW) for confirmatory PCR testing. Patients with negative antigen tests were still risk-stratified for admission to isolation areas based on epidemiological risk and clinical syndromes.

2.3. Dengue Diagnostics

Our institution utilized the SD Bioline Dengue Duo (Abbott Diagnostics, Santa Clara, CA) for dengue diagnostic testing in the ED on blood specimens. This is a commercially available rapid immunochromatographic test that comes in a combo of two joint cassettes, one for nonstructural protein 1 (NS1) antigen (Ag) and another for IgM/IgG. Previous studies have indicated a combined sensitivity of 82.4% (95% CI: 76.8–87.1), with a specificity of 87.4% (95% CI: 82.8–91.2) [6]. Dengue NS1 Ag and IgM test using enzyme-linked immunosorbent assay (EIA) is also available inpatient, which has better sensitivity and specificity but a longer turnaround time due to batch testing. Reverse transcription-PCR for dengue virus from blood and urine specimens is also available at our institution as part of an in-house triplex PCR assay (testing for dengue, chikungunya and zikavirus).

2.4. COVID-19 Testing

SARS-CoV-2 testing was initially performed on respiratory specimens (nasopharyngeal, oropharyngeal, sputum or bronchoalveolar lavage specimens) using in-house qualitative real-time RT-PCR assays targeting E gene and ORF1b-nsp14 for SARS-CoV-2 [20]. Subsequently, with the availability of commercial assays, PCR testing was performed using the Cepheid Xpert Xpress SARS-CoV-2 assay or the Roche cobas SARS-CoV-2 test [21]. All samples were chemically inactivated for 30 min prior to transfer to the GeneXpert Infinity (Cepheid) in biosafety level 2 containment, or cobas 6800 System (Roche) in biosafety level 2 plus containment, for the SARS-CoV-2 tests. RAD testing for SARS-CoV-2 was performed using the Veritor SARS-CoV-2 antigen rapid test kit (Becton Dickinson, Franklin Lakes, NJ,

USA), with a positive percentage agreement of ≥80% and a negative percentage agreement of 99.5% compared to PCR testing [8,22]. Confirmatory SARS-CoV-2 PCR-testing was performed for all positive RAD tests at our institution.

2.5. Statistical Methods

Differences in the proportion of dengue hospitalisations requiring high-dependency/ intensive-care-unit admission, as well as the proportions of ED admissions presenting with fever during the pre-pandemic and pandemic periods were compared using chi-square test. Length-of-stay for dengue hospitalisations during the pre-pandemic and pandemic periods, and amongst dengue cases initially admitted to isolation areas (versus cases admitted outside of isolation areas) were compared using *t*-test. SPSS (Version 20.0. Armonk, NY, USA: IBM Corp) was used for statistical analysis and a cutoff of $p < 0.05$ was set for statistical significance.

3. Results

Over the COVID-19 pandemic period, a total of 6103 cases of COVID-19 and 1251 cases of dengue were admitted at our institution, comprising a total of 3.9% (6103/155,452) and 0.8% (1251/155,452) of admissions, respectively. A surge in the number of dengue hospitalisations in mid-2020 corresponded closely with the imposition of a community-wide lockdown period in 2020 as part of public health measures for COVID-19 containment. Conversely, despite a surge in COVID-19 cases in end-2021 driven by the SARS-CoV-2 delta variant, there was no surge in dengue hospitalisations in 2021 (Figure 1). Mortality amongst dengue hospitalisations remained low. Pre-pandemic, 0.51% (3/580) of dengue hospitalisations resulted in mortality; during the pandemic period, 0.40% (5/1251) of dengue hospitalisations resulted in mortality. There was no significant difference in mortality amongst dengue hospitalisations during the pandemic period when compared with the pre-pandemic period (incidence-rate-ratio, IRR = 0.77, 95%CI = 0.15–4.98, $p = 0.716$). There was also no significant difference in the odds of high-dependency/intensive-care-unit admission amongst dengue hospitalisations during the pandemic period, when compared with the pre-pandemic period (2.2% (28/1251) vs. 2.9% (17/580), odds-ratio, OR = 0.76, 95%CI = 0.42–1.40). However, average length-of-stay for dengue inpatients during the pandemic period was 7.53 days (standard-deviation, S.D = 7.30), compared with 6.27 days (S.D = 9.59) during the pre-pandemic period; the difference was statistically significant (difference in means = 1.27 days, 95%CI = 0.47–2.07, $p = 0.002$). Average length-of-stay for dengue cases initially admitted to isolation areas during the pandemic period was 8.35 days (S.D = 6.53), compared with 6.91 days (S.D = 8.61) for dengue cases admitted outside of isolation areas; the difference was statistically significant (difference in means = 1.44 days, 95%CI = 0.58–2.30, $p = 0.001$). Pre-pandemic, only 1.6% (9/580) of dengue cases were admitted initially to isolation areas; in contrast, during the pandemic period, 66.6% (833/1251) of dengue cases were initially admitted to isolation areas while awaiting the results of SARS-CoV-2 PCR-testing, due to epidemiological risk (e.g., contact with COVID-19 cases) or overlapping clinical syndromes.

While undifferentiated fever (≥37.8 °C) accounted for a significant proportion of ED admissions, the proportion of ED admissions presenting with fever decreased significantly in the pandemic period, compared to the pre-pandemic period. During the COVID-19 pandemic, 9.0% (8976/99,784) of ED admissions had concomitant fever, compared with 14.3% (15,097/105,435) of ED admissions in the pre-pandemic period (OR = 0.59, 95%CI = 0.57–0.61, $p < 0.001$). In the pre-pandemic period, dengue accounted for only 3.8% (573/15,097) of fever cases admitted via the ED, compared with 11.3% (1018/8976) during the pandemic period (OR = 3.24, 95%CI = 2.92–3.60, $p < 0.001$. In contrast, COVID-19 accounted for 6.1% (6103/99,784) of ED admissions and 17.2% (1548/8976) of fever cases admitted via the ED during the pandemic period. Amongst patients diagnosed with COVID-19, 25.3% (1548/6103) presented with fever (≥37.8 °C) at ED triage. In contrast, fever was present amongst 81.3% (1018/1251) of patients diagnosed with dengue at ED triage during the COVID-19 pandemic. The odds of concomitant fever amongst ED admissions diagnosed with COVID-19 were lower compared to ED admissions diagnosed with dengue (OR = 0.08, 95%CI = 0.07–0.09, $p < 0.001$).

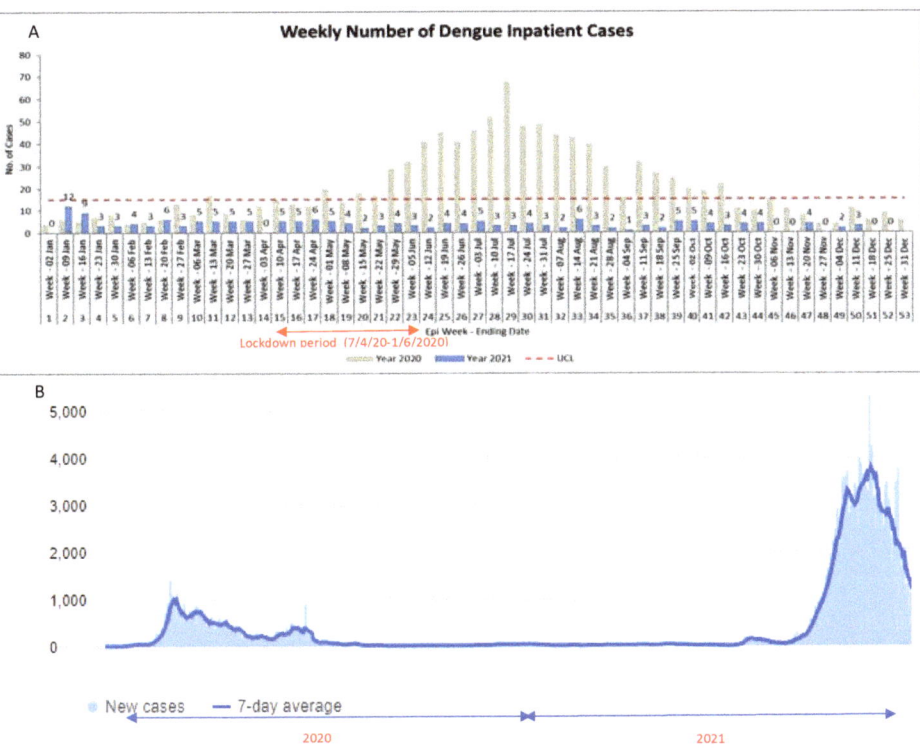

Figure 1. Rates of dengue hospitalisations in a Singaporean tertiary hospital over a 2-year study period during successive waves of community transmission in the COVID-19 pandemic. (**A**) Number of dengue admissions in a Singaporean tertiary hospital from January 2020 to December 2021; (**B**) Epidemic curve of COVID-19 cases in Singapore from January 2020 to December 2021.

A small proportion (15.9%, 974/6103) of PCR-confirmed COVID-19 cases were concurrently tested for dengue due to a compatible overlapping clinical syndrome. A total of 23 cases of PCR-proven COVID-19 infection with positive dengue serology were identified over the 2-year pandemic period; the large majority of these cases were deemed to have false-positive dengue serology on subsequent review (Table 1).

Table 1. Cases of PCR-proven COVID-19 infection with positive dengue serology at a Singaporean tertiary hospital during the COVID-19 pandemic, 2020–2021.

Case Number	Biodata	Presenting Symptoms	Pulmonary Infiltrates on Chest Radiograph	Thrombocytopenia at Presentation (10^9/L)	Dengue Tests (Serology and/or PCR)	Diagnosis	Outcome	Infection Prevention Consequences
1	31 yo male	Fever, sore throat, headache, myalgia, ageusia	No	Yes (nadir 109)	NS1 +ve, IgM −ve	COVID-19 URTI with probable dengue coinfection (NS1 +ve)	Full recovery	None. Managed in isolation from admission due to epidemiological risk factors for COVID-19
2	31 yo male	Fever, headache, myalgia, cough	No	Yes (nadir 122)	NS1 −ve, IgM +ve	COVID-19 URTI with likely false-positive dengue IgM	Full recovery	None. Managed in isolation from admission due to epidemiological risk factors for COVID-19
3	38 yo male	Fever, sore throat, headache, myalgia	No	No	NS1 −ve, IgM +ve	COVID-19 URTI with likely false-positive dengue IgM	Full recovery	None. Managed in isolation from admission due to epidemiological risk factors for COVID-19
4	34 yo male	Vomiting, diarrhea	No	No	NS1 −ve, IgM +ve	COVID-19 URTI with likely false-positive dengue IgM	Full recovery	None. Managed in isolation from admission due to epidemiological risk factors for COVID-19

Table 1. Cont.

Case Number	Biodata	Presenting Symptoms	Pulmonary Infiltrates on Chest Radiograph	Thrombocytopenia at Presentation (10^9/L)	Dengue Tests (Serology and/ or PCR)	Diagnosis	Outcome	Infection Prevention Consequences
5	29 yo male	Fever, headache, myalgia, cough, diarrhea	No	No	NS1 –ve, IgM +ve	COVID-19 URTI with likely false-positive dengue IgM	Full recovery	None. Managed in isolation from admission due to epidemiological risk factors for COVID-19
6	69 yo female	Fever	Yes	Yes (nadir 120)	NS1 –ve, IgM +ve	COVID-19 URTI with likely false-positive dengue IgM	Full recovery but needed ICU admission	None. Managed in isolation from admission due to epidemiological risk factors for COVID-19
7	38 yo male	Fever, headache, sore throat, myalgia, vomiting, diarrhea	No	No	NS1 –ve, IgM +ve; blood PCR at day 4 of illness –ve	COVID-19 URTI with false-positive dengue IgM (PCR negative)	Full recovery	None. Managed in isolation from admission due to epidemiological risk factors for COVID-19
8	34 yo male	Fever, headache, vomiting, dysgeusia	No	Yes (nadir 125)	NS1 –ve, IgM +ve; blood PCR at day 4 of illness –ve	COVID-19 URTI with false-positive dengue IgM (PCR negative)	Full recovery	Initially spent 14 hrs outside of isolation. 11 HCW and 2 inpatient close-contacts, none tested positive for SARS-CoV-2 on 14d surveillance
9	48 yo male	Fever, myalgia	No	Yes (nadir 82)	NS1 –ve, IgM +ve; blood PCR at day 7 of illness –ve	COVID-19 URTI with false-positive dengue IgM (PCR negative)	Full recovery	Initially spent 14.5 hrs outside of isolation. 10 HCW and 1 inpatient close-contacts, none tested positive for SARS-CoV-2 on 14d surveillance
10	43 yo male	Asymptomatic	No	Yes (nadir 100)	NS1 –ve, IgM +ve	COVID-19 URTI with likely false-positive dengue IgM	Full recovery	None. Managed in isolation from admission due to epidemiological risk factors for COVID-19
11	26 yo male	Cough, rhinorrhea	No	Yes (nadir 110)	NS1 –ve, IgM +ve	COVID-19 URTI with likely false-positive dengue IgM	Full recovery	None. Managed in isolation from admission due to epidemiological risk factors for COVID-19
12	30 yo male	Fever, myalgia	No	Yes (nadir 75)	NS1 +ve, IgM –ve	COVID-19 URTI with probable dengue coinfection (NS1 +ve)	Full recovery	None. Managed in isolation from admission due to epidemiological risk factors for COVID-19
13	49 yo male	Fever, cough, sore throat, rhinorrhea	Yes	No	NS1 –ve, IgM +ve	COVID-19 pneumonia with likely false-positive dengue IgM	Full recovery	None. Managed in isolation from admission due to epidemiological risk factors for COVID-19
14	89 yo male	Myalgia	No	No	NS1 –ve, IgM +ve	COVID-19 URTI with likely false-positive dengue IgM	Full recovery	None. Managed in isolation from admission due to positive rapid-antigen-detection test for COVID-19
15	73 yo male	Myalgia	No	Yes (nadir 100)	NS1 –ve, IgM +ve	COVID-19 URTI with likely false-positive dengue IgM	Full recovery	None. Managed in isolation from admission due to positive rapid-antigen-detection test for COVID-19
16	57 yo male	Fever, cough, dyspnea	Yes	Yes (nadir 105)	NS1 –ve, IgM +ve	COVID-19 pneumonia with likely false-positive dengue IgM	Full recovery	None. Managed in isolation from admission due to positive rapid-antigen-detection test for COVID-19
17	68 yo male	Fever, cough	Yes	Yes (nadir 96)	NS1 –ve, IgM +ve	COVID-19 pneumonia with likely false-positive dengue IgM	Full recovery	None. Managed in isolation from admission due to positive rapid-antigen-detection test for COVID-19
18	67 yo male	Fever, cough	No	Yes (nadir 110)	NS1 –ve, IgM +ve	COVID-19 pneumonia with likely false-positive dengue IgM	Full recovery	None. Managed in isolation from admission due to positive rapid-antigen-detection test for COVID-19
19	76 yo male	Fever, dyspnea	Yes	Yes (nadir 105)	NS1 –ve, IgM +ve	COVID-19 pneumonia with likely false-positive dengue IgM	Demised at D32 of illness, required ICU admission	None. Managed in isolation from admission due to epidemiological risk factors for COVID-19
20	57 yo male	Fever, cough, rhinorrhea, sore throat	Yes	No	NS1 –ve, IgM +ve	COVID-19 pneumonia with likely false-positive dengue IgM	Full recovery	None. Managed in isolation from admission as though rapid-antigen-detection test for COVID-19 was negative, patient had epidemiological risk factors for COVID-19
21	65 yo female	Fever, cough	No	Yes (nadir 105)	NS1 –ve, IgM +ve; blood PCR at day 4 of illness –ve	COVID-19 URTI with false-positive dengue IgM (PCR negative)	Full recovery	None. Managed in isolation from admission due to positive rapid-antigen-detection test for COVID-19
22	69 yo male	Fever, cough, dyspnea, diarrhea	Yes	Yes (nadir 106)	NS1 –ve, IgM +ve	COVID-19 pneumonia with likely false-positive dengue IgM	Full recovery	None. Managed in isolation from admission due to epidemiological risk factors for COVID-19
23	56 yo male	Fever, rhinorrhea, maculopapular rash	No	Yes (nadir 52)	NS1 –ve, IgM +ve; blood PCR at day 4 of illness –ve	COVID-19 URTI with false-positive dengue IgM (PCR negative)	Full recovery. Case of acute HIV seroconversion	None. Managed in isolation from admission due to epidemiological risk factors for COVID-19

Only 2 cases were deemed to have COVID-19 URTI with probable dengue coinfection (NS1-positive; compatible clinical syndrome with fever, myalgia and thrombocytopenia); both cases were managed in isolation from admission due to epidemiological risk factors for COVID-19. Amongst the remaining 21 cases of PCR-proven COVID-19 infection with likely false-positive dengue IgM, only 2 cases were managed outside of isolation areas initially; there was no evidence of onward healthcare-associated transmission to exposed HCWs or patients (Table 1). The remaining cases were isolated from onset due to either epidemiological risk factors or a positive RAD test for SARS-CoV-2, which prompted pre-emptive isolation despite a positive dengue IgM and a potential alternative diagnosis for undifferentiated fever.

4. Discussion

During the COVID-19 pandemic, successive waves of both COVID-19 and dengue in a dengue-endemic country placed significant burden on healthcare services; almost 5% of admissions at our institution were concomitantly diagnosed with either COVID-19 or dengue over a 2-year pandemic period. Other studies attributed an increase of over 37.2% in dengue cases from baseline to the introduction of social distancing measures aimed at curbing the spread of SARS-CoV-2 in Singapore; [13] indeed, lockdown measures during the COVID-19 pandemic coincided with a spike in dengue hospitalisations at our institution. This further exacerbated the diagnostic challenge posed by undifferentiated febrile illness during a "twindemic" of both COVID-19 and dengue, as both illnesses could potentially present with febrile syndromes. Over the 2-year pandemic period, COVID-19 and dengue together accounted for almost 30% of patients admitted from our hospital's ED with fever. Due to infection prevention challenges posed by SARS-CoV-2 and turnaround time required for diagnostic PCR-testing, a large proportion of dengue cases diagnosed via point-of-care testing in our hospital's ED still required admission to isolation areas while awaiting the return of SARS-CoV-2 PCR-testing. Pre-pandemic, $\leq$2% of dengue cases required initial admission to isolation areas while awaiting the return of diagnostic testing for other infections; in contrast, during the pandemic period, two-thirds of dengue cases were admitted initially to isolation areas. While there was no significant difference in mortality or odds of requiring high-dependency/intensive-care amongst dengue inpatients at our institution during the pandemic, there was a significant increase in length-of-stay, compared with the pre-pandemic period. This was potentially attributed to the requirement for isolation while awaiting the result of SARS-CoV-2 PCR-testing.

The requirement for isolation of febrile cases with positive dengue serology was driven by concern regarding COVID-19 cases masquerading as dengue with false-positive IgM as well as shared clinical and laboratory features between COVID-19 infection and dengue [1]. This is a clinical conundrum unique to dengue-endemic countries grappling with the COVID-19 pandemic; indeed, the first reports of patients incorrectly diagnosed with dengue due to a false-positive dengue rapid serological test who were subsequently diagnosed with COVID-19 originated from Singapore [9]. Misdiagnosis of COVID-19 as dengue with failure to isolate such patients could potentially trigger outbreaks in healthcare settings. Cases of potential nosocomial transmission have been reported amongst HCWs attending to such patients without appropriate PPE, due to the misplaced reassurance of a false-positive dengue serology test [10,11]. In addition, dengue and SARS-CoV-2 co-infection has been reported, providing an additional diagnostic challenge [23]. However, there is little information on the prevalence of dengue and SARS-CoV-2 co-infection; our experience suggests that both false-positive dengue IgM and co-infection with dengue are uncommon scenarios for COVID-19 infection, even in a dengue-endemic county. Over a two-year period, despite widespread availability of diagnostic testing for both dengue and COVID-19, only 21 cases of COVID-19 infection with false-positive dengue IgM and 2 cases of dengue and SARS-CoV-2 co-infection were identified at our centre, forming <0.5% of all COVID-19 cases admitted over the same time period. The infection prevention consequences of COVID-19 cases masquerading as dengue with false-positive IgM need to be balanced against the low likelihood, in practice, of encountering such cases, as well as the resources required to pre-emptively isolate all patients with undifferentiated febrile illness while awaiting the return of PCR-testing for COVID-19. Point-of-care tests, such as RAD testing for SARS-CoV-2, may potentially offer the clinician some additional reassurance with a faster clinical turnaround, though issues of sensitivity and specificity remain [22].

The limitations of our study are as follows. As this was a single-centre study, direct extrapolation of our observations to other contexts is difficult; nevertheless, the long study period allowed us to observe the prevalence of both dengue and COVID-19 at our institution through successive pandemic waves, given the seasonal nature of both dengue and COVID-19 infection. Prolonged length-of-stay during the pandemic period might have been due to other contributory factors associated with the challenges of care delivery during a pandemic, not just isolation requirements; nevertheless, throughout the pandemic our hospital continued to function as normal and did not require temporary closures due to nosocomial COVID-19 outbreaks, in part due to stringent inpatient and HCW surveillance [18]. Despite the stress placed on clinical laboratories during the COVID-19 pandemic [2], diagnostic testing for both COVID-19 and dengue continued to be made available at our institution throughout the pandemic period, with no delay in turnaround times. While false-positive dengue serology could be ruled out via PCR testing, the possibility of cross-reactivity with a different flavivirus could not be completely excluded. However, there were no outbreaks of zikavirus reported in Singapore during the study period, and Japanese encephalitis is not endemic in Singapore. Additionally, the prevalence of dengue may be underestimated since the sensitivity of NS1 detection with rapid diagnostic tests is lower during secondary infections, and dengue PCR was only performed in selected samples to confirm infection.

5. Conclusions

During successive COVID-19 pandemic waves in a dengue-endemic country, dengue was established as an alternative diagnosis in a minority of COVID-19 suspects. Coinfection with dengue and COVID-19 was uncommon. A triage strategy of routine COVID-19 testing for febrile patients with viral prodromes was successful in containing the potential infection-prevention risk from COVID-19 cases masquerading as dengue with false-positive IgM. While there was no significant difference in mortality amongst dengue hospitalisations during the pandemic, there was a significant increase in length-of-stay, especially amongst dengue cases initially admitted to isolation while awaiting results of SARS-CoV-2 testing.

Author Contributions: Conceptualization, L.E.W.; methodology, L.E.W. and E.P.C.; formal analysis, L.E.W. and E.P.C.; investigation, M.K.A., A.M.O., Y.Y. and S.A.; writing—original draft preparation, L.E.W.; writing—review and editing, J.X.-Y.S., M.K.A., A.M.O., Y.Y., S.A. and I.V.; supervision, I.V. All authors have read and agreed to the published version of the manuscript.

Funding: This research received no external funding.

Institutional Review Board Statement: As both dengue and COVID-19 are infectious diseases notifiable to our national MOH, in-formation presented in this paper was based on data routinely collected by our institution's epidemiology department as part of outbreak-investigation; ethics approval was not required under our institutional-review-board guidelines.

Informed Consent Statement: For clinical data on cases of COVID-19 with concurrent positive dengue serology, data was collected as part of surveillance and outbreak management, waiver of informed consent was approved by our hospital's institutional review board (CIRB Ref 2020/2436).

Data Availability Statement: The datasets for this study are available from the authors on reasonable request.

Acknowledgments: We thank our colleagues for their unstinting support in the COVID-19 pandemic.

Conflicts of Interest: The authors declare no conflict of interest.

References

1. Wilder-Smith, A.; Tissera, H.; Ooi, E.E.; Coloma, J.; Scott, T.W.; Gubler, D.J. Preventing Dengue Epidemics during the COVID-19 Pandemic. *Am. J. Trop. Med. Hyg.* **2020**, *103*, 570–571. [CrossRef] [PubMed]
2. Waterman, S.H.; Paz-Bailey, G.; San Martin, J.L.; Gutierrez, G.; Castellanos, L.G.; Mendez-Rico, J.A. Diagnostic Laboratory Testing and Clinical Preparedness for Dengue Outbreaks during the COVID-19 Pandemic. *Am. J. Trop. Med. Hyg.* **2020**, *103*, 1339–1340. [CrossRef] [PubMed]
3. Harapan, H.; Ryan, M.; Yohan, B.; Abidin, R.S.; Nainu, F.; Rakib, A.; Jahan, I.; Emran, T.B.; Ullah, I.; Panta, K.; et al. COVID-19 and dengue: Double punches for dengue-endemic countries in Asia. *Rev. Med. Virol.* **2021**, *31*, e2161. [CrossRef] [PubMed]

4. Lu, X.; Bambrick, H.; Pongsumpun, P.; Dhewantara, P.W.; Toan, D.T.T.; Hu, W. Dengue outbreaks in the COVID-19 era: Alarm raised for Asia. *PLoS Negl. Trop. Dis.* **2021**, *15*, e0009778. [CrossRef]
5. Hossain, M.S.; Amin, R.; Mosabbir, A.A. COVID-19 onslaught is masking the 2021 dengue outbreak in Dhaka, Bangladesh. *PLoS Negl. Trop. Dis.* **2022**, *16*, e0010130. [CrossRef]
6. Chong, Z.L.; Sekaran, S.D.; Soe, H.J.; Peramalah, D.; Rampal, S.; Ng, C.W. Diagnostic accuracy and utility of three dengue diagnostic tests for the diagnosis of acute dengue infection in Malaysia. *BMC Infect. Dis.* **2020**, *20*, 210. [CrossRef]
7. Van Honacker, E.; Van Vaerenbergh, K.; Boel, A.; De Beenhouwer, H.; Leroux-Roels, I.; Cattoir, L. Comparison of five SARS-CoV-2 rapid antigen detection tests in a hospital setting and performance of one antigen assay in routine practice: A useful tool to guide isolation precautions? *J. Hosp. Infect.* **2021**, *114*, 144–152. [CrossRef]
8. Wee, L.E.; Conceicao, E.P.; Sim, J.X.; Venkatachalam, I.; Wan, P.W.; Zakaria, N.D.; Tan, K.B.; Wijaya, L. Utilization of rapid antigen assays for detection of severe acute respiratory coronavirus virus 2 (SARS-CoV-2) in a low-incidence setting in emergency department triage: Does risk-stratification still matter? *Infect. Control Hosp. Epidemiol.* **2021**, *15*, 1–2. [CrossRef]
9. Yan, G.; Lee, C.K.; Lam, L.T.M.; Yan, B.; Chua, Y.X.; Lim, A.Y.N.; Phang, K.F.; Kew, G.S.; Teng, H.; Ngai, C.H.; et al. Covert COVID-19 and false-positive dengue serology in Singapore. *Lancet Infect. Dis.* **2020**, *20*, 536. [CrossRef]
10. Prasitsirikul, W.; Pongpirul, K.; Pongpirul, W.A.; Panitantum, N.; Ratnarathon, A.C.; Hemachudha, T. Nurse infected with COVID-19 from a provisional dengue patient. *Emerg. Microbes Infect.* **2020**, *9*, 1354–1355. [CrossRef]
11. Ratnarathon, A.C.; Pongpirul, K.; Pongpirul, W.A.; Charoenpong, L.; Prasithsirikul, W. Potential dual dengue and SARS-CoV-2 infection in Thailand: A case study. *Heliyon* **2020**, *6*, e04175. [CrossRef] [PubMed]
12. Clapham, H.E.; Chia, W.N.; Tan, L.W.L.; Kumar, V.; Lim, J.M.; Shankar, N.; Tun, Z.M.; Zahari, M.; Hsu, L.Y.; Sun, L.J.; et al. Contrasting SARS-CoV-2 epidemics in Singapore: Cohort studies in migrant workers and the general population. *Int. J. Infect. Dis.* **2022**, *115*, 72–78. [CrossRef] [PubMed]
13. Lim, J.T.; Chew, L.Z.X.; Choo, E.L.W.; Dickens, B.S.L.; Ong, J.; Aik, J.; Ng, L.C.; Cook, A.R. Increased Dengue Transmissions in Singapore Attributable to SARS-CoV-2 Social Distancing Measures. *J. Infect. Dis.* **2021**, *223*, 399–402. [CrossRef] [PubMed]
14. Ang, L.W.; Thein, T.L.; Ng, Y.; Boudville, I.C.; Chia, P.Y.; Lee, V.J.M.; Leo, Y.S. A 15-year review of dengue hospitalizations in Singapore: Reducing admissions without adverse consequences, 2003 to 2017. *PLoS Negl. Trop. Dis.* **2019**, *13*, e0007389. [CrossRef]
15. Thein, T.L.; Ang, L.W.; Young, B.E.; Chen, M.I.; Leo, Y.S.; Lye, D.C.B. Differentiating coronavirus disease 2019 (COVID-19) from influenza and dengue. *Sci. Rep.* **2021**, *11*, 19713. [CrossRef]
16. Wee, L.E.; Cherng, B.P.Z.; Conceicao, E.P.; Goh, K.C.-M.; Wan, W.Y.; Ko, K.K.K.; Aung, M.K.; Sim, X.Y.J.; Wijaya, L.; Ling, M.L.; et al. Experience of a Tertiary Hospital in Singapore with Management of a Dual Outbreak of COVID-19 and Dengue. *Am. J. Trop. Med. Hyg.* **2020**, *103*, 2005–2011. [CrossRef]
17. Wee, L.E.; Hsieh, J.Y.C.; Phua, G.C.; Tan, Y.; Conceicao, E.P.; Wijaya, L.; Tan, T.T.; Tan, B.H. Respiratory surveillance wards as a strategy to reduce nosocomial transmission of COVID-19 through early detection: The experience of a tertiary-care hospital in Singapore. *Infect. Control Hosp. Epidemiol.* **2020**, *41*, 820–825. [CrossRef]
18. Wee, L.E.I.; Conceicao, E.P.; Aung, M.K.; Aung, M.O.; Yong, Y.; Venkatachalam, I.; Sim, J.X. Rostered routine testing for healthcare workers and universal inpatient screening: The role of expanded hospital surveillance during an outbreak of coronavirus disease 2019 (COVID-19) in the surrounding community. *Infect. Control Hosp. Epidemiol.* **2021**, *6*, 1–3. [CrossRef]
19. Wee, L.E.; Fua, T.P.; Chua, Y.Y.; Ho, A.F.W.; Sim, X.Y.J.; Conceicao, E.P.; Venkatachalam, I.; Tan, K.B.; Tan, B.H. Containing COVID-19 in the Emergency Department: The Role of Improved Case Detection and Segregation of Suspect Cases. *Acad. Emerg. Med.* **2020**, *27*, 379–387. [CrossRef]
20. Corman, V.M.; Landt, O.; Kaiser, M.; Molenkamp, R.; Meijer, A.; Chu, D.K.; Bleicker, T.; Brünink, S.; Schneider, J.; Schmidt, M.L.; et al. Detection of 2019 novel coronavirus (2019-nCoV) by real-time RT-PCR. *Eurosurveillance* **2020**, *25*, 2000045. [CrossRef]
21. Yingtaweesittikul, H.; Ko, K.; Rahman, N.A.; Tan, S.Y.L.; Nagarajan, N.; Suphavilai, C. CalmBelt: Rapid SARS-CoV-2 Genome Characterization for Outbreak Tracking. *Front. Med.* **2021**, *8*, 790662. [CrossRef] [PubMed]
22. Young, S.; Taylor, S.N.; Cammarata, C.L.; Varnado, K.G.; Roger-Dalbert, C.; Montano, A.; Griego-Fullbright, C.; Burgard, C.; Fernandez, C.; Eckert, K.; et al. Clinical Evaluation of BD Veritor SARS-CoV-2 Point-of-Care Test Performance Compared to PCR-Based Testing and versus the Sofia 2 SARS Antigen Point-of-Care Test. *J. Clin. Microbiol.* **2020**, *59*, e02338-20. [CrossRef] [PubMed]
23. Carosella, L.M.; Pryluka, D.; Maranzana, A.; Barcan, L.; Cuini, R.; Freuler, C.; Martinez, A.; Equiza, T.R.; Peria, C.R.; Yahni, D.; et al. Characteristics of Patients Co-infected with Severe Acute Respiratory Syndrome Coronavirus 2 and Dengue Virus, Buenos Aires, Argentina, March–June 2020. *Emerg. Infect. Dis.* **2021**, *27*, 348–351. [CrossRef] [PubMed]

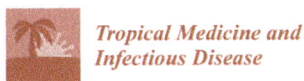

Article

Transmission of SARS-CoV-2 in the Population Living in High- and Low-Density Gradient Areas in Dhaka, Bangladesh

Syed Moinuddin Satter [1,*], Taufiqur Rahman Bhuiyan [1], Zarin Abdullah [1], Marjahan Akhtar [1], Aklima Akter [1], S. M. Zafor Shafique [1], Muhammad Rashedul Alam [1], Kamal Ibne Amin Chowdhury [1], Arifa Nazneen [1], Nadia Ali Rimi [1], A. S. M. Alamgir [2], Mahbubur Rahman [2], Farzana Islam Khan [2], Tahmina Shirin [2], Meerjady Sabrina Flora [3], Sayera Banu [1], Mustafizur Rahman [1], Mahmudur Rahman [4] and Firdausi Qadri [1]

1. Programme for Emerging Infections, Infectious Diseases Division, icddr,b, Dhaka 1212, Bangladesh; taufiqur@icddrb.org (T.R.B.); zarin.abdullah@icddrb.org (Z.A.); marjahan.akhtar@icddrb.org (M.A.); aklima17@gmail.com (A.A.); zafor.shafique@icddrb.org (S.M.Z.S.); rashedul.alam@icddrb.org (M.R.A.); kiachowdhury@icddrb.org (K.I.A.C.); arifa.nazneen@icddrb.org (A.N.); nadiarimi@icddrb.org (N.A.R.); sbanu@icddrb.org (S.B.); mustafizur@icddrb.org (M.R.); fqadri@icddrb.org (F.Q.)
2. Institute of Epidemiology, Disease Control & Research, 44 Mohakhali, Dhaka 1212, Bangladesh; dr.alamgir@iedcr.gov.bd (A.S.M.A.); dr.mahbub@iedcr.gov.bd (M.R.); dr.farzana@iedcr.gov.bd (F.I.K.); director@iedcr.gov.bd (T.S.)
3. Directorate General of Health Services (DGHS), Mohakhali, Dhaka 1212, Bangladesh; adgplanning@ld.dghs.gov.bd
4. Global Health Development, EMPHNET, 69 Mohakhali, Dhaka 1212, Bangladesh; mrahman@globalhealthdev.org
* Correspondence: dr.satter@icddrb.org; Tel.: +88-0179-066-5868

Abstract: Community transmission of SARS-CoV-2 in densely populated countries has been a topic of concern from the beginning of the pandemic. Evidence of community transmission of SARS-CoV-2 according to population density gradient and socio-economic status (SES) is limited. In June–September 2020, we conducted a descriptive longitudinal study to determine the community transmission of SARS-CoV-2 in high- and low-density areas in Dhaka city. The Secondary Attack Rate (SAR) was 10% in high-density areas compared to 20% in low-density areas. People with high SES had a significantly higher level of SARS-CoV-2-specific Immunoglobulin G (IgG) antibodies on study days 1 ($p = 0.01$) and 28 ($p = 0.03$) compared to those with low SES in high-density areas. In contrast, the levels of seropositivity of SARS-CoV-2-specific Immunoglobulin M (IgM) were comparable ($p > 0.05$) in people with high and low SES on both study days 1 and 28 in both high- and low-density areas. Due to the similar household size, no differences in the seropositivity rates depending on the population gradient were observed. However, people with high SES showed higher seroconversion rates compared to people with low SES. As no difference was observed based on population density, the SES might play a role in SARS-CoV-2 transmission, an issue that calls for further in-depth studies to better understand the community transmission of SARS-CoV-2.

Keywords: COVID-19; SARS-CoV-2; community transmission; population density gradient; Dhaka; Bangladesh

1. Introduction

The COVID-19 pandemic, caused by the novel severe acute respiratory syndrome coronavirus 2 (SARS-CoV-2), has affected 450 million people, with 6.01 million deaths, worldwide up to 8 March 2022. The transmission of SARS-CoV-2 from an index case has been documented to occur following close contact through infected secretions such as saliva and respiratory secretions or respiratory droplets, as well as other body fluids [1,2]. Secondary attack rates, which indicate how interactions relate to the transmission risk, have been estimated at 3.3% for SARS-CoV-2, 16.1% of which following household contacts, and 1.1% following social contacts [3]. The basic reproduction number (R0) of SARS-CoV-2, an indication of the virus's initial transmissibility, was estimated to be 4.71 (range of 4.50–4.92) when the pandemic started in December 2019 [4]. In recent publications, the basic reproduction numbers of SARS-CoV-2 were observed to vary in the range of 1.0011–2.7936 for different countries [5]. Worldwide, the parameters of transmission dynamics of SARS-CoV-2 have been estimated mostly among household or social contacts. However, evidence on transmission dynamics of SARS-CoV-2 according to population density gradients in low- and middle-income countries was scarce when this study was started. Bangladesh is a densely populated country, with 1116 people living per square kilometer, and in Dhaka, the capital, it is estimated that 220,246 persons live per square kilometer (km) in high-density areas like slums [3], and 29,857 persons live per square kilometer (km) in low-density areas such as non-slums [6]. On 8 March 2020, the Government of Bangladesh reported the first case of SARS-CoV-2, and as of May 2021, close to a million people have tested positive for SARS-CoV-2 in Bangladesh, with over 12,549 confirmed deaths [7]. From the data of the Bangladesh Bureau of Statistics, it has been observed that there are significant differences in population density in different areas of Dhaka city. Therefore, we assumed that the transmission dynamics of SARS-CoV-2 might be diverse according to population density gradients. Moreover, people in Bangladesh mostly maintain a robust social network, and community members interact with each other often. This practice might also contribute to the community transmission of SARS-CoV-2 but may differ according to the population density. From mid-April 2020 up to December 2020, a nationwide community-based transmission study on "Transmission Dynamics of COVID-19 in Bangladesh" was carried out both in rural and urban areas to estimate the secondary attack rate (SAR) and the basic reproduction number (R0) among household contacts. At that time, we were not aware that the parameters of transmission dynamics of SARS-CoV-2 may differ among contacts of SARS-CoV-2 index cases according to the population density gradient of Dhaka city. Therefore, we initiated this study intending to estimate the secondary attack rate (SAR) and basic reproduction number (R0) among contacts in high- and low-density areas of Dhaka city. Our hypothesis was that SAR would be higher in high-density areas because of the local social structure and behavior patterns. For a long time, the Government of Bangladesh implemented area-wise lock-down or mobility restrictions depending upon the level of risk of infection in different communities. The findings of this study aim to supplement governmental policies for future outbreaks of SARS-CoV-2. To gain a comprehensive understanding of the susceptible population, we also tested for sero-positivity people who reported household or neighborhood contacts with a laboratory-confirmed case. We also collected qualitative data on risk perception and prevention practices such as masking and social distancing in high- and low-density populations in Bangladesh, which will be reported in a subsequent article. Here, we report key epidemiological and laboratory-based data from a longitudinal study of SARS-CoV-2 transmission among household and neighborhood contacts.

2. Materials and Methods
2.1. Study Design and Settings

The study design was longitudinal, and its duration was 6 months, commencing on 27 June 2020. In the beginning, we located laboratory-confirmed index cases in high-density communities of six slums and low-density communities of seven wards of Dhaka city through the "Transmission Dynamics of COVID-19 in Bangladesh" study. The detailed methodology of symptomatic and asymptomatic index case enrollment was described elsewhere [8]. Then, the cases were interviewed to trace their home and neighborhood contacts. We followed World Health Organization (WHO) contact definition considering our study and country context. We considered an individual as a contact who experienced any of the following exposures during the 2 days before and the 14 days after the onset of symptoms of a laboratory-confirmed COVID-19 case: (1) face-to-face contact with a confirmed case within 1 m and for more than 15 min (including travel, gossips, tea stall) or (2) direct physical contact with a confirmed COVID-19 case. The contacts were communicated by the team for verification of the exposure to the case and possible enrollment. After enrollment, collection of epidemiological data and specimens was done. Nasopharyngeal samples were collected on day 1, day 7, day 14, and day 28 for RT-PCR. Blood samples were collected on day 1 and day 28 for ELISA antibody test for seropositivity. The contacts were followed up for 14 days for signs and symptoms. The distance from the index case household to their neighbor was determined using a Global Positioning System (GPS) tracker.

2.2. Participants and Procedures

We used operational definitions to describe high- and low-density neighborhoods (see Appendix A). In high-density neighborhoods, considering an overall SAR at a neighborhood of 20% with a 95% confidence interval, a 5% desired precision, and a 1.5 design (household cluster) effect, it was estimated that 365 exposed contacts were required [9]. After considering a 10% loss to follow-up and a 15% non-response rate (refusal/non-availability), an estimated 460 neighborhood contacts had to be enrolled. In low-density neighborhoods, a similar methodology was followed, with an overall SAR per neighborhood of 5%; we estimated that 143 contacts needed to be enrolled. We assumed that one case would yield 15–20 contacts [10]. We estimated to approach 31 cases in high-density neighborhoods and 10 cases in low-density neighborhoods to enroll the estimated number of contacts. However, during the fieldwork, we stopped after the enrollment of the 14th index case, as we reached the target number of contacts (n = 460). On the other hand, we had to enroll more cases (n = 23) to reach the estimated target number of controls (n = 143).

2.3. Laboratory Testing

2.3.1. SARS-CoV-2 RT-PCR

Viral RNA was extracted and purified from nasopharyngeal swab samples using the Invimag Pathogen kit and an automatic extractor (KingFisher Flex96 system). SARS-CoV-2 detection was performed using a semi-quantitative, matrix gene-specific, probe-based real-time reverse-transcription polymerase chain reaction (RT-qPCR) assay.

2.3.2. SARS-CoV-2-Specific Enzyme-Linked Immunosorbent Assay (ELISA)

The Receptor Binding Domain (RBD) of the spike protein of SARS-CoV-2 was used as an antigen to detect antibody responses as discussed previously (Akter et al., 2021, manuscript in review). RBD-specific IgG and IgM antibody responses were measured using a monoclonal antibody (CR3022) of known concentration, specific to SARS-CoV-2 RBD. This ELISA procedure was validated and described previously [11] (Akter et al., 2021, manuscript in review). Using serum from pre-pandemic healthy controls, we determined the concentration of 500 ng/mL (0.5 µg/mL) as a cut-off value for seropositivity for both RBD-specific IgG and IgM antibodies.

2.4. Statistical Analysis

We summarized all categorical variables using frequency and percentage, and all symmetric continuous variables using mean and standard deviation. All variables not having a normal distribution are presented using a median and inter-quartile range. The results from the seroprevalence data were used for the calculation of the fraction of the population that was susceptible.

The secondary attack rate was calculated by dividing the number of positive SARS-CoV-2 contacts on any day of sample collection by the number of contacts enrolled and is presented as a proportion. The basic reproduction number was calculated by dividing the positive SARS-CoV-2 contacts during 14 days of follow-up by the number of index cases. χ^2 tests were used to compare proportions, and Wilcoxon rank-sum test was used for continuous variables.

We analyzed seroprevalence data based on socioeconomic status in high- and low-density areas as we did not observe any difference in the seroprevalence level depending on the density gradient. Statistical differences in the antibody levels between high- and low-SES groups were analyzed using the Mann–Whitney U test. p-values < 0.05 were considered statistically significant.

Written informed consent was obtained from the enrolled cases and contacts. The study protocol was reviewed and approved by icddr,b's Research Review and Ethical Review Committees.

3. Results

3.1. Epidemiological Findings

From 27 June 2020 to 26 September 2020, 14 and 23 index cases were enrolled from high- and low-density areas, respectively. During this period, 497 contacts were enrolled from high-density areas, and 187 contacts from low-density areas. The average number of contacts per case was 36 in high-density areas and 8 in low-density areas (Figure 1).

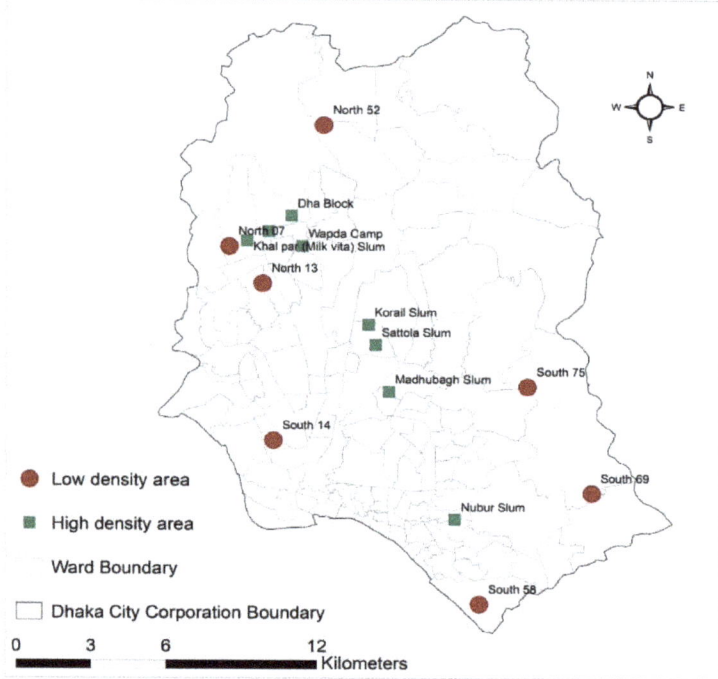

Figure 1. Map showing the location of the selected high- and low-density areas of Dhaka city.

The total number of refusals was 107 in high-density areas and 40 in low-density areas. The primary reasons for not being able to collect the samples were absence from home (47%), refusal (38%), and migration (15%). Most of the enrolled contacts were in the 11–30 age groups in high- and low-density areas (Table 1). Enrollment of female contacts was higher in both high- (54%) and low-density (53%) areas (Table 1). The contacts had mostly a primary education level in both high- (40%) and low-density (52%) areas (Table 1). Ten percent of the contacts (10%, 50/497) were SARS-CoV-2-positive in high-density areas, and 20% (37/187) were SARS-CoV-2-positive in low-density areas. SARS-CoV-2 was identified at least in one of four nasopharyngeal specimens, collected on days 1, 7, 14, and 28.

Table 1. Distribution of the demographic characteristics of contacts in high-density and low-density areas.

Characteristic	High-Density N = 497		Low-Density N = 187	
	n	(%)	n	(%)
Median Age (range) in years	25	(0 *–95) ψ	27	(3–75) ψ
Age Distribution				
<5 years	7	(1)	1	(1)
6–10 years	33	(7)	9	(5)
11–20 years	141	(28)	42	(22)
21–30 years	120	(24)	67	(36)
31–40 years	92	(19)	24	(13)
41–50 years	60	(12)	22	(12)
51–60 years	32	(6)	13	(7)
>60 years	12	(2)	9	(5)
Sex				
Male	228	(46)	88	(47)
Female	269	(54)	99	(53)
Education				
No education	141	(28)	20	(11)
Primary	201	(40)	98	(52)
Secondary	131	(26)	49	(26)
Higher Secondary	18	(4)	10	(5)
Tertiary	6	(1)	10	(5)
Household †				
Household size (Median, range)	4	(1–14)	4	(1–9)
No. of bedrooms (Median, range)	1	(1–4)	2	(1–6)
Size of bedroom, sft (Median, range)	110	(12–289)	140	(13–400)
Sharing bedroom	462	(97)	136	(94)
No. of family members sharing one bedroom (Median, Range)	3	(0–7)	3	(0–12)
Income and Expenditure †				
Monthly income, BDT (mean, SD±)	16,942	(±12,691)	20,881	(±13,549)
Monthly expenditure, BDT (mean, SD±)	14,098	(±8284)	18,852	(±16,267)

ψ Range, * 8 months, † Neighborhood contacts (N = 623).

In high-density areas, 91% (452/497) of the contacts were asymptomatic during enrollment, compared to 75% (141/187) in low-density areas. Among them, 7% (31/452) developed symptoms within 14 days of follow-up, and 13% (4/31) were diagnosed as SARS-CoV-2-positive in high-density areas. Eleven percent (16/141) of the contacts later developed symptoms in low-density areas, and 31% (5/16) became SARS-CoV-2-positive. The detection of new positive contacts was highest on day 1 in both high-density (48%) and low-density (54%) areas compared to the follow-up days at 7, 14, and 28.

The highest proportions of SARS-CoV-2-positive subjects were detected among contacts aged between 21 and 30 years in both high- (30%) and low-density (46%) areas. In high-density areas, 40% of males were infected with SARS-CoV-2, whereas in low-density areas, 32% of males were infected with SARS-CoV-2.

Overall, the secondary attack rate (SAR) was 13% (87/684), and the SAR among contacts was 10% in high-density areas compared to 20% in low-density areas (Table 2). The basic reproduction number (R0) was 2.7 in high-density areas and 1 in low-density areas (Table 3).

Table 2. Secondary attack rate (SAR) in high-density and low-density areas in Dhaka city.

	Secondary Case				Uninfected Contacts				Secondary Attack Rate		p-Value
	High		Low		High		Low		High	Low	
	n	%	n	%	n	%	n	%	%	%	
Contact type											
Household	1	(2)	12	(32)	19	(4)	29	(19)	5	29	<0.05
Neighborhood	49	(98)	25	(68)	428	(96)	121	(81)	10	17	<0.05
Overall	50	(100)	37	(100)	447	(100)	150	(100)	10	20	<0.05
Seropositivity at day 1											
Positive	27	(54)	23	(62)	277	(62)	85	(57)	9	21	<0.05
Negative	23	(46)	14	(38)	170	(38)	65	(43)	12	18	>0.05
Age, years											
<18	11	(22)	6	(16)	122	(27)	25	(17)	8	19	>0.05
18–49	31	(62)	25	(68)	279	(62)	103	(69)	10	20	<0.05
≥50	8	(16)	6	(16)	46	(10)	22	(15)	15	21	>0.05
Sex											
Male	20	(40)	12	(32)	208	(47)	76	(51)	9	14	<0.05
Female	30	(60)	25	(68)	239	(53)	74	(49)	11	25	<0.05
Education											
No education	9	(18)	2	(5)	132	(30)	18	(12)	6	10	>0.05
Primary	26	(52)	24	(65)	175	(39)	74	(49)	13	24	<0.05
Secondary	14	(28)	9	(24)	117	(26)	40	(27)	11	18	>0.05
Higher Secondary	1	(2)	1	(3)	17	(4)	9	(6)	6	10	>0.05
Tertiary	0	(0)	1	(3)	6	(1)	9	(6)	0	10	>0.05
Household size †											
<6 members	43	(88)	19	(76)	332	(79)	96	(79)	11	17	>0.05
≥6 members	6	(12)	6	(24)	96	(23)	25	(21)	6	19	<0.05
Sharing bedroom †											
Yes	46	(94)	25	(100)	417	(97)	112	(93)	10	18	<0.05
No	2	(4)	0	(0)	11	(3)	9	(7)	15	0	>0.05
Monthly income, BDT ** †											
≤10,000	14	(29)	7	(28)	115	(27)	19	(16)	11	27	<0.05
>10,000	35	(71)	18	(72)	313	(73)	102	(86)	10	15	>0.05
Monthly expenditure, BDT ** †											
≤10,000	22	(45)	11	(44)	169	(39)	25	(21)	12	31	<0.05
>10,000	27	(55)	14	(56)	259	(61)	96	(79)	9	13	>0.05

** BDT, Bangladeshi Taka. † Neighborhood contacts (N = 623).

The effective reproduction number was higher than 1 in high-density areas (1.4), whereas it was lower than 1 in low-density areas (0.71). By using a GPS tracker, a total of 497 contacts from 268 households in high-density areas and of 187 contacts from 92 households in low-density areas were identified. We observed that the average distance between an index case household and a contact household was 35 m in high-density areas, whereas it was 44 m in low-density areas. We found positive contacts up to a distance of 250 m from an index case household in high-density areas and of up to 440 m away from an index case household in low-density areas (Figures A1 and A2).

Table 3. Estimation of the basic reproduction number (Ro) in high-density and low-density areas in Dhaka city.

	Secondary Case within 14 Days		Index Case	
	High (n = 39)	Low (n = 34)	High (n = 14)	Low (n = 23)
	n	n	Basic Reproduction Number (Ro)	
Contact type				
Household	1	11	0.1	0.5
Neighborhood	38	23	**2.7**	1
Age, years				
<18	9	6	0.6	0.3
18–49	24	24	1.7	1.0
≥50	6	4	0.4	0.2
Overall	39	34	2.8	1.5
Sex				
Male	16	10	1.1	0.4
Female	23	24	1.6	1
Education				
No education	8	1	0.6	0
Primary	20	23	1.4	1
Secondary	10	8	0.7	0.3
Higher Secondary	1	1	0.1	0
Tertiary	0	1	0	0
Household size †				
<6 members	33	18	**2.4**	0.8
≥6 members	5	5	0.4	0.2
Sharing bedroom †				
Yes	35	23	**2.5**	0.3
No	3	0	0.2	0.7
Monthly income, ** †				
≤10,000	13	6	0.9	0.3
>10,000	25	17	**1.8**	0.7
Monthly expenditure, ** †				
≤10,000	19	10	1.4	0.4
>10,000	19	13	1.4	0.6

** BDT, Bangladeshi Taka. † Neighborhood contacts (N = 623).

3.2. SARS-CoV-2-Specific Antibody Responses in Relation to High and Low SES

Primarily, we analyzed the seroprevalence of SARS-CoV-2 antibodies in high- and low-density areas of Dhaka city. However, there was no difference in the magnitude and frequencies ($p > 0.05$; data not shown) in the level of SARS-CoV-2 antibodies between people in high- and low-density areas of Dhaka. Thereafter, we performed additional seroprevalence analyses for SARS-CoV-2 antibodies comparing people with high and low socioeconomic status living within high- and low-density areas. We determined SARS-CoV-2-specific IgG and IgM seropositivity in all individuals on study day 1 and day 28. People living in high-density areas with high SES had significantly higher levels of SARS-CoV-2-specific IgG antibodies on both study day 1 ($p = 0.011$) and study day 28 ($p = 0.005$) compared to the people with low SES. In contrast, this effect was not observed in the low-density areas (Table 4). IgG seropositivity was also significantly higher in high-SES people living in high-density areas than in low-SES participants on both study day 1 (73% vs. 59%, $p = 0.011$) and study day 28 (74% vs. 59%, $p = 0.005$). In contrast, the level of seropositivity for SARS-CoV-2-specific IgM was comparable ($p > 0.05$) in people with high and low socioeconomic status on both study day 1 and study day 28 (Table 4).

Table 4. Seropositivity and level of SARS-CoV-2 antibodies in high- and low-SES people living in high- and low-density areas of Dhaka city.

	Day 1						Day 28					
	High Density			Low Density			High Density			Low Density		
	High SES (n = 119)	Low SES (n = 323)	p Value	High SES (n = 47)	Low SES (n = 71)	p Value	High SES (n = 119)	Low SES (n = 323)	p Value	High SES (n = 47)	Low SES (n = 71)	p Value
IgG												
[a] Seropositivity, n (%)	87 (73)	192 (59)	0.011 *	31 (66)	41 (58)	0.482	88 (74)	192 (59)	0.005 **	34 (72)	43 (61)	0.237
[b] GM (ng/mL)	827	448	0.015 *	478	460	0.783	627	365	0.029 *	525	453	0.694
IgM												
[a] Seropositivity, n (%)	61 (51)	153 (47)	0.536	18 (38)	35 (49)	0.324	48 (40)	128 (40)	0.913	14 (30)	24 (34)	0.691
[b] GM (ng/mL)	443	441	0.562	345	490	0.129	365	381	0.949	296	356	0.098

[a] Statistical analysis for seropositivity in high- and low-SES groups was performed using the chi-square test. [b] Statistical difference in the geometric mean conc. of antibodies between high- and low-SES groups was analyzed using the Mann-Whitney U test. * p = <0.05; ** p = <0.01.

Next, we analyzed seropositivity among RT-PCR-positive contacts found on days 1, 7, 14, and 28. Overall, individuals with both low and high SES who were RT-PCR-positive on day 1 had increased levels of IgG antibodies on day 28 (Table A1). IgG seropositivity also rose from 62–69% (day 1) to 100% (day 28), but no statistically significant differences were observed between high- and low-SES participants. In contrast, when considering the RT-PCR-positive individuals on day 7, high-SES participants had significantly higher ($p < 0.005$) seropositivity on day 1 compared to low-SES individuals (70% vs. 45%). A similar trend was observed among high-SES individuals who were RT-PCR-positive on study days 14 and 28 (Table A1).

No apparent increase in IgM seropositivity was observed between study day 1 and day 28 among RT-PCR-positive individuals. Higher, but not significant, IgM antibody levels were found on day 28 in RT-PCR-positive participants compared to day 1. Among RT-PCR-positive individuals on day 14, high-SES participants had significantly higher ($p = 0.006$) seropositivity on day 1 compared to low-SES subjects (67% vs. 47%) (Table A1).

4. Discussion

To our knowledge, this is the first population-based study on secondary attack rate (SAR) and prevalence of antibodies in people affected by COVID-19 in Bangladesh as well as in South East Asia. In Bangladesh, particularly, a second wave of the pandemic started just a year after the first case was detected in In March 2020. Interestingly, in our study, we did not observe any difference in the frequencies of SARS-CoV-2-specific antibodies in people living in areas with different density gradients in Dhaka city. Since we followed up active cases from randomly chosen areas with similar population densities, the number of household members, age distribution, and collection of biological specimens from the high and low-density areas were also important factors when analyzing the data. This study was carried out to observe differences in the SAR and seroprevalence level in people living in high- and low-density areas.

We found that 10% (50/497) of contacts were SARS-CoV-2-positive as determined by RT-PCR in high-density areas, compared to 20% (37/187) in low-density areas. Studies conducted on SARS-CoV-2 transmission reported an attack rate ranging from 17 to 18.9%, which is comparable with the findings of our study conducted in low-density neighborhoods [12–15]. At the beginning of the study, it was assumed that SAR would be higher in high-density areas because of the local social structure and behavior patterns. Studies conducted on the correlation of population density and SARS-CoV-2 transmission also suggested an influence of population density. One study conducted in the United States reported that a lower population density was associated with decreased community transmission [16]. In our study, we observed that most of the high-density population lost their job or income source due to the lockdown and therefore had to migrate back to villages. Therefore, this might be one reason why the low-density population SAR was higher than that measured for the high-density population. When considering age groups, the highest levels of SARS-CoV-2 positivity were detected among contacts aged between 18 and 49 years in both high- and low-density areas (30%). This result is consistent with other reports since, in most countries, the age group between 20 and 59 years is the most numerous [9,17,18]. Males were more frequently infected, which is in contrast to what was observed in China [9]. Overall, the SAR among contacts was 13% (87/684), similar to what was observed in China and Denmark, [9,12]. We observed that the SAR was higher among people who received primary education, shared a bedroom, and earned less than 10,000 BDT (~USD 119), similar to what was found in a study conducted in Singapore, where sharing a bedroom was associated with SARS-CoV-2 transmission [17]. Basic reproduction rates were higher in high-density areas than in low-density ones. Asymptomatic contacts, who were followed up for 14 days and developed symptoms, had a similar SARS-CoV-2 positivity rate compared to other studies [12]. We found higher frequencies of seropositive participants for SARS-CoV-2 IgG antibodies in areas with a high socioeconomic level on day 1 and day 28 in comparison to areas with a low socioeconomic level. A similar study conducted in Cape Town, South Africa [18], reported a higher seroprevalence of SARS-CoV-2 antibodies in participants with a low standardized income, which is opposite to our study findings.

Moreover, participants who were working in low-income occupations and living in informal accommodations more likely tested positive for antibody responses [18]. Nearly half of Khayelitsha participants, who belonged to a partially informal township in Cape Town, were affected by overcrowding and poverty and tested positive for SARS-CoV-2 antibodies [18]. This discrepancy may be due to differences in the definition of these countries' low and high socioeconomic status. Another limitation of the study may be linked to the small number of participants in the high socioeconomic status, which skewed the analyses. Similar disparities were observed in high-income countries like the USA. In New York City, the number of laboratory-confirmed COVID-19 cases was significantly associated with multiple socioeconomic factors, e.g., population density, dependent children, and median household income [19]. In another study, the number of laboratory-confirmed COVID-19 cases and deaths was compared to the poverty index of each USA county. It was observed that, at the beginning of the pandemic, the counties with a higher poverty index yielded a higher number of cases and deaths, and this trend was confirmed throughout the pandemic [20]. In Leicester, UK, the likelihood of testing SARS-CoV-2-positive by RT-PCR was higher in the population with a larger household and belonging to an ethnic minority [21]. Smartphone tracking data in the USA demonstrated that the 'stay at home' orders were less followed in low-income areas compared to high-income areas [22]. In that study, participants from low-income districts reported facing multiple physical barriers to social distancing and stay-at-home orders, which may explain the higher seroprevalence in these areas [22].

Not only antibodies levels but also the levels of SARS-CoV-2-specific memory T cells may reflect a previous infection and can be important for the establishment of a long-term immunity to COVID-19. Recently, SARS-CoV-2-specific T-cells have been identified in a subset of seronegative individuals, and, importantly, SARS-CoV-2-specific T-cells were more commonly detected in close contacts of confirmed SARS-CoV-2 patients than in blood donors [23]. Using the identification of SARS-CoV-2 RNA by PCR as a marker of infection, we may have underestimated the true prevalence of COVID-19 in our cohort in comparison to seroconversion analysis. Participants may have been infected by SARS-CoV-2, as evident by seropositivity, though remaining asymptomatic. In addition, dampened immune responses in the low-SES people may be related to the lack of T cell immune responses. Therefore, prospective seroprevalence studies in different settings (high- and low-density areas) of Dhaka city are needed to establish infection control guidelines, along with in-depth studies for measuring SARS-CoV-2-specific T-cell responses.

This study has several limitations. First, we conducted it at the beginning of the pandemic (June–September 2020). Second, we cannot claim that COVID-19-positive neighborhood contacts had not been infected by other index cases rather than by the enrolled index cases. Third, the transmission of infection could also have been possible from our defined contacts to cases. Fourth, we observed no differences related to the socio-economic conditions between high- and low-density areas among the study population for any of the variables tested. To mitigate this limitation, we further analyzed our data using the Modified Kuppuswamy Socioeconomic Scale.

5. Conclusions

We observed that the secondary attack rate for COVID-19 infection was higher in low-density areas. On the other hand, the basic reproduction number (R0) was higher in high-density areas in the same period. Our study shows that people with a higher socioeconomic status seroconvert significantly compared to those with a lower socioeconomic status. More in-depth studies are needed, following this cohort longitudinally and observing their nutrition patterns, behavioral practices, and household size, so to better understand the mechanism of COVID-19 infection, its nature, and its transmission process.

Author Contributions: Conceptualization, S.M.S., T.R.B., A.N., N.A.R., T.S., S.B., M.R. (Mustafizur Rahman), M.R. (Mahmudur Rahman) and F.Q.; Data curation, Z.A., M.A., S.M.Z.S. and M.R.A.; Formal analysis, S.M.S., T.R.B., Z.A., M.A. and A.A.; Funding acquisition, S.M.S., T.S., S.B., M.R. (Mustafizur Rahman) and F.Q.; Investigation, S.M.S., T.R.B., Z.A., M.A., K.I.A.C., M.R. (Mustafizur Rahman) and F.Q.; Methodology, S.M.S., T.R.B., S.B., M.R. (Mustafizur Rahman), M.R. (Mahmudur Rahman) and F.Q.; Project administration, S.M.S., Z.A., S.M.Z.S. and K.I.A.C.; Resources, S.M.S., S.B. and F.Q.; Software, Z.A., S.M.Z.S. and M.R.A.; Supervision, S.M.S., Z.A. and K.I.A.C.; Validation, Z.A., A.A. and K.I.A.C.; Visualization, S.M.S.; Writing—original draft, S.M.S., T.R.B., Z.A., M.A., A.A. and F.Q.; Writing—review & editing, A.S.M.A., M.R. (Mahbubur Rahman), F.I.K., T.S., M.S.F., M.R. (Mustafizur Rahman) and M.R. (Mahmudur Rahman). All authors have read and agreed to the published version of the manuscript.

Funding: This research was funded by the Bill and Melinda Gates Foundation, grant number INV-017556.

Institutional Review Board Statement: The study protocol was reviewed and approved by icddr,b's Research Review and Ethical Review Committees (PR-20066).

Informed Consent Statement: Informed consent was obtained from all subjects involved in the study.

Data Availability Statement: Data cannot be shared publicly because they are confidential. Data are available from the respective department of icddr,b for researchers who meet the criteria for access to confidential data.

Acknowledgments: The authors would like to thank the Bill and Melinda Gates Foundation, the Ministry of Health and Family Welfare (MOHFW) of Bangladesh, the Institute of Epidemiology, Disease Control and Research (IEDCR) for their continuous support. The authors would also like to express their sincere thanks to the staff members of icddr, b for their dedicated work in the field and laboratory during this pandemic situation; icddr,b is supported by the Governments of Bangladesh, Canada, Sweden, and UK. We thank Jason Harris from Harvard Medical School for providing the SARS-CoV-2 RBD antigen.

Conflicts of Interest: The authors declare no conflict of interest.

Appendix A

Appendix A.1. Definition of Secondary Attack Rate (SAR)

In this study, secondary attack rate (SAR) was defined as a measure of the frequency of new infections of COVID-19 among neighboring contacts of confirmed cases in a defined period and their household members (as per WHO, exposure begins 2 days prior to symptoms), determined by a positive COVID-19 result [24].

Appendix A.2. Definition of Basic Reproduction Number (R0)

R-naught (R0) was defined as the basic reproduction number of COVID-19, the confirmed number of cases among the contacts directly generated by one case in a population where all individuals are susceptible to infection [25].

Appendix A.3. Definition of Effective Reproduction Number (Rt)

The effective reproduction number (Rt or R) was estimated by the product of the basic reproductive number of COVID-19 and the fraction of the host population susceptible to COVID-19 infection [26].

Appendix A.4. Definition of Serologic Response or Seroconversion

Sero-conversion can be defined as $\geq$two-fold increase in antibody titer in sera between enrolment and later time points (e.g., at day 1 and day 28) of neighborhood contacts [27–32].

Appendix A.5. Operational Definition of High-Density and Low-Density Areas

High-density areas are slums which are horizontally shared spaces with more than 5 people living in a 9–12 feet by 6–8 feet room.

Low-density areas are non-slum wards, which have high-rise buildings and apartments.

Table A1. Response rate and levels of SARS-CoV-2 antibodies in RT-PCR-positive contacts with high-SES and low-SES in Dhaka city.

RT-PCR Positive on	SARS-CoV-2 IgG				SARS-CoV-2 IgM			
	Day 1		Day 28		Day 1		Day 28	
	High SES	Low SES	High SES	Low SES	High SES	Low SES	High SES	Low SES
Day 1								
Seropositivity, n	11/16	13/21	14/14	16/16	8/16	10/21	7/14	6/16
(%)	(69)	(62)	(100)	(100)	(50)	(48)	(50)	(38)
# GM (ng/mL)	501	695	1509	2141	528	501	485	440
Day 7								
Seropositivity, n	7/10	9/20	10/10	10/16	6/10	7/20	5/10	7/16
(%)	(70) ***	(45)	(100) ***	(63)	(60)	(35)	(50)	(44)
GM (ng/mL)	517	736	1556	2432	563	604	539	630
Day 14								
Seropositivity, n	1/3	6/15	3/3	10/11	2/3	7/15	2/3	7/11
(%)	(33)	(40)	(100) **	(91)	(67) **	(47)	(67)	(64)
GM (ng/mL)	602	313	1918	2078	476	528	509	619
Day 28								
Seropositivity, n	1/3	1/12	2/3	4/12	1/3	5/12	1/3	6/12
(%)	(33) ***	(8)	(67) ***	(33)	(33)	(42)	(33)	(50) *
GM (ng/mL)	183	61	842	150	230	396	509	490

Statistically significant differences were observed between RT-PCR-positive participants with high and low SES. Statistical analysis was performed using Fisher's exact test. * $p < 0.05$, ** $p < 0.01$, *** $p < 0.001$. # No statistical differences were observed for Geometric mean (GM) concs. of IgG and IgM antibodies between people with high and low SES.

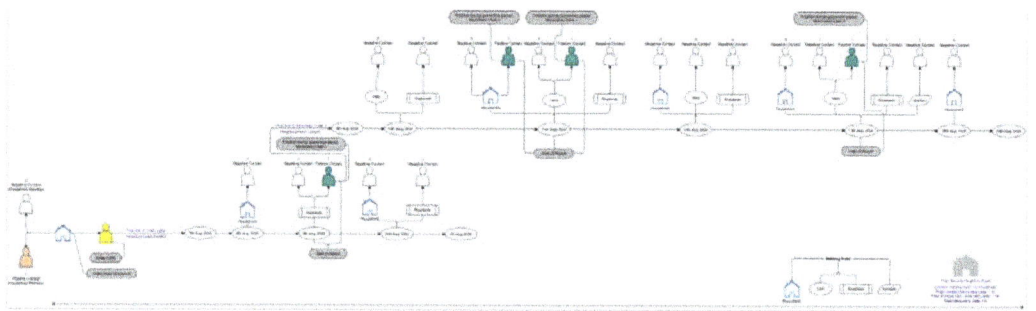

Figure A1. Diagram showing the setting of exposure and the direction of transmission from index case to household and neighborhood contacts in high-density areas in Dhaka city.

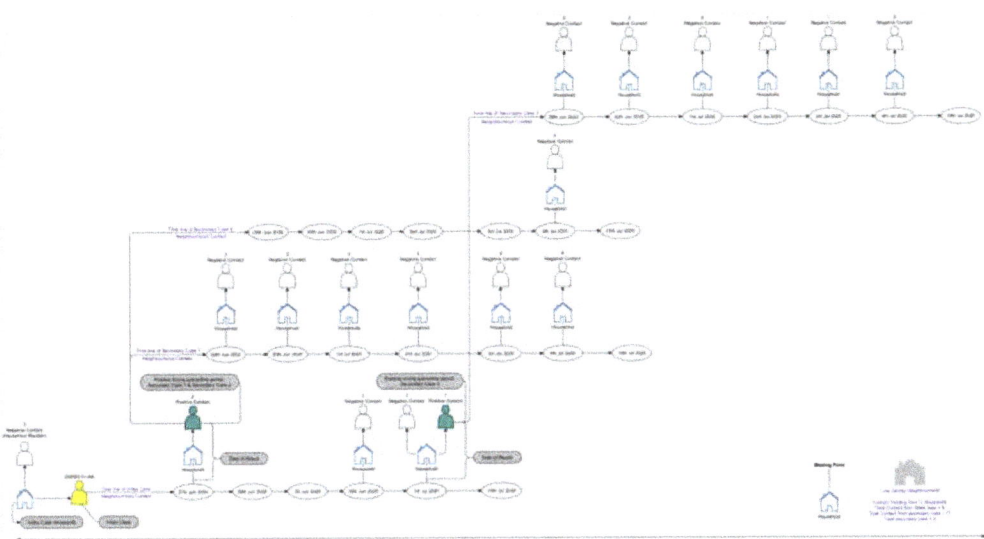

Figure A2. Diagram showing the setting of exposure and the direction of transmission from index case to household and neighborhood contacts in low-density areas in Dhaka city.

References

1. Transmission of SARS-CoV-2: Implications for Infection Prevention Precautions. Available online: https://www.who.int/news-room/commentaries/detail/transmission-of-sars-cov-2-implications-for-infection-prevention-precautions (accessed on 4 January 2021).
2. Kutti-Sridharan, G.; Vegunta, R.; Vegunta, R.; Mohan, B.P.; Rokkam, V. SARS-CoV2 in different body fluids, risks of transmission, and preventing COVID-19: A comprehensive evidence-based review. *Int. J. Prev. Med.* **2020**, *11*, 97. [PubMed]
3. Ahmed, I. Factors in building resilience in urban slums of Dhaka, Bangladesh. *Procedia Econ. Financ.* **2014**, *18*, 745–753. [CrossRef]
4. Rahman, B.; Sadraddin, E.; Porreca, A. The basic reproduction number of SARS-CoV-2 in Wuhan is about to die out, how about the rest of the World? *Rev. Med. Virol.* **2020**, *30*, e2111. [CrossRef]
5. Al-Raeei, M. The basic reproduction number of the new coronavirus pandemic with mortality for India, the Syrian Arab Republic, the United States, Yemen, China, France, Nigeria and Russia with different rate of cases. *Clin. Epidemiol. Glob. Health* **2021**, *9*, 147–149. [CrossRef] [PubMed]
6. Hossain, S. The production of space in the negotiation of water and electricity supply in a bosti of Dhaka. *Habitat Int.* **2012**, *36*, 68–77. [CrossRef]
7. Available online: https://news.google.com/covid19/map?hl=en-US&mid=%2Fm%2F0162b&gl=US&ceid=US%3Aen (accessed on 2 June 2021).
8. Nazneen, A.; Sultana, R.; Rahman, M.; Rahman, M.; Qadri, F.; Rimi, N.A.; Hossain, K.; Alam, M.R.; Rahman, M.; Chakraborty, N.; et al. Prevalence of COVID-19 in Bangladesh, April to October 2020—A cross-sectional study. *IJID Reg.* **2021**, *1*, 92–99. [CrossRef]
9. Jing, Q.-L.; Liu, M.-J.; Zhang, Z.-B.; Fang, L.-Q.; Yuan, J.; Zhang, A.-R.; E Dean, N.; Luo, L.; Ma, M.-M.; Longini, I.; et al. Household secondary attack rate of COVID-19 and associated determinants in Guangzhou, China: A retrospective cohort study. *Lancet Infect. Dis.* **2020**, *20*, 1141–1150. [CrossRef]
10. Burke, R.M.; Midgley, C.M.; Dratch, A.; Fenstersheib, M.; Haupt, T.; Holshue, M.; Ghinai, I.; Jarashow, M.C.; Lo, J.; McPherson, T.D.; et al. Active Monitoring of Persons Exposed to Patients with Confirmed COVID-19—United States, January–February 2020. *MMWR Morb. Mortal. Wkly. Rep.* **2020**, *69*, 245–246. [CrossRef]
11. Akter, A.; Ahmed, T.; Tauheed, I.; Akhtar, M.; Rahman, S.I.A.; Khaton, F.; Ahmmed, F.; Ferdous, J.; Afrad, M.H.; Kawser, Z.; et al. Disease characteristics and serological responses in patients with differing severity of COVID-19 infection: A longitudinal cohort study in Dhaka, Bangladesh. *PLoS Negl. Trop. Dis.* **2022**, *16*, e0010102. [CrossRef]
12. Lyngse, F.P.; Kirkeby, C.; Halasa, T.; Andreasen, V.; Skov, R.L.; Møller, F.T.; Krause, T.G.; Mølbak, K. Nationwide study on SARS-CoV-2 transmission within households from lockdown to reopening, Denmark, 27 February 2020 to 1 August 2020. *Eur. Commun. Dis. Bull.* **2022**, *27*, 2001800. [CrossRef]
13. Madewell, Z.J.; Yang, Y.; Longini, I.M., Jr.; Halloran, M.E.; Dean, N.E. Household Transmission of SARS-CoV-2: A Systematic Review and Meta-analysis. *JAMA Netw. Open* **2020**, *3*, e2031756. [CrossRef] [PubMed]

14. Fung, H.F.; Martinez, L.; Alarid-Escudero, F.; Salomon, J.A.; Studdert, D.M.; Andrews, J.R.; Goldhaber-Fiebert, J.D.; Stanford-CIDE Coronavirus Simulation Model (SC-COSMO) Modeling Group. The Household Secondary Attack Rate of Severe Acute Respiratory Syndrome Coronavirus 2 (SARS-CoV-2): A Rapid Review. *Clin. Infect. Dis.* **2021**, *73* (Suppl. S2), S138–S145. [CrossRef] [PubMed]
15. Madewell, Z.J.; Yang, Y.; Longini, I.M., Jr.; Halloran, M.E.; Dean, N.E. Factors Associated With Household Transmission of SARS-CoV-2: An Updated Systematic Review and Meta-analysis. *JAMA Netw. Open* **2021**, *4*, e2122240. [CrossRef] [PubMed]
16. Smith, T.P.; Flaxman, S.; Gallinat, A.S.; Kinosian, S.P.; Stemkovski, M.; Unwin, H.J.T.; Watson, O.J.; Whittaker, C.; Cattarino, L.; Dorigatti, I.; et al. Temperature and population density influence SARS-CoV-2 transmission in the absence of nonpharmaceutical interventions. *Proc. Natl. Acad. Sci. USA* **2021**, *118*, e2019284118. [CrossRef]
17. Salzberger, B.; Buder, F.; Lampl, B.; Ehrenstein, B.; Hitzenbichler, F.; Holzmann, T.; Schmidt, B.; Hanses, F. Epidemiology of SARS-CoV-2. *Infection* **2021**, *49*, 233–239. [CrossRef]
18. Paireau, J.; Mailles, A.; Eisenhauer, C.; de Laval, F.; Delon, F.; Bosetti, P.; Salje, H.; Pontiès, V.; Cauchemez, S. Early chains of transmission of COVID-19 in France, January to March 2020. *Eur. Commun. Dis. Bull.* **2022**, *27*, 2001953. [CrossRef]
19. Ng, O.T.; Marimuthu, K.; Koh, V.; Pang, J.; Linn, K.Z.; Sun, J.; De Wang, L.; Chia, W.N.; Tiu, C.; Chan, M.; et al. SARS-CoV-2 seroprevalence and transmission risk factors among high-risk close contacts: A retrospective cohort study. *Lancet Infect. Dis.* **2021**, *21*, 333–343. [CrossRef]
20. Shaw, J.A.; Meiring, M.; Cummins, T.; Chegou, N.N. Higher SARS-CoV-2 seroprevalence in workers with lower socioeconomic status in Cape Town, South Africa. *PLoS ONE* **2021**, *16*, e0247852. [CrossRef]
21. Whittle, R.S.; Diaz-Artiles, A. An ecological study of socioeconomic predictors in detection of COVID-19 cases across neighborhoods in New York City. *BMC Med.* **2020**, *18*, 271. [CrossRef]
22. Finch, W.H.; Finch, M.E.H. Poverty and COVID-19: Rates of Incidence and Deaths in the United States During the First 10 Weeks of the Pandemic. *Front. Sociol.* **2020**, *5*, 47. [CrossRef]
23. Martin, C.A.; Jenkins, D.R.; Minhas, J.S.; Gray, L.J.; Tang, J.; Williams, C.; Sze, S.; Pan, D.; Jones, W.; Verma, R.; et al. Sociodemographic heterogeneity in the prevalence of COVID-19 during lockdown is associated with ethnicity and household size: Results from an observational cohort study. *EClinicalMedicine* **2020**, *25*, 100466. [CrossRef] [PubMed]
24. Jay, J.; Bor, J.; Nsoesie, E.O.; Lipson, S.K.; Jones, D.K.; Galea, S.; Raifman, J. Neighbourhood income and physical distancing during the COVID-19 pandemic in the United States. *Nat. Hum. Behav.* **2020**, *4*, 1294–1302. [CrossRef] [PubMed]
25. Sekine, T.; Perez-Potti, A.; Rivera-Ballesteros, O.; Strålin, K.; Gorin, J.B.; Olsson, A.; Llewellyn-Lacey, S.; Kamal, H.; Bogdanovic, G.; Muschiol, S.; et al. Robust T Cell Immunity in Convalescent Individuals with Asymptomatic or Mild COVID-19. *Cell* **2020**, *183*, 158–168.e14. [CrossRef] [PubMed]
26. Halloran, M. Secondary Attack Rate. In *Encyclopedia of Biostatistics*; Wiley Online Library: Hoboken, NJ, USA, 2005.
27. Delamater, P.; Street, E.; Leslie, T.; Yang, Y.T.; Jacobsen, K. Complexity of the Basic Reproduction Number (R_0). *Emerg. Infect. Dis. J.* **2019**, *25*, 1. [CrossRef]
28. Hridoy, A.-E.; Naim, M.; Alam, E.; Laam, N.U.; Tipo, I.; Tusher, S.; Alam, S.; Islam, M.S. Estimation of Effective Reproduction Number for COVID-19 in Bangladesh and its districts. *medRxiv* **2020**, *6*. [CrossRef]
29. Qadri, F.; Ryan, E.T.; Faruque, A.S.; Ahmed, F.; Khan, A.I.; Islam, M.M.; Akramuzzaman, S.M.; Sack, D.A.; Calderwood, S.B. Antigen-specific immunoglobulin A antibodies secreted from circulating B cells are an effective marker for recent local immune responses in patients with cholera: Comparison to antibody-secreting cell responses and other immunological markers. *Infect. Immun.* **2003**, *71*, 4808–4814. [CrossRef]
30. Asaduzzaman, M.; Ryan, E.T.; John, M.; Hang, L.; Khan, A.I.; Faruque, A.S.; Taylor, R.K.; Calderwood, S.B.; Qadri, F. The major subunit of the toxin-coregulated pilus TcpA induces mucosal and systemic immunoglobulin A immune responses in patients with cholera caused by Vibrio cholerae O1 and O139. *Infect. Immun.* **2004**, *72*, 4448–4454. [CrossRef]
31. Johnson, R.A.; Uddin, T.; Aktar, A.; Mohasin, M.; Alam, M.M.; Chowdhury, F.; Harris, J.B.; Larocque, R.C.; Bufano, M.K.; Yu, Y.; et al. Comparison of immune responses to the O-specific polysaccharide and lipopolysaccharide of Vibrio cholerae O1 in Bangladeshi adult patients with cholera. *Clin. Vaccine Immunol. CVI* **2012**, *19*, 1712–1721. [CrossRef]
32. Qadri, F.; Ahmed, T.; Ahmed, F.; Bhuiyan, M.S.; Mostofa, M.G.; Cassels, F.J.; Helander, A.; Svennerholm, A.-M. Mucosal and Systemic Immune Responses in Patients with Diarrhea Due to CS6-Expressing Enterotoxigenic *Escherichia coli*. *Infect. Immun.* **2007**, *75*, 2269. [CrossRef]

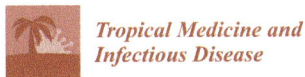

Article

The Effectiveness of the Use of Regdanvimab (CT-P59) in Addition to Remdesivir in Patients with Severe COVID-19: A Single Center Retrospective Study

Ganghee Chae [1], Aram Choi [1], Soyeoun Lim [2], Sooneun Park [3], Seungjun Lee [3], Youngick Ahn [3], Jinhyoung Kim [1], Seungwon Ra [1], Yangjin Jegal [1], Jongjoon Ahn [1], Eunji Park [4], Jaebum Jun [1], Woonjung Kwon [2,*,†] and Taehoon Lee [1,*,†]

[1] Department of Internal Medicine, Ulsan University Hospital, University of Ulsan College of Medicine, Ulsan 44033, Korea; margiela07@naver.com (G.C.); 0735483@uuh.ulsan.kr (A.C.); 0733808@uuh.ulsan.kr (J.K.); docra@docra.pe.kr (S.R.); yjjegal@uuh.ulsan.kr (Y.J.); jjahn@uuh.ulsan.kr (J.A.); jjb@uuh.ulsan.kr (J.J.)
[2] Department of Radiology, Ulsan University Hospital, University of Ulsan College of Medicine, Ulsan 44033, Korea; soyeoun.lim.xr@uuh.ulsan.kr
[3] Department of Anesthesiology and Pain Medicine, Ulsan University Hospital, University of Ulsan College of Medicine, Ulsan 44033, Korea; gamju@uuh.ulsan.kr (S.P.); 0735496@uuh.ulsan.kr (S.L.); 0735495@uuh.ulsan.kr (Y.A.)
[4] Big Data Center, Ulsan University Hospital, University of Ulsan College of Medicine, Ulsan 44033, Korea; 0735779@uuh.ulsan.kr
* Correspondence: becareful123@uuh.ulsan.kr (W.K.); tleepulalg@uuh.ulsan.kr (T.L.); Tel.: +82-52-250-2871 (W.K.); +82-52-250-7029 (T.L.); Fax: +82-52-250-7048 (W.K. & T.L.)
† These authors contributed equally to this work.

Abstract: Introduction: Coronavirus disease 2019 (COVID-19) still has a high mortality rate when it is severe. Regdanvimab (CT-P59), a neutralizing monoclonal antibody that has been proven effective against mild to moderate COVID-19, may be effective against severe COVID-19. This study was conducted to determine the effectiveness of the combined use of remdesivir and regdanvimab in patients with severe COVID-19. Methods: From March to early May 2021, 124 patients with severe COVID-19 were admitted to Ulsan University Hospital (Ulsan, Korea) and received oxygen therapy and remdesivir. Among them, 25 were also administered regdanvimab before remdesivir. We retrospectively compared the clinical outcomes between the remdesivir alone group [n = 99 (79.8%)] and the regdanvimab/remdesivir group [n = 25 (20.2%)]. Results: The oxygen-free days on day 28 (primary outcome) were significantly higher in the regdanvimab/remdesivir group [mean ± SD: 19.36 ± 7.87 vs. 22.72 ± 3.66, p = 0.003]. The oxygen-free days was also independently associated with use of regdanvimab in the multivariate analysis, after adjusting for initial pulse oximetric saturation (SpO_2)/fraction of inspired oxygen (FiO_2) ratio (severity index). Further, in the regdanvimab/remdesivir group, the lowest SpO_2/FiO_2 ratio during treatment was significantly higher (mean ± SD: 237.05 ± 89.68 vs. 295.63 ± 72.74, p = 0.003), and the Kaplan-Meier estimates of oxygen supplementation days in surviving patients (on day 28) were significantly shorter [mean ± SD: 8.24 ± 7.43 vs. 5.28 ± 3.66, p = 0.024]. Conclusions: In patients with severe COVID-19, clinical outcomes can be improved by administering regdanvimab, in addition to remdesivir.

Keywords: regdanvimab; remdesivir; COVID-19; severe

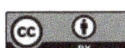

1. Introduction

Coronavirus disease 2019 (COVID-19) is an infectious disease caused by severe acute respiratory syndrome coronavirus 2 (SARS-CoV-2) virus infection [1]. Following the first epidemic that occurred in Wuhan, China in December 2019, there have been 180,654,652 globally confirmed cases until June 2021, of which 3,920,463 have resulted in fatality (case-fatality rate: 2.17%) [2]. In Korea, the first case occurred in January 2020, and by June 2021, 155,572 people were infected, with there being 2015 deaths (case-fatality rate: 1.29%) [2].

Regarding the clinical course of COVID-19 (based on data before remdesivir and systemic corticosteroids were administered) [3], 80% of patients are asymptomatic or have a mild clinical course, 20% develop severe COVID-19 requiring oxygen therapy, and 5% of patients (a quarter of severe COVID-19 cases) progress to critical COVID-19, which requires tracheal intubation or high-flow oxygen therapy, eventually leading to death in 2.3% of all COVID-19 patients [3].

Through large-scale prospective studies conducted in early 2020, it was recognized that the use of remdesivir and systemic corticosteroids was somewhat effective in reducing this mortality rate [4,5]. Accordingly, since September 2020, remdesivir and systemic corticosteroids have been actively used to treat patients with severe COVID-19 in Korea. Korea's COVID-19 case fatality rate was 1.58% from January 2020 to August 2020 (deaths/cases = 334/21,177) and 1.25% from September 2020 to June 2021 (deaths/cases = 1681/134,395) [2]. As such, it seems that there is a slight reduction in mortality after the use of both drugs. A recent meta-analysis also revealed a decrease in mortality in patients with severe COVID-19 requiring oxygen therapy, after the use of both drugs; however, the degree of mortality reduction was not sufficient [6].

According to the recent Korea Disease Control and Prevention Agency (KDCA) data, which reviewed 8949 COVID-19 patients in Korea, severe COVID-19 with oxygen treatment requirement was observed in 9.1% (816/8949) of cases, of which 29.2% (238/816) resulted in death [7]. Depending on the study, the mortality rate of severe COVID-19 has been reported to be as low as 10% and as high as 36% [3–5,7–9]. Deaths occur mainly in the elderly (over 60 years of age) and patients with underlying diseases (diabetes mellitus, hypertension, obesity, and chronic heart/kidney/lung disease). In this high-risk group, new drugs other than remdesivir and systemic corticosteroids are urgently needed.

Recently, a monoclonal antibody (mAb) called regdanvimab (CT-P59) was developed by a domestic pharmaceutical company (Celltrion Inc., Incheon, Korea) [10]. Safety and potential antiviral efficacy were confirmed in the phase 1 study [11], and a notable clinical effectivity was confirmed in a phase 2/3 clinical trial, for treatment of mild or moderate COVID-19 patients (reducing hospitalization and oxygen therapy requirement by half, from 8.7% to 4.0%) [12]. It also showed an effect on recently emerged variants [13]. In Korea, regdanvimab has been actively used to treat high-risk patients with mild-to-moderate COVID-19 since March 2021.

Currently, regdanvimab has no clinical usage for treating patients with severe COVID-19, but it has the potential to be effective such cases, when used early in the course of infection. In this study, we evaluated the clinical outcomes of severe COVID-19, when regdanvimab is used in addition to remdesivir and systemic corticosteroids (the current standard of care for severe COVID-19).

2. Material and Methods

2.1. Study Patients

We retrospectively recruited all severe COVID-19 patients who were admitted and treated with remdesivir and oxygen supplementation at Ulsan University Hospital (UUH) (Ulsan, Korea) from 1 March to 11 May 2021. The recruitment start time was set to 1 March 2021 because regdanvimab has been supplied since the end of February. Since then, regdanvimab has been administered to patients with non-severe COVID-19. Severe COVID-19 patients received remdesivir, and some remdesivir-treated patients had previously been administered regdanvimab because their condition had been non-severe immediately after hospitalization (but progressed to severe COVID-19 during hospitalization). Inclusion criteria and exclusion criteria of the present study were as follows: inclusion criteria (i) those who were diagnosed with COVID-19 and received inpatient treatment at Ulsan University Hospital (UUH) (Ulsan, Korea) from 1 March to 11 May 2021, and (ii) those classified as severe COVID-19 and received remdesivir during the study period; exclusion criteria (i) those who did not received oxygen therapy.

The diagnosis of COVID-19 was made using the real-time polymerase chain reaction (RT-PCR) test for SARS-CoV-2 using the swab sample obtained from the oropharynx and nasopharynx. Severe COVID-19 was defined as the presence of pneumonia and hypoxia [room air pulse oximetric saturation (SpO_2) $\leq$ 94%], with laboratory-confirmed SARS-CoV-2 infection. Pneumonia was identified radiologically [via chest X-ray (CXR) or computed tomography] by the presence of an infiltrate. Remdesivir (200 mg IV on the first day, and 100 mg IV from the next day, for a total of 5 days) was administered to patients with symptoms for less than 10 days, among patients with severe COVID-19, according to the KDCA guidelines [14]. Regdanvimab (a single IV dose of 40 mg/kg) was administered to patients with non-severe COVID-19 (room air SpO_2 > 94%) with laboratory-confirmed SARS-CoV-2 infection, according to the following KDCA guidelines: within 7 days of symptom onset and over 60 years of age, underlying diseases (cardiovascular disease, chronic lung disease, diabetes mellitus, or hypertension), or radiologically identified pneumonia (via CXR or computed tomography) [15].

2.2. Study Design

Data were obtained via medical record review from the time of remdesivir initiation to 8 weeks after. After gathering baseline demographic and clinical data at the time of initiation of remdesivir, the following indicators related to clinical outcomes were collected: oxygen use (including the on/off date), type of respiratory support: oxygen with nasal prong or simple mask, or advanced respiratory support [mask with reservoir bag, high flow nasal cannula (HFNC), non-invasive ventilation, invasive ventilation, or extracorporeal membrane oxygenation (ECMO)], SpO_2/fraction of inspired oxygen (FiO_2) ratio [16] at the time of initiation of remdesivir, the highest FiO_2 during treatment, the lowest SpO_2/FiO_2 ratio during treatment, CXR scores [17], and survival and hospital discharge.

When a patient was oxygenated via nasal prong, the FiO_2 values were calculated as 0.24 at 1 L/min, 0.28 at 2 L/min, 0.32 at 3 L/min, 0.36 at 4 L/min, and 0.4 at 5 L/min. When the patient wore a simple oxygen mask, the FiO_2 value was calculated to be 0.4 for 5–6 L/min. A FiO_2 value of 0.8 was calculated if the patient was receiving oxygen > 10 L/min with a mask with a reservoir bag [18]. CXR scoring was performed by two thoracic radiologists (W. J. Kwon and S. Lim), with two CXRs at the time around remdesivir start and hospital discharge using the method described in a recent paper [17]. If not discharged until 28 days after starting remdesivir, a CXR around 28 days after remdesivir start was selected as the second point.

After the above investigation, patients were divided into a remdesivir alone group and a regdanvimab/remdesivir group. The outcomes were then analyzed. The present study was approved by the Institutional Review Board of Ulsan University Hospital (IRB number: UUH 2021-06-028).

2.3. Primary and Secondary Outcomes

The primary outcome was oxygen-free days on day 28, which was defined as the number of days that a patient was alive and free from oxygen, calculated from the time of initiation of remdesivir. The concept of oxygen-free days is an application of ventilator-free days [19] and has been used in many recent studies [20,21].

As the secondary outcomes, we analyzed the oxygen-free days (on days 14 and 56), days of oxygen supplementation in surviving patients (on days 14, 28, and 56), the highest FiO_2 and lowest SpO_2/FiO_2 ratio during treatment, CXR improvement, duration of hospital stay, and mortality (on days 14, 28, and 56).

2.4. Statistical Analysis

Chi-square test and Fisher's exact test were used to compare the categorical variables. An independent Student's t-test was used to compare the continuous variables. To identify independent factors associated with oxygen-free days on day 28, multiple linear regression analysis was performed using basic demographic variables [age, sex, and body mass index

(BMI)], baseline severity index (SpO$_2$/FiO$_2$ ratio at the time of initiation of remdesivir), and regdanvimab use. The oxygen supplementation days in surviving patients were estimated using the Kaplan-Meier method and log-rank test. All statistical analyses were performed using SPSS version 24 (IBM Corporation, Armonk, NY, USA). Statistical significance was set at $p < 0.05$.

3. Results

3.1. Enrolled Patients and Baseline Characteristics

From 1 March to 11 May 2021, 390 symptomatic or high-risk COVID-19 patients were admitted to the UUH. Of these, 74 patients received regdanvimab. Of the 390 patients, 127 were diagnosed with severe COVID-19 and received remdesivir, but three of them did not receive oxygen supplementation at the start of remdesivir administration and were excluded from the analysis. Accordingly, 124 severe COVID-19 patients who received remdesivir and oxygen therapy were included in the present study. Of these, 25 received both regdanvimab and remdesivir (regdanvimab/remdesivir group) and 99 received only remdesivir (remdesivir alone group) (Figure 1).

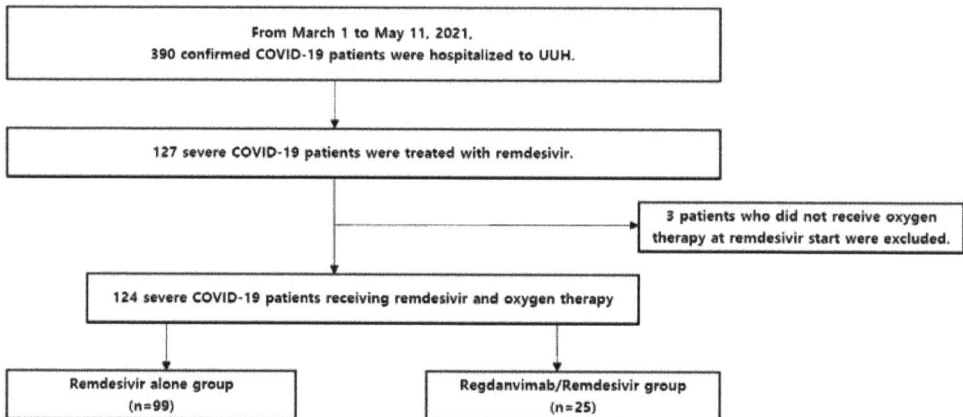

Figure 1. Flowchart of the present study. 390 symptomatic or high-risk COVID-19 patients were hospitalized to UUH from 1 March 1 to 11 May 2021. Of these, 74 patients received regdanvimab. Among 390 hospitalized patients, those receiving remdesivir were selected (n = 127). Remdesivir was administered to severe COVID-19 patients with pneumonia (determined via chest imaging) and room air SpO2 ≤ 94%. Three patients were excluded from the study because they did not receive oxygen therapy at the start of remdesivir administration, and finally, 124 severe COVID-19 patients were selected for the current study. Of these, 99 patients were administered only remdesivir, and 25 patients were treated using regdanvimab before remdesivir administration. Regdanvimab was used when room air SpO2 > 94% and chest imaging showed pneumonia, over the age of 60 years, or those with underlying diseases (cardiovascular disease, chronic lung disease, diabetes mellitus, or hypertension). Among the patients who were treated with regdanvimab, remdesivir was administered owing to the change in status to severe COVID-19 during hospitalization. Abbreviations: COVID-19, coronavirus disease 2019; UUH, Ulsan University Hospital; SpO2, pulse oximetric saturation.

Table 1 shows the baseline characteristics of the two groups. The mean age was 57.59 years, and 43.5% were male. There was no significant difference in demographic characteristics between the two groups, except for BMI, with that of the regdanvimab/remdesivir group being higher than that of the remdesivir alone group [kg/m^2, mean ± standard deviation (SD): 24.94 ± 3.19 vs. 26.79 ± 3.83, p = 0.014]. Hypertension was the most common underlying disease (25.8%), followed by dyslipidemia (16.1%), diabetes mellitus (12.9%), neurological disease (4.8%), chronic kidney disease (4.0%), and chronic liver disease

(4.0%). There was no statistically significant difference in the distribution of underlying diseases between the two groups. The period from symptom onset to hospitalization was slightly shorter in the regdanvimab/remdesivir group (days, mean ± SD: 3.19 ± 3.14 vs. 1.76 ± 3.21, $p = 0.045$), but there was no difference in the period from symptom onset to remdesivir administration (days, mean ± SD: 5.21 ± 3.29 vs. 5.00 ± 3.12, $p = 0.772$). In the regdanvimab/remdesivir group, regdanvimab was administered at 3.68 and 1.92 days, on average, from symptom onset and admission, respectively, and the administration of remdesivir was performed at 1.32 days, on average, after regdanvimab administration. Respiratory support at the start of remdesivir administration showed a tendency to receive less advanced support in the regdanvimab/remdesivir group (10.1% vs. 4.0%, $p = 0.460$), and the SpO_2/FiO_2 ratio was significantly higher in the regdanvimab/remdesivir group (290.09 ± 69.76 vs. 326.63 ± 62.39, $p = 0.018$). There was no difference in the baseline CXR severity, and systemic corticosteroids were used in nearly all patients.

Table 1. Baseline characteristics at initiation of remdesivir administration.

Variables		Total ($n = 124$)	Remdesivir Alone ($n = 99$)	Regdanvimab/ Remdesivir ($n = 25$)	p-Value
Age (years)		57.59 ± 12.24	56.64 ± 12.13	61.36 ± 12.20	0.085
Age (years), distribution					0.413
	20–29	2 (1.6)	2 (2.0)	0 (0.0)	
	30–39	8 (6.5)	8 (8.1)	0 (0.0)	
	40–49	18 (14.5)	14 (14.1)	4 (16.0)	
	50–59	36 (29.0)	29 (29.3)	7 (28.0)	
	60–69	47 (37.9)	37 (37.4)	10 (40.0)	
	70–79	7 (5.6)	6 (6.1)	1 (4.0)	
	80–89	6 (4.8)	3 (3.0)	3 (12.0)	
Sex					1.000
	Male	54 (43.5)	43 (43.4)	11 (44.0)	
	Female	70 (56.5)	56 (56.6)	14 (56.0)	
Body weight (kg)		68.56 ± 12.68	67.66 ± 11.78	72.12 ± 15.52	0.116
Height (cm)		164.17 ± 8.52	164.35 ± 8.04	163.47 ± 10.34	0.645
BMI (kg/m^2)		25.31 ± 3.40	24.94 ± 3.19	26.79 ± 3.83	0.014
Race					1.000
	Asian	123 (99.2)	98 (99.0)	25 (100.0)	
	White	1 (0.8)	1 (1.0)	0 (0.0)	
Underlying diseases					
	Hypertension	32 (25.8)	25 (25.3)	7 (28.0)	0.779
	Diabetes	16 (12.9)	12 (12.1)	4 (16.0)	0.738
	Dyslipidemia	20 (16.1)	15 (15.2)	5 (20.0)	0.551
	Chronic heart disease	3 (2.4)	2 (2.0)	1 (4.0)	0.494
	Chronic lung disease	3 (2.4)	2 (2.0)	1 (4.0)	0.494
	Chronic kidney disease	5 (4.0)	4 (4.0)	1 (4.0)	1.000
	Chronic liver disease	5 (4.0)	3 (3.0)	2 (8.0)	0.264
	Rheumatologic disease	2 (1.6)	2 (2.0)	0 (0.0)	1.000
	Neurologic disease	6 (4.8)	5 (5.1)	1 (4.0)	1.000
	Psychiatiric disease	2 (1.6)	2 (2.0)	0 (0.0)	1.000
	Active malignancy	3 (2.4)	2 (2.0)	1 (4.0)	0.494
Days from symptom onset					
	To admission	2.90 ± 3.19	3.19 ± 3.14	1.76 ± 3.21	0.045
	To regdanvimab	NA	NA	3.68 ± 3.00	NA
	To remdesivir	5.17 ± 3.25	5.21 ± 3.29	5.00 ± 3.12	0.772
Days from admission					
	To regdanvimab	NA	NA	1.92 ± 2.08	NA
	To remdesivir	2.27 ± 2.84	2.02 ± 2.89	3.24 ± 2.47	0.055
Days from regdanvimab					
	To remdesivir	NA	NA	1.32 ± 1.77	NA
Respiratory support at the time of initiation of remdesivir					0.460
	Oxygen with nasal prong or simple mask	113 (91.1)	89 (89.9)	24 (96.0)	
	Advanced respiratory support	11 (8.9)	10 (10.1)	1 (4.0)	
	Mask with reservoir bag	2 (1.6)	2 (2.0)	0 (0.0)	
	HFNC	9 (7.3)	8 (8.1)	1 (4.0)	
	NIV	0 (0.0)	0 (0.0)	0 (0.0)	
	Invasive ventilation	0 (0.0)	0 (0.0)	0 (0.0)	
	ECMO	0 (0.0)	0 (0.0)	0 (0.0)	

Table 1. Cont.

Variables		Total (n = 124)	Remdesivir Alone (n = 99)	Regdanvimab/ Remdesivir (n = 25)	p-Value
FiO_2 at the time of initiation of remdesivir		0.34 ± 013	0.35 ± 0.14	0.30 ± 0.08	0.078
SpO_2/FiO_2 ratio at the time of initiation of remdesivir		297.46 ± 69.67	290.09 ± 69.76	326.63 ± 62.39	0.018
SpO_2/FiO_2 ratio distribution at the time of initiation of remdesivir					0.213
	0–99	3 (2.4)	3 (3.0)	0 (0.0)	
	100–199	8 (6.5)	7 (7.1)	1 (4.0)	
	200–299	39 (31.5)	33 (33.3)	6 (24.0)	
	300–399	69 (55.6)	54 (54.5)	15 (60.0)	
	400–499	5 (4.0)	2 (2.0)	3 (12.0)	
CXR score at the time of initiation of remdesivir		5.16 ± 4.31	5.42 ± 4.42	4.16 ± 3.75	0.194
Systemic corticosteroids use		122 (98.4)	97 (98.0)	25 (100.0)	1.000
	Dexamethasone	121 (97.6)	97 (98)	24 (96.0)	
	Prednisolone	1 (0.8)	0 (0.0)	1 (4.0)	

Data are presented as mean ± standard deviation or number (%). BMI: body mass index; CXR: chest X-ray; NA: not applicable; HFNC: high flow nasal cannula; NIV: non-invasive ventilation; ECMO: extracorporeal membrane oxygenation; FiO2: fraction of inspired oxygen; SpO2: pulse oximetric saturation.

3.2. Primary Outcome

28 days after the initiation of remdesivir administration, the regdanvimab/remdesivir group showed significantly longer oxygen-free days than the remdesivir alone group (days, mean ± SD: 19.36 ± 7.87 vs. 22.72 ± 3.66, p = 0.003) (Table 2).

Table 2. Clinical outcomes of the remdesivir alone group and the regdanvimab/remdesivir group.

Variables	Total (n = 124)	Remdesivir Alone (n = 99)	Regdanvimab/ Remdesivir (n = 25)	p-Value
Primary outcome				
Oxygen-free days on day 28				0.003
Mean ± SD	20.04 ± 7.33	19.36 ± 7.87	22.72 ± 3.66	
Median (IQR)	22.0 (20.0–24.5)	22.0 (19.0–24.0)	23.0 (22.0–25.0)	
Secondary outcomes				
Oxygen-free days on day 14				0.074
Mean ± SD	7.48 ± 4.15	7.14 ± 4.26	8.80 ± 3.43	
Median (IQR)	8.0 (6.0–10.5)	8.0 (5.0–10.0)	9.0 (8.0–11.0)	
Oxygen-free days on day 56				0.001
Mean ± SD	46.85 ± 11.52	45.87 ± 12.59	50.72 ± 3.66	
Median (IQR)	50.0 (48.0–52.5)	50.0 (47.0–52.0)	51.0 (50.0–53.0)	
Oxygen off and live on day 14	104 (83.9)	80 (80.8)	24 (96.0)	0.074
Oxygen off and live on day 28	116 (93.5)	91 (91.9)	25 (100.0)	0.357
Oxygen off and live on day 56	119 (96.0)	94 (94.9)	25 (100.0)	0.582
The highest FiO_2 during treatment	0.45 ± 0.24	0.48 ± 0.26	0.34 ± 0.15	0.001
The lowest SpO_2/FiO_2 ratio during treatment	248.86 ± 89.43	237.05 ± 89.68	295.63 ± 72.74	0.003
The lowest SpO_2/FiO_2 ratio distribution during treatment				0.087
0–99	15 (12.1)	15 (15.2)	0 (0.0)	
100–199	17 (13.7)	14 (14.1)	3 (12.0)	
200–299	41 (33.1)	34 (34.3)	7 (28.0)	
300–399	50 (40.3)	35 (35.4)	15 (60.0)	
400–499	1 (0.8)	1 (1.0)	0 (0.0)	
The highest degree of respiratory support during treatment				0.077
Oxygen with nasal prong or simple mask	92 (74.2)	70 (70.7)	22 (88.0)	
Advanced respiratory support	32 (25.8)	29 (29.3)	3 (12.0)	
Mask with Reservoir bag	0 (0.0)	0 (0.0)	0 (0.0)	
HFNC	20 (16.1)	18 (18.2)	2 (8.0)	
NIV	0 (0.0)	0 (0.0)	0 (0.0)	
Invasive ventilation	12 (9.7)	11 (11.1)	1 (4.0)	
ECMO	0 (0.0)	0 (0.0)	0 (0.0)	

Table 2. Cont.

Variables	Total (n = 124)	Remdesivir Alone (n = 99)	Regdanvimab/ Remdesivir (n = 25)	p-Value
Changes in CXR				
Days from the first scored CXR	10.93 ± 6.69	11.45 ± 7.03	8.96 ± 4.80	0.098
Difference between the two CXR scores (initial minus post)	1.36 ± 4.66	1.58 ± 4.59	0.48 ± 4.95	0.294
Duration of hospital stay (days)	15.40 ± 10.38	15.67 ± 11.12	14.32 ± 6.78	0.563
Mortality *				
Death at day 14	1 (0.8)	1 (1.0)	0 (0.0)	1.000
Death at day 28	2 (1.6)	2 (2.0)	0 (0.0)	1.000
Death at day 56	2 (1.6)	2 (2.0)	0 (0.0)	1.000
All-cause mortality	2 (1.6)	2 (2.0)	0 (0.0)	1.000

Data are presented as mean ± standard deviation or number (%). SD: standard deviation; IQR: interquartile range; FiO_2: fraction of inspired oxygen; SpO_2: pulse oximetric saturation; HFNC: high flow nasal cannula; NIV: non-invasive ventilation; ECMO: extracorporeal membrane oxygenation; CXR: chest X-ray. * Two deaths occurred: a 78-year-old male and an 83-year-old female died on days 15 and 12, respectively. Their cause of death was COVID-19.

3.3. Secondary Outcomes

In line with the primary outcome, oxygen-free days on days 14 (days, mean ± SD: 7.14 ± 4.26 vs. 8.80 ± 3.43, $p = 0.074$) and 56 (days, mean ± SD: 45.87 ± 12.59 vs. 50.72 ± 3.66, $p = 0.001$) were longer in the regdanvimab/remdesivir group. Survivors for whom oxygen supplementation was stopped also showed a higher tendency in the regdanvimab/remdesivir group on days 14 (80.8% vs. 96.0%, $p = 0.074$), 28 (91.9% vs. 100.0%, $p = 0.357$), and 56 (94.9% vs. 100.0%, $p = 0.582$). The regdanvimab/remdesivir group had a lower FiO_2 and higher SpO_2/FiO_2 ratio during treatment (highest FiO_2 during treatment, mean ± SD: 0.48 ± 0.26 vs. 0.34 ± 0.15, $p = 0.001$; lowest SpO_2/FiO_2 ratio during treatment, mean ± SD: 237.05 ± 89.68 vs. 295.63 ± 72,74, $p = 0.003$). Respiratory support during treatment tended to receive less advanced support in the regdanvimab/remdesivir group (29.3% vs. 12.0%, $p = 0.077$). There were no statistical differences in the degree of CXR change, length of hospitalization, and mortality (Table 2).

According to Kaplan-Meier estimates, the durations of oxygen supplementation in survivors were significantly shorter in the regdanvimab/remdesivir group on days 14 (days, mean ± SD: 6.71 ± 4.18 vs. 5.20 ± 3.43, $p = 0.046$), 28 (days, mean ± SD: 6.71 ± 4.18 vs. 5.20 ± 3.43, $p = 0.046$), and 56 (days, mean ± SD: 9.31 ± 11.41 vs. 5.28 ± 3.66, $p = 0.024$), as compared to the remdesivir alone group (Figure 2).

3.4. Independent Factors Associated with Oxygen-Free Days on Day 28

Independent factors associated with oxygen-free days on day 28, identified through multiple linear regression analysis, included regdanvimab use [B: 3.568; 95% confidence interval (CI): 0.596–6.539, $p = 0.019$], age (per year, B: −0.254; 95% CI: −0.352–−0.156, $p < 0.001$), and baseline SpO_2/FiO_2 ratio (B: 0.029; 95% CI: 0.013–0.046, $p = 0.001$) (Table 3).

3.5. Adverse Events Associated with Regdanvimab Use

Of the 25 regdanvimab users, 14 (56%) had no adverse events. However, some users had the following events: fever in 5 patients (20%), dyspnea in 7 patients (28%), nausea in 1 patient (4%), and delirium in 1 patient (4%). However, these adverse events may be a presentation of COVID-19 itself.

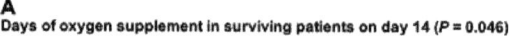
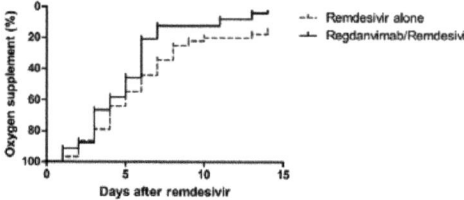
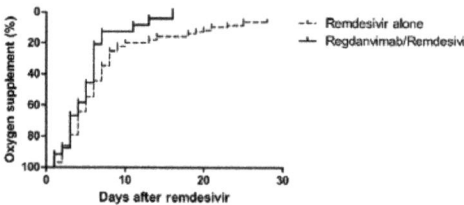
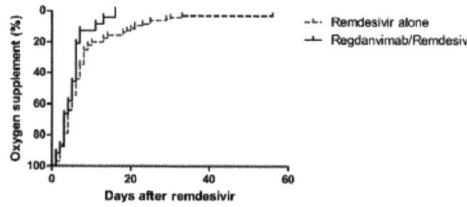

Figure 2. Kaplan-Meier estimates of the remdesivir alone and regdanvimab/remdesivir groups. (**A**) Days of oxygen supplementation, in surviving patients on day 14, were shorter in the regdanvimab/remdesivir group (days, mean ± SD: 6.71 ± 4.18 vs. 5.20 ± 3.43, p = 0.046). (**B**) Days of oxygen supplementation, in surviving patients on day 28, were shorter in the regdanvimab/remdesivir group (days, mean ± SD: 8.24 ± 7.43 vs. 5.28 ± 3.66, p = 0.024). (**C**) Days of oxygen supplementation, in surviving patients on day 56, were shorter in the regdanvimab/remdesivir group (days, mean ± SD: 9.31 ± 11.41 vs. 5.28 ± 3.66, p = 0.024). Abbreviations: SD, standard deviation.

Table 3. Factors associated with oxygen-free days on day 28.

Variables	Simple Linear Regression							Multiple Linear Regression						
	B	SE	β	t	p-Value	95% CI for B		B	SE	β	t	p-Value	95% CI for B	
						Lower	Upper						Lower	Upper
Regdanvimab use	3.356	1.619	0.184	2.073	0.040	0.151	6.562	3.568	1.501	0.196	2.377	0.019	0.596	6.539
Age (per year)	−0.246	0.049	−0.411	−4.981	<0.001	−0.344	−0.148	−0.254	0.049	−0.424	−5.126	<0.001	−0.352	−0.156
Female sex	2.761	1.309	0.188	2.109	0.037	0.169	5.353	1.742	1.140	0.118	1.528	0.129	−0.516	4.000
BMI (per kg/m^2)	0.306	0.193	0.142	1.585	0.116	−0.076	0.689	−0.043	0.181	−0.020	−0.238	0.812	−0.402	0.316
Baseline SpO$_2$/FiO$_2$ ratio	0.040	0.009	0.383	4.582	<0.001	0.023	0.058	0.029	0.009	0.280	3.461	0.001	0.013	0.046

CI: Confidence Interval; SE: standard error; BMI: body mass index; SpO$_2$: pulse oximetric saturation; FiO$_2$: fraction of inspired oxygen, SpO$_2$: pulse oximetric saturation.

4. Discussion

In severe COVID-19 patients, the use of regdanvimab, in addition to remdesivir, increased the number of oxygen-free days. The oxygen-free days was also independently associated with use of regdanvimab, as determined via multiple linear regression analysis with adjustment of baseline severity and demographic variables including age. In addition, the FiO$_2$ requirement was lower, the SpO$_2$/FiO$_2$ ratio was higher, and oxygen dependence was shorter, in patients using regdanvimab. These findings suggest that the use of regdanvimab, in addition to remdesivir, has a significantly favorable impact on the clinical outcomes of severe COVID-19. Our small-scale retrospective study needs to be validated via a prospective, large-scale study. However, given the current high mortality rate of severe COVID-19, the simultaneous use of regdanvimab and remdesivir could be considered in severe COVID-19.

Hospital admissions or deaths due to COVID-19 have been decreasing with the use of vaccines, and vaccines are effective against recently emerged variants [22]. However, once a person develops COVID-19 severe enough to be hospitalized, the mortality rate is very high, ranging from 10–36% [3–5,7–9]. Although remdesivir and systemic corticosteroids are somewhat effective against severe COVID-19, the associated decrease in mortality rate is insufficient [6]. Deaths from severe COVID-19 occur primarily in people over the age of 60 years and those with underlying medical conditions, and additional new drugs are needed for treating these individuals [3–5,7–9].

Among several candidate drugs, anti-SARS-CoV-2 mAbs against the receptor-binding domain (RBD) of the spike glycoprotein can be effective in severe COVID-19. This is because they have been proven effective in mild and moderate conditions of the same disease [23,24]. When used early in the course of the disease, such drugs inhibit the progression of mild or moderate COVID-19 to severe COVID-19, which requires hospitalization or oxygen supplementation. As of June 2021, anti-SARS-CoV-2 mAbs that have proven their effectiveness through early phase clinical trials and have secured emergency or conditional use authorization include bamlanivimab (Eli Lily and Company, Indianapolis, IN, USA), a combination of bamlanivimab and etesevimab (Eli Lily and Company, Indianapolis, IN, USA), and a combination of casirivimab and imdevimab (Regeneron Pharmaceuticals, Eastview/Tarrytown, NY, USA) in the United States, as well as regdanvimab (Celltrion Inc., Incheon, Korea) in Korea [23,24].

Regdanvimab is a potent neutralizing antibody against various SARS-CoV-2 isolates, which blocks the interaction regions of the RBD [meant for binding angiotensin-converting enzyme 2 (ACE2)] of SARS-CoV-2 spike protein [10]. Regdanvimab was found to be effective at reducing viral load and ameliorating clinical symptoms in animal experiments [10], and safety and virologic efficacy were confirmed through two randomized phase 1 clinical trials in healthy adults and patients with mild SARS-CoV-2 infection [11]. A recent phase 2/3 clinical trial demonstrated that the progression rates to severe COVID-19 were reduced by 54% (from 8.7% to 4.0%) for patients with mild to moderate COVID-19 and 68% (from 23.7% to 7.5%) for moderate COVID-19 patients aged 50 years and over. Furthermore, the clinical recovery time was 3.4 to 6.4 days faster in patients treated with regdanvimab, compared to those treated with placebo [12]. Recently published retrospective studies also demonstrated that regdanvimab treatment prevented progression to severe disease [25,26]. Accordingly, in February 2021, the Korean Ministry of Food and Drug Safety approved the conditional marketing authorization for the emergency use of regdanvimab for adult ($\geq$18 years) patients with mild to moderate COVID-19, when the following conditions were met: within 7 days of symptom onset and over 60 years of age, underlying disease (cardiovascular disease, chronic lung disease, diabetes mellitus, or hypertension), or radiologically identified pneumonia (either by CXR or computed tomography) [15].

Regdanvimab has been supplied to our hospital (UUH) since the end of February 2021. Since then, regdanvimab has been administered to indicated patients with non-severe COVID-19. Severe COVID-19 patients received remdesivir according to indications, and some remdesivir-treated patients had been treated with regdanvimab because their condition had been non-severe immediately after hospitalization (but progressed to severe COVID-19 during hospitalization). We extracted severe COVID-19 patients who received remdesivir and oxygen therapy after regdanvimab had been supplied and divided them into a group using only remdesevir and a group using both regdanvimab and remdesivir to investigate clinical outcomes.

In our study, the use of regdanvimab in patients with severe COVID-19 significantly increased the number of oxygen-free days, compared to the remdesivir alone group. The use of regdanvimab and increase in oxygen-free days (on day 28) were also significantly associated, as per multiple linear regression analysis that included important clinical indicators such as age, sex, BMI, and baseline SpO_2/FiO_2 ratio at the time of initiation of remdesivir administration, which represent the initial severity. Furthermore, the use of regdanvimab was associated with lower FiO_2 requirement, higher SpO_2/FiO_2 ratio during treatment, and a shorter duration of oxygen supplementation. These results suggest that the use of regdanvimab in combination with remdesivir has a significant beneficial effect on the clinical outcomes of severe COVID-19.

Some clinical trials involving targeting of severe COVID-19 by mAbs have already been conducted. In the ACTIV-3 trial (n = 326, 1:1 randomization), administration of bamlanivimab, in combination with the standard of care (typically being remdesivir administration), did not demonstrate additional clinical benefits in hospitalized patients with severe COVID-19 [27]. However, in the REGN-COV2 trial (n = 9785, 1:1 randomization), a combination of two mAbs (casirivimab and imdevimab), in addition to usual care (not fully disclosed yet), reduced the risk of death by 20%, in patients hospitalized with COVID-19 [28]. The full report of the REGN-COV2 trial has not yet been published, so it is difficult to interpret its results, but the difference between the two conflicting results is presumed to be the timing of mAb injection. In the REGN-COV2 trial, mAbs were administered to early phase patients who were seronegative (before developing an immune response to SARS-COV-2). In the ACTIV-3 trial, which showed negative results, mAb administration took a median of 7 (interquartile range: 5–9) days after symptom onset [27]. In our study, it took an average of 3.68 days for regdanvimab to be administered after symptom onset. For mAbs to be effective in viral infectious diseases, they must be administered in the early stages of infectious diseases, when the viral load is high, but before seroconversion occurs [23]. It is difficult to expect the effect of mAbs in the post-viral phase, wherein a secondary immune response is induced after the initial virally driven phase [23].

There were no serious adverse drug reactions related to the administration of regdanvimab. Fewer than 50% of patients had fever and dyspnea while using regdanvimab, which could be symptoms of COVID-19 itself. None of the users stopped taking the drug due to side effects, and all 25 patients were administered the full dose of regdanvimab without any major events. Also in a previous phase 2/3 trial, there were no reports of serious adverse events associated with the use of regdanvimab [12].

Our study has some important limitations. First, patients with relatively mild COVID-19 might have been included in the regdanvimab/remdesivir group, and patients with relatively severe COVID-19 might have been included in the remdesivir alone group; as the baseline SpO_2/FiO_2 ratio was higher in the regdanvimab/remdesivir group, this is a reasonable deduction. However, we found a significant correlation between regdanvimab administration and oxygen-free days, as per the multivariate analysis, adjusted for the SpO_2/FiO_2 ratio. And it is also possible that the use of regdanvimab resulted in a relatively mild degree of severe COVID-19. Second, the number of patients was small. Although the results of this study had statistical significance, it is a retrospective, small sample-sized, single-center study; thus, there might be selection bias. Despite these limitations, our study has a novelty in attempting to elucidate the effectiveness of regdanvimab in severe COVID-19.

5. Conclusions

Administration of regdanvimab, in addition to remdesivir, significantly improved clinical outcomes in severe COVID-19. Although results of the present study require confirmation via a large-scale, prospective, randomized study, active consideration of regdanvimab administration in severe COVID-19 is needed to facilitate the reduction of high mortality rate associated with severe COVID-19 and the mild adverse drug reaction associated with regdanvimab administration.

Author Contributions: Conceptualization, G.C., A.C., W.K. and T.L.; Methodology, A.C., E.P. and T.L.; Formal Analysis, A.C., E.P. and T.L.; Data Curation, A.C. and T.L.; Writing—Original Draft Preparation, T.L.; Writing—Review & Editing, G.C., S.L., S.P., S.L., Y.A., J.K., S.R., Y.J., J.A. and J.J. All authors have read and agreed to the published version of the manuscript.

Funding: This research did not receive any specific grant from funding agencies in the public, commercial, or not-for-profit sectors.

Institutional Review Board Statement: The present study was approved by the Institutional Review Board of Ulsan University Hospital (IRB number: UUH 2021-06-028).

Informed Consent Statement: Patient consent was waived due to the retrospective nature of the study.

Data Availability Statement: No new data were created or analyzed in this study. Data sharing is not applicable to this article.

Conflicts of Interest: The authors declare no conflict of interest.

References

1. Park, S.E. Epidemiology, virology, and clinical features of severe acute respiratory syndrome -coronavirus-2 (SARS-CoV-2; Coronavirus Disease-19). *Clin. Exp. Pediatr.* **2020**, *63*, 119–124. [CrossRef] [PubMed]
2. World Health Organization. WHO Coronavirus (COVID-19) Dashboard. Available online: https://covid19.who.int (accessed on 30 June 2021).
3. Wu, Z.; McGoogan, J.M. Characteristics of and important lessons from the coronavirus disease 2019 (COVID-19) outbreak in China: Summary of a report of 72314 cases from the Chinese Center for Disease Control and Prevention. *JAMA* **2020**, *323*, 1239–1242. [CrossRef]
4. RECOVERY Collaborative Group; Horby, P.; Lim, W.S.; Emberson, J.R.; Mafham, M.; Bell, J.L.; Linsell, L.; Staplin, N.; Brightling, C.; Ustianowski, A.; et al. Dexamethasone in hospitalized patients with COVID-19. *N. Engl. J. Med.* **2021**, *384*, 693–704. [CrossRef] [PubMed]
5. Beigel, J.H.; Tomashek, K.M.; Dodd, L.E.; Mehta, A.K.; Zingman, B.S.; Kalil, A.C.; Hohmann, E.; Chu, H.Y.; Luetkemeyer, A.; Kline, S.; et al. Remdesivir for the treatment of COVID-19—final report. *N. Engl. J. Med.* **2020**, *383*, 1813–1826. [CrossRef] [PubMed]
6. Lee, T.C.; McDonald, E.G.; Butler-Laporte, G.; Harrison, L.B.; Cheng, M.P.; Brophy, J.M. Remdesivir and systemic corticosteroids for the treatment of COVID-19: A Bayesian re-analysis. *Int. J. Infect. Dis.* **2021**, *104*, 671–676. [CrossRef]
7. Lee, J.; Lim, D.S.; Hong, S.O.; Park, M.-J.; Kim, G.; Lim, N.-K.; Lee, S.Y.; Park, J.K.; Song, D.S.; Chai, H.y.; et al. The primary report of clinical data analysis on the COVID-19 in the Republic of Korea. *Public Health Wkly. Rep.* **2020**, *13*, 2054–2058.
8. Olivas-Martínez, A.; Cárdenas-Fragoso, J.L.; Jiménez, J.V.; Lozano-Cruz, O.A.; Ortiz-Brizuela, E.; Tovar-Méndez, V.H.; Medrano-Borromeo, C.; Martínez-Valenzuela, A.; Román-Montes, C.M.; Martínez-Guerra, B.; et al. In-hospital mortality from severe COVID-19 in a tertiary care center in Mexico City; causes of death, risk factors and the impact of hospital saturation. *PLoS ONE* **2021**, *16*, e0245772. [CrossRef]
9. Wang, Z.; Wang, Z. Identification of risk factors for in-hospital death of COVID-19 pneumonia – lessions from the early outbreak. *BMC Infect. Dis.* **2021**, *21*, 113. [CrossRef] [PubMed]
10. Kim, C.; Ryu, D.K.; Lee, J.; Kim, Y.I.; Seo, J.M.; Kim, Y.G.; Jeong, J.H.; Kim, M.; Kim, J.I.; Kim, P.; et al. A therapeutic neutralizing antibody targeting receptor binding domain of SARS-CoV-2 spike protein. *Nat. Commun.* **2021**, *12*, 288. [CrossRef]
11. Kim, J.Y.; Jang, Y.R.; Hong, J.H.; Jung, J.G.; Park, J.H.; Streinu-Cercel, A.; Streinu-Cercel, A.; Săndulescu, O.; Lee, S.J.; Kim, S.H.; et al. Safety, Virologic Efficacy, and Pharmacokinetics of CT-P59, a Neutralizing Monoclonal Antibody Against SARS-CoV-2 Spike Receptor-Binding Protein: Two Randomized, Placebo-Controlled, Phase I Studies in Healthy Individuals and Patients With Mild SARS-CoV-2 Infection. *Clin. Ther.* **2021**, *43*, 1706–1727. [CrossRef]
12. Eom, J.S.; Ison, M.; Streinu-Cercel, A.; Săndulescu, O.; Preotescu, L.-L.; Kim, Y.-S.; Kim, J.Y.; Cheon, S.H.; Jang, Y.R.; Lee, S.J.; et al. Efficacy and safety of CT-P59 plus standard of care: A phase 2/3 randomized, double-blind, placebo-controlled trial in outpatients with mild-to-moderate SARS-CoV-2 infection. *Res. Sq.* **2021**, *in preprint*. [CrossRef]
13. Ryu, D.K.; Kang, B.; Noh, H.; Woo, S.J.; Lee, M.H.; Nuijten, P.M.; Kim, J.I.; Seo, J.M.; Kim, C.; Kim, M.; et al. The in vitro and in vivo efficacy of CT-P59 against Gamma, Delta and its associated variants of SARS-CoV-2. *Biochem. Biophys. Res. Commun.* **2021**, *578*, 91–96. [CrossRef]
14. Ministry of Health and Welfare; Korea Disease Control and Prevention Agency (KDCA). Supplying Remdesivir for the Treatment of COVID-19 (Korean). Available online: http://www.mohw.go.kr/react/al/sal0301vw.jsp?PAR_MENU_ID=04&MENU_ID=0403&page=1&CONT_SEQ=355233 (accessed on 9 July 2021).
15. Ministry of Health and Welfare; Korea Disease Control and Prevention Agency (KDCA). Guide to Administration Management Plan for COVID-19 Antibody Treatment (Regkirona) (Ver.02) (Release Date: FEB 14, 2021) (Korean). Available online: http://ncov.mohw.go.kr/upload/ncov/file/202108/1627978032143_20210803170712.pdf (accessed on 14 February 2021).

16. Rice, T.W.; Wheeler, A.P.; Bernard, G.R.; Hayden, D.L.; Schoenfeld, D.A.; Ware, L.B.; National Institutes of Health, National Heart, Lung, and Blood Institute ARDS Network. Comparison of the SpO_2/FIO_2 ratio and the PaO_2/FIO_2 ratio in patients with acute lung injury or ARDS. *Chest* **2007**, *132*, 410–417. [CrossRef]
17. Borghesi, A.; Maroldi, R. COVID-19 outbreak in Italy: Experimental chest X-ray scoring system for quantifying and monitoring disease progression. *Radiol. Med.* **2020**, *125*, 509–513. [CrossRef]
18. Choi, K.J.; Hong, H.L.; Kim, E.J. The association between mortality and the oxygen saturation and fraction of inhaled oxygen in patients requiring oxygen therapy due to COVID-19-associated pneumonia. *Tuberc. Respir. Dis.* **2021**, *84*, 125–133. [CrossRef]
19. Simonis, F.D.; Serpa Neto, A.; Binnekade, J.M.; Braber, A.; Bruin, K.C.M.; Determann, R.M.; Goekoop, G.J.; Heidt, J.; Horn, J.; Innemee, G.; et al. Effect of a low vs intermediate tidal volume strategy on ventilator-free days in intensive care unit patients without ARDS: A randomized clinical trial. *JAMA* **2018**, *320*, 1872–1880. [CrossRef]
20. Waghmare, A.; Xie, H.; Kimball, L.; Yi, J.; Özkök, S.; Leisenring, W.; Cheng, G.S.; Englund, J.A.; Watkins, T.R.; Chien, J.W.; et al. Supplemental oxygen-free days in hematopoietic cell transplant recipients with respiratory syncytial virus. *J. Infect. Dis.* **2017**, *216*, 1235–1244. [CrossRef]
21. Ulrich, R.J.; Troxel, A.B.; Carmody, E.; Eapen, J.; Bäcker, M.; DeHovitz, J.A.; Prasad, P.J.; Li, Y.; Delgado, C.; Jrada, M.; et al. Treating COVID-19 with hydroxychloroquine (TEACH): A multicenter, double-blind randomized controlled trial in hospitalized patients. *Open Forum Infect. Dis.* **2020**, *7*, ofaa446. [CrossRef]
22. Sheikh, A.; McMenamin, J.; Taylor, B.; Robertson, C.; Public Health Scotland and the EAVE II Collaborators. SARS-CoV-2 Delta VOC in Scotland: Demographics, risk of hospital admission, and vaccine effectiveness. *Lancet* **2021**, *397*, 2461–2462. [CrossRef]
23. Taylor, P.C.; Adams, A.C.; Hufford, M.M.; de la Torre, I.; Winthrop, K.; Gottlieb, R.L. Neutralizing monoclonal antibodies for treatment of COVID-19. *Nat. Rev. Immunol.* **2021**, *21*, 382–393. [CrossRef]
24. Kim, S.B.; Kim, J.; Huh, K.; Choi, W.S.; Kim, Y.J.; Joo, E.J.; Kim, Y.J.; Yoon, Y.K.; Heo, J.Y.; Seo, Y.B.; et al. Korean Society of Infectious Diseases/National Evidence-based Healthcare Collaborating Agency recommendations for anti-SARS-CoV-2 monoclonal antibody treatment of patients with COVID-19. *Infect. Chemother.* **2021**, *53*, 395–403. [CrossRef] [PubMed]
25. Lee, S.; Lee, S.O.; Lee, J.E.; Kim, K.H.; Lee, S.H.; Hwang, S.; Kim, S.W.; Chang, H.H.; Kim, Y.; Bae, S.; et al. Regdanvimab in patients with mild-to-moderate SARS-CoV-2 infection: A propensity score-matched retrospective cohort study. *Int. Immunopharmacol.* **2022**, *106*, 108570. [CrossRef] [PubMed]
26. Lee, J.Y.; Lee, J.Y.; Ko, J.H.; Hyun, M.; Kim, H.A.; Cho, S.; Lee, Y.D.; Song, J.; Shin, S.; Peck, K.R. Effectiveness of Regdanvimab Treatment in High-Risk COVID-19 Patients to Prevent Progression to Severe Disease. *Front. Immunol.* **2021**, *12*, 772320. [CrossRef] [PubMed]
27. ACTIV-3/TICO LY-CoV555 Study Group; Lundgren, J.D.; Grund, B.; Barkauskas, C.E.; Holland, T.L.; Gottlieb, R.L.; Sandkovsky, U.; Brown, S.M.; Knowlton, K.U.; Self, W.H.; et al. A neutralizing monoclonal antibody for hospitalized patients with COVID-19. *N. Engl. J. Med.* **2021**, *384*, 905–914. [CrossRef]
28. Regeneron. REGEN-COV™ (Casirivimab and Imdevimab) Phase 3 Recovery Trial Meets Primary Outcome, Improving Survival in Hospitalized COVID-19 Patients Lacking an Immune Response to SARS-COV-2. Available online: https://investor.regeneron.com/news-releases/news-release-details/regen-covtm-casirivimab-and-imdevimab-phase-3-recovery-trial (accessed on 21 January 2022).

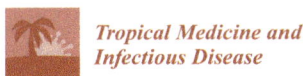

Tropical Medicine and Infectious Disease

Article

Analysis of Excess All-Cause Mortality and COVID-19 Mortality in Peru: Observational Study

Max Carlos Ramírez-Soto [1,*] and Gutia Ortega-Cáceres [2]

1 Facultad de Ciencias de la Salud, Universidad Tecnológica del Perú, Lima 15046, Peru
2 Escuela de Posgrado, Universidad Ricardo Palma, Lima 15039, Peru; gutiaortega@gmail.com
* Correspondence: maxcrs22@gmail.com

Citation: Ramírez-Soto, M.C.; Ortega-Cáceres, G. Analysis of Excess All-Cause Mortality and COVID-19 Mortality in Peru: Observational Study. *Trop. Med. Infect. Dis.* **2022**, *7*, 44. https://doi.org/10.3390/tropicalmed7030044

Academic Editors: Peter A. Leggat, John Frean and Lucille Blumberg

Received: 25 January 2022
Accepted: 2 March 2022
Published: 5 March 2022

Publisher's Note: MDPI stays neutral with regard to jurisdictional claims in published maps and institutional affiliations.

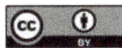

Copyright: © 2022 by the authors. Licensee MDPI, Basel, Switzerland. This article is an open access article distributed under the terms and conditions of the Creative Commons Attribution (CC BY) license (https://creativecommons.org/licenses/by/4.0/).

Abstract: During the COVID-19 pandemic, an excess of all-cause mortality has been recorded in several countries, including Peru. Most excess deaths were likely attributable to COVID-19. In this study, we compared the excess all-cause mortality and COVID-19 mortality in 25 Peruvian regions to determine whether most of the excess deaths in 2020 were attributable to COVID-19. Excess deaths were calculated as the difference between the number of observed deaths from all causes during the COVID-19 pandemic (in 2020) and the number of expected deaths in 2020 based on a historical from recent years (2017–2019). Death data were retrieved from the Sistema Informatico Nacional de Defunciones (SINADEF) at the Ministry of Health of Peru from January 2017 to December 2020. Population counts were obtained from projections from Peru's Instituto Nacional de Estadística e Informática (INEI). All-cause excess mortality and COVID-19 mortality were calculated by region per 100,000 population. Spearman's test and linear and multiple regression models were used to estimate the correlation between excess all-cause mortality and COVID-19 mortality per 100,000 population. Excess all-cause death rates varied widely among regions (range: 115.1 to 519.8 per 100,000 population), and COVID-19 mortality ranged between 83.8 and 464.6 per 100,000 population. There was a correlation between the all-cause excess mortality and COVID-19 mortality ($r = 0.90$; $p = 0.00001$; $y = 0.8729x + 90.808$; $R^2 = 0.84$). Adjusted for confounding factors (mean age in the region, gender balance, and number of intensive care unit (ICU) beds), the all-cause excess mortality rate was correlated with COVID-19 mortality rate ($\beta = 0.921$; $p = 0.0001$). These findings suggest that most of the excess deaths in Peru are related to COVID-19. Therefore, these findings can help decision-makers to understand the high COVID-19 mortality rates in Peru.

Keywords: excess mortality; COVID-19; mortality; Peru

1. Introduction

During the COVID-19 pandemic, an all-cause mortality excess has been recorded in several countries, including Peru [1–4]. This all-cause mortality excess varied substantially across countries [1–3] because of measures taken to handle the COVID-19 pandemic, demographic and socio-economic characteristics, and capacity of health care systems [5–8]. Excess deaths are the difference between the number of observed deaths from all causes during a given time period, and the number of expected deaths from the same time period, based on a historical from recent years (often estimated using the average over several preceding years) [8]. Excess all-cause mortality can also be standardized for age, sex, region, or population size in a geographical region to aid comparisons. Mortality below the expected levels is called "avoided mortality", whereas the mortality above the expected levels is known as "excess deaths" [3]. Assessing the direct and indirect effects of the COVID-19 pandemic on overall mortality requires the measurement of excess deaths since most excess deaths are likely attributable to COVID-19 [3,8].

Worldwide, Peru is the country with the highest number of COVID-19 deaths per 100,000 population [9]. In 2020, 93,851 COVID-19 deaths were registered in the country, and by 26 December 2021, the total had reached 202,524 deaths [10]. Because of the Peruvian national healthcare system's limited capacity, the collapse of health services in the first wave, limited number of intensive care unit (ICU) beds, lack of oxygen [11,12], and the high COVID-19 death rate, excess all-cause mortality is likely attributable to COVID-19. Therefore, our objective was to compare the all-cause excess mortality with the COVID-19 mortality in 25 Peruvian regions to determine whether most of the excess deaths in 2020 were attributable to COVID-19. These findings could be used to determine the indirect impact of the COVID-19 pandemic on the overall mortality rate in Peru.

2. Materials and Methods

This cross-sectional, geographical time-series study was performed according to the Strengthening the Reporting of Observational Studies in Epidemiology (STROBE) reporting guidelines [13]. We retrieved disaggregated region-level data on confirmed COVID-19 deaths and all-cause mortality, as of 31 December 2020, from the Sistema Informatico Nacional de Defunciones (SINADEF) at the Ministry of Health of Peru [14,15]. We used death registers from 1 January through to 31 December 2020 (1–52 epidemiological weeks) and from the preceding 3 years (2017–2019) [14,15]. Data regarding the populations of Peruvian regions were obtained from the projections of the Instituto Nacional de Estadística e Informática (INEI) [16]. Confounding factors included the mean age, gender balance, and number of ICU beds for each region (from 2020). The mean age and gender balance in the regions were obtained from INEI (from 2016 to 2020) [16]. The number of ICU beds was obtained from the Superintendencia Nacional de Salud, Peru (SUSALUD) via App. F500.2 [17].

Statistical Analysis

The average numbers of all-cause deaths for the years 2017–2019 were used to estimate expected deaths in 2020 [8,18]. Observed deaths were the deaths reported from 1 January through to 31 December 2020. Excess all-cause deaths during the pandemic period were estimated as the difference between observed deaths and expected deaths in 2020 [8,18]. We calculated the excess all-cause mortality rate and COVID-19 mortality rate by region per 100,000 population. Excess deaths attributable to COVID-19 were calculated (%) by dividing COVID-19 deaths per 100,000 by excess deaths per 100,000 population. Spearman's test and a linear regression model were used to estimate the correlation between excess all-cause mortality rate and COVID-19 mortality rate per 100,000 population. Multiple regression analysis was also used for confounding factors (mean age in the region, gender balance, and number of ICU beds). Values of $p < 0.05$ were considered significant. Results were displayed using a scatterplot. All analyses were performed using StataSE 16.0 for Windows.

This descriptive study was based on public-use datasets. Therefore, it was exempt from Institutional Review Board review and approval, and no informed consent was required.

3. Results

All Peruvian regions experienced an all-cause mortality excess in 2020, compared with expected deaths (determined from the mean between 2017 and 2019). Excess all-cause death rates varied widely among regions (range: 115.1 to 519.8 per 100,000 population). The ratio of observed to expected all-cause deaths ranged between 1.5 and 2.8. COVID-19 death rates ranged between 83.8 and 464.6 per 100,000 population, and excess deaths (%) ranged between 48.8 and 108.3% (Table 1). In the general population of Peru, the excess all-cause mortality exceeded COVID-19 mortality (371.9 vs. 287.7 population, respectively). There were variations in excess all-cause mortality and COVID-19 mortality by region. The highest excess all-cause mortality per 100,000 habitants was reported in the Callao region, followed by Lima, Moquegua, and Piura regions. The highest COVID-19 mortality rates per 100,000 habitants were reported in Moquegua, Lima, Ica, and Lambayeque. In 19 Peruvian regions, the ratio of excess all-cause deaths to COVID-19 deaths was almost 1 (Table 1). In six Peruvian regions, there was a gap between the all-cause excess mortality and COVID-19 mortality, e.g., in the Apurimac, Huancavelica, and Pasco regions, the ratio of excess all-cause deaths to COVID-19 deaths was 2.0, while in the Ayacucho, Cajamarca, and Puno regions it was almost 2.0 (Table 1).

There was a correlation between the all-cause excess mortality rate and the COVID-19 mortality rate ($r = 0.90$; $p = 0.00001$; $y = 0.8729x + 90.808$; $R^2 = 0.84$) (Figure 1). Adjusted for confounding factors (mean age in the region, gender balance, and number of ICU beds), the all-cause excess mortality rate was correlated with the COVID-19 mortality rate ($\beta = 0.921$; $p = 0.0001$) (Table 2). The model was statistically significant ($F\ (4,20) = 37.46$, $p = 0.00001$, Adj. $R^2 = 0.882$).

Table 1. Excess all-cause deaths and COVID-19 mortality, 1 January to 31 December 2020, 25 Peruvian regions.

Region	Observed Deaths in 2020 [15]	Expected Deaths in 2020 [15]	Ratio of Observed to Expected	Population in 2020 [16]	Excess Deaths	Excess Deaths per 100,000	Total Deaths COVID-19 [14]	COVID-19 Deaths per 100,000	Excess Deaths Attributable to COVID-19, % [a]	Ratio of Excess Deaths to COVID-19 Deaths	Mean Age (Years) in the Regions in 2020 [16]	Gender Balance (Men/Women) in 2020 [16]	No. of ICU Beds [b]
Amazonas	1309	818	1.6	426,806	491	115.1	585	137.1	119.1	0.8	30.95	1.1	10
Ancash	8800	5143	1.7	1,180,638	3657	309.7	2889	244.7	79.0	1.3	32.36	1.0	18
Apurimac	2242	1502	1.5	430,736	740	171.7	361	83.8	48.8	2.0	29.99	1.1	10
Arequipa	11,634	5655	2.1	1,497,438	5979	399.3	4260	284.5	71.2	1.4	32.45	1.0	22
Ayacucho	3097	1713	1.8	668,213	1384	207.1	836	125.1	60.4	1.7	30.04	1.0	15
Cajamarca	6041	3116	1.9	1,453,711	2925	201.2	1615	111.1	55.2	1.8	30.71	1.0	18
Callao	10,124	4327	2.3	1,129,854	5797	513.1	5249	464.6	90.5	1.1	32.36	0.9	16
Cusco	7857	5775	1.4	1,357,075	2082	153.4	1594	117.5	76.5	1.3	30.34	1.0	14
Huancavelica	2457	1680	1.5	365,317	777	212.6	393	107.6	50.6	2.0	30.28	1.0	12
Huanuco	4268	2768	1.5	760,267	1500	197.3	1070	140.7	71.3	1.4	30.01	1.0	25
Ica	7785	4105	1.9	975,182	3680	377.4	3796	389.3	103.2	1.0	30.93	1.0	26
Junin	8573	5347	1.6	1,361,467	3226	236.9	2423	178.0	75.1	1.3	31.18	1.0	42
La Libertad	13,800	7594	1.8	2,016,771	6206	307.7	4891	242.5	78.8	1.3	31.55	1.0	26
Lambayeque	8421	3447	2.4	1,310,785	4974	379.5	4631	353.3	93.1	1.1	32.24	0.9	22
Lima	87,139	31,889	2.7	10,628,470	55,250	519.8	42,182	396.9	76.3	1.3	33.05	0.9	367
Loreto	5102	2050	2.5	1,027,559	3052	297.0	2832	275.6	92.8	1.1	28.50	1.1	2
Madre de Dios	1089	512	2.1	173,811	577	332.2	446	256.6	77.3	1.3	27.48	1.4	7
Moquegua	1574	757	2.1	192,740	817	423.9	885	459.2	108.3	0.9	32.85	1.2	6
Pasco	1234	564	2.2	271,904	670	246.3	331	121.7	49.4	2.0	30.12	1.1	6
Piura	13,974	4992	2.8	2,047,954	8982	438.6	6345	309.8	70.6	1.4	30.42	1.0	26
Puno	8173	5192	1.6	1,237,997	2981	240.8	1535	124.0	51.5	1.9	29.72	1.0	14
San Martin	4361	2409	1.8	899,648	1952	217.0	1579	175.5	80.9	1.2	29.89	1.1	14
Tacna	2167	1274	1.7	370,974	893	240.8	791	213.2	88.5	1.1	31.91	1.0	20
Tumbes	1796	895	2.0	251,521	901	358.4	774	307.7	85.9	1.2	29.91	1.2	8
Ucayali	3533	1706	2.1	589,110	1827	310.1	1558	264.5	85.3	1.2	28.00	1.1	12
Peru	226,550	105,229	2.2	32,625,948	121,321	371.9	93,851	287.7	77.4	1.3	NA	1.0	758

[a] Excess deaths attributable to COVID-19 calculated (%) by dividing COVID-19 deaths per 100,000 by excess deaths per 100,000 population. [b] SICOVID App. F500.2, SUSALUD (accessed on 30 September 2020). COVID-19, coronavirus disease 2019; NA, not aplicable; ICU, intensive care unit.

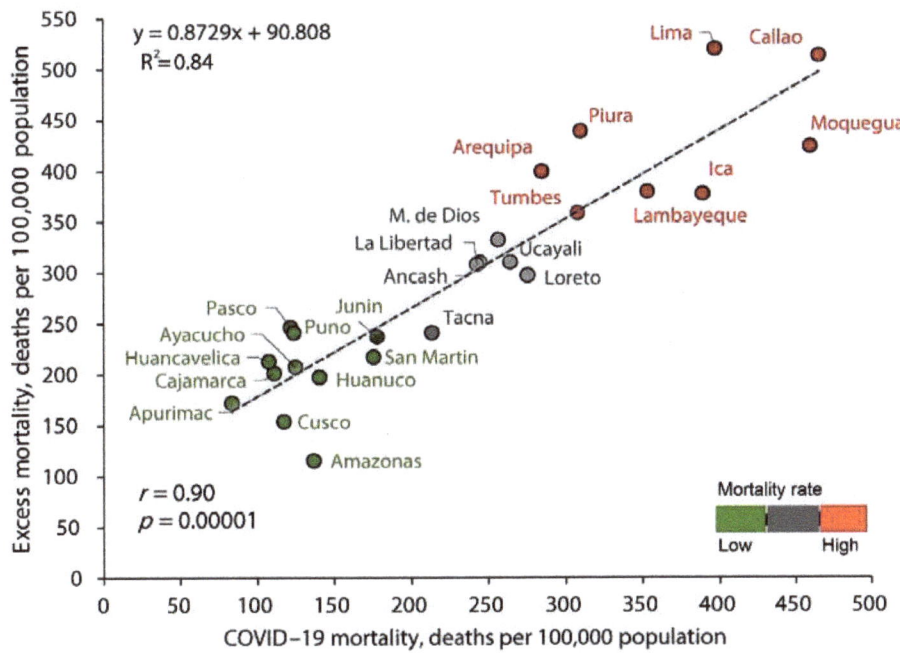

Figure 1. Correlation between the all-cause excess mortality and COVID-19 mortality in Peru.

Table 2. Multiple regression analysis of mortality all-cause excess rate and COVID-19 mortality rate adjusted.

Variable	Coef.	SE	Beta	t	p-Value
Mortality all-cause excess and COVID-19 mortality					
COVID-19 mortality rate	0.875	0.088	0.921	9.89	0.0001
Mean age (years) in the region	−9.500	8.673	−0.126	−1.10	0.286
Gender balance	−138.9	114.4	−0.128	−1.21	0.239
Number of ICU beds	0.257	0.132	0.167	1.95	0.065

COVID-19, coronavirus disease 2019; SE, standard error; ICU, intensive care unit.

4. Discussion

Worldwide, Peru is the country with the highest number of COVID-19 deaths per 100,000 population [9]. This has caused an excess of all-cause mortality [4] and compared with other countries, in 2020 Peru experienced the largest excess mortality among 103 countries studied [1]. This excess all-cause mortality recorded in 2020 is clearly related to the health crisis caused by the COVID-19 pandemic. This was shown by the ratio of excess all-cause deaths to COVID-19 deaths and the adjusted analysis of death rates reported in the same period in most Peruvian regions. In addition, we found that COVID-19 mortality as excess all-causes mortality varied widely between Peruvian regions. Similar to Peru, some Brazilian states, Iran, and Belgium reported an excess all-cause mortality during the first wave proportional to the number of people who died of COVID-19 in the same period [19–21].

Excess mortality during the COVID-19 pandemic can be the sum of distinct factors. These factors include: (1) deaths directly caused by COVID-19 infection, (2) medical system collapse due to COVID-19 pandemic, (3) excess deaths from other natural causes, (4) unnatural causes, or (5) extreme events [1]. Compared with other factors, most excess deaths are likely attributable to COVID-19 infection [1,8]. In that setting, the literature has described some factors that directly or indirectly impact COVID-19 mortality in Peru [1,11,12], and therefore on excess all-cause mortality (Figure 2).

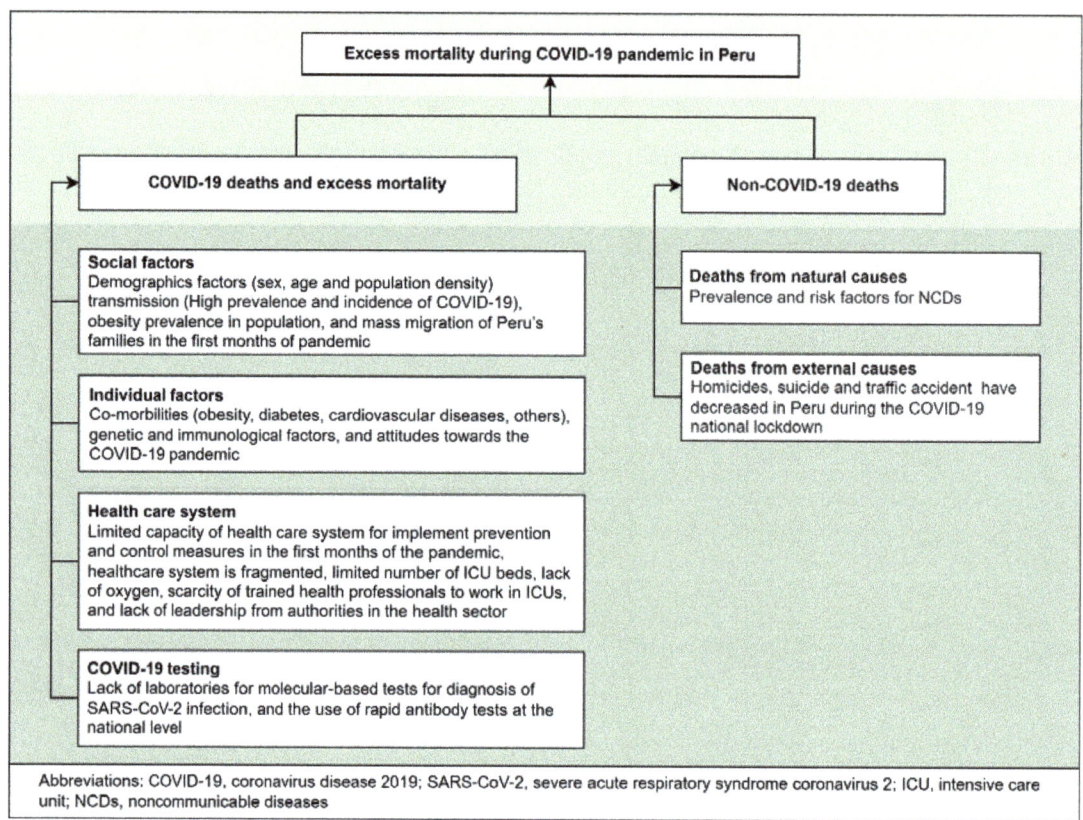

Figure 2. Factors that directly or indirectly impact excess all-cause mortality and COVID-19 mortality [1,8,11,12].

The factors that may have contributed to the causal relationship between all-cause excess mortality and COVID-19 mortality in Peru and the large differences in excess mortality from one region of Peru to another could have several explanations. First, mortality rates depend on social factors such as demographic and socio-economic characteristics, including age, population structure, population size, lifestyles, obesity prevalence, ethnicity, and the mobility of populations across between regions, as was observed in several countries, including Peru [2,12,22,23]. Second, mortality rates also depend on the probability of being infected, prevalence and incidence rates, and mortality among the infected population, since worldwide, Peru was the country with the highest number of COVID-19 deaths per 100,000 population [9]. Third, because of the Peruvian national healthcare system's limited capacity, excess all-cause mortality may be a more comprehensive and robust indicator than COVID-19 mortality. Thus, the collapse of the health services in Peru, the fragmented health system, the limited number of ICU beds, and lack of oxygen during the first wave may have also contributed directly or indirectly to the increased relationship between the death rate due to COVID-19 and the excess all-cause mortality [11,12]. A recent study found a gap between excess mortality and COVID-19 deaths in 67 countries, including Peru [24]. Their findings revealed that the countries where COVID-19 mortality exceeded excess all-cause mortality had an extremely high testing capacity and effective response measures against the COVID-19 pandemic. In contrast, the excess all-cause mortality exceeded COVID-19 mortality in the general population of Peru, because there was a low rate of RT-PCR testing for COVID-19 in Peru in 2020; therefore, most of the cases were diagnosed using rapid tests, the sensitivity limits of which are low compared with molecular tests. Because of this, it is possible that some of the deaths recorded as other causes might have been due to COVID-19; consequently, the excess all-cause death rate increased and was greater than the COVID-19 mortality. Fourth, individual factors such as comorbidities and genetic and immunological factors also directly or indirectly impact COVID-19 mortality [25], and therefore the excess all-cause mortality can be seen as an indirect consequence of COVID-19 mortality. In addition, the COVID-19 mortality in Peru was highest in men 60 years of age or older [26], and with co-morbidities [27]. This could have caused difficulty in identifying the basic cause of death, and therefore an underreporting of COVID-19 deaths that increased the excess all-cause mortality. Finally, COVID-19 is a new disease and physicians have limited experience in certifying these deaths, which may have resulted in deaths being underreported in the first months of 2020.

During the COVID-19 pandemic, it is likely that deaths from non-COVID-19 causes may also have increased due to the medical system being overloaded. However, to date, in Peru, there are no studies on excess mortality from non-COVID-19 causes. The restrictive measures adopted in Peru to control the COVID-19 pandemic in the first months of 2020 (COVID-19 lockdown) also could have caused changes in mortality rates due to external causes such as injuries or accidents, as was reported previously in England [28]; however, this did not happen in Peru, since in 2020 there was a decrease in the mortality rates by homicides, suicides, and traffic accidents during the COVID-19 lockdown [29].

The main limitation of our study was the method used to estimate excess mortality. In the literature, the methods for estimating excess mortality vary from simple estimates to modeled studies, making it difficult to compare results across studies. Another limitation in this observational study is the retrospective design; we used several different information sources (SINADEF, INEI, and SUSALUD) which may have resulted in a possible bias. Despite these limitations, the strengths of this study include: (1) the used method allows for transparency and reproducibility of the findings; (2) the simplicity in the analysis of excess mortality (all-cause and COVID-19 mortality) allows for the opportunity to use the findings in epidemiological surveillance and their interpretation by the health authorities; (3) the large number of deaths included for estimating the excess all-cause mortality and COVID-19 mortality and the multiple regression analyses for confounding factors; and (4) the findings add further evidence for policymakers in Peru.

5. Conclusions

This study provides the first causal relationship analysis between excess all-cause mortality and COVID-19 mortality for 2020 across 25 Peruvian regions, adjusted for confounding factors. Our findings suggest that most of the excess deaths in Peru in 2020 were related to COVID-19. Therefore, our findings could be used to explain the indirect impact of the COVID-19 pandemic on the overall mortality rate up to the point where vaccination against SARS-CoV-2 started to become available in Peru.

Author Contributions: Conceptualization, M.C.R.-S.; methodology, M.C.R.-S. and G.O.-C.; software, M.C.R.-S. and G.O.-C.; validation, M.C.R.-S.; formal analysis, M.C.R.-S. and G.O.-C.; investigation, M.C.R.-S. and G.O.-C.; data curation, M.C.R.-S.; writing—original draft preparation, M.C.R.-S.; writing—review and editing, M.C.R.-S. and G.O.-C. All authors have read and agreed to the published version of the manuscript.

Funding: This manuscript had no funding. The APC was funded by the Universidad Tecnologica del Peru.

Institutional Review Board Statement: This descriptive study was based on public use datasets. Therefore, it was exempt from Institutional Review Board review and approval, and no informed consent was required.

Informed Consent Statement: Not applicable.

Data Availability Statement: The data presented in this study are publicly available at: COVID-19 deaths. National System of Deaths (SINADEF). Available online: https://www.datosabiertos.gob.pe/dataset/fallecidos-por-covid-19-ministerio-de-salud-minsa (accessed on 26 December 2021); Deaths. National System of Deaths (SINADEF). Available online: https://www.datosabiertos.gob.pe/dataset/informaci%C3%B3n-de-fallecidos-del-sistema-inform%C3%A1tico-nacional-de-defunciones-sinadef-ministerio (accessed on 26 December 2021); INEI, Peruvian population: https://www.inei.gob.pe/estadisticas/indice-tematico/population-estimates-and-projections/ (accessed on 26 December 2021); Daily Report on Form F500.2, app. for centralized management of the availability of Hospitalization and ICU beds at the national level and of all subsystems (Application F500.2): http://portal.susalud.gob.pe/seguimiento-del-registro-de-camas-f500-2/ (accessed on 26 December 2021).

Conflicts of Interest: The authors declare no conflict of interest.

References

1. Karlinsky, A.; Kobak, D. Tracking excess mortality across countries during the COVID-19 pandemic with the World Mortality Dataset. *Elife* **2021**, *10*, e69336. [CrossRef] [PubMed]
2. Kontis, V.; Bennett, J.E.; Rashid, T.; Parks, R.M.; Pearson-Stuttard, J.; Guillot, M.; Asaria, P.; Zhou, B.; Battaglini, M.; Corsetti, G.; et al. Magnitude, demographics and dynamics of the effect of the first wave of the Covid-19 pandemic on all-cause mortality in 21 industrialized countries. *Nat. Med.* **2020**, *26*, 1919–1928. [CrossRef]
3. Islam, N.; Shkolnikov, V.M.; Acosta, R.J.; Klimkin, I.; Kawachi, I.; Irizarry, R.A.; Alicandro, G.; Khunti, K.; Yates, T.; Jdanov, D.A.; et al. Excess deaths associated with covid-19 pandemic in 2020: Age and sex disaggregated time series analysis in 29 high income countries. *BMJ* **2021**, *373*, n1137. [CrossRef] [PubMed]
4. Sempé, L.; Lloyd-Sherlock, P.; Martínez, R.; Ebrahim, S.; McKee, M.; Acosta, E. Estimation of all-cause excess mortality by age-specific mortality patterns for countries with incomplete vital statistics: A population-based study of the case of Peru during the first wave of the COVID-19 pandemic. *Lancet Reg. Health Am.* **2021**, *2*, 100039. [CrossRef]
5. Islam, N.; Sharp, S.J.; Chowell, G.; Shabnam, S.; Kawachi, I.; Lacey, B.; Massaro, J.M.; D'Agostino, R.B.; White, M. Physical distancing interventions and incidence of coronavirus disease 2019: Natural experiment in 149 countries. *BMJ* **2020**, *370*, m2743. [CrossRef] [PubMed]
6. Chu, D.K.; Akl, E.A.; Duda, S.; Solo, K.; Yaacoub, S.; Schünemann, H.J.; COVID-19 Systematic Urgent Review Group Effort (SURGE) Study Authors. Physical distancing, face masks, and eye protection to prevent person-to-person transmission of SARS-CoV-2 and COVID-19: A systematic review and meta-analysis. *Lancet* **2020**, *395*, 1973–1987. [CrossRef]
7. Legido-Quigley, H.; Asgari, N.; Teo, Y.Y.; Leung, G.M.; Oshitani, H.; Fukuda, K.; Cook, A.R.; Hsu, L.Y.; Shibuya, K.; Heymann, D. Are high-performing health systems resilient against the COVID-19 epidemic? *Lancet* **2020**, *395*, 848–850. [CrossRef]
8. Beaney, T.; Clarke, J.M.; Jain, V.; Golestaneh, A.K.; Lyons, G.; Salman, D.; Majeed, A. Excess mortality: The gold standard in measuring the impact of COVID-19 worldwide? *J. R. Soc. Med.* **2020**, *113*, 329–334. [CrossRef] [PubMed]
9. Johns Hopkins University School of Medicine. Mortality Analyses: Cases and Mortality by Country. In *Baltimore, MD: Coronavirus Resource Center*; Johns Hopkins University School of Medicine: Baltimore, MD, USA, 2021. Available online: https://coronavirus.jhu.edu/data/mortality (accessed on 21 July 2021).
10. Peruvian Ministry of Health (MINSA). *COVID-19 in Peru*; MINSA: Lima, Peru, 2022. Available online: https://covid19.minsa.gob.pe/ (accessed on 2 January 2022).
11. Schwalb, A.; Seas, C. The COVID-19 Pandemic in Peru: What Went Wrong? *Am. J. Trop. Med. Hyg.* **2021**, *104*, 1176–1178. [CrossRef]
12. Taylor, L. Covid-19: Why Peru suffers from one of the highest excess death rates in the world. *BMJ* **2021**, *372*, n611. [CrossRef] [PubMed]
13. Vandenbroucke, J.P.; von Elm, E.; Altman, D.G.; Gøtzsche, P.C.; Mulrow, C.D.; Pocock, S.J.; Poole, C.; Schlesselman, J.J.; Egger, M.; STROBE Initiative. Strengthening the Reporting of Observational Studies in Epidemiology (STROBE): Explanation and elaboration. *PLoS Med.* **2007**, *4*, e297. [CrossRef]
14. Peruvian Ministry of Health (MINSA). *COVID-19 Deaths. National System of Deaths (SINADEF)*; MINSA: Lima, Peru, 2021. Available online: https://www.datosabiertos.gob.pe/dataset/fallecidos-por-covid-19-ministerio-de-salud-minsa (accessed on 26 December 2021).
15. Peruvian Ministry of Health (MINSA). *Deaths. National System of Deaths (SINADEF)*; MINSA: Lima, Peru, 2021. Available online: https://www.datosabiertos.gob.pe/dataset/informaci%C3%B3n-de-fallecidos-del-sistema-inform%C3%A1tico-nacional-de-defunciones-sinadef-ministerio (accessed on 26 December 2021).

16. National Institute of Statistics and Informatics (INEI). *Peruvian Population*; INEI: Lima, Peru, 2020. Available online: https://www.inei.gob.pe/estadisticas/indice-tematico/population-estimates-and-projections/ (accessed on 26 December 2021).
17. Superintendencia Nacional de Salud, Peru (SUSALUD). *Daily Report on Form F500.2, App. for Centralized Management of the Availability of Hospitalization and ICU Beds at the National Level and of All Subsystems (Application F500.2)*; SUSALUD: Lima, Peru, 2020. Available online: http://portal.susalud.gob.pe/seguimiento-del-registro-de-camas-f500-2/ (accessed on 26 December 2021).
18. Hannah Ritchie, Edouard Mathieu, Lucas Rodés-Guirao, Cameron Appel, Charlie Giattino, Esteban Ortiz-Ospina, Joe Hasell, Bobbie Macdonald, Diana Beltekian and Max Roser (2020)—"Coronavirus Pandemic (COVID-19)". Excess Mortality during the Coronavirus Pandemic (COVID-19). Published online at OurWorldInData.org. Available online: https://ourworldindata.org/coronavirus (accessed on 26 December 2021).
19. dos Santos, A.M.; de Souza, B.F.; de Carvalho, C.A.; Garcia Campos, M.A.; Alves de Oliveira, B.L.C.; Diniz, E.M.; Freitas Carvalho Branco, M.R.; de Sousa Queiroz, R.C.; de Carvalho, V.A.; Machado Araújo, W.R.; et al. Excess deaths from all causes and by COVID-19 in Brazil in 2020. *Rev. Saude Publica* **2021**, *55*, 71. [CrossRef]
20. Tadbiri, H.; Moradi-Lakeh, M.; Naghavi, M. All-cause excess mortality and COVID-19-related deaths in Iran. *Med. J. Islam. Repub Iran* **2020**, *34*, 80. [CrossRef]
21. Bustos Sierra, N.; Bossuyt, N.; Braeye, T.; Leroy, M.; Moyersoen, I.; Peeters, I.; Scohy, A.; Van der Heyden, J.; Van Oyen, H.; Renard1, F. All-cause mortality supports the COVID-19 mortality in Belgium and comparison with major fatal events of the last century. *Arch. Public Health* **2020**, *78*, 117. [CrossRef] [PubMed]
22. Sarmadi, M.; Ahmadi-Soleimani, S.M.; Fararouei, M.; Dianatinasab, M. COVID-19, body mass index and cholesterol: An ecological study using global data. *BMC Public Health* **2021**, *21*, 1712. [CrossRef] [PubMed]
23. Ramírez-Soto, M.C.; Alarcón-Arroyo, M.; Chilcon-Vitor, Y.; Chirinos-Pérez, Y.; Quispe-Vargas, G.; Solsol-Jacome, K.; Quintana-Zavaleta, E. Association between Obesity and COVID-19 Mortality in Peru: An Ecological Study. *Trop. Med. Infect. Dis.* **2021**, *6*, 182. [CrossRef]
24. Sanmarchi, F.; Golinelli, D.; Lenzi, J.; Esposito, F.; Capodici, A.; Reno, C.; Gibertoni, D. Exploring the Gap Between Excess Mortality and COVID-19 Deaths in 67 Countries. *JAMA. Netw. Open* **2021**, *4*, e2117359. [CrossRef] [PubMed]
25. Dhama, K.; Khan, S.; Tiwari, R.; Sircar, S.; Bhat, S.; Malik, Y.S.; Singh, K.P.; Chaicumpa, W.; Bonilla-Aldana, D.K.; Rodriguez-Morales, A.J. Coronavirus Disease 2019-COVID-19. *Clin. Microbiol. Rev.* **2020**, *33*, e00028-20. [CrossRef]
26. Ramírez-Soto, M.C.; Arroyo-Hernández, H.; Ortega-Cáceres, G. Sex differences in the incidence, mortality, and fatality of COVID-19 in Peru. *PLoS ONE* **2021**, *16*, e0253193. [CrossRef] [PubMed]
27. Díaz-Vélez, C.; Urrunaga-Pastor, D.; Romero-Cerdán, A.; Peña-Sánchez, E.R.; Fernández Mogollon, J.L.; Cossio Chafloque, J.D.; Marreros Ascoy, G.C.; Benites-Zapata, V.A. Risk factors for mortality in hospitalized patients with COVID-19 from three hospitals in Peru: A retrospective cohort study. *F1000Research* **2021**, *10*, 224. [CrossRef] [PubMed]
28. Davies, N.G.; Kucharski, A.J.; Eggo, R.M.; Gimma, A.; Edmunds, W.J. Centre for the Mathematical Modelling of Infectious Diseases COVID-19 Working Group. Effects of non-pharmaceutical interventions on COVID-19 cases, deaths, and demand for hospital services in the UK: A modelling study. *Lancet Public Health* **2020**, *5*, e375–e385. [CrossRef]
29. Calderon-Anyosa, R.J.C.; Bilal, U.; Kaufman, J.S. Variation in Non-external and External Causes of Death in Peru in Relation to the COVID-19 Lockdown. *Yale J. Biol. Med.* **2021**, *94*, 23–40. [PubMed]

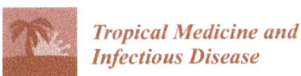

Article

Depression, Anxiety and Associated Factors among Frontline Hospital Healthcare Workers in the Fourth Wave of COVID-19: Empirical Findings from Vietnam

Quoc-Hung Doan [1,2,3], Nguyen-Ngoc Tran [3,4,5,*], Manh-Hung Than [6], Hoang-Thanh Nguyen [7,*], Van-San Bui [3,4,5,*], Dinh-Hung Nguyen [8], Hoang-Long Vo [9], Trong-Thien Do [4], Ngoc-Thach Pham [10], Tuan-Khanh Nguyen [10], Duc-Chinh Cao [11], Vu-Trung Nguyen [11], Thin-Mai T. Tran [12], Ba-Hien Pham [12], Anh-Long Tran [13], Van-Thuong Nguyen [13], Van-Thanh Nguyen [14], Xuan-Thang Tran [14], Duc-Truong Lai [15], Quang-Hieu Vu [15] and Satoko Otsu [15]

1 Department of Surgery, Hanoi Medical University, Hanoi 100000, Vietnam; hung.doanquoc@hmu.edu.vn
2 Department of Cardiovascular and Thoracic Surgery, Viet Duc University Hospital, Hanoi 100000, Vietnam
3 Hanoi Medical University Hospital, Hanoi Medical University, Hanoi 100000, Vietnam
4 Department of Psychiatry, Hanoi Medical University, Hanoi 100000, Vietnam; dotrongthien1794@gmail.com
5 National Institute of Mental Health, Bach Mai Hospital, Hanoi 100000, Vietnam
6 Emergency Department, National Hospital of Tropical Diseases, Hanoi 100000, Vietnam; hungykhoa@gmail.com
7 Office of Postgraduate Management, Hanoi Medical University, Hanoi 100000, Vietnam
8 Hanoi Department of Health, Hanoi 100000, Vietnam; ndhung71@gmail.com
9 Institute for Preventive Medicine and Public Health, Hanoi Medical University, Hanoi 100000, Vietnam; vohoanglonghmu@gmail.com
10 National Hospital of Tropical Diseases, Hanoi 100000, Vietnam; phamngocthachnhtd@gmail.com (N.-T.P.); ntkhanhdp@gmail.com (T.-K.N.)
11 Ha Dong General Hospital, Hanoi 100000, Vietnam; dr.chinh68hd@gmail.com (D.-C.C.); vutrungy2e@gmail.com (V.-T.N.)
12 Dong Da General Hospital, Hanoi 100000, Vietnam; hoasythanoi@gmail.com (T.-M.T.T.); phambahien.bvdd@gmail.com (B.-H.P.)
13 Duc Giang General Hospital, Hanoi 100000, Vietnam; trananhlong64@gmail.com (A.-L.T.); thuongnhixanhpon@gmail.com (V.-T.N.)
14 North Thang Long Hospital, Hanoi 100000, Vietnam; bsnguyenthanhbvbtl@gmail.com (V.-T.N.); xuanthangbvbtl@gmail.com (X.-T.T.)
15 Disease Control and Health Emergency Program, World Health Organization Vietnam Country Office, Hanoi 100000, Vietnam; laiD@who.int (D.-T.L.); vuh@who.int (Q.-H.V.); otsus@who.int (S.O.)
* Correspondence: trannguyenngoc@hmu.edu.vn (N.-N.T.); Nguyenhoangthanh@hmu.edu.vn (H.-T.N.); buivansan@hmu.edu.vn (V.-S.B.)

Abstract: (1) Background: This study aims to assess the magnitude of, and factors associated with, depression and anxiety among Vietnamese frontline hospital healthcare workers in the fourth wave of COVID-19; (2) Methods: A hospital based cross-sectional study was carried out within two weeks, October 2020, at a central COVID-19 treatment hospital. Depression and anxiety were measured with PHQ-9 and GAD-7, respectively. Bivariate and multivariate logistic regression analysis were applied to recognize variables related to depression and anxiety, respectively; (3) Results: Among 208 frontline hospital healthcare workers, overall prevalence of depressive symptoms, anxiety symptoms, and both symptoms of depression and anxiety was 38.94%, 25.48% and 24.04%, respectively, in healthcare workers. In a reduced model after using multivariate stepwise logistic regression, age (OR = 0.9, p = 0.001), marital status (OR = 7.84, p = 0.027), profession (OR = 0.39, p = 0.028), having experienced traumatic stress following a work event (OR = 46.24, p < 0.001), feeling at very high risk for COVID-19 (OR = 0.02, p < 0.04), and affected by workplace conditions (OR = 5.36, p < 0.001) were associated with the symptoms of depression. With regard to symptoms of anxiety, single status (OR: 12.18, p = 0.002), being medical technician (OR: 68.89, p < 0.001), alcohol use (OR: 6.83, p = 0.014), using pain relief medications (OR: 25.50, p = 0.047), having experienced traumatic stress following a family event (OR: 130.32, p = 0.001), having experienced traumatic stress following a work event (OR: 181.55, p = 0.002), reporting at very high risk for COVID-19 (OR: 29.64, p = 0.011), treating moderate (OR: 6.46, p = 0.038) and severe (OR: 18.96, p = 0.004) COVID-19 patients, and being significantly

Citation: Doan, Q.-H.; Tran, N.-N.; Than, M.-H.; Nguyen, H.-T.; Bui, V.-S.; Nguyen, D.-H.; Vo, H.-L.; Do, T.-T.; Pham, N.-T.; Nguyen, T.-K.; et al. Depression, Anxiety and Associated Factors among Frontline Hospital Healthcare Workers in the Fourth Wave of COVID-19: Empirical Findings from Vietnam. *Trop. Med. Infect. Dis.* **2022**, *7*, 3. https://doi.org/10.3390/tropicalmed7010003

Academic Editors: Peter A. Leggat, John Frean and Lucille Blumberg

Received: 8 November 2021
Accepted: 22 December 2021
Published: 23 December 2021

Publisher's Note: MDPI stays neutral with regard to jurisdictional claims in published maps and institutional affiliations.

Copyright: © 2021 by the authors. Licensee MDPI, Basel, Switzerland. This article is an open access article distributed under the terms and conditions of the Creative Commons Attribution (CC BY) license (https://creativecommons.org/licenses/by/4.0/).

affected by the community (OR: 6.33, p = 0.003) were increased risk factors for the symptoms of anxiety. Meanwhile, those living with 4–5 people (OR: 0.15, p = 0.011), specializing in infectious disease (OR: 0.13, p = 0.044)/resuscitation and emergency medicine (OR: 0.04, p = 0.046), and having knowledge preparation before participating in COVID-19 (OR: 0.008, p = 0.014) were less associated with the symptoms of anxiety; (4) Conclusions: There was a relatively high prevalence among Vietnamese hospital healthcare workers exhibiting symptoms of depression and anxiety during the ongoing pandemic. Greater attention to training in psychological skills should be suggested for those belonging to a younger age group, being single/widowed/divorced, treating moderate and severe COVID-19 patients, feeling at very high risk for COVID-19, being significantly affected a lot the community or workplace conditions, or experiencing traumatic stress following a family/work event in the past week.

Keywords: COVID-19; psychological impacts; public health; preparedness

1. Introduction

With the rapid spread of SARS-CoV-2, health care resource responsiveness challenges are posed to health systems globally [1]. Especially when high rates of COVID-19 infection are reported among healthcare workers [2–4], with the increase in SARS-CoV-2-related mortalities in the general population, anxiety and depression tended to be common psychological problems in healthcare workers [5]. Medical staff not only have to work overtime compared to their working time as before the COVID-19 epidemic, but also have a high risk of virus infection during the care and treatment of COVID-19 patients [6,7]. Besides, prolonged stress also contributes to an increased likelihood of depression or other mental disorder, leading to an increased risk of infection and disease severity [8,9]. In a recent systematic review of updated prevalence estimates for depression and anxiety from 65 studies, Yufei Li showed a high prevalence of moderate depression and anxiety among health care workers across 21 countries during the COVID-19 pandemic [10], which can negatively impact on the quality of COVID-19 patient care [11]. In Southeast Asia alone, recent evidence has revealed that there seems to be an increasing trend for anxiety and depression over time among healthcare workers compared to the first wave of COVID-19 [12–16].

Frontline healthcare workers are at high-risk of acquiring SARS-CoV-2 infection during medical procedures due to their close contact with highly infectious patients, particularly those who are in COVID-19 patient-treatment isolation zones [17–19]. There is currently no clarity regarding the estimates of the prevalence of depression and anxiety among medical staff working in isolation treatment facilities for COVID-19 patients, who known as frontline hospital healthcare workers, limiting the possibility of informing action in policy and practice to perform targeted psychological interventions for health care workers during this time of crisis. The impact of the fourth wave of COVID-19 in Vietnam was extremely severe with the emergence of the dangerous Delta variant of the SARS-CoV-2 virus, which reversed Vietnam's epidemic prevention and control achievements in previous COVID-19 waves. The recent wave of the COVID-19 pandemic in Vietnam significantly exceeded the aforementioned previous three pandemic phases in many aspects. There are few studies from different settings of the psychological burden of the Vietnamese healthcare workforce during early national waves of the COVID-19 pandemic, indicating moderately severe depression symptoms, anxiety symptoms, stress and insomnia in healthcare professionals [20–22], suggesting initial negative psychological responses among the healthcare workforce; nevertheless, there was no understanding of the psychological issues surrounding the medical staff involved in direct treatment of COVID-19 patients. Moreover, continuous monitoring of the psychological consequences for this high-risk population should become routine as part of targeted interventions during times of crisis because unforeseen changes and the impact of psychological problems are different in each particular context. In the face of long work shifts (that reach 16 h per day on average), the risk of getting infected by a highly infectious disease and the lack of sufficient biological protection measures, mental suffering among health professionals suddenly became evident. Due to this situation in the fourth national COVID-19 wave, we conducted a cross-sectional study at a central COVID-19 treatment hospital in the Northern region of Vietnam to evaluate the prevalence of the symptoms of anxiety and depression of frontline hospital healthcare workers who are working in COVID-19 treatment isolation zones. We further explore the risk factors and protective factors for symptoms of anxiety and depression.

2. Methods

2.1. Study Design and Participants

We carried out a hospital-based cross-sectional study of the healthcare workforce who worked at the National Hospital of Tropical Diseases (base 2, Hanoi, Vietnam) between 1 October 2021 and 20 October 2021. To foster the engagement of the healthcare workforce, a convenience sampling method was employed for this study, appropriate due to its rapid nature and low-cost given our resource-scarce research setting. Eligibility criteria specified that participants in the study should be: (1) aged from 18 and over; (2) hospital healthcare workers who had obtained a contract to work full-time or part-time at the hospitals, including medical doctors, nurses, midwives, and technicians; (3) involved in the direct treatment of COVID-19 patients and (4) agreed to participate in the survey by providing an informed consent.

2.2. Outcome Measurements

The study questionnaire was developed by a group of psychiatrists from the National Institute of Mental Health (Hanoi, Vietnam) and public health experts from the Hanoi Medical University (Hanoi, Vietnam) to collect potential data on profession-related and socio-demographic characteristics, psychological trauma in the past week, COVID-19 control and prevention-related characteristics and psychological status of these hospital healthcare workers. Participants's psychological problems were assessed with the use of the Vietnamese versions of the 9-item Patient Health Questionnaire (PHQ-9), and the 7-item Generalized Anxiety Disorder-7 (GAD-7) scale. PHQ-9 and GAD-7 are common instruments and easily used to measure and screen the overall presence and level of depression and anxiety.

Then, the developed questionnaire was piloted on a sample of 20 respondents to test its validity. The primary data was collected via sending the invitation directly to the participants, utilizing structured self-completed questionnaires in the Vietnamese version. No material incentives were suggested to the respondents for their engagement in the survey to avoid them from answering more than once. Final analysis did not include the data from the pilot survey.

- PHQ-9

Depression and degree of depression severity were measured using the PHQ-9, a shorter version of the complete PHQ, where individuals were asked how often they were bothered by various problems within the past two weeks. The nine items of PHQ-9 were 'Little interest or pleasure in doing things', 'Feeling down, depressed, or hopeless', 'Trouble falling or staying asleep, or sleeping too much', 'Feeling tired or having little energy', 'Poor appetite or overeating', 'Feeling bad about yourself—or that you are a failure or have let yourself or your family down', 'Trouble concentrating on things, such as reading the newspaper or watching television', 'Moving or speaking so slowly that other people could have noticed, or so fidgety or restless that you have been moving a lot more than usual', 'Thoughts that you would be better off dead, or thoughts of hurting yourself in some way'. Each item was selected, with four-point-scale based answers ranging from 0 (not at all) to 3 (nearly every day). The total score of the PHQ-9 scale after self-reported response ranges from 0 to 27, and more severe depression symptoms are shown by a higher score. Symptom severity was based on the total score and was categorized as follows: absence of depression (0–4), mild depression (5–9), moderate depression (10–14), and severe depression (15–27). In various medical settings, the validated depression scale was reported with good reliability (Cronbach's α = 0.86–0.89).

- GAD-7

Anxiety was measured using the GAD-7. The GAD-7 scale is a self-reported anxiety questionnaire including seven items 'Feeling nervous, anxious or on edge', 'Not being able to stop or control worrying', 'Worrying too much about different things', 'Trouble relaxing', 'Being so restless that it is hard to sit still', 'Becoming easily annoyed or irritable', 'Feeling afraid as if something awful might happen'. All the items were rated on a four-point scale scoring from 0 (not at all) to 3 (nearly every day). The total score ranges from 0 to 21, and symptom severity was interpreted as follows: absence of anxiety (0–4), mild anxiety (5–9), moderate anxiety (10–14), and severe anxiety (15–21). Though initially designed to identify generalized anxiety disorder (GAD), the GAD-7 has also been considered as a good screening tool for other common anxiety disorders. The GAD-7 was proved valid with high reliability (Cronbach's α = 0.89).

2.3. Dependent and Independent Variables

We considered clinically significant depression and clinically significant anxiety as binary dependent variables. Clinically significant depression was defined as that in which an individual had a PHQ-9 score of ≥ 5. Clinically significant anxiety was defined as that in which an individual had a GAD-7 score of ≥ 5.

Description of independent variables is presented in Table 1. The list of independent variables was based on psychiatric judgment and a literature review.

Profession-related and socio-demographic variables included age, gender, marital status, number of people lived with, family household with own children under 18 years, family household with older person above 60 years, education, profession, medical specialty, alcohol, smoking, comorbidities, and using pain relief medications.

Psychological trauma-related characteristics: hospital health workers were asked whether they had experienced traumatic stress in the past week, including due to family, work, academic, social, disease and economic events.

COVID-19 control and prevention-related characteristics included the severity of the COVID-19 patients who treated, duration of participation in COVID-19 control, knowledge preparation before participation, full equipment in current workplace, being affected by workplace conditions, being affected by the community, feelings regarding COVID-19 infection risk, and having a relative/friend/colleague positive for COVID-19.

2.4. Data Analysis

The data obtained was entered in EpiData 3.1, and responses were coded appropriately before being exported to Stata® 15 (StataCorp LLC, College Station, TX, USA) for analysis. Descriptive statistical analysis was first used to characterize the samples of hospital healthcare workers by profession-related and socio-demographic variables, psychological trauma-related characteristics and COVID-19 control and prevention work-related characteristics. Frequencies and proportions for each categorical variable were calculated and described, while quantitative variables were expressed as mean, standard deviation (SD) and interquartile range (IQR). Bivariate logistic regression analyses were used to examine the associations between all variables of interest and the two outcomes. Both univariate and multivariate logistic regression models were used to identify the associations between profession-related and socio-demographic variables, psychological trauma-related characteristics and COVID-19 control and prevention-related characteristics and the two outcome variables of clinically significant depression and anxiety, respectively. Finally, a total of valid variables that were considered as independent variables (work-related and socio-demographic variables, psychological trauma-related characteristics and COVID-19 control and prevention-related characteristics) were put into a full model for multivariate logistic regression analysis. A stepwise backward selection strategy with p values < 0.2 was applied, and then two reduced models with multivariable logistic regression were established for clinically significant depression and anxiety, respectively. A p-value < 0.05 was considered to be statistically significant.

Table 1. Description of independent variables.

Variable Name	Variable Label	Value Label	Types of Variable
	Profession-Related and Socio-Demographic Variables		
A1	Age	Years	Quantitative variable (Discrete)
A2	Gender	1 = male; 2 = female	Qualitative variable (Binary)
A3	Marital status	1 = married; 2 = single; 3 = widowed/divorced	Qualitative variable (Nominal)
A4	Number of people living with	People	Quantitative variable (Discrete)
A5	Family household with own children under 18 years	1 = no; 2 = yes	Qualitative variable (Binary)
A6	Family household with own older person above 60 years	1 = no; 2 = yes	Qualitative variable (Binary)
A7	Education	1 = lower secondary/upper secondary; 2 = college; 3 = university; 4 = postgraduation	Qualitative variable (Nominal)
A8	Profession	1 = medical doctor; 2 = nurse and midwife; 3 = others	Qualitative variable (Nominal)
A9	Medical specialty	1 = internal medicine; 2 = surgery; 3 = infectious disease; 4 = resuscitation and emergency medicine; 5 = anesthesiology; 6 = others	Qualitative variable (Nominal)
A10	Alcohol	1 = no; 2 = yes	Qualitative variable (Binary)
A11	Smoking	1 = no; 2 = yes	Qualitative variable (Binary)
A12	Comorbidities	1 = no; 2 = yes	Qualitative variable (Binary)
A13	Using pain relief medications	1 = no; 2 = yes	Qualitative variable (Binary)
	Psychological trauma-related characteristics		
B1	Having experienced traumatic stress following a family event	1 = no; 2 = yes	Qualitative variable (Binary)
B2	Having experienced traumatic stress following a work event	1 = no; 2 = yes	Qualitative variable (Binary)
B3	Having experienced traumatic stress following an academic event	1 = no; 2 = yes	Qualitative variable (Binary)
B4	Having experienced traumatic stress following a social event	1 = no; 2 = yes	Qualitative variable (Binary)
B5	Having experienced traumatic stress following a disease event	1 = no; 2 = yes	Qualitative variable (Binary)
B6	Having experienced traumatic stress following an economic event	1 = no; 2 = yes	Qualitative variable (Binary)

Table 1. Cont.

Variable Name	Variable Label	Value Label	Types of Variable
COVID-19 control and prevention-related characteristics			
C1	Severity of COVID-19 patients who were treated	1 = normal level; 2 = mild level; 3 = moderate level; 4 = severe level	Qualitative variable (Ordinal)
C2	Duration participating in COVID-19 control	Months	Quantitative variable (Discrete)
C3	Knowledge preparation before participating in COVID-19	1 = no; 2 = yes	Qualitative variable (Binary)
C4	Full equipment in current workplace conditions	1 = no; 2 = yes	Qualitative variable (Binary)
C5	Affected by workplace conditions	1 = no; 2 = yes	Qualitative variable (Binary)
C6	Affected a lot by the community	1 = no; 2 = yes	Qualitative variable (Binary)
C7	Feeling with COVID-19 infection risk	1 = no risk; 2 = low risk; 3 = average risk; 4 = high risk; 5 = very high risk; 6 = infected	Qualitative variable (Ordinal)
C8	Having a relative/friend/colleague with positive COVID-19	1 = no; 2 = yes	Qualitative variable (Binary)

3. Results

In total, the responses of 208 hospital healthcare workers were included in the final analysis between 1 October 2021 and 20 October 2021.

Table 2 summarizes the profession-related and socio-demographic characteristics of the hospital healthcare workers. There were 79 (37.98%) male and 129 (62.02%) female respondents. The majority of the participants were married (75.00%), were a medical doctor or nurse/midwife (85.09%), and had an educational level of university and post-graduate (49.52%). Respectively, 67.31% and 27.40% reported a family household with own children under 18 years, and with older relative above 60 years. The distribution of medical speciality groups included 28.37% infectious disease, 9.13% resuscitation and emergency medicine, 11.54% surgery, 7.69% internal medicine, and 5.29% anesthesiology. Most were living with 1–5 people (75.48%). Self-reported alcohol and smoking were documented in 50.00% and 13.94%, respectively. The prevalence of non-psychiatric comorbidities was 48.08% in participants, and 2.88% had been using pain relief medications.

Regarding COVID-19 control and prevention work-related characteristics, a total of 61 of 208 healthcare workers (29.33%) participated in the treatment of severe COVID-19 patients, and 74 (35.58%) were involved in the treatment of moderate patients. Most had participated in controlling COVID-19 for over 1 month (85.10%). The majority of healthcare workers had obtained relevant knowledge before participating in COVID-19 care (94.23%), and reported with full equipment in the current workplace conditions (93.75%). Of healthcare workers, 38.46% were affected by workplace conditions, and 37.98% were influenced significantly by the community. A feeling of high and very high risk from COVID-19 was common in participants (62.98%) and 52.88% of healthcare workers had a relative/friend/colleague with positive COVID-19 (Table 2). As was shown in Table 2, the most common traumatic stress among medical staff followed an economic event (17.79%) or a family event (10.58%).

Table 2. Profession-related and socio-demographic characteristics of hospital health workers.

Profession-Related and Socio-Demographic Characteristics		N = 208	Percentage (%)
Age—Mean; SD (IQR)		33.20; 6.77 (22–60)	
Gender	Male	79	37.98
	Female	129	62.02
Marital status	Married	156	75.00
	Single	42	20.19
	Widowed/Divorced	10	4.81
Number of people living with (people)	1–3 people	43	20.67
	4–5 people	114	54.81
	>5 people	51	24.52
Family household with own children under 18 years	No	68	32.69
	Yes	140	67.31
Family household with own older person above 60 years	No	151	72.60
	Yes	57	27.40
Education	Lower secondary/upper secondary	10	4.81
	College	95	45.67
	University	64	30.77
	Postgraduation	39	18.75
Profession	Medical doctor	57	27.40
	Nurse and midwife	120	57.69
	Medical technician	31	14.90
Medical specialty	Internal medicine	16	7.69
	Surgery	24	11.54
	Infectious disease	59	28.37
	Resuscitation and emergency medicine	19	9.13
	Anesthesiology	11	5.29
	Others	79	37.98
Alcohol	No	104	50.00
	Yes	104	50.00
Smoking	No	179	86.06
	Yes	29	13.94
Comorbidities	No	108	51.92
	Yes	100	48.08
Using pain relief medications	No	202	97.12
	Yes	6	2.88
COVID-19 control and prevention-related characteristics			
Severity of COVID-19 patient	Normal level	32	15.38
	Mild level	41	19.71
	Moderate level	74	35.58
	Severe level	61	29.33
Duration participating in COVID-19 control (months)	<1 month	31	14.90
	1–3 month(s)	62	29.81
	>3 months	115	55.29
Knowledge preparation before participating in COVID-19	No	12	5.77
	Yes	196	94.23
Full equipment in current workplace conditions	No	13	6.25
	Yes	195	93.75
Affected by workplace conditions	No	128	61.54
	Yes	80	38.46

Table 2. Cont.

Profession-Related and Socio-Demographic Characteristics		N = 208	Percentage (%)
Affected a lot by the community	No	129	62.02
	Yes	79	37.98
Feeling with COVID-19 infection risk	No risk	22	10.58
	Low risk	55	26.44
	Average risk	54	25.96
	High risk	49	23.56
	Very high risk	26	12.50
	Infected	2	0.96
Having a relative/friend/colleague with positive COVID-19	No	98	47.12
	Yes	110	52.88
Psychological trauma-related characteristics in the past one week			
Having experienced traumatic stress following a family event	No	186	89.42
	Yes	22	10.58
Having experienced traumatic stress following a work event	No	177	85.10
	Yes	31	14.90
Having experienced traumatic stress following an academic event	No	198	95.19
	Yes	10	4.81
Having experienced traumatic stress following a social event	No	193	92.79
	Yes	15	7.21
Having experienced traumatic stress following a disease event	No	201	96.63
	Yes	7	3.37
Having experienced traumatic stress following an economic event	No	171	82.21
	Yes	37	17.79

SD: standard deviation; IQR: interquartile range.

Table 3. Prevalence of depression and anxiety among hospital health workers.

		N = 208
Depression by PHQ-9—Frequency (%)	Absence of depression	127 (61.06)
	Mild depression	57 (27.40)
	Moderate depression	16 (7.69)
	Severe depression	8 (3.85)
Total score by PHQ-9—Mean, SD (IQR)		4.31, 4.83 (0–27)
Anxiety by GAD-7	Absence of anxiety	155 (74.52)
	Mild anxiety	44 (21.15)
	Moderate anxiety	7 (3.37)
	Severe anxiety	2 (0.96)
Total score by GAD-7—Mean, SD (IQR)		2.67, 3.76 (0–21)
Both depression and anxiety—Frequency (%)		50 (24.04)

SD: standard deviation; IQR: interquartile range.

3.1. Mental Health Status

Table 3 depicts the percentage of respondents by level of depression and anxiety during the fourth wave of COVID-19 in Vietnam. Of the 208 participants, 38.94% of them reported symptoms of depression, 25.48% reported symptoms of anxiety, and 24.04% reported both symptoms of depression and anxiety. Results found that 3.85% of the hospital healthcare workers reported severe depression, 7.69% reported moderately severe depression and more than one-fourth (27.40%) reported mildly severe depression. Of the participants, 24.52% had mild and severe anxiety symptoms, and only 2 (0.96%) respondents had severe depression symptoms. 24.04% had undergone both depression and anxiety.

Especially, statistically significant difference in total score by PHQ-9 (p = 0.0202) and total score by GAD-7 (p = 0.0011) were observed amongst the severity levels of COVID-19 patients. Both depression score by PHQ-9 and anxiety score by GAD-7 were highest in the severe group (Figure 1).

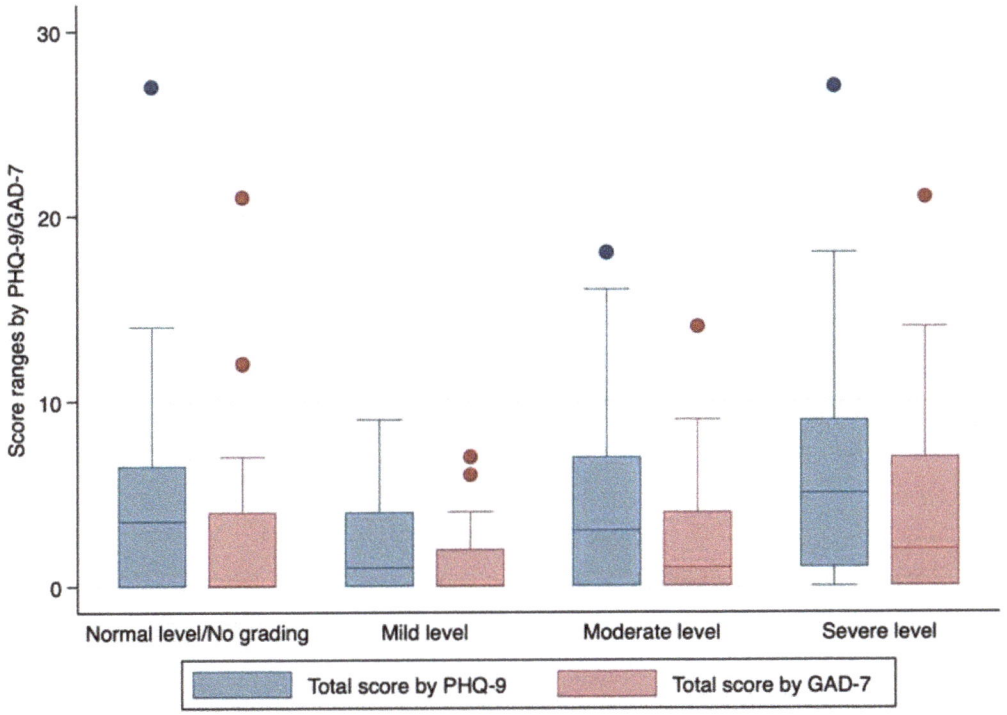

Figure 1. Measurement of total score by PHQ-9 and total score by GAD-7 according to the severity of COVID-19 patient who were treated by hospital health workers.

3.2. Association with Symptoms of Depression

Table 4 indicates analysis result of factors associated with depression using univariable and multivariable logistic regression. Statistically significant variables which were associated with depression in both logistic regressions included medical staff's age (OR univariable: 0.93, 95%CI 0.88–0.97; OR multivariable: 0.88, 95%CI 0.81–0.97), having experienced traumatic stress following a work event in the past week (OR univariable: 11.53, 95%CI 4.20–31.62; OR multivariable: 298.08, 95%CI 14.99–5926.01), having experienced traumatic stress following a disease event in the past week (OR univariable: 10.08, 95%CI 1.19–85.35; OR multivariable: 136.42, 95%CI 1.57–11,792.85), duration of participation in COVID-19 control within 1–3 months (OR univariable: 0.29, 95%CI 0.12–0.72; OR multivariable: 0.21, 95%CI 0.05–0.86), and being affected by workplace conditions (OR univariable: 3.93, 95%CI 2.17–7.12; OR multivariable: 4.50, 95%CI 1.63–12.39).

3.3. Association of the Symptoms of Anxiety

In the reduced model after using multivariate stepwise logistic regression (Table 5), we found age, marial status, profession, having experienced traumatic stress following a work event, feeling at very high risk for COVID-19, and being affected by workplace conditions were associated with clinically significant depression in hospital healthcare workers. Older age was associated with a lower risk of depression (OR = 0.9, 95%CI: 0.85–0.96, p = 0.001). The prevalence of depression symptoms in the widowed/divorced group was higher than in the married group (OR = 7.84, 95%CI: 1.26–48.60, p = 0.027). Compared to respondents who were medical doctors, those being a medical technician was associated with lower risks of depression (OR = 0.39, 95%CI: 0.17–0.90, p = 0.028). Those with traumatic stress following a work event in the past week had higher risk of depression than those without traumatic stress following a work event (OR = 46.24, 95%CI: 9.12–234.28, p < 0.001). Those who felt at very high risk for COVID-19 had lower risk of depression compared to those reporting no infected risk (OR = 0.02, 95%CI: 0.0005–0.83, p < 0.04). Individuals affected by workplace conditions had an elevated risk for depression (OR = 5.36, 95%CI: 2.41–11.92, p < 0.001).

In both univariate and multivariable analysis (Table 6), single status (OR univariable: 2.44, 95%CI 1.18–5.03; OR multivariable: 7.28, 95%CI 1.03–51.24), having experienced traumatic stress following a family event (OR univariable: 10.73, 95%CI 3.93–29.33; OR multivariable: 153.97, 95%CI 5.43–4362.13), having experienced traumatic stress following a work event (OR univariable: 17.49, 95%CI 6.89–44.40; OR multivariable: 265.42, 95%CI 8.39–8389.72), and being significantly affected by the community (OR univariable: 4.90, 95%CI 2.51–9.55; OR multivariable: 6.13, 95%CI 1.40–26.84) were found to be associated with the symptoms of anxiety.

The results from the multivariate stepwise logistic regression are presented in Table 6. Single status (OR: 12.18, 95%CI 2.48–59.85, p = 0.002), being a medical technician (OR: 68.89, 95%CI 7.33–646.98, p < 0.001), alcohol intake (OR: 6.83, 95%CI 1.48–31.58, p = 0.014), using pain relief medication (OR: 25.50, 95%CI 1.04–620.52, p = 0.047), having experienced traumatic stress following a family event (OR: 130.32, 95%CI 7.06–2404.04, p = 0.001), having experienced traumatic stress following a work event (OR: 181.55, 95%CI 8.80–3745.22, p = 0.002), reporting at very high risk for COVID-19 (OR: 29.64, 95%CI 2.20–398.16, p = 0.011), treating moderate (OR: 6.46, p = 0.038) and severe (OR: 18.96, p = 0.004) COVID-19 patients, and being significantly affected by the community (OR: 6.33, 95%CI 1.89–21.19, p = 0.003) were increasing risk factors for the symptoms of anxiety in hospital healthcare workers. Meanwhile, those living with 4–5 people (OR: 0.15, 95%CI 0.03–0.65, p = 0.011), specializing in infectious diseases (OR: 0.13, 95%CI 0.01–0.94, p = 0.044)/resuscitation and emergency medicine (OR: 0.04, 95%CI 0.002–0.94, p = 0.046), and obtaining relevant knowledge before participating in COVID-19 treatment (OR: 0.008, 95%CI 0.0002–0.37, p = 0.014) were less associated with the symptoms of anxiety.

Table 4. Analysis of factors associated with the symptoms of depression: univariable and multivariable logistic regression.

		Clinically Significant Depression		Univariable				Multivariable			
		No (N = 127)	Yes (N = 81)	OR	p-Value	Confidence Interval 95%		OR	p-Value	Confidence Interval 95%	
						Lower	Upper			Lower	Upper
Work-Related and Socio-Demographic Variables											
Age (Mean; SD)		34.35 (6.80)	31.41 (6.39)	0.93	0.003 **	0.88	0.97	0.88	0.010 *	0.81	0.97
Gender	Male (ref)	44	35								
	Female	83	46	0.69	0.215	0.39	1.23	1.83	0.310	0.56	5.90
Marital status	Married (ref)	100	56								
	Single	23	19	1.47	0.270	0.73	2.94	0.53	0.316	0.15	1.83
	Widowed/Divorced	4	6	2.67	0.139	0.72	9.89	13.34	0.032 *	1.25	142.10
Number of people living with (people)	1–3 people (ref)	22	21								
	4–5 people	73	41	0.58	0.143	0.28	1.19	0.87	0.834	0.24	3.06
	>5 people	32	19	0.62	0.259	0.27	1.41	1.25	0.765	0.27	5.68
Family household with own children under 18 years	No (ref)	37	31								
	Yes	90	50	0.66	0.172	0.36	1.19	0.87	0.805	0.29	2.57
Family household with own older person above 60 years	No (ref)	89	62								
	Yes	38	19	0.71	0.309	0.37	1.35	0.56	0.316	0.18	1.72
Education	Lower secondary/upper secondary (ref)	7	3								
	College	54	41	1.77	0.427	0.43	7.27	1.05	0.965	0.07	14.13
	University	42	22	1.22	0.786	0.28	5.19	0.62	0.719	0.04	8.05
	Postgraduation	24	15	1.45	0.622	0.32	6.52	0.60	0.729	0.03	10.14
Profession	Medical doctor (ref)	30	27								
	Nurse and midwife	77	43	0.62	0.144	0.32	1.17	0.244	0.137	0.03	1.56
	Medical technician	20	11	0.61	0.284	0.24	1.50	0.82	0.860	0.10	6.78

Table 4. Cont.

		Clinically Significant Depression		Univariable				Multivariable			
		No (N = 127)	Yes (N = 81)	OR	p-Value	Confidence Interval 95%		OR	p-Value	Confidence Interval 95%	
						Lower	Upper			Lower	Upper
Medical specialty	Internal medicine (ref)	12	4								
	Surgery	9	15	4.99	0.024	1.23	20.30	3.10	0.280	0.39	24.20
	Infectious disease	41	18	1.31	0.668	0.37	4.64	0.60	0.618	0.08	4.43
	Resuscitation and emergency medicine	9	10	3.33	0.103	0.78	14.15	1.35	0.806	0.12	14.88
	Anesthesiology	5	6	3.59	0.126	0.69	18.55	0.86	0.917	0.06	11.88
	Others	51	28	1.64	0.423	0.48	5.58	1.31	0.779	0.19	9.14
Alcohol	No (ref)	67	37								
	Yes	60	44	1.32	0.320	0.75	2.32	1.75	0.305	0.59	5.15
Smoking	No (ref)	110	69								
	Yes	17	12	1.12	0.772	0.50	2.49	1.25	0.742	0.31	4.99
Comorbidities	No (ref)	70	38								
	Yes	57	43	1.38	0.249	0.79	2.43	1.35	0.578	0.46	3.93
Using pain relief medications	No (ref)	126	76								
	Yes	1	5	8.28	0.056	0.95	72.29	9.56	0.176	0.36	251.95
Psychological trauma-related variables in the past one week											
Having experienced traumatic stress following a family event	No (ref)	120	66								
	Yes	7	15	3.89	0.005 **	1.51	10.03	0.35	0.423	0.02	4.53
Having experienced traumatic stress following a work event	No (ref)	122	55								
	Yes	5	26	11.53	0.000 ***	4.20	31.62	298.08	0.000 ***	14.99	5926.01
Having experienced traumatic stress following an academic event	No (ref)	123	75								
	Yes	4	6	2.46	0.174	0.67	9.00	0.03	0.096	0.0006	1.82
Having experienced traumatic stress following a social event	No (ref)	122	71								
	Yes	5	10	3.43	0.030 *	1.12	10.45	0.220	0.278	0.01	3.38

Table 4. Cont.

		Clinically Significant Depression		Univariable				Multivariable			
		No (N = 127)	Yes (N = 81)	OR	p-Value	Confidence Interval 95% Lower	Upper	OR	p-Value	Confidence Interval 95% Lower	Upper
Having experienced traumatic stress following a disease event	No (ref)	126	75								
	Yes	1	6	10.08	0.034 *	1.19	85.35	136.42	0.031 *	1.57	11,792.85
Having experienced traumatic stress following an economic event	No (ref)	115	56								
	Yes	12	25	4.28	0.000 ***	2.00	9.13	1.42	0.677	0.26	7.66
COVID-19 control and prevention-related variables											
Severity of COVID-19 patient	Normal level (ref)	21	11								
	Mild level	31	10	0.61	0.352	0.22	1.70	0.77	0.757	0.14	3.99
	Moderate level	45	29	1.23	0.639	0.51	2.92	1.30	0.713	0.31	5.37
	Severe level	30	31	1.97	0.133	0.81	4.78	2.43	0.259	0.51	11.46
Duration participating in COVID-19 control (months)	<1 month (ref)	13	18								
	1–3 month(s)	44	18	0.29	0.008 **	0.12	0.72	0.21	0.030 *	0.05	0.86
	>3 months	70	45	0.46	0.062	0.20	1.03	0.396	0.200	0.09	1.63
Knowledge preparation before participating in COVID-19	No (ref)	4	8								
	Yes	123	73	0.29	0.054	0.08	1.01	0.12	0.091	0.01	1.38
Full equipment in current workplace conditions	No (ref)	7	6								
	Yes	120	75	0.72	0.583	0.23	2.25	1.38	0.746	0.18	10.16
Affected by workplace conditions	No (ref)	94	34								
	Yes	33	47	3.93	0.000 ***	2.17	7.12	4.50	0.004 **	1.63	12.39
Affected a lot by the community	No (ref)	93	36								
	Yes	34	45	3.41	0.000 ***	1.89	6.15	1.47	0.416	0.57	3.79

Table 4. Cont.

		Clinically Significant Depression		Univariable				Multivariable			
		No (N = 127)	Yes (N = 81)	OR	p-Value	Confidence Interval 95%		OR	p-Value	Confidence Interval 95%	
						Lower	Upper			Lower	Upper
Feeling with COVID-19 infection risk	No risk (ref)	15	7								
	Low risk	35	20	1.22	0.706	0.42	3.50	3.99	0.166	0.56	28.29
	Average risk	31	23	1.58	0.385	0.55	4.52	3.228	0.221	0.49	21.05
	High risk	32	17	1.13	0.813	0.38	3.32	2.77	0.311	0.38	20.00
	Very high risk	13	13	2.14	0.206	0.65	6.98	3.05	0.352	0.28	32.28
	Infected	1	1	2.14	0.608	0.11	39.46	0.06	0.264	0.0005	7.843
Having a relative/friend/colleague with positive COVID-19	No (ref)	64	34								
	Yes	63	47	1.40	0.236	0.80	2.46	0.53	0.216	0.19	1.44
Pseudo R2									0.4054		

OR: odd ratio; *, **, ***: significant at 0.05, 0.01 and 0.001.

Table 5. Analysis of factors associated with the symptoms of depression and anxiety, respectively: multivariate stepwise logistic regression.

		Clinically Significant Depression				Clinically Significant Anxiety			
		OR	p-Value	Confidence Interval 95%		OR	p-Value	Confidence Interval 95%	
				Lower	Upper			Lower	Upper
Profession-Related and Socio-Demographic Variables									
Age		0.90	0.001 **	0.85	0.96				
Marital status	Married (ref)								
	Single					12.18	0.002 **	2.48	59.85
	Widowed/Divorced	7.84	0.027 *	1.26	48.60	15.03	0.089	0.66	341.68
Number of people living with (people)	1–3 people (ref)								
	4–5 people								
	>5 people					0.15	0.011 *	0.03	0.65

Table 5. Cont.

		Clinically Significant Depression				Clinically Significant Anxiety			
				Confidence Interval 95%				Confidence Interval 95%	
		OR	p-Value	Lower	Upper	OR	p-Value	Lower	Upper
Family household with own older person above 60 years	No (ref)								
	Yes	0.51	0.14	0.21	1.24				
Education	Lower secondary/upper secondary (ref)								
	College								
	University					0.20	0.054	0.04	1.02
	Postgraduation								
Profession	Medical doctor (ref)								
	Nurse and midwife	0.39	0.028*	0.17	0.90	68.89	0.000 ***	7.33	646.98
	Medical technician								
Medical specialty	Internal medicine (ref)								
	Surgery	3.22	0.05	1.00	10.35	0.13	0.044 *	0.01	0.94
	Infectious disease	0.51	0.162	0.20	1.30				
	Resuscitation and emergency medicine	37.61	0.066	0.79	1787.41	0.04	0.046 *	0.002	0.94
	Anesthesiology					0.15	0.179	0.01	2.32
	Others					0.07	0.01 *	0.009	0.53
Alcohol	No (ref)								
	Yes					6.83	0.014 *	1.48	31.58
Smoking	No (ref)								
	Yes					0.16	0.101	0.02	1.41
Comorbidities	No (ref)								
	Yes					0.36	0.168	0.08	1.53
Using pain relief medications	No (ref)								
	Yes	9.83	0.111	0.59	163.55	25.50	0.047 *	1.04	620.52
Psychological trauma-related variables in the past one week									
Having experienced traumatic stress following a family event	No (ref)								
	Yes					130.32	0.001 **	7.06	2404.04

Table 5. Cont.

		Clinically Significant Depression				Clinically Significant Anxiety			
		OR	p-Value	Confidence Interval 95%		OR	p-Value	Confidence Interval 95%	
				Lower	Upper			Lower	Upper
Having experienced traumatic stress following a work event	No (ref)								
	Yes	46.24	0.000 ***	9.12	234.28	181.55	0.001 **	8.80	3745.22
Having experienced traumatic stress following an academic event	No (ref)								
	Yes	0.06	0.053	0.004	1.03	0.01	0.113	0.00004	2.90
Having experienced traumatic stress following a social event	No (ref)								
	Yes								
Having experienced traumatic stress following a disease event	No (ref)								
	Yes	26.04	0.058	0.89	754.53				
Having experienced traumatic stress following an economic event	No (ref)								
	Yes					4.79	0.164	0.52	43.53
COVID-19 control and prevention-related variables									
Feeling with COVID-19 infection risk	No risk (ref)								
	Low risk					5.05	0.071	0.87	29.28
	Average risk								
	High risk					3.89	0.128	0.67	22.45
	Very high risk					29.64	0.011 *	2.20	398.16
	Infected	0.02	0.04 *	0.0005	0.83				
Knowledge preparation before participating in COVID-19	No (ref)								
	Yes	0.19	0.053	0.03	1.02	0.008	0.014 *	0.0002	0.37
Severity of COVID-19 patient	Normal level (ref)								
	Mild level								
	Moderate level	2.16	0.09	0.88	5.27	6.46	0.038 *	1.10	37.78
	Severe level					18.96	0.004 **	2.52	142.41
Full equipment in current workplace conditions	No (ref)								
	Yes					26.68	0.061	0.86	825.40
Duration participating in COVID-19 control (months)	<1 month (ref)								
	1–3 month(s)	0.52	0.147	0.22	1.25	0.16	0.089	0.02	1.30
	>3 months					0.22	0.14	0.03	1.62
Affected a lot by the community	No (ref)								
	Yes					6.33	0.003 **	1.89	21.19

Table 5. Cont.

		Clinically Significant Depression				Clinically Significant Anxiety			
		OR	p-Value	Confidence Interval 95%		OR	p-Value	Confidence Interval 95%	
				Lower	Upper			Lower	Upper
Affected by workplace conditions	No (ref) Yes	5.36	0.000 ***	2.41	11.92		0.5654		
Pseudo R2		0.3520							

OR: odd ratio; *, **, ***: significant at 0.05, 0.01 and 0.001.

Table 6. Analysis of factors associated with the symptoms of anxiety: univariable and multivariable logistic regression.

		Clinically Significant Anxiety		Univariate				Multivariate			
		No (N = 155)	Yes (N = 53)	OR	p-Value	Confidence Interval 95%		OR	p-Value	Confidence Interval 95%	
						Lower	Upper			Lower	Upper
Profession-Related and Socio-Demographic Variables											
Age (Mean; SD)		33.74 (6.87)	31.62 (6.27)	0.95	0.051	0.90	1.00	0.95	0.56	0.83	1.10
Gender	Male (ref) Female	55 100	24 29	0.66	0.206	0.35	1.25	0.68	0.668	0.12	3.85
Marital status	Married (ref) Single Widowed/Divorced	122 25 8	34 17 2	2.44 0.89	0.016 * 0.894	1.18 0.18	5.03 4.42	7.28 18.90	0.046 * 0.162	1.03 0.30	51.24 1159.24
Number of people living with (people)	1–3 people (ref) 4–5 people >5 people	28 90 37	15 24 14	0.49 0.70	0.077 0.438	0.23 0.29	1.07 1.70	0.22 2.26	0.119 0.494	0.03 0.21	1.47 23.67
Family household with own children under 18 years	No (ref) Yes	44 111	24 29	0.47	0.025*	0.25	0.91	0.62	0.625	0.09	4.19
Family household with own older person above 60 years	No (ref) Yes	112 43	39 14	0.93	0.852	0.46	1.89	0.50	0.438	0.08	2.84

Table 6. Cont.

		Clinically Significant Anxiety		Univariate				Multivariate			
		No (N = 155)	Yes (N = 53)	OR	p-Value	Confidence Interval 95% Lower	Upper	OR	p-Value	Confidence Interval 95% Lower	Upper
Education	Lower secondary/upper secondary (ref)	8	2								
	College	65	30	1.84	0.455	0.36	9.22	0.81	0.918	0.01	43.69
	University	50	14	1.12	0.893	0.21	5.88	0.11	0.328	0.001	8.51
	Postgraduation	32	7	0.87	0.881	0.15	5.04	0.22	0.5	0.003	16.92
Profession	Medical doctor (ref)	43	14								
	Nurse and midwife	89	31	1.06	0.856	0.51	2.21	0.67	0.792	0.03	12.96
	Medical technician	23	8	1.06	0.897	0.39	2.91	42.46	0.058	0.87	2054.21
Medical specialty	Internal medicine (ref)	13	3								
	Surgery	14	10	3.09	0.138	0.69	13.80	1.34	0.865	0.04	39.44
	Infectious disease	47	12	1.106	0.888	0.27	4.51	0.21	0.391	0.006	7.05
	Resuscitation and emergency medicine	13	6	2.00	0.391	0.40	9.75	0.03	0.164	0.0004	3.77
	Anesthesiology	7	4	2.47	0.312	0.42	14.34	0.20	0.476	0.002	15.44
	Others	61	18	1.27	0.723	0.32	4.98	0.07	0.155	0.002	2.67
Alcohol	No (ref)	81	23								
	Yes	74	30	1.42	0.266	0.76	2.67	6.61	0.058	0.93	46.79
Smoking	No (ref)	132	47								
	Yes	23	6	0.73	0.525	0.28	1.90	0.14	0.102	0.01	1.46

Table 6. Cont.

		Clinically Significant Anxiety		Univariate				Multivariate			
		No (N = 155)	Yes (N = 53)	OR	p-Value	Confidence Interval 95%		OR	p-Value	Confidence Interval 95%	
						Lower	Upper			Lower	Upper
Comorbidities	No (ref)	82	26								
	Yes	73	27	1.16	0.629	0.62	2.17	0.29	0.214	0.04	2.03
Using pain relief medications	No (ref)	154	48								
	Yes	1	5	16.04	0.012 *	1.82	140.68	50.00	0.061	0.83	2993.35
Psychological trauma-related variables in the past one week											
Having experienced traumatic stress following a family event	No (ref)	149	37								
	Yes	6	16	10.73	0.000 ***	3.93	29.33	153.97	0.003	5.43	4362.13
Having experienced traumatic stress following a work event	No (ref)	148	29								
	Yes	7	24	17.49	0.000 ***	6.89	44.40	265.42	0.002 **	8.39	8389.72
Having experienced traumatic stress following an academic event	No (ref)	152	46								
	Yes	3	7	7.71	0.004 **	1.91	31.02	0.01	0.14	0.00002	4.44
Having experienced traumatic stress following a social event	No (ref)	149	44								
	Yes	6	9	5.07	0.003 **	1.71	15.05	0.003	0.014 *	0.00004	0.32
Having experienced traumatic stress following a disease event	No (ref)	154	47								
	Yes	1	6	19.65	0.006 **	2.30	167.43	N/A			
Having experienced traumatic stress following an economic event	No (ref)	141	30								
	Yes	14	23	7.72	0.000 ***	3.56	16.71	5.28	0.174	0.47	58.26
COVID-19 control and prevention-related variables											
Severity of COVID-19 patient	Normal level (ref)	25	7								
	Mild level	38	3	0.28	0.086	0.06	1.19	0.40	0.57	0.01	9.11
	Moderate level	56	18	1.14	0.785	0.42	3.09	3.57	0.37	0.22	58.05
	Severe level	36	25	2.48	0.070	0.92	6.61	15.56	0.052	0.97	248.97

Table 6. Cont.

		Clinically Significant Anxiety		Univariate				Multivariate			
		No (N = 155)	Yes (N = 53)	OR	p-Value	Confidence Interval 95%		OR	p-Value	Confidence Interval 95%	
						Lower	Upper			Lower	Upper
Duration participating in COVID-19 control (months)	<1 month (ref)	21	10								
	1–3 month(s)	52	10	0.40	0.079	0.14	1.11	0.09	0.062	0.008	1.12
	>3 months	82	33	0.84	0.700	0.35	1.98	0.11	0.088	0.009	1.38
Knowledge preparation before participating in COVID-19	No (ref)	5	7								
	Yes	150	46	0.21	0.013 *	0.06	0.72	0.02	0.101	0.0002	2.11
Full equipment in current workplace conditions	No (ref)	10	3								
	Yes	145	50	1.14	0.837	0.30	4.34	20.60	0.106	0.52	803.78
Affected by workplace conditions	No (ref)	106	22								
	Yes	49	31	3.04	0.001 **	1.60	5.79	1.60	0.521	0.37	6.75
Affected a lot by the community	No (ref)	111	18								
	Yes	44	35	4.90	0.000 ***	2.51	9.55	6.13	0.016 *	1.40	26.84
Feeling with COVID-19 infection risk	No risk (ref)	17	5								
	Low risk	45	10	0.75	0.650	0.22	2.53	5.59	0.286	0.23	132.36
	Average risk	41	13	1.07	0.900	0.33	3.49	1.46	0.814	0.06	35.46
	High risk	36	13	1.22	0.734	0.37	4.00	5.41	0.299	0.22	131.15
	Very high risk	14	12	2.91	0.096	0.82	10.27	33.29	0.078	0.67	1647.01
	Infected	2	0	N/A				N/A			
Having a relative/friend/colleague with positive COVID-19	No (ref)	76	22								
	Yes	79	31	1.35	0.344	0.72	2.54	0.87	0.875	0.17	4.51
Pseudo R2									0.5838		

OR: odd ratio; *, **, ***: significant at 0.05, 0.01 and 0.001.

4. Discussion

Despite the research regarding the various impact of COVID-19 on healthcare worker wellness, little is currently known about psychological impacts of the COVID-19 pandemic on the medical staff involved in direct treatment of COVID-19 patients in isolation treatment zones which can be aggregated to assess prevalence accurately and to provide a complete understanding of the effectiveness of psychological interventional strategies. The present study, promptly carried out during the ongoing COVID-19 pandemic in Vietnam, investigated the prevalence of and risk/protective factors associated with depression and anxiety symptoms among hospital healthcare workers who are working in COVID-19 treatment facilities based on a health facility convenient-sample survey. Approximately two-fifth (38.94%) and one-fourth (25.48%) of healthcare workers exhibited symptoms of depression and anxiety, respectively, while nearly one-fourth (24.04%) of them documented both symptoms of depression and anxiety. In fact, the rates of depression and anxiety in this study were not higher than those reported previously. This can be understood due to the long-term adaptive response to the fight against the COVID-19 epidemic of the Vietnamese health system in general, as well as frontline medical staff in particular. Especially, the healthcare workforce who have been working at the National Hospital of Tropical Diseases were involved in the treatment of COVID-19 from the first cases in the first wave of COVID-19 pandemic, and so by the current fourth COVID-19 wave in Vietnam had extensive experience in managing COVID-19 patients in isolation treatment areas. Several psychologically vulnerable populations were also identified, such as individuals with single/widowed/divorced status, those who had experienced traumatic stress following a work event in the past week, those who were treating moderate and severe COVID-19 patients, and those who were significantly affected by the community. These findings contributed to the building of clear strategies to support and appropriately manage hospital healthcare workers involved in the treatment of COVID-19 patients, essential to ensure effective staff management and to engender trust in isolation treatment zones.

The result suggests that feeling at very high risk for COVID-19 is a critical factor in understanding the increased prevalence of depression and anxiety among participants who were working in isolation COVID-19 treatment zones. This finding is in accord with previous evidence reporting that doctors and nurses working in high-risk departments had higher risk of at least one mental health problem [23]. With the rapid increase in the number of hospitalized COVID-19 patients, medical staffs have to face enormous workload and high-risk of infection [24], which easily leads to work trauma for the COVID-19 treatment staff team. One of our findings was consistent with this statement, as higher levels of anxiety/depression were also documented among those who reported with traumatic stress following a work event in the past week.

Our findings indicate that advanced age was a protective factor for depression symptoms, but this age variable is not statistically significant for anxiety related models in all present analyses. In the Egyptian population, age was reported to show a significantly negative correlation with depression during the COVID 19 outbreak [25]. A systematic review of Jiaqi Xiong also showed that those from the younger age group ($\leq$40 years) presented with more depressive symptoms [26]. Compared healthcare workers only, our finding was consistent with previous reports [27]. In addition, with respect to marital status, this was identified as associated with the prevalence of depression and anxiety in hospital healthcare workers. Herein, the prevalence of depression/anxiety symptoms in those being widowed/divorced was higher than in those who were married. There was an association of marital status with depressive symptoms in healthcare workers in Di Tella's study [28], while one other study reported that married people had higher levels of anxiety when compared to those unmarried [29].

Usually, most medical staff working in hospitals had not receivedd mental health training, and consequently daily working hours were positively associated with all psychological disorders in frontline healthcare workers, such as depression and anxiety, [27,30], especially worrisome in hospital health professionals who were involved in treating moderate and severe COVID-19 patients. We found that treating moderate and severe COVID-19 patients was a predictor for clinically significant anxiety. The reason may be that hospital medical staffs facing severely infected patients must regularly monitor, as well as worry about the worsening of, these severe cases, which is clearly different to healthcare workers who managed mild cases with no symptoms.

Several implications can be inferred from these results. It seems that the symptoms of depression and anxiety during the COVID-19 pandemic for frontline healthcare workers are mainly caused as a response to the life-threatening situation and being placed under significant pressure. At the family and social level, a psychological counseling hotline should be widely opened with the support of family members, psychological doctors, social workers, and volunteers.

The strengths of the current study are determined by several issues. To date, no updated report of the prevalence of anxiety and depression during the fourth wave of COVID-19 has been published in Vietnam. Despite caveats, the present study provides insights into the work-related and socio-demographic factors, psychological trauma-related factors and COVID-19 control and prevention work-related factors and the symptoms of depression, and is the first study in Vietnam indicating relative prevalence of clinically significant depression and anxiety in a particular healthcare population.

The study limitations should, however, also be noted before interpretation. First, the PHQ-9 and GAD-7 have been, in fact, less commonly applied to ascertain population or community prevalence of depression symptoms or generalised anxiety symptoms. The present study did not establish the sensitivity, specificity and positive and negative predictive values of cut-off scores using the PHQ-9 and GAD-7 with health workers. Second, self-reported alcohol and tobacco consumption, in addition, comes with an inherent limitation due to no measurement with specific instruments for the two variables. Third, owing to the COVID-19 urgency and the time limit, the frontline medical staff involved in direct treatment of COVID-19 patients in isolation treatment zones might have expressed less depression and anxiety than the actual condition, due to social desirability factors. Fourth, the survey's timing may limit generalization to all hospital healthcare workers who were working during fourth COVID-19 epidemic period and in other parts of Vietnam where the pandemic situation was more severe such as Ho Chi Minh City and western provinces of Vietnam. Finally, our sample size is not large enough to represent COVID-19 treatment facilities with the cross-sectional design used, which may also have limited statistical power to detect differential associations with the severity of depressive and anxiety symptoms. Given the time-sensitivity of the COVID-19 outbreak and limited resources available, the study was not distributed to wider, similar populations in other COVID-19 hotspots.

5. Conclusions

This study provides the first empirical evidence of the relative prevalence among Vietnamese hospital healthcare workers of symptoms of depression and anxiety during the ongoing pandemic. Training in psychological skills for individuals belonging to younger age groups, being single/widowed/divorced, treating moderate and severe COVID-19 patients, feeling very high COVID-19 infection risk, being significantly affected a lot by community/workplace conditions, and experiencing traumatic stress following a family/work event in the past week should be studied further to ensure the continuous involvement of the hospital healthcare workforce in COVID-19 patient management and treatment in isolation health facilities.

Author Contributions: Conceptualization, Q.-H.D. and N.-N.T.; methodology, Q.-H.D., N.-N.T., H.-T.N., V.-S.B. and H.-L.V.; Formal analysis, N.-N.T., H.-T.N., V.-S.B. and H.-L.V.; investigation, Q.-H.D., N.-N.T., M.-H.T., H.-T.N., V.-S.B., H.-L.V., T.-T.D., N.-T.P., T.-K.N., D.-C.C., V.-T.N. (Vu-Trung Nguyen), T.-M.T.T., B.-H.P., A.-L.T., V.-T.N. (Van-Thuong Nguyen), V.-T.N. (Van-Thanh Nguyen), X.-T.T., D.-T.L., Q.-H.V. and S.O.; resources, Q.-H.D. and N.-N.T.; data curation, Q.-H.D., N.-N.T., H.-T.N., V.-S.B., D.-H.N. and H.-L.V.; Supervision, Q.-H.D.; Writing—original draft, N.-N.T., H.-T.N.,

V.-S.B. and H.-L.V.; Writing—review and editing, all authors. All authors have read and agreed to the published version of the manuscript.

Funding: This research was supported by the National Hospital of Tropical Diseases (base 2, Hanoi, Vietnam) and the Hanoi Medical University (Hanoi, Vietnam). The project was funded by a re-search grant from the World Health Organization (WHO reference: 2021/1161468-0; Date: 1 October 2021).

Institutional Review Board Statement: The study was conducted according to the guidelines of the Declaration of Helsinki, and approved by the Institutional Review Board of Hanoi Medical University (ethics code: No. 5092/QĐ-ĐHYHN).

Informed Consent Statement: Informed consent was obtained from all subjects involved in the study.

Data Availability Statement: The data used to support the findings of this study are available from the author Hoang-Long Vo (H.-L.V.) upon request (Email: vohoanglonghmu@gmail.com).

Acknowledgments: We sincerely thank board of directors and medical staffs from National Hospital of Tropical Diseases (base 2, Hanoi, Vietnam) for supporting data collection. We also thank Minh-Tam Duong for his constructive insights and the participating medical students (Vu Kim Duy and Tuyet Trinh) at Hanoi Medical University.

Conflicts of Interest: The authors declare no conflict of interest.

References

1. Tanne, J.H.; Hayasaki, E.; Zastrow, M.; Pulla, P.; Smith, P.; Rada, A.G. COVID-19: How doctors and healthcare systems are tackling coronavirus worldwide. *BMJ* **2020**, *368*. [CrossRef] [PubMed]
2. Chen, W.; Huang, Y. To Protect Health Care Workers Better, To Save More Lives with COVID-19. *Anesthesia Analg.* **2020**, *131*, 97–101. [CrossRef]
3. Giannis, D.; Geropoulos, G.; Matenoglou, E.; Moris, D. Impact of coronavirus disease 2019 on healthcare workers: Beyond the risk of exposure. *Postgrad. Med. J.* **2021**, *97*, 326–328. [CrossRef] [PubMed]
4. Nguyen, L.H.; Drew, D.A.; Graham, M.S.; Joshi, A.D.; Guo, C.-G.; Ma, W.; Mehta, R.S.; Warner, E.T.; Sikavi, D.R.; Lo, C.-H.; et al. Risk of COVID-19 among front-line health-care workers and the general community: A prospective cohort study. *Lancet Public Health* **2020**, *5*, e475–e483. [CrossRef]
5. Taghizadeh, F.; Cherati, J.Y. Procrastination and self-efficacy among intravenous drug users on a methadone maintenance program in Sari City, Iran, 2013. *Iran. J. Psychiatry Behav. Sci.* **2015**, *9*, e3738. [CrossRef]
6. The Lancet. COVID-19: Protecting health-care workers. *Lancet* **2020**, *395*, 922. [CrossRef]
7. Almaghrabi, R.H.; Alfaradi, H.; Al Hebshi, W.A.; Albaadani, M.M. Healthcare workers experience in dealing with Coronavirus (COVID-19) pandemic. *Saudi Med. J.* **2020**, *41*, 657–660. [CrossRef] [PubMed]
8. Khan, S.; Khan, R.A. Chronic stress leads to anxiety and depression. *Ann. Psychiatry Ment. Health* **2017**, *5*, 1091.
9. Yang, L.; Zhao, Y.; Wang, Y.; Liu, L.; Zhang, X.; Li, B.; Cui, R. The Effects of Psychological Stress on Depression. *Curr. Neuropharmacol.* **2015**, *13*, 494–504. [CrossRef] [PubMed]
10. Li, Y.; Scherer, N.; Felix, L.; Kuper, H. Prevalence of depression, anxiety and post-traumatic stress disorder in health care workers during the COVID-19 pandemic: A systematic review and meta-analysis. *PLoS ONE* **2021**, *16*, e0246454. [CrossRef]
11. Tawfik, D.S.; Scheid, A.; Profit, J.; Shanafelt, T.; Trockel, M.; Adair, K.C.; Sexton, J.B.; Loannidis, J.P.A. Evidence Relating Health Care Provider Burnout and Quality of Care: A Systematic Review and Meta-analysis. *Ann. Intern Med.* **2019**, *171*, 555–567. [CrossRef]
12. Chow, S.; Francis, B.; Ng, Y.; Naim, N.; Beh, H.; Ariffin, M.; Yusuf, M.; Lee, J.; Sulaiman, A. Religious Coping, Depression and Anxiety among Healthcare Workers during the COVID-19 Pandemic: A Malaysian Perspective. *Health* **2021**, *9*, 79. [CrossRef] [PubMed]
13. Norhayati, M.N.; Yusof, R.C.; Azman, M.Y. Depressive symptoms among frontline and non-frontline healthcare providers in response to the COVID-19 pandemic in Kelantan, Malaysia: A cross sectional study. *PLoS ONE* **2021**, *16*, e0256932. [CrossRef]
14. Sunjaya, D.K.; Herawati, D.M.D.; Siregar, A.Y.M. Depressive, anxiety, and burnout symptoms on health care personnel at a month after COVID-19 outbreak in Indonesia. *BMC Public Health* **2021**, *21*, 227. [CrossRef]
15. Lugito, N.P.H.; Kurniawan, A.; Lorens, J.O.; Sieto, N.L. Mental Health Problems in Indonesian Internship Doctors during the COVID-19 Pandemic. *J. Affect. Disord. Rep.* **2021**, *6*, 100283. [CrossRef] [PubMed]
16. Lum, A.; Goh, Y.-L.; Wong, K.S.; Seah, J.; Teo, G.; Ng, J.Q.; Abdin, E.; Hendricks, M.M.; Tham, J.; Nan, W.; et al. Impact of COVID-19 on the mental health of Singaporean GPs: A cross-sectional study. *BJGP Open* **2021**, *5*. [CrossRef] [PubMed]
17. Rivett, L.; Sridhar, S.; Sparkes, D.; Routledge, M.; Jones, N.K.; Forrest, S.; Young, J.; Pereira-Dias, J.; Hamilton, W.L.; Ferris, M.; et al. Screening of healthcare workers for SARS-CoV-2 highlights the role of asymptomatic carriage in COVID-19 transmission. *Elife* **2020**, *9*, e58728. [CrossRef] [PubMed]

18. Gómez-Ochoa, S.A.; Franco, O.H.; Rojas, L.Z.; Raguindin, P.F.; Roa-Díaz, Z.M.; Wyssmann, B.M.; Guevara, S.L.R.; Echeverría, L.E.; Glisic, M.; Muka, T. COVID-19 in Healthcare Workers: A Living Systematic Review and Meta-analysis of Prevalence, Risk Factors, Clinical Characteristics, and Outcomes. *Am. J. Epidemiol.* **2020**, *190*, 161–175. [CrossRef]
19. Wang, X.; Zhang, X.; He, J. Challenges to the system of reserve medical supplies for public health emergencies: Reflections on the outbreak of the severe acute respiratory syndrome coronavirus 2 (SARS-CoV-2) epidemic in China. *Biosci. Trends* **2020**, *14*, 3–8. [CrossRef] [PubMed]
20. Tuan, N.Q.; Phuong, N.D.; Co, D.X.; Son, D.N.; Chinh, L.Q.; Dung, N.H.; Thach, P.T.; Thai, N.Q.; Thu, T.A.; Tuan, N.A.; et al. Prevalence and Factors Associated with Psychological Problems of Healthcare Workforce in Vietnam: Findings from COVID-19 Hotspots in the National Second Wave. *Healthcare* **2021**, *9*, 718. [CrossRef]
21. Than, H.M.; Nong, V.M.; Nguyen, C.T.; Dong, K.P.; Ngo, H.T.; Doan, T.T.; Do, N.T.; Nguyen, T.H.T.; Van Do, T.; Dao, C.X.; et al. Mental Health and Health-Related Quality-of-Life Outcomes Among Frontline Health Workers During the Peak of COVID-19 Outbreak in Vietnam: A Cross-Sectional Study. *Risk Manag. Healthc. Policy* **2020**, *13*, 2927–2936. [CrossRef]
22. Nguyen, T.T.; Le, X.T.T.; Nguyen, N.T.T.; Nguyen, Q.N.; Le, H.T.; Pham, Q.T.; Ta, N.K.T.; Nguyen, Q.T.; Nguyen, A.N.; Hoang, M.T.; et al. Psychosocial Impacts of COVID-19 on Healthcare Workers During the Nationwide Partial Lockdown in Vietnam in April 2020. *Front. Psychiatry* **2021**, *12*. [CrossRef] [PubMed]
23. Liu, Z.; Han, B.; Jiang, R.; Huang, Y.; Ma, C.; Wen, J.; Zhang, T.; Wang, Y.; Chen, H.; Ma, Y. Mental health status of doctors and nurses during COVID-19 epidemic in China. *SSRN* **2020**. [CrossRef]
24. Kang, L.; Li, Y.; Hu, S.; Chen, M.; Yang, C.; Yang, B.X.; Wang, Y.; Hu, J.; Lai, J.; Ma, X.; et al. The mental health of medical workers in Wuhan, China dealing with the 2019 novel coronavirus. *Lancet Psychiatry* **2020**, *7*, e14. [CrossRef]
25. Shehata, G.A.; Gabra, R.; Eltellawy, S.; Elsayed, M.; Gaber, D.E.; Elshabrawy, H.A. Assessment of Anxiety, Depression, Attitude, and Coping Strategies of the Egyptian Population during the COVID-19 Pandemic. *J. Clin. Med.* **2021**, *10*, 3989. [CrossRef]
26. Xiong, J.; Lipsitz, O.; Nasri, F.; Lui, L.M.W.; Gill, H.; Phan, L.; Chen-Li, D.; Iacobucci, M.; Ho, R.; Majeed, A.; et al. Impact of COVID-19 pandemic on mental health in the general population: A systematic review. *J. Affect. Disord.* **2020**, *277*, 55–64. [CrossRef]
27. Zhou, Y.; Wang, W.; Sun, Y.; Qian, W.; Liu, Z.; Wang, R.; Qi, L.; Yang, J.; Song, X.; Zhou, X.; et al. The prevalence and risk factors of psychological disturbances of frontline medical staff in china under the COVID-19 epidemic: Workload should be concerned. *J. Affect. Disord.* **2020**, *277*, 510–514. [CrossRef]
28. Di Tella, M.; Romeo, A.; Benfante, A.; Castelli, L. Mental health of healthcare workers during the COVID-19 pandemic in Italy. *J. Eval. Clin. Pract.* **2020**, *26*, 1583–1587. [CrossRef]
29. Gao, J.; Zheng, P.; Jia, Y.; Chen, H.; Mao, Y.; Chen, S.; Wang, Y.; Fu, H.; Dai, J. Mental health problems and social media exposure during COVID-19 outbreak. *PLoS ONE* **2020**, *15*, e0231924. [CrossRef]
30. Lima, C.K.T.; Carvalho, P.M.D.M.; Lima, I.D.A.A.S.; Nunes, J.V.A.D.O.; Saraiva, J.S.; de Souza, R.I.; da Silva, C.G.L.; Neto, M.L.R. The emotional impact of Coronavirus 2019-nCoV (new Coronavirus disease). *Psychiatry Res.* **2020**, *287*, 112915. [CrossRef]

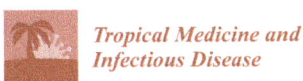

Tropical Medicine and Infectious Disease

Article

Association between Obesity and COVID-19 Mortality in Peru: An Ecological Study

Max Carlos Ramírez-Soto *, Miluska Alarcón-Arroyo, Yajaira Chilcon-Vitor, Yelibeth Chirinos-Pérez, Gabriela Quispe-Vargas, Kelly Solsol-Jacome and Elizabeth Quintana-Zavaleta

Facultad de Ciencias de la Salud, Universidad Tecnologica del Peru, 15046 Lima, Peru; U18205082@utp.edu.pe (M.A.-A.); U19102232@utp.edu.pe (Y.C.-V.); U18301301@utp.edu.pe (Y.C.-P.); U18305711@utp.edu.pe (G.Q.-V.); U18302765@utp.edu.pe (K.S.-J.); U19205940@utp.edu.pe (E.Q.-Z.)
* Correspondence: maxcrs22@gmail.com or max.ramirez@upch.pe

Citation: Ramírez-Soto, M.C.; Alarcón-Arroyo, M.; Chilcon-Vitor, Y.; Chirinos-Pérez, Y.; Quispe-Vargas, G.; Solsol-Jacome, K.; Quintana-Zavaleta, E. Association between Obesity and COVID-19 Mortality in Peru: An Ecological Study. *Trop. Med. Infect. Dis.* **2021**, *6*, 182. https://doi.org/10.3390/tropicalmed6040182

Academic Editors: Peter A. Leggat, John Frean and Lucille Blumberg

Received: 12 August 2021
Accepted: 21 September 2021
Published: 7 October 2021

Publisher's Note: MDPI stays neutral with regard to jurisdictional claims in published maps and institutional affiliations.

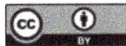

Copyright: © 2021 by the authors. Licensee MDPI, Basel, Switzerland. This article is an open access article distributed under the terms and conditions of the Creative Commons Attribution (CC BY) license (https://creativecommons.org/licenses/by/4.0/).

Abstract: There is a gap in the epidemiological data on obesity and COVID-19 mortality in low and middle-income countries worst affected by the COVID-19 pandemic, including Peru. In this ecological study, we explored the association between body mass index (BMI), the prevalence of overweight and obesity, and the COVID-19 mortality rates in 25 Peruvian regions, adjusted for confounding factors (mean age in the region, mean income, gender balance and number of Intensive Care Unit (ICU) beds) using multiple linear regression. We retrieved secondary region-level data on the BMI average and prevalence rates of overweight and obesity in individuals aged $\geq$ 15 years old, from the Peruvian National Demographics and Health Survey (ENDES 2020). COVID-19 death statistics were obtained from the National System of Deaths (SINADEF) from the Peruvian Ministry of Health and were accurate as of 3 June 2021. COVID-19 mortality rates (per 100,000 habitants) were calculated among those aged $\geq$ 15 years old. During the study period, a total of 190,046 COVID-19 deaths were registered in individuals aged $\geq$ 15 years in 25 Peruvian regions. There was association between the BMI (r = 0.74; p = 0.00001) and obesity (r = 0.76; p = 0.00001), and the COVID-19 mortality rate. Adjusted for confounding factors, only the prevalence rate of obesity was associated with COVID-19 mortality rate (β = 0.585; p = 0.033). These findings suggest that as obesity prevalence increases, the COVID-19 mortality rates increase in the Peruvian population $\geq$ 15 years. These findings can help to elucidate the high COVID-19 mortality rates in Peru.

Keywords: COVID-19; pandemic; overweight; obesity; Peru

1. Introduction

Overweight and obesity are global public health problems [1]. Their prevalence has increased rapidly during recent decades [2,3], and studies have shown an association between obesity and infectious diseases [4]. During the COVID-19 pandemic, studies in high-income countries have shown that obesity increases the risk for hospitalization and death among patients with COVID-19 [5,6]. Most studies included patients with COVID-19 symptoms admitted to hospital, where obesity itself and the severity of the disease increase the risk of death [7,8]. Avoiding this bias, one recent study showed that excess weight linearly increased the risk of severe COVID-19, leading to admission to hospital and death (body mass index > 28 kg/m^2) [9]. In other observational studies, obesity prevalence was significantly correlated with both infection and/or COVID-19 mortality [10–13]. Despite these findings, to date, there is a gap of epidemiological data on obesity and COVID-19 mortality in low- and middle-income countries.

In Latin American, Peru has been one of the worst-affected countries by the COVID-19 pandemic [14,15]. Despite the rapid implementation of control measures, by the end of June 2021, more than two million cases and over 190,000 deaths were confirmed, with a case fatality rate of 9.31% [16]. In addition, a study in the first months of the COVID-19 pandemic found a correlation between the prevalence of obesity and COVID-19 mortality, although its findings are limited [13]. Despite this, it has not been documented how COVID-19 mortality rates vary according to body mass index (BMI) and the prevalence of overweight and obesity. Here, we explored the association between body mass index (BMI), the prevalence of overweight and obesity, and COVID-19 mortality in 25 Peruvian regions, adjusted by for possible confounding factors.

2. Materials and Methods

2.1. Study Design and Setting

We performed an ecological study following the Strengthening the Reporting of Observational Studies in Epidemiology (STROBE) reporting guidelines [17]. For this study, we retrieved secondary region-level data on the BMI average and prevalence rates of overweight and obesity in individuals aged ≥ 15 years old from the Peruvian National Demographics and Health Survey (ENDES 2020) [18]. ENDES 2020 includes a sample of 32,197 men and women aged 15 years or more, from 25 Peruvian regions (Figure 1), from January to December 2020. COVID-19 deaths were obtained from the National System of Deaths (SINADEF) from the Peruvian Ministry of Health (MINSA), accurate as of 3 June 2021 [19]. The SINADEF database records all deaths that occur in Peru and generates the death certificates and statistical reports. Death records with COVID-19 as the underlying cause of death were included in the study. Data on the mean age in the region, mean income and gender balance were retrieved obtained from the National Institute of Statistics and Informatics (INEI). The number of Intensive Care Unit (ICU) beds was obtained of App. F500.2 from at the Superintendencia Nacional de Salud, Perú (SUSALUD).

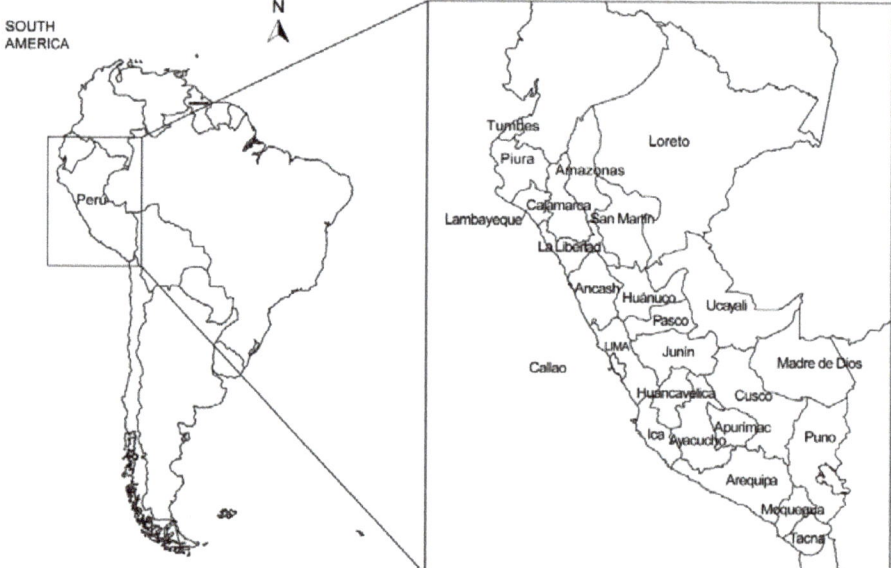

Figure 1. Location of Peru within South American.

2.2. Statistical Analysis

COVID-19 mortality rates (per 100,000 habitants) among those aged ≥ 15 years old were calculated by dividing the number of COVID-19 deaths per department by the estimated population of each department. Population counts for calculating mortality rates were obtained from the INEI, Peru [20]. Spearman's test and linear regression models were used to estimate correlations between the BMI, the prevalence of overweight and obesity, and COVID-19 mortality rates. Multiple regression analysis was also used for possible confounding factors. p-values < 0.05 were considered significant. Confounding factors included the mean age in the region (years), mean monthly income (PEN), gender balance and number of ICU beds. Statistical analyses were conducted using StataSE 16.0 Software.

This study was based on public use data that do not include personal information; therefore, it was exempt from institutional review board approval.

3. Results

During the study period, a total of 190,046 COVID-19 deaths were registered in individuals aged ≥ 15 years in 25 Peruvian regions. Among the individuals aged ≥ 15 years old, the highest prevalence rates of overweight and obesity were registered in Tacna, Moquegua, and Ica regions. The five regions with the highest COVID-19 mortality rates were Ica (1083.6 per 100,000 habitants), Callao (1071.3 per 100,000 habitants), Lima (979.9 per 100,000 habitants), Moquegua (883.3 per 100,000 habitants), and Lambayeque (811.4 per 100,000 habitants) (Table 1).

Table 1. BMI average, prevalence of overweight and obesity, and COVID-19 mortality rate in ≥15-year-olds in 25 Peruvian regions, March 2020 to June 2021.

Region	BMI (kg/m^2) [18]	Prevalence of Overweight (%) [18]	Prevalence of Obesity (%) [18]	COVID-19 Deaths [19]	Population [20]	COVID-19 Mortality Rate (per 100,000 Habitants)	Mean Age (Years)	Mean Monthly Income (PEN)	Gender Balance (Men/Women) [20]	No. of ICU Beds
Amazonas	26.2	36.1	15.8	1135.0	289,802.0	391.6	30.95	1014.0	1.07	19
Ancash	26.9	35.6	21.8	6373.0	876,703.0	726.9	32.36	1230.9	1.01	62
Apurimac	25.8	33.2	14.7	1401.0	300,395.0	466.4	29.99	1123.8	1.05	38
Arequipa	28.0	36.8	28.8	8519.0	1,187,931.0	717.1	32.45	1703.1	0.95	92
Ayacucho	25.9	33.9	15.5	1949.0	464,136.0	419.9	30.04	970.6	1.04	20
Cajamarca	25.9	38.6	13.9	3839.0	1,016,792.0	377.6	30.71	954.4	0.98	61
Callao	28.4	35.3	31.8	9670.0	902,609.0	1071.3	32.36	1579.6	0.94	113
Cusco	26.2	36.6	16.8	4390.0	988,897.0	443.9	30.34	1234.1	1.02	50
Huancavelica	24.9	30.8	9.6	1079.0	236,955.0	455.4	30.28	742.1	1.01	21
Huanuco	26.2	36.9	15.9	2558.0	524,371.0	487.8	30.01	1007.1	1.01	44
Ica	28.4	36.5	33.5	7863.0	725,610.0	1083.6	30.93	1507.5	0.99	84
Junin	26.4	39.3	17.0	6570.0	982,199.0	668.9	31.18	1206.3	0.98	77
La Libertad	27.9	38.5	27.8	9778.0	1,531,668.0	638.4	31.55	1307.5	0.97	96
Lambayeque	27.5	39.5	25.0	8042.0	991,121.0	811.4	32.24	1203.6	0.93	86
Lima	28.1	37.0	28.9	85,748.0	8,750,417.0	979.9	33.05	1885.9	0.91	845
Loreto	26.4	29.6	22.1	3977.0	680,927.0	584.1	28.50	1231.5	1.08	52
Madre de Dios	28.5	43.9	32.4	727.0	135,428.0	536.8	27.48	1665.0	1.37	25
Moquegua	28.7	37.7	35.8	1374.0	155,545.0	883.3	32.85	1801.5	1.17	28
Pasco	26.3	37.7	17.2	961.0	195,114.0	492.5	30.12	1172.0	1.07	31
Piura	27.2	34.2	25.0	11,414.0	1,535,433.0	743.4	30.42	1146.0	1.01	109
Puno	26.8	37.9	20.4	3603.0	904,267.0	398.4	29.72	876.1	0.96	42
San Martin	26.4	36.5	19.9	2833.0	639,533.0	443.0	29.89	1159.2	1.14	49
Tacna	28.7	38.7	34.4	1821.0	303,701.0	599.6	31.91	1392.3	1.04	32
Tumbes	27.8	40.0	27.6	1489.0	191,850.0	776.1	29.91	1264.3	1.20	17
Ucayali	26.9	37.7	22.0	2933.0	416,932.0	703.5	28.00	1174.4	1.13	37

BMI: body mass index (kg/m^2). ICU: Intensive Care Unit.

There was an association between BMI ($r = 0.74$; $p = 0.00001$) and obesity ($r = 0.76$; $p = 0.00001$) and the COVID-19 mortality rate (per 100,000 habitants) (Figure 2A–C). Adjusted by possible confounding factors (mean age in the region, mean monthly income, gender balance and number of ICU beds), only the prevalence rate of obesity was associated with COVID-19 mortality rate ($\beta = 0.585$; $p = 0.033$) (Table 2). The model was statistically significant ($F\ (5,19) = 8.89$, $p < 0.0002$, Adj. $R^2 = 0.60$).

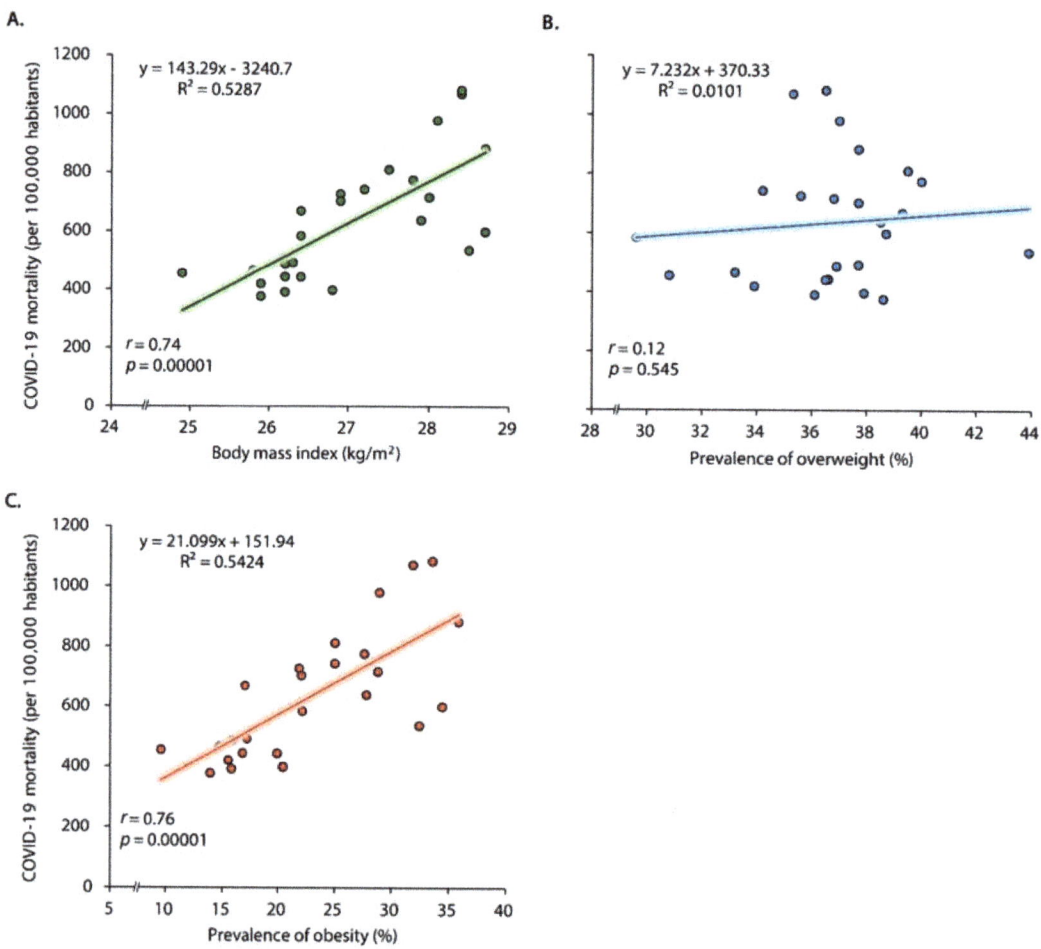

Figure 2. Correlation between body mass index (BMI) average (**A**), prevalence of overweight (**B**) and obesity (**C**) and mortality rates due to COVID-19 in Peru, March 2020 to June 2021.

Table 2. Multiple regression analysis of prevalence of obesity and COVID-19 mortality adjusted.

Variable	Coef.	SE	Beta	t	p-Value
BMI and COVID-19 mortality					
BMI (kg/m^2)	94.49	51.60	0.479	1.83	0.083
Mean age in the region (years)	−5.58	32.62	−0.038	−0.17	0.866
Mean monthly income (PEN)	0.262	0.23	0.359	1.10	0.285
Gender balance (men/women)	−707.0	482.3	−0.336	−1.47	0.159
No. of ICU beds	0.028	0.251	0.021	0.11	0.911
Obesity and COVID-19 mortality					
Prevalence of obesity (%)	16.76	7.28	0.585	2.3	0.033
Mean age in the region (years)	−2.52	31.2	−0.017	−0.08	0.937
Mean monthly income (PEN)	0.17	0.23	0.240	0.75	0.464
Gender balance (men/women)	−693.81	462.6	−0.330	−1.5	0.15
No. of ICU beds	0.08	0.24	0.068	0.36	0.72

BMI: body mass index (kg/m^2). ICU: Intensive Care Unit.

4. Discussion

During the COVID-19 pandemic, older adults and people with co-morbidities, including patients with obesity, have experienced the highest risk of COVID-19 death [6–8,21]. A previous cohort study reported that, compared with patients with a BMI of 18.5–24 kg/m^2, patients with BMI $\geq$ 40 kg/m^2 had a higher risk of COVID-19 death [7]. Recently, another study reported that the risk of COVID-19 death was more strongly associated with people with a BMI of more than 28 kg/m^2 [9]. Our findings, despite being correlational, support this observation, because in the Peruvian regions where the BMI was higher (i.e., Tacna, Moquegua and Ica), we found higher COVID-19 mortality rates. However, adjusted by possible confounding factors, there was not association between the BMI and COVID-19 mortality rates. To date, there is little evidence on the mechanisms attributable to BMI effects on COVID-19 mortality. A possible explanation is that excess weight can cause the metabolic impairment of organ functioning [22]. Other possible explanations for BMI increasing COVID-19 mortality could be associated with the severity of COVID-19, male sex, increasing age, and other factors that were not investigated in this study.

In our study, there was correlation between the prevalence of obesity and COVID-19 mortality, i.e., as the obesity prevalence increased, the COVID-19 mortality rates increased in the population aged $\geq$ 15 years. These findings are consistent with correlational studies which found that, as the obesity prevalence increased, the COVID-19 deaths increased [10–13]. Cohort studies and meta-analyses on the effect of excess weight on COVID-19 clinical outcomes also reported that obesity was independently associated with the severity of COVID-19 and the risk of death increased [7,8]. The increase in COVID-19 mortality in patients with obesity could be explained by associations with hypertension, diabetes, or respiratory distress syndrome [7,9]; however, to date, the mechanisms explaining the association between obesity and COVID-19 mortality remain limited. In Peru, obesity and high COVID-19 mortality also could be explained by other external factors, such as infrastructure, overload of the health system, medicines, and available intensive care unit beds [14,15].

As with any observational study, the limitations of our study include its ecological design, because we used several different information sources (ENDES 2020, SINADEF, INEI, and SUSALUD); therefore, our findings could have resulted in a possible bias. In our findings, there could also have been an overestimation due to unmeasured covariates, such as the population density, and delayed COVID-19 death registration. On the other hand, the ecological design (group level variables) made it difficult to determine causality between the obesity and the COVID-19 mortality, i.e., we cannot make causal inference with the average characteristics of the group about individual risk. Therefore, our findings should be interpreted at the population level, not the individual-level. Finally, the ecological design is not able to account for changes that impact transmission dynamics, such as the appearance of new variants of concern or the introduction of vaccination. Despite these limitations, the main strengths of our study were the large number of deaths included (n = 190,046, as of June 2021) for estimating the COVID-19 mortality and the multiple regression analyses for possible confounding factors (mean age in the region, mean monthly income, gender balance and number of ICU beds), compared with a previous study that included a total of 51,789 deaths (as of July 2020) [13].

5. Conclusions

Our findings suggest that, as the obesity prevalence increases, the COVID-19 mortality rates increase in Peruvian populations aged $\geq$ 15 years. Interventions for obesity improve weight loss; however, we cannot assure that these interventions might reduce COVID-19 mortality. In the long term, there is a need to strive towards achieving healthy weights in the Peruvian population and to decrease the risk of death from other infections in future.

Author Contributions: Conceptualization, Y.C.-V.; methodology, G.Q.-V. and M.C.R.-S.; software, Y.C.-P. and M.C.R.-S.; validation, M.A.-A. and M.C.R.-S.; formal analysis, K.S.-J., E.Q.-Z. and M.C.R.-S.; investigation, all authors; data curation, M.C.R.-S.; writing—original draft preparation, M.C.R.-S.; writing—review and editing, M.C.R.-S.; visualization, M.C.R.-S.; supervision, M.C.R.-S. All authors have read and agreed to the published version of the manuscript.

Funding: The publication of this study was funded at the Universidad Tecnologica del Peru, Lima, Peru.

Institutional Review Board Statement: Not applicable.

Informed Consent Statement: Not applicable.

Data Availability Statement: The data presented in this study are publicly available at: Demographic and Health Survey (ENDES) 2020. Noncommunicable and Communicable Diseases. 2020. Available online: https://proyectos.inei.gob.pe/endes/2020/SALUD/ENFERMEDADES_ENDES_2020.pdf (accessed on 14 September 2021); COVID-19 deaths. National System of Deaths (SINADEF). Available online: https://www.datosabiertos.gob.pe/dataset/fallecidos-por-covid-19-ministerio-de-salud-minsa (accessed on 3 June 2021); INEI, Peruvian population: http://censos2017.inei.gob.pe/redatam/ (accessed on 3 June 2021); Daily Report on Form F500.2, app. for centralized management of the availability of Hospitalization and ICU beds at the national level and of all subsystems (Application F500.2): http://portal.susalud.gob.pe/seguimiento-del-registro-de-camas-f500-2/ (accessed on 17 September 2021); Mean monthly income (PEN): https://www.inei.gob.pe/estadisticas/indice-tematico/income/ (accessed on 17 September 2021).

Acknowledgments: The publication of this study was funded at the Universidad Tecnologica del Peru, Lima, Peru.

Conflicts of Interest: The authors declare no conflict of interest.

References

1. Blüher, M. Obesity: Global epidemiology and pathogenesis. *Nat. Rev. Endocrinol.* **2019**, *15*, 288–298. [CrossRef] [PubMed]
2. GBD 2015 Obesity Collaborators. Health Effects of Overweight and Obesity in 195 Countries over 25 Years. *N. Engl. J. Med.* **2017**, *377*, 13–27.
3. Dai, H.; Alsalhe, T.A.; Chalghaf, N.; Riccò, M.; Bragazzi, N.L.; Wu, J. The global burden of disease attributable to high body mass index in 195 countries and territories, 1990–2017: An analysis of the Global Burden of Disease Study. *PLoS. Med.* **2020**, *17*, e1003198. [CrossRef] [PubMed]
4. Huttunen, R.; Syrjänen, J. Obesity and the risk and outcome of infection. *Int. J. Obes.* **2013**, *37*, 333–340. [CrossRef] [PubMed]
5. Huang, Y.; Lu, Y.; Huang, Y.M.; Wang, M.; Ling, W.; Sui, Y.; Zhao, H.L. Obesity in patients with COVID-19: A systematic review and meta-analysis. *Metabolism* **2020**, *113*, 154378. [CrossRef] [PubMed]

6. Hoong, C.W.S.; Hussain, I.; Aravamudan, V.M.; Phyu, E.E.; Lin, J.H.X.; Koh, H. Obesity is Associated with Poor Covid-19 Outcomes: A Systematic Review and Meta-Analysis. *Horm. Metab. Res.* **2021**, *53*, 85–93. [PubMed]
7. Tartof, S.Y.; Qian, L.; Hong, V.; Wei, R.; Nadjafi, R.F.; Fischer, H.; Li, Z.; Shaw, S.F.; Caparosa, S.L.; Nau, C.L.; et al. Obesity and mortality among patients diagnosed with COVID-19: Results from an Integrated Health Care Organization. *Ann. Intern. Med.* **2020**, *173*, 773–781. [CrossRef] [PubMed]
8. Wang, J.; Zhu, L.; Liu, L.; Zhao, X.A.; Zhang, Z.; Xue, L.; Yan, X.; Huang, S.; Li, Y.; Cheng, J.; et al. Overweight and Obesity are Risk Factors of Severe Illness in Patients with COVID-19. *Obesity* **2020**, *28*, 2049–2055. [CrossRef] [PubMed]
9. Gao, M.; Piernas, C.; Astbury, N.M.; Hippisley-Cox, J.; O'Rahilly, S.; Aveyard, P.; Jebb, S.A. Associations between body-mass index and COVID 19 severity in 6·9 million people in England: A prospective, community-based, cohort study. *Lancet Diabetes Endocrinol.* **2021**, *9*, 350–359. [CrossRef]
10. Jayawardena, R.; Jeyakumar, D.T.; Misra, A.; Hills, A.P.; Ranasinghe, P. Obesity: A potential risk factor for infection and mortality in the current COVID-19 epidemic. *Diabetes Metab. Syndr.* **2020**, *14*, 2199–2203. [CrossRef] [PubMed]
11. Ekiz, T.; Pazarlı, A.C. Relationship between COVID-19 and obesity. *Diabetes Metab. Syndr.* **2020**, *14*, 761–763. [CrossRef] [PubMed]
12. Carneiro, R.A.V.D.; Hillesheim, D.; Hallal, A.L.C. Correlation of overweight condition and obesity with mortality by COVID-19 in Brazil's state capitals. *Arch. Endocrinol. Metab.* **2021**, *65*. [CrossRef]
13. Seclén, S.N.; Nunez-Robles, E.; Yovera-Aldana, M.; Arias-Chumpitaz, A. Incidence of COVID-19 infection and prevalence of diabetes, obesity and hypertension according to altitude in Peruvian population. *Diabetes Res. Clin. Pract.* **2020**, *169*, 108463. [CrossRef] [PubMed]
14. Schwalb, A.; Seas, C. The COVID-19 pandemic in Peru: What went wrong? *Am. J. Trop. Med. Hyg.* **2021**, *104*, 1176–1178. [CrossRef] [PubMed]
15. Taylor, L. Covid-19: Why Peru suffers from one of the highest excess death rates in the world. *BMJ* **2021**, *372*, n611. [CrossRef] [PubMed]
16. Peruvian Ministry of Health (MINSA). COVID-19 in Peru. Available online: https://covid19.minsa.gob.pe/ (accessed on 27 July 2021).
17. Vandenbroucke, J.P.; von Elm, E.; Altman, D.G.; Gøtzsche, P.C.; Mulrow, C.D.; Pocock, S.J.; Poole, C.; Schlesselman, J.J.; Egger, M.; STROBE Initiative. Strengthening the Reporting of Observational Studies in Epidemiology (STROBE): Explanation and elaboration. *PLoS Med.* **2007**, *4*, e297. [CrossRef] [PubMed]
18. National Institute of Statistics and Informatics (INEI); Peru—National Demographic and Health Survey (ENDES) 2020. Non-communicable and Communicable Diseases. 2020. Available online: https://proyectos.inei.gob.pe/endes/2020/SALUD/ENFERMEDADES_ENDES_2020.pdf (accessed on 14 September 2021).
19. Peruvian Ministry of Health (MINSA). COVID-19 deaths. National System of Deaths (SINADEF). Available online: https://www.datosabiertos.gob.pe/dataset/fallecidos-por-covid-19-ministerio-de-salud-minsa (accessed on 3 June 2021).
20. National Institute of Statistics and Informatics (INEI). Peruvian Population. Available online: https://www.inei.gob.pe/estadisticas/indice-tematico/population-estimates-and-projections/ (accessed on 3 June 2021).
21. Singh, A.K.; Gillies, C.L.; Singh, R.; Singh, A.; Chudasama, Y.; Coles, B.; Seidu, S.; Zaccardi, F.; Davies, M.J.; Khunti, K. Prevalence of co-morbidities and their association with mortality in patients with COVID-19: A systematic review and meta-analysis. *Diabetes Obes. Metab.* **2020**, *22*, 1915–1924. [CrossRef] [PubMed]
22. Shulman, G.I. Ectopic fat in insulin resistance, dyslipidemia, and cardiometabolic disease. *N. Engl. J. Med.* **2014**, *371*, 1131–1141. [CrossRef] [PubMed]

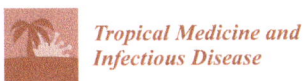

Article

An Autochthonous Outbreak of the SARS-CoV-2 P.1 Variant of Concern in Southern Italy, April 2021

Daniela Loconsole [1], Anna Sallustio [2], Francesca Centrone [1], Daniele Casulli [2], Maurizio Mario Ferrara [3], Antonio Sanguedolce [3], Marisa Accogli [1] and Maria Chironna [1,*]

[1] Department of Biomedical Sciences and Human Oncology-Hygiene Section, University of Bari, 70124 Bari, Italy; daniela.loconsole@uniba.it (D.L.); francesca.centrone.fc@gmail.com (F.C.); accoisa@gmail.com (M.A.)
[2] Hygiene Unit, University Hospital Consortium Policlinico, 70124 Bari, Italy; annasallustio@libero.it (A.S.); daniele.casulli@hotmail.com (D.C.)
[3] Local Health Unit of Bari, Department of Prevention, 70132 Bari, Italy; mauriziomario.ferrara@asl.bari.it (M.M.F.); antonio.sanguedolce@asl.bari.it (A.S.)
* Correspondence: maria.chironna@uniba.it; Tel.: +39-080-5592328

Abstract: The SARS-CoV-2 P.1 variant of concern (VOC) was first identified in Brazil and is now spreading in European countries. It is characterized by the E484K mutation in the receptor-binding domain, which could contribute to the evasion from neutralizing antibodies. In Italy, this variant was first identified in January 2021. Here, we report an autochthonous outbreak of SARS-CoV-2 P.1 variant infections in southern Italy in subjects who had not travelled to endemic areas or outside the Apulia region. The outbreak involved seven subjects, three of whom had received a COVID-19 vaccine (one had received two doses and two had received one dose). Four patients had a mild clinical presentation. Laboratory investigations of nasopharyngeal swabs revealed that all strains were S-gene target failure-negative and molecular tests revealed they were the P.1 variant. Whole-genome sequencing confirmed that five subjects were infected with closely related strains classified as the P.1 lineage. The circulation of VOCs highlights the importance of strictly monitoring the spread of SARS-CoV-2 variants through genomic surveillance and of investigating local outbreaks. Furthermore, public health measures including social distancing, screening, and quarantine for travelers are key tools to slow down the viral transmission and to contain and mitigate the impact of VOC diffusion, and rapid scaling-up of vaccination is crucial to avoid a possible new epidemic wave.

Keywords: outbreak; P.1 variant; Gamma variant; SARS-CoV-2 infection; COVID-19; whole-genome sequencing

Citation: Loconsole, D.; Sallustio, A.; Centrone, F.; Casulli, D.; Ferrara, M.M.; Sanguedolce, A.; Accogli, M.; Chironna, M. An Autochthonous Outbreak of the SARS-CoV-2 P.1 Variant of Concern in Southern Italy, April 2021. *Trop. Med. Infect. Dis.* **2021**, *6*, 151. https://doi.org/10.3390/tropicalmed6030151

Academic Editors: Peter A. Leggat, John Frean and Lucille Blumberg

Received: 3 August 2021
Accepted: 11 August 2021
Published: 12 August 2021

Publisher's Note: MDPI stays neutral with regard to jurisdictional claims in published maps and institutional affiliations.

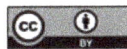

Copyright: © 2021 by the authors. Licensee MDPI, Basel, Switzerland. This article is an open access article distributed under the terms and conditions of the Creative Commons Attribution (CC BY) license (https://creativecommons.org/licenses/by/4.0/).

1. Introduction

In December 2020, the European Center for Disease Control and Prevention (ECDC) first reported the spread of a new SARS-CoV-2 variant of concern (VOC) characterized by multiple spike protein mutations and mutations in other genomic regions, called VOC 202012/01—lineage B.1.1.7, in the UK, and labeled Alpha variant by the World Health Organization [1,2]. A few weeks later, a new ECDC risk assessment described the emergence of two new VOCs, namely, the 501Y.V2 variant (Beta variant), which was isolated in South Africa, and the P.1 variant (Gamma variant), which was identified in Brazil, mostly in the Amazonas state [3]. The overall risk associated with the introduction and community spread of these VOCs was assessed as being high/very high [3]. In May 2021, the SARS-CoV-2 B.1.617.2 Delta variant emerged in India and has spread all over the world [4]. At the time of writing, all these lineages seem to have almost replaced the previous circulating viruses in the geographic regions and the Delta VOC, in particular, shows very high probability of becoming the dominant circulating strain in the EU/EAA [4–7]. The spread of VOCs with a high transmission potential poses a serious risk in terms of virulence, potential reinfections, and antibody responses to and efficacies of vaccines [4,8].

The P.1 variant is characterized by 11 amino acid changes in the spike protein, three of which are located in the receptor-binding domain (RBD) [3]. These amino acid changes are L18F, T20N, P26S, D138Y, R190S, K417T, E484K, N501Y, H655Y, T1027I, and V1176F [3]. The 501Y.V2 and P.1 variants are both characterized by the E484K mutation in the RBD, which could contribute to the evasion from neutralizing antibodies [9,10]. Cases of reinfection caused by SARS-CoV-2 strains carrying the E484K mutation have been described [11]. The P.1 variant was first identified in Japan in four travelers from Brazil, but there was no indication it was associated with more severe disease [8]. However, recent studies reported evidence that disease severity is increased with this variant [12]. Moreover, an impact on transmissibility has also been demonstrated [13]. Retrospective analyses of samples collected in Manaus (Brazil) demonstrated the presence of the P.1 variant from November 2020, when case numbers of COVID-19 were high, and a rise of this variant from 0% to 87% in 7 weeks [13]. Moreover, a statistically significant association between P.1 infection and a lower Cycle threshold (Ct) value in real-time PCR, which is an indirect index of viral load in different specimens [14], was reported [13].

In Europe, infections of the P.1 variant, as well as the B.1.1.7, B.1.351, and B.1.617.2 VOCs, have been associated with a higher risk of hospitalization and intensive care unit admission [4,12]. In Italy, the P.1 variant was first reported in January 2021 in three patients returning from Brazil [15]. Monthly national flash surveys conducted in Italy to estimate the prevalence of VOCs from February 2021, reported that the estimated prevalence of the P.1 variant increased from 0% in February 2021 to 11.8% in June 2021 [16]. In the Apulia region, the estimated prevalence of the P.1 variant remained below 1% [16].

Here, we report an autochthonous outbreak of SARS-CoV-2 P.1 variant infections in southern Italy occurred in April 2021, when strict non-pharmaceutical interventions (NPI) were mandatory and travels outside the regions were forbidden.

2. Results

Of the seven patients involved in the outbreak, six were members of the same family and one was a friend of the index case. The demographic and clinical characteristics of the patients are shown in Table 1.

Table 1. Demographic and clinical characteristics of seven cases of SARS-CoV-2 P.1 variant infections.

Patient Number	Relationship with the Index Case	Age (Years)	Sex	Comorbidities	Date of Onset of Symptoms	Date of Diagnosis	Clinical Presentation	Vaccinated
1	Index case	45	Male	No	20 April 2021	21 April 2021	Mild	No
2	Wife	31	Female	No	-	29 April 2021	Asymptomatic	No
3	Father-in-law	73	Male	Diabetes, Hypertension	28 April 2021	28 April 2021	Mild	Yes, BNT162b2 (second dose on 30 March 2021)
4	Mother-in-law	69	Female	No	-	28 April 2021	Asymptomatic	Yes, BNT162b2 (first dose on 19 April 2021)
5	Brother-in-law	53	Male	No	21 April 2021	22 April 2021	Mild	No
6	Nephew	16	Male	No	-	12 May 2021	Asymptomatic	No
7	Friend	37	Male	No	26 April 2021	27 April 2021	Mild	Yes, ChAdOx1-S (first dose on 29 March 2021)

The index case (patient 1) was a healthy 45-year-old man who resided in a small town with about 13,000 inhabitants in the province of Bari, Italy, and presented with high-grade fever (>39 °C), sore throat, diarrhea, anosmia, and ageusia on 20 April 2021. He reported no history of travel in any area endemic for the SARS-CoV-2 P.1 variant or travel out of the Apulia region because travel was forbidden by national health authorities, nor contacts with any SARS-CoV-2 positive case. The patient tested positive for SARS-CoV-2 on 21 April 2021. His wife and other household members also tested positive for SARS-CoV-2 and were promptly quarantined. Contact tracing revealed that 30 subjects were contacts of the index case and his household members. All of them were tested for SARS-CoV-2 infection. Among these contacts, only a friend of the index case who showed symptoms on 26 April 2021, tested positive (patient 7). Epidemiological investigation revealed that the contact with the index case occurred on 20 April 2021 during football training. Patients 3, 5, and 7 had mild clinical presentation, with symptoms developing between 21 and 26 April 2021. Patient 3 was fully vaccinated with two doses of the BNT162b2 COVID-19 vaccine. The first dose was administered on 8 March 2021, and the second dose was administered on 30 March 2021, in accordance with the recommended schedule. Patients 4 had received one dose of the BNT162b2 COVID-19 vaccine on 19 April 2021, and patient 7 had received one dose of the ChAdOx1-S COVID-19 vaccine on 29 March 2021 (Table 1).

The seven patients involved in the outbreak tested positive for SARS-CoV-2 by real-time PCR and all were S-gene target failure (SGTF)-negative. Therefore, samples were subjected to molecular screening for variants and designated the P.1 variant because of the presence of the K417T, E484K, and N501Y spike mutations. Whole-genome sequencing was performed of all seven strains, but high-quality SARS-CoV-2 genome sequences were only obtained for patients 1, 3, 4, 5, and 7. These were imputed into the PANGOLIN tool for lineage classification [17] and classified as the P.1 lineage. The sequences were deposited in the GISAID database (www.gisaid.com, accessed on 11 August 2021). The accession numbers are reported in Figure 1. The phylogenetic tree showed closely related strains, thus suggesting a common source of exposure (Figure 1).

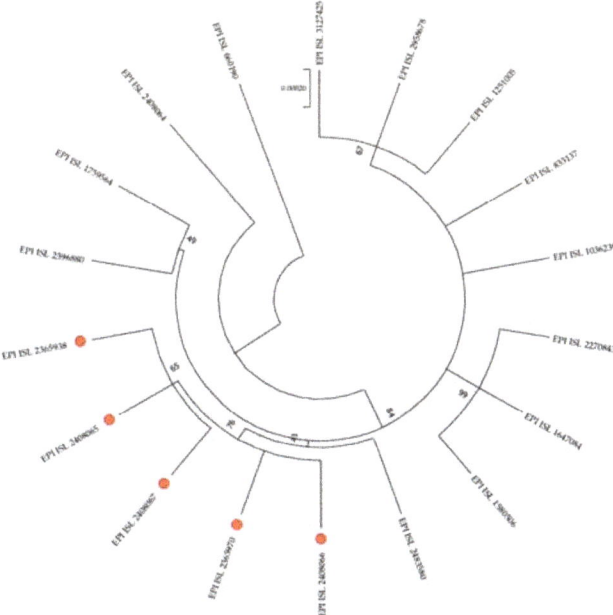

Figure 1. Phylogenetic tree of 18 SARS-CoV-2 full genome sequences, including the five genomes examined in this study (red dots). The reference SARS-CoV-2 genome (GISAID accession number: EPI_ISL_660190) was included to root the tree. P.1 reference strain has been used to construct the tree (GISAID accession numbers: EPI_ISL_833137). Other Italian P.1 SARS-CoV-2 sequences have been used for comparison (GISAID accession numbers: EPI_ISL_2408064, EPI_ISL_1759564, EPI_ISL_2396880, EPI_ISL_2483580, EPI_ISL_1580506, EPI_ISL_1647084, EPI_ISL_2270843, EPI_ISL_1036239, EPI_ISL_1251005, EPI_ISL_2958678, EPI_ISL_3127425). Evolutionary analyses were conducted in MEGAX by using the maximum likelihood method and Tamura-Nei model. The robustness of branching pattern was tested by 1000 bootstrap replications. Bootstrap values are reported. The scale bar indicates nucleotides substitutions per site.

3. Discussion

Virus importation associated with travel has been the key driver of viral spread since the first wave of the COVID-19 pandemic in Italy [18]. Cases of imported SARS-CoV-2 variant P.1 infection were first reported on 7 January 2021 in Central Italy in travelers returning from Brazil, and this variant was also subsequently identified in northern and southern Italy [15]. All direct flights from Brazil to Italy were cancelled on 16 January 2021. Another case of P.1 infection was identified in a traveler returning from Brazil on 17 January 2021, thus confirming the risk of introducing variants via indirect flights [19]. An in-depth molecular epidemiological analysis performed by Di Giallonardo et al. showed intensive local transmission of the P.1 variant in Italy after its travel-linked introduction [20]. In the Apulia region, the P.1 variant was first identified through a flash national survey on 20 April 2021 [21]. It was identified in a patient without risk factors for P.1 variant infection (i.e., travel or contact with a P.1 variant-positive case). Thereafter, we documented the circulation of the P.1 variant in two more provinces of the Apulia region (data not published). The present study reports an outbreak of the SARS-CoV-2 P.1 VOC in southern Italy. Among cases, no subjects with known travel history, nor contacts with other SARS-CoV-2 positive subjects were identified. Therefore, despite lockdown restrictions being imposed in Italy from December 2020, the cluster described here is concerning and suggests a local ongoing transmission, although at a low level, of this variant in the Apulia region.

The symptomatic cases of the outbreak here described showed a mild clinical presentation. Recently, de Siqueira et al. also reported a familial cluster of five cases, with three having severe disease, one of whom died [22]. We could speculate that the difference in clinical presentation between this previous study and the cases described here could be related to the fact that three of our seven cases had received at least one dose of a COVID-19 vaccine, which may have protected them against severe disease. Of note, patient 4 received the first vaccine dose only a few days before being diagnosed and was asymptomatic, while patient 3 was fully vaccinated and received the second dose 1 month before the clinical onset of symptoms. As previously reported for the B.1.1.7 lineage VOC in the Apulia region [23], the P.1 variant raises concerns about such strains causing possible symptomatic post-vaccination infections. Some studies demonstrated that samples of vaccinated and convalescent people exhibit lower neutralization activity against SARS-CoV-2 strains harboring the E484K spike mutation [24], showing the need to induce the highest neutralization titers through vaccination. According to the European approach, the Italian national guidelines indicate that the booster vaccination should be postponed to provide more subjects with a first vaccination [25]. However, this approach will result in a lower level of neutralizing antibodies and could leave some vaccinees unprotected in the context of the rising spread of SARS-CoV-2 variants [24,26].

This study has some limitations. First, only five in seven samples were successfully subjected to WGS. However, the molecular screening for variants and the epidemiological linkage suggested the presence of SARS-CoV-2 P.1 lineage in all cases. Second, serum samples after vaccination and before symptom onset for anti-spike IgG detection were not available. Nevertheless, due to the incomplete vaccination schedule for two subjects, we could hypothesize a low humoral response to vaccination.

In Italy, where the vaccination campaign is accelerating but has not yet reached sufficient coverage, the spread of variants with higher transmissibility may have a significant impact, also in the light of the reduction of NPI. The current scenario characterized by the circulation of multiple VOCs and, in particular, of the Delta VOC [4], highlights the importance of closely monitoring the spread of SARS-CoV-2 variants through genomic surveillance and of investigating local outbreaks. Furthermore, maintaining public health measures including social distancing, screening, and quarantine for travelers are key tools to slow down the viral transmission and to contain and mitigate the impact of VOCs diffusion on the National Health Service. Finally, rapid up scaling of vaccination in Italy is crucial to avoid a possible new epidemic wave, particularly in younger people who have not yet been vaccinated.

4. Materials and Methods

Seven patients were involved in the outbreak. Their clinical presentations were classified according to the National Institute of Health (NIH) clinical staging of COVID-19 disease [27]. Nasopharyngeal swabs were collected from all patients at the Local Health Unit of Bari (Italy) and were processed at the Laboratory of Molecular Epidemiology and Public Health of the Hygiene Unit (A.O.U.C. Policlinico Bari), which is the coordinator of the Regional Laboratory Network for SARS-CoV-2 diagnosis in the Apulia region. RNA was extracted using a MagMAX Viral/Pathogen Nucleic Acid Isolation Kit (Thermo Fisher Scientific, Waltham, MA, USA). The molecular test was performed using a three-target commercial multiplex real-time PCR assay targeting the N, ORF1ab, and S genes (TaqPath RT-PCR COVID-19 Assay; Thermo Fisher Scientific). SGTF was assessed to rule out the B.1.1.7 lineage VOC because SGTF can be considered a robust proxy of VOC 202012/01 [26,28]. SGTF-negative samples were screened for the presence of notable types of spike protein mutations (HV 69-70 deletion, N501Y, K417N, E484K, and K417T) using a commercial multiplex real-time PCR kit (Seegene Allplex SARS-CoV-2 Variants I Assay, Arrows Diagnostics, Genova, Italy). Whole-genome sequencing was performed using the Ion Torrent platform (Thermo Fisher Scientific, Monza, Italy). The library was prepared using an Ion AmpliSeq Library Kit Plus according to the manufacturer's instructions and the Ion AmpliSeq SARS-CoV-2 RNA custom primer panel (Thermo Fisher Scientific, Monza, Italy). Quality control of AmpliSeq reads and their alignment to the complete genome of the SARS-CoV-2 Wuhan-Hu-1 isolate were performed using the Torrent Server of the Ion Torrent S5 sequencer with default settings. The aligned reads were utilized for both reference-guided assembly and variant calling. The quality metrics for the reference-based assemblies are as follows: 784,477 sequence reads (average length 149 bp), 674,160 mapped reads, GC% 40, and an average base coverage depth of 3222. The total genome size was 29,780 bp. Assembly was performed using the Iterative Refinement Meta-Assembler (IRMA) v.1.3.0.2, which produced a consensus sequence for the sample using a cut-off of >50% for calling single nucleotide polymorphisms. The whole-genome sequences have been deposited in the GISAID database (https://www.gisaid.com, accessed on 11 August 2021). Phylogenetic analysis was performed using MEGAX software.

Author Contributions: Conceptualization, M.C. and D.L.; methodology, A.S. (Anna Sallustio); formal analysis, A.S. (Anna Sallustio) and M.A.; investigation, M.M.F. and A.S. (Antonio Sanguedolce); data curation, F.C. and D.C.; writing—original draft preparation, D.L. and M.A.; writing—review and editing, M.C. All authors have read and agreed to the published version of the manuscript.

Funding: This research did not receive any specific grant from funding agencies in the public, commercial, or not-for-profit sectors.

Institutional Review Board Statement: Ethical review and approval were waived for this study because all the activities were conducted as part of the legislated mandate of the Health Promotion and Public Health Department of Apulia. All procedures were carried out in accordance with the Declaration of Helsinki, as revised in 2013, for human subjects.

Informed Consent Statement: Informed written consent was obtained from all subjects involved in the study.

Data Availability Statement: All data regarding the patients and laboratory tests are available from the corresponding author by e-mail request.

Conflicts of Interest: The authors declare no conflict of interest.

References

1. European Center for Disease Control and Prevention. Threat Assessment Brief: Rapid Increase of a SARS-CoV-2 Variant with Multiple Spike Protein Mutations Observed in the United Kingdom. *Risk Assessment*. 2020. Available online: https://www.ecdc.europa.eu/en/publications-data/threat-assessment-brief-rapid-increase-sars-cov-2-variant-united-kingdom (accessed on 30 May 2021).
2. World Health Organization. Tracking SARS-CoV-2 Variants. 2021. Available online: https://www.who.int/en/activities/tracking-SARS-CoV-2-variants/ (accessed on 15 July 2021).
3. European Center for Disease Control and Prevention. Risk Related to the Spread of New SARS-CoV-2 Variants of Concern in the EU/EEA—First Update. 2021. Available online: https://www.ecdc.europa.eu/en/publications-data/covid-19-risk-assessment-spread-new-variants-concern-eueea-first-update (accessed on 28 January 2021).
4. European Center for Disease Control and Prevention. Risk Assessment: Implications for the EU/EEA on the Spread of the SARS-CoV-2 Delta (B.1.617.2) Variant of Concern. 2021. Available online: https://www.ecdc.europa.eu/en/publications-data/threat-assessment-emergence-and-impact-sars-cov-2-delta-variant (accessed on 15 July 2021).
5. O'Toole, Á.; Hill, V.; Pybus, O.G.; Watts, A.; Bogoch, I.I.; Khan, K.; Messina, J.P.; Tegally, H.; Lessells, R.R.; Giandhari, J.; et al. Tracking the international spread of SARS-CoV-2 lineages B.1.1.7 and B.1.351/501Y-V2. *Wellcome Open Res.* **2021**, *6*, 121. [CrossRef] [PubMed]
6. Walensky, R.P.; Walke, H.T.; Fauci, A.S. SARS-CoV-2 variants of concern in the United States—Challenges and opportunities. *JAMA* **2021**, *325*, 1037. [CrossRef] [PubMed]
7. Sabino, E.C.; Buss, L.F.; Carvalho, M.P.S.; Prete, C.A.; Crispim, M.A.E.; Fraiji, N.A.; Pereira, R.H.M.; Parag, K.V.; Peixoto, P.D.S.; Kraemer, M.U.G.; et al. Resurgence of COVID-19 in Manaus, Brazil, despite high seroprevalence. *Lancet* **2021**, *397*, 452–455. [CrossRef]
8. Fujino, T.; Nomoto, H.; Kutsuna, S.; Ujiie, M.; Suzuki, T.; Sato, R.; Fujimoto, T.; Kuroda, M.; Wakita, T.; Ohmagari, N. Novel SARS-CoV-2 variant in travelers from Brazil to Japan. *Emerg. Infect. Dis.* **2021**, *27*, 1243–1245. [CrossRef] [PubMed]
9. Weisblum, Y.; Schmidt, F.; Zhang, F.; DaSilva, J.; Poston, D.; Lorenzi, J.C.C.; Muecksch, F.; Rutkowska, M.; Hoffmann, H.H.; Michailidis, E.; et al. Escape from neutralizing antibodies by SARS-CoV-2 spike protein variants. *bioRxiv* **2020**. [CrossRef] [PubMed]
10. Greaney, A.J.; Loes, A.N.; Crawford, K.H.; Starr, T.N.; Malone, K.D.; Chu, H.Y.; Bloom, J.D. Comprehensive mapping of mutations in the SARS-CoV-2 receptor-binding domain that affect recognition by polyclonal human plasma antibodies. *Cell Host Microbe* **2021**, *29*, 463–476. [CrossRef] [PubMed]
11. Nonaka, C.K.V.; Franco, M.M.; Gräf, T.; Barcia, C.A.L.; Mendonça, R.N.; de Sousa, K.A.F.; Neiva, L.M.C.; Fosenca, V.; Mendes, A.V.A.; de Aguiar, R.S.; et al. Genomic evidence of SARS-CoV-2 reinfection involving E484K spike mutation, Brazil. *Emerg. Infect. Dis.* **2021**, *27*, 1522–1524. [CrossRef] [PubMed]
12. Funk, T.; Pharris, A.; Spiteri, G.; Bundle, N.; Melidou, A.; Carr, M.; Gonzalez, G.; Garcia-Leon, A.; Crispie, F.; O'Connor, L.; et al. Characteristics of SARS-CoV-2 variants of concern B.1.1.7, B.1.351 or P.1: Data from seven EU/EEA countries, weeks 38/2020 to 10/2021. *Eurosurveillance* **2021**, *26*, 2100348. [CrossRef] [PubMed]
13. Faria, N.R.; Mellan, T.A.; Whittaker, C.; Claro, I.M.; Candido, D.D.S.; Mishra, S.; Crispim, M.A.E.; Sales, F.C.S.; Hawryluk, I.; McCrone, J.T.; et al. Genomics and epidemiology of the P.1 SARS-CoV-2 lineage in Manaus, Brazil. *Science* **2021**, *372*, 815–821. [CrossRef] [PubMed]
14. Romero-Gómez, M.P.; Gómez-Sebastian, S.; Cendejas-Bueno, E.; Montero-Vega, M.D.; Mingorance, J.; García-Rodríguez, J. Ct value is not enough to discriminate patients harbouring infective virus. *J. Infect.* **2020**, *82*, e35–e37. [CrossRef] [PubMed]
15. Compagni, E.D.; Jurisic, L.; Caporale, M.; Bacà, F.; Scialabba, S.; Fanì, S.; Perullo, A.; Toro, M.; Marchegiano, A.; Martino, M.; et al. Genome sequences of three SARS-CoV-2 P.1 strains identified from patients returning from Brazil to Italy. *Microbiol. Resour. Announc.* **2021**, *10*. [CrossRef]
16. Istituto Superiore di Sanità. Prevalenza delle Varianti VOC (Variant of Concern) Appartenenti ai Lignaggi B.1.1.7, P.1, B.1.617.2 e B.1.351 e di Altre Varianti in Italia. *Indagine del 22/06/2021*. Available online: https://www.epicentro.iss.it/coronavirus/pdf/sars-cov-2-monitoraggio-varianti-indagini-rapide-22-giugno-2021.pdf (accessed on 10 July 2021).
17. Rambaut, A.; Holmes, E.C.; O'Toole, A.; Hill, V.; McCrone, J.T.; Ruis, C.; du Plessis, L.; Pybus, O.G. A dynamic nomenclature proposal for SARS-CoV-2 lineages to assist genomic epidemiology. *Nat. Microbiol.* **2020**, *5*, 1403–1407. [CrossRef] [PubMed]
18. Di Giallonardo, F.; Duchene, S.; Puglia, I.; Curini, V.; Profeta, F.; Cammà, C.; Marcacci, M.; Calistri, P.; Holmes, E.C.; Lorusso, A. Genomic epidemiology of the first wave of SARS-CoV-2 in Italy. *Viruses* **2020**, *12*, 1438. [CrossRef] [PubMed]
19. Maggi, F.; Novazzi, F.; Genoni, A.; Baj, A.; Spezia, P.G.; Focosi, D.; Zago, C.; Colombo, A.; Cassani, G.; Pasciuta, R.; et al. Imported SARS-CoV-2 variant, P.1 in traveler returning from Brazil to Italy. *Emerg. Infect. Dis.* **2021**, *27*, 1249–1251. [CrossRef] [PubMed]
20. Di Giallonardo, F.; Puglia, I.; Curini, V.; Cammà, C.; Mangone, I.; Calistri, P.; Cobbin, J.; Holmes, E.; Lorusso, A. Emergence and spread of SARS-CoV-2 lineages, B.1.1.7 and P.1 in Italy. *Viruses* **2021**, *13*, 794. [CrossRef]
21. Istituto Superiore di Sanità. Prevalenza delle VOC (Variant of Concern) del Virus SARS-CoV-2 in Italia: Lineage B.1.1.7, P.1 e B.1.351, e Altre Varianti (Variant of Interest, VOI) Tra cui Lineage P.2 e Lineage B.1.525. *Indagine del 20/4/2021*. Available online: https://www.iss.it/documents/20126/0/Relazione+tecnica+indagine+rapida+varianti+SARS-COV-2.pdf/f425e647-efdb-3f8c-2f86-87379d56ce8d?t=1620232350272 (accessed on 28 May 2021).

22. De Siqueira, I.C.; Camelier, A.A.; Maciel, E.A.; Nonaka, C.K.V.; Neves, M.C.L.; Macêdo, Y.S.F.; de Sousa, K.A.F.; Araujo, V.C.; Paste, A.A.; Souza, B.S.D.F.; et al. Early detection of P.1 variant of SARS-CoV-2 in a cluster of cases in Salvador, Brazil. *Int. J. Infect. Dis.* **2021**, *108*, 252–255. [CrossRef]
23. Loconsole, D.; Sallustio, A.; Accogli, M.; Leaci, A.; Sanguedolce, A.; Parisi, A.; Chironna, M. Investigation of an outbreak of symptomatic SARS-CoV-2 VOC 202012/01-lineage B.1.1.7 infection in healthcare workers, Italy. *Clin. Microbiol. Infect.* **2021**, *27*, 1174. [CrossRef] [PubMed]
24. Jangra, S.; Ye, C.; Rathnasinghe, R.; Stadlbauer, D.; Krammer, F.; Simon, V.; Martinez-Sobrido, L.; García-Sastre, A.; Schotsaert, M.; Alshammary, H.; et al. SARS-CoV-2 spike E484K mutation reduces antibody neutralisation. *Lancet Microbe* **2021**. [CrossRef]
25. Ministero della Salute. Circolare 0019748-05/05/2021-DGPRE-DGPRE-P. Trasmissione Parere del CTS in Merito alla Estensione dell'Intervallo Tra le Due Dosi dei Vaccini a mRNAe alla Seconda Dose del Vaccino Vaxzevria. Available online: https://www.trovanorme.salute.gov.it/norme/renderNormsanPdf?anno=2021&codLeg=80236&parte=1%20&serie=null (accessed on 30 May 2021).
26. Loconsole, D.; Centrone, F.; Morcavallo, C.; Campanella, S.; Sallustio, A.; Accogli, M.; Fortunato, F.; Parisi, A.; Chironna, M. Rapid spread of the SARS-CoV-2 variant of concern 202012/01 in southern Italy (December 2020–March 2021). *Int. J. Environ. Res. Public Health* **2021**, *18*, 4766. [CrossRef]
27. National Institute of Health (NIH). Coronavirus Disease 2019 (COVID-19) Treatment Guidelines. Available online: https://files.covid19treatmentguidelines.nih.gov/guidelines/covid19treatmentguidelines.pdf (accessed on 30 May 2021).
28. Investigation of Novel SARS-CoV-2 Variant: Variant of Concern 202012/01—Technical Briefing 7. Available online: https://assets.publishing.service.gov.uk/government/uploads/system/uploads/attachment_data/file/968581/Variants_of_Concern_VOC_Technical_Briefing_7_England.pdf (accessed on 15 March 2021).

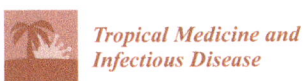

Tropical Medicine and Infectious Disease

Article

Newly Diagnosed Diabetes in Patients with COVID-19: Different Types and Short-Term Outcomes

Alaa A. Farag [1,*], Hassan M. Hassanin [1], Hanan H. Soliman [2], Ahmad Sallam [3], Amany M. Sediq [3], Elsayed S. Abd elbaser [4] and Khaled Elbanna [1]

1. Internal Medicine Department, Faculty of Medicine, Zagazig University, Zagazig 44519, Egypt; drhassan_h99@yahoo.com (H.M.H.); aboamro76@yahoo.com (K.E.)
2. Community Medicine Department, Faculty of Medicine, Suez Canal University, Ismailia 41522, Egypt; hananhasan81@yahoo.com
3. Clinical Pathology Department, Faculty of Medicine, Zagazig University, Zagazig 44519, Egypt; nancyabdelhamid@yahoo.com (A.S.); amany_mohy2006@yahoo.com (A.M.S.)
4. Tropical Medicine Department, Faculty of Medicine, Zagazig University, Zagazig 44519, Egypt; dr.sayedsaad79@gmail.com
* Correspondence: dr_alaafarag@yahoo.com or AAFaraj@medicine.zu.edu.eg

Abstract: A great global concern is currently focused on the coronavirus disease 2019 (COVID-19) pandemic and its associated morbidities. The goal of this study was to determine the frequency of newly diagnosed diabetes mellitus (DM) and its different types among COVID-19 patients, and to check the glycemic control in diabetic cases for three months. After excluding known cases of DM, 570 patients with confirmed COVID-19 were studied. All participants were classified as non-diabetic or newly discovered diabetic. According to hemoglobin A1c (HbA1c) and fasting insulin, newly discovered diabetic patients were further classified into pre-existing DM, new-onset type 1 DM, and new-onset type 2 DM. Glycemic control was monitored for three months in newly diagnosed diabetic patients. DM was diagnosed in 77 patients (13.5%); 12 (2.1%) with pre-existing DM, 7 (1.2%) with new-onset type 1 DM, and 58 (10.2%) with new-onset type 2 DM. Significantly higher rates of severe infection and mortality ($p < 0.001$ and $p = 0.046$) were evident among diabetic patients. Among survived diabetic patients ($n = 63$), hyperglycemia and the need for anti-diabetic treatment persisted in 73% of them for three months. COVID-19 was associated with a new-onset of DM in 11.4% of all participants and expression of pre-existing DM in 2.1% of all participants, both being associated with severe infection. COVID-19 patients with newly diagnosed diabetes had high risk of mortality. New-onset DM persisted for at least three months in more than two-thirds of cases.

Keywords: COVID-19; new-onset DM; severe infection; mortality

1. Introduction

In December 2019, in Wuhan (China), the first cases of severe pneumonia of unknown origin were reported [1]. The causative organism has been identified as a new enveloped RNA beta-coronavirus, and it was later named severe acute respiratory syndrome coronavirus 2 (SARS-CoV-2) [2]. Early in 2020, the World Health Organization (WHO) declared coronavirus disease 2019 (COVID-19) as a global pandemic. Globally, as of 7 July 2021, there have been 184,324,026 confirmed cases of COVID-19, including 3,992,680 deaths, reported to WHO [3].

Diabetes is a common chronic metabolic disease, and one of the major causes of morbidity and mortality, which leads to huge health and financial burden worldwide. Patients with diabetes have an increased risk of severe complications, including severe acute respiratory syndrome (SARS) and multi-organ failure [4].

There is a two-way relationship between COVID-19 and DM [5]. In the first way, diabetes is associated with a poor COVID-19 prognosis [6]. In the other way, new-onset

Citation: Farag, A.A.; Hassanin, H.M.; Soliman, H.H.; Sallam, A.; Sediq, A.M.; Abd elbaser, E.S.; Elbanna, K. Newly Diagnosed Diabetes in Patients with COVID-19: Different Types and Short-Term Outcomes. *Trop. Med. Infect. Dis.* **2021**, *6*, 142. https://doi.org/10.3390/tropicalmed6030142

Academic Editors: John Frean, Peter A. Leggat and Lucille Blumberg

Received: 7 July 2021
Accepted: 30 July 2021
Published: 2 August 2021

Publisher's Note: MDPI stays neutral with regard to jurisdictional claims in published maps and institutional affiliations.

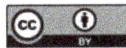

Copyright: © 2021 by the authors. Licensee MDPI, Basel, Switzerland. This article is an open access article distributed under the terms and conditions of the Creative Commons Attribution (CC BY) license (https://creativecommons.org/licenses/by/4.0/).

DM and severe complications of pre-existing DM, including diabetic ketoacidosis (DKA) and hyperosmolarity, have been reported in patients with COVID-19 [7].

Severe acute respiratory syndrome coronavirus 2 may enter the pancreatic beta cells through the expression of angiotensin-converting enzyme 2 (ACE2) receptors, impairing insulin production, and consequently, either worsening DM or developing new-onset DM [8]. Insulin resistance due to higher levels of interleukin-6 and tumor necrosis factor-alpha in patients with severe COVID-19 could be another probable explanation for developing DM [9].

Despite this, many recently published data entailed the effect of previously diagnosed DM on the clinical course and outcome of COVID-19 [5,8]. Only a few data are available regarding the new-onset of DM among COVID-19 patients, its different types, its clinical course, and its outcome after the recovery from COVID-19. The purpose of this work was to determine the frequency of newly diagnosed DM and its different types among COVID-19 patients, and to assess the infection outcome and glycemic control during the study.

2. Methods

2.1. Study Population and Recruitment

In this biphasic cross-sectional/prospective study, after excluding known cases of DM, we included 570 confirmed COVID-19 patients who were admitted to Zagazig University Hospital and Zagazig General Hospital, from 1 April 2020 to 31 May 2020. Exclusion criteria included age <18 years old, pregnancy, unconfirmed cases of COVID-19, and previously diagnosed cases of DM.

2.2. Patient Assessment

All patients underwent thorough clinical and laboratory assessment and chest computerized tomography (CT). The following laboratory measures were recorded in all participants on admission: complete blood count measured using Sysmex XN-2000 autoanalyzer (Siemens Diagnostic, Erlangen, Germany) and erythrocyte sedimentation rate (ESR) measured using Vision B analyzer (YHLO Biotech diagnostic, Shenzhen, China). Biochemical blood tests included FPG, HbA1c, C-reactive protein (CRP), serum total bilirubin, albumin, Transaminases (ALT, AST), LDH, creatinine, and urea nitrogen measured using dedicated reagent on Cobas c702/8000 (Roche diagnostic, Mannheim, Germany), and D-dimer measured on Cobas c501/6000 (Roche diagnostic, Germany). Serum ferritin, serum fasting insulin, and C-peptide were measured on Cobas c602/8000 (Roche diagnostic, Germany) in newly diagnosed diabetic subjects. COVID-19 diagnosis was confirmed by reverse transcription-polymerase chain reaction (RT-PCR) using nasal and pharyngeal swabs.

2.3. Study Design and Setting

According to Chinese National Health Committee diagnostic guidelines for COVID-19, disease severity was graded as either mild/moderate (minimal symptoms and negative chest CT findings) or severe (extensive clinical manifestations and positive CT findings) [10]. According to the American Diabetes Association, newly diagnosed DM was defined as either new-onset DM (no preceding history of DM with fasting plasma glucose [FPG] $\geq$ 126 mg/dL or random blood glucose [RBG] $\geq$ 200 mg/dL and HbA1c < 6.5%) or previously undiagnosed DM (FPG $\geq$ 126 mg/dL or RBG $\geq$ 200 mg/dL and HbA1c $\geq$ 6.5% or HbA1c $\geq$ 6.5% only [11]. In the first (cross-sectional) phase of the study, based on mean readings of FPG on the first day of hospital admission, all participants were classified into two main groups: group I (non-diabetic, FPG < 126 mg/dL) or group II (newly discovered diabetic, FPG $\geq$ 126 mg/dL). According to measurements of HbA1c and serum fasting insulin and C-peptide on admission, group II patients were further classified into group IIA (newly discovered pre-existing DM; HbA1c $\geq$ 6.5), group IIB (new-onset type 1 DM; HbA1c < 6.5, low fasting insulin and low C-peptide), or group IIC (new-onset type 2 DM; HbA1c < 6.5, normal fasting insulin and normal C-peptide). The outcome of COVID-19 infection was recorded either as recovery or mortality in different groups. In the second (prospective) phase of the study, patients with new-onset DM (groups II B,C) were followed for three months (from diagnosis of DM), even after discharge from the hospital, with weekly based outpatient visits, repeated testing of FPG, and recording of anti-diabetic treatment.

2.4. Statistical Analysis

Statistical calculations were conducted using SPSS version 21.0 for Windows (SPSS Inc., Chicago, IL, USA). If the continuous variables were parametric, they were expressed as mean ± SD, meanwhile if they were nonparametric, the median was the method of expression. In addition, categorical variables were expressed as numbers and percentages. Student's t-test, Mann–Whitney U test, Fisher's exact test, Pearson's Chi-squared test, and logistic regression model were among the appropriate tests utilized. Statistical significance was considered at $p < 0.05$.

3. Results

3.1. Cross-Sectional Phase

This study comprised 570 confirmed COVID-19 patients. The mean age of the study population was 47.9 ± 10.9 years, and 317 patients (55.5%) were males. Diabetes was newly defined in 77 (13.5%) patients. Our results showed that there were significant differences between newly diagnosed diabetic patients and non-diabetic patients regarding body mass index (BMI) and family history of DM ($p < 0.001$, for both). Fasting blood glucose (208.3 ± 109.9) and glycated hemoglobin (5.7 ± 0.8) were found to be significantly higher in the newly diagnosed diabetic patients ($p < 0.001$). In terms of onset symptoms in the newly diagnosed diabetic patients, 70 (90.9%) patients exhibited symptoms of fever; the other common symptoms were cough in 70 (90.9%), dyspnea in 66 (85.7%), and diarrhea in 11 (14.3%) patients. There were several differences in laboratory findings between newly diagnosed diabetic patients and non-diabetic patients, including higher levels of C-reactive protein (CRP), lactate dehydrogenase (LDH), ferritin, and D-dimer in newly diagnosed DM ($p < 0.001$, for all). The study enrolled 297 severe COVID-19 cases (52.1%) and 273 mild/moderate cases (47.9%). Out of all cases of newly diagnosed DM, 89.6% had a severe infection (69/77), which was significantly higher than that among non-diabetic patients ($p < 0.001$). A total number of 62 patients died during the study (10.9%) from COVID-19 sequelae. Mortality was significantly higher among diabetic subjects (18.2%) than non-diabetic subjects (9.7%) ($p < 0.001$) (Table 1).

Out of 77 diabetic patients, newly discovered pre-existing DM was defined in 12 (2.1%) patients, new-onset type 1 DM developed in seven (1.2%) patients, and 58 (10.2%) patients had new-onset type 2 DM (Figure 1).

As displayed in Table 2, HbA1C level was significantly elevated in group IIA (7.2 ± 0.4), compared with group IIB (5.3 ± 0.5) and group IIC (5.4 ± 0.5) ($p < 0.001$). However, fasting insulin and C-peptide levels were much lower in group IIB (3.6 ± 1.3, 0.3 ± 0.1) compared with group IIA (33.4 ± 9.2, 3.5 ± 1) and group IIC (38.1 ± 9.1, 3.6 ± 0.8) ($p < 0.001$). There were significant differences among groups IIA, IIB, and IIC regarding age, BMI, FPG, HbA1c, fasting insulin, and C-peptide ($p < 0.001$, for all). Four cases (57.1%) in group IIB showed positive urinary acetone with DKA on presentation. There were several differences in laboratory findings between groups IIA, IIB, and IIC, including higher levels of CRP, serum ferritin, and D-dimer in group IIB.

Serum CRP, ferritin, LDH, and D-dimer had significant positive correlations with newly diagnosed DM. In addition, age, BMI, severe COVID-19, and positive chest CT findings had significant positive correlations with newly diagnosed DM ($p < 0.001$, for all) (Table 3).

Table 4 shows the independent significant predictors of the presence of newly diagnosed DM among COVID-19 patients as determined by logistic regression analyses. Older age, higher BMI, elevated CRP, and elevated ferritin were the significant predictors ($p < 0.001$, for each).

Table 1. Comparison between diabetic and non-diabetic groups regarding clinical, laboratory, and radiological differences.

Variables	All Participants (n = 570)	Non-Diabetic Patients (Group I, n = 493)	Newly Diagnosed Diabetic Patients (Group II, n = 77)	p
Age (years)	47.9 ± 10.9	46.4 ± 10	57.7 ± 11.4	<0.001
Male gender	317 (55.5%)	276 (56%)	41(53.2)	0.712 *
BMI	26 ± 5.9	25 ± 4.5	32 ± 9	<0.001 **
Hypertensive	45 (7.9%)	36 (7.3%)	9 (11.7%)	0.178 *
IHD	19 (3.3%)	12 (2.4%)	7 (9.1%)	0.008 *
Family history of DM	56 (9.8%)	22 (4.5%)	34 (44.2%)	<0.001 *
Severe COVID-19	297 (52.1%)	228 (46.2%)	69 (89.6%)	<0.001 *
Fever	327 (57.4%)	257 (52.1%)	70 (90.9%)	<0.001 *
Cough	312 (54.7%)	242 (49.1%)	70 (90.9%)	<0.001 *
Dyspnea	301 (52.8%)	235 (47.7%)	66 (85.7%)	<0.001 *
Diarrhea	78 (13.7%)	67 (13.6%)	11 (14.3%)	0.859 *
FPG (mg/dL)	105.9 ± 57.9	89.9 ± 10.3	208.3 ± 109.9	<0.001 **
HbA1C	5.4 ± 0.6	5.4 ± 0.6	5.7 ± 0.8	<0.001
Positive urinary acetone	4 (0.7%)	0	4 (5.2%)	<0.001 *
DKA on presentation	4 (0.7%)	0	4 (5.2%)	<0.001 *
Hemoglobin (g/dL)	11.8 ± 1.4	11.7 ± 1.4	11.9 ± 1.4	0.234
Platelets count ($\times 10^3/mm^3$)	191.3 ± 50.6	192.3 ± 50.1	184.9 ± 53.1	0.230
WBCs ($\times 10^3/mm^3$)	6.4 ± 2.5	6.4 ± 2.6	6.2 ± 2.3	0.511
Lymphocytes ($\times 10^3/mm^3$)	2.1 ± 1.1	2.2 ± 1.1	1.5 ± 0.8	<0.001 **
Absolute lymphopenia (<1 × $10^3/mm^3$)	169 (29.6%)	123 (24.9%)	46 (59.7%)	<0.001 **
CRP (mg/dL)	38.8 ± 23.8	36.3 ± 19.9	55.4 ± 37.2	0.009 **
ESR (mm/h)	41.3 ± 14	41.1 ± 13.9	42.6 ± 14.5	0.389
Serum ferritin (ng/mL)	236 ± 170.3	217.9 ± 150.4	351.7 ± 234.6	<0.001 **
LDH (IU/L)	246.2 ± 80.5	239.9 ± 77.4	287 ± 88.7	<0.001 **
D-dimer (µg/mL)	1 ± 1.4	0.9 ± 1.2	1.5 ± 2	<0.001 **
Serum creatinine (mg/dL)	1 ± 0.3	1 ± 0.3	1 ± 0.2	0.727
Blood urea (mg/dL)	36.6 ± 25.5	36.5 ± 25.3	37 ± 26.3	0.893
INR	1.1 ± 0.2	1.1 ± 0.2	1.1 ± 0.1	0.098
Serum albumin (g/dL)	3.6 ± 0.5	3.6 ± 0.5	3.7 ± 0.4	0.352
Serum total bilirubin (g/dL)	1.1 ± 0.2	1.1 ± 0.2	1.1 ± 0.1	0.058 **
ALT (IU/L)	33.9 ± 23.7	33.4 ± 23.2	36.6 ± 26.7	0.278
AST (IU/L)	56.2 ± 37.7	55.4 ± 36.8	60.8 ± 43	0.249
Positive chest CT findings	297 (52.1%)	228 (46.2%)	69 (89.6%)	<0.001 *
Deceased	62 (10.9%)	48 (9.7%)	14 (18.2%)	0.046 *

Unless otherwise indicated, data represent the mean ± SD with the range in parenthesis. No: number; SD: standard deviation; BMI: body mass index; IHD: ischemic heart disease; WBCs: white blood cells; CRP: C-reactive protein; ESR: erythrocyte sedimentation rate; LDH: lactate dehydrogenase; IU: international unit; INR: international normalized ratio; ALT: alanine aminotransferase; AST: aspartate aminotransferase; CT: computerized tomography. *: Fisher's Exact Test; **: Mann–Whitney Test.

Table 2. Clinical, laboratory, and radiological differences among different diabetic subgroups (n = 77).

Variables	Pre-Existing DM (Group IIA, n = 12)	New-Onset Type 1 DM (Group IIB, n = 7)	New-Onset Type 2 DM (Group IIC, n = 58)	p
Age (years)	58.3 ± 8.7	36 ± 8.6	60.1 ± 9.3	<0.001
Male patients	7 (58.3%)	4 (57.1%)	30 (51.7%)	0.895
BMI	29.1 ± 6.7	21.4 ± 2.4	33.9 ± 9	<0.001 **
Hypertensive	1 (8.3%)	0	8 (13.8%)	0.520
IHD	0	0	7 (12.1%)	0.283
Family history of DM	5 (41.7%)	2 (28.6%)	27 (46.6%)	0.652
Severe COVID-19	8 (66.7%)	7 (100%)	54 (93.1%)	0.015
FPG (mg/dL)	194.3 ± 64.3	473.4 ± 124.4	179.2 ± 64.5	<0.001 **
HbA1C	7.2 ± 0.4	5.3 ± 0.5	5.4 ± 0.5	<0.001
Fasting insulin (mIU/L)	33.4 ± 9.2	3.6 ± 1.3	38.1 ± 9.1	<0.001
C-peptide (ng/mL)	3.5 ± 1	0.3 ± 0.1	3.6 ± 0.8	<0.001 **
Positive urinary acetone	0	4 (57.1%)	0	<0.001
DKA on presentation	0	4 (57.1%)	0	<0.001
Hemoglobin (g/dL)	12.2 ± 1.9	10.9 ± 1.4	12 ± 1.3	0.119

Table 2. Cont.

Variables	No. (%), Mean ± SD or Median.			p
	Pre-Existing DM (Group IIA, n = 12)	New-Onset Type 1 DM (Group IIB, n = 7)	New-Onset Type 2 DM (Group IIC, n = 58)	
Platelets count ($\times 10^3$/mm^3)	154.9 ± 32.4	190.1 ± 88.2	190.4 ± 50.1	0.103
WBCs ($\times 10^3$/mm^3)	6.3 ± 2.5	6.9 ± 2.9	6.2 ± 2.3	0.747
Lymphocytes (mean ± SD, $\times 10^3$/mm^3)	1.7 ± 0.9	1 ± 0.3	1.5 ± 0.8	0.282
Absolute lymphopenia (<1 $\times 10^3$/mm^3)	6 (50%)	6 (85.7%)	34 (58.6%)	0.291
CRP (mg/L)	55.7 ± 31	113.1 ± 56.9	48.4 ± 29.2	0.004 **
ESR ((mm/h)	39.5 ± 15.3	52.7 ± 14.4	42 ± 14.1	0.130
Serum ferritin (ng/mL)	318.9 ± 177.9	832 ± 252.7	300.6 ± 171.2	0.002 **
LDH (IU/L)	256.1 ± 82.5	360 ± 100.8	284.6 ± 85.1	0.100 **
D-dimer (µg/mL)	0.9 ± 0.5	5 ± 5.3	1.2 ± 0.9	0.007 s**
Serum creatinine (mg/dL)	1 ± 1.3	1.1 ± 0.3	1 ± 0.2	0.336
Blood urea (mg/dL)	29 ± 19	49.3 ± 37.6	37.1 ± 26	0.272
Positive chest CT findings	8 (66.7%)	7 (100%)	54 (93.1%)	0.015
Deceased	3 (25%)	3 (42.9%)	8 (13.8%)	0.136

Unless otherwise indicated, data represent the mean ± SD with the range in parenthesis. No: number; SD: standard deviation; BMI: body mass index; IHD: ischemic heart disease; WBCs: white blood cells; CRP: C-reactive protein; ESR: erythrocyte sedimentation rate; LDH: lactate dehydrogenase; IU: international unit; CT: computerized tomography. **: Kruskal–Wallis Test.

Table 3. Correlation between presence of newly diagnosed DM and different clinical and laboratory parameters (n = 570).

Variables	R	p
Age (years)	0.354	<0.001 *
BMI	0.312	<0.001 **
Severe COVID-19	0.297	<0.001 **
Lymphocytes ($\times 10^3$/mm^3)	−0.236	<0.001 *
Absolute lymphopenia (<1 $\times 10^3$/mm^3)	0.260	<0.001 *
CRP (mg/L)	0.186	<0.001 **
Serum ferritin (ng/mL)	0.222	<0.001 **
LDH	0.191	<0.001 **
D-dimer (µg/mL)	0.202	<0.001 **
Positive chest CT findings	0.297	<0.001 **

r: correlation coefficient; BMI: body mass index; CRP: C-reactive protein; LDH: lactate dehydrogenase; IU: international unit; CT: computerized tomography. *: Pearson's correlation; **: Spearman's correlation.

Table 4. Logistic regression analysis for predictors of presence of newly diagnosed DM among COVID-19 patients (n = 570).

Variables	B	Exp (B)	95% C.I. for Exp (B)		p
			Lower	Upper	
COVID-19 severity	−1.300	0.272	0.096	0.776	0.015
Age	0.081	1.084	1.047	1.123	<0.001
BMI	0.175	1.192	1.123	1.265	<0.001
Lymphocytes	−0.562	0.570	0.329	0.988	0.045
Lymphopenia	0.975	2.650	0.859	8.176	0.090
CRP	0.023	1.024	1.010	1.037	<0.001
Ferritin	0.003	1.003	1.001	1.004	<0.001
LDH	−0.002	0.998	0.994	1.003	0.456
D. dimer	0.020	1.020	0.824	1.264	0.854

CI: confidence interval; BMI: body mass index; CRP: C-reactive protein; LDH: lactate dehydrogenase.

Predictors of mortality among COVID-19 patients (62/570, 10.9%) comprised older age, hypertension, ischemic heart disease (IHD), development of DM, DKA on presentation, severe COVID-19 infection, positive Chest CT findings, elevated CRP, elevated ferritin, lymphopenia, and elevated D-dimer ($p < 0.001$, for each) (Table 5).

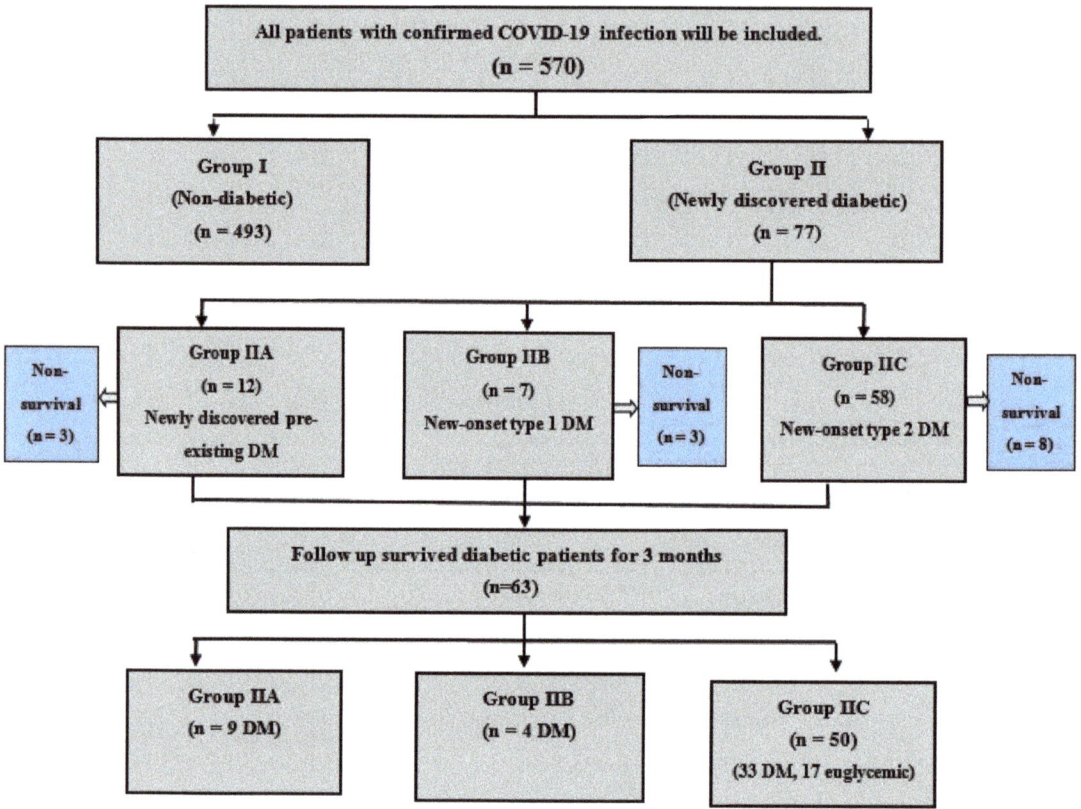

Figure 1. Flow diagram of study participants.

Table 5. Predictors of mortality among all participants (62/570, 10.9%).

Variables	No. (%), Mean ± SD or Median.		p
	Survived Patients (n = 508)	Died Patients (n = 62)	
Age (years)	47.4 ± 10.9	52.2 ± 9.6	<0.001
Male gender	279 (54.9%)	38 (61.3)	0.341
BMI	25.9 ± 5.6	26.7 ± 7.8	0.284
Hypertensive	33 (6.5%)	12 (19.4%)	<0.001 *
IHD	14 (2.8%)	5 (8.1%)	0.028 *
Newly discovered DM	63 (12.4%)	14 (22.6%)	0.027
Type of DM			
Pre-existing DM	9 (1.8%)	3 (4.8%)	
DM type 1	4 (0.8%)	3 (4.8%)	0.012 *
DM type 2	50 (9.8%)	8 (12.9%)	
Severe COVID-19	247 (48.6%)	50 (80.6%)	<0.001
FPG (mg/dL)	103.5 ± 49.9	125.5 ± 100.5	0.179 **
HbA1C	5.4 ± 0.6	5.4 ± 0.6	0.966
DKA on presentation	2 (0.4%)	2 (3.2%)	<0.012 *
Hemoglobin (g/dL)	11.8 ± 1.4	11.7 ± 1.1	0.455

Table 5. Cont.

Variables	No. (%), Mean ± SD or Median.		p
	Survived Patients (n = 508)	Died Patients (n = 62)	
Platelets count ($\times 10^3$/mm^3)	192.1 ± 50.5	185.1 ± 51.2	0.305
WBCs ($\times 10^3$/mm^3)	6.5 ± 2.6	5.9 ± 2.4	0.113
Lymphocytes ($\times 10^3$/mm^3)	2.3 ± 1.1	1.2 ± 0.9	<0.001 **
Absolute lymphopenia (<1 × 10^3/mm^3)	116 (22.8%)	53 (85.5%)	<0.001 *
CRP (mg/dL)	36.2 ± 20.2	60.9 ± 36.9	<0.001 **
ESR (mm/h)	41.4 ± 14.1	40.0 ± 13.4	0.458
Serum ferritin (ng/mL)	223.4 ± 157.2	338.7 ± 230.5	<0.001 **
LDH (IU/L)	237.7 ± 75.5	316.2 ± 86.6	<0.001 **
D-dimer (µg/mL)	0.9 ± 0.9	1.9 ± 3.1	<0.001 **
Serum creatinine (mg/dL)	1 ± 0.3	1 ± 0.3	0.610
Blood urea (mg/dL)	36.1 ± 24.8	40.3 ± 30.5	0.367 **
INR	1.1 ± 0.2	1.2 ± 0.2	0.321
Serum albumin (g/dL)	3.6 ± 0.5	3.6 ± 0.5	0.328
Serum total bilirubin (g/dL)	1.1 ± 0.2	1.1 ± 0.2	0.764 **
ALT (IU/L)	34.4 ± 24.1	29.6 ± 19.5	0.269 **
AST (IU/L)	56.9 ± 38.7	50.2 ± 27.7	0.435 **
Positive chest CT findings	247 (48.6%)	50 (80.6%)	<0.001

Unless otherwise indicated, data represent the mean ± SD with the range in parenthesis. No: number; SD: standard deviation; BMI: body mass index; IHD: ischemic heart disease; WBCs: white blood cells; CRP: C-reactive protein; ESR: erythrocyte sedimentation rate; LDH: lactate dehydrogenase; IU: international unit; INR: international normalized ratio; ALT: alanine aminotransferase; AST: aspartate aminotransferase; CT: computerized tomography. *: Fisher's Exact Test; **: Mann–Whitney Test.

3.2. Follow-Up Phase (for DM)

All patients with newly diagnosed DM (n = 77) were given the appropriate anti-diabetic treatment (starting with insulin therapy). Four cases of DKA were diagnosed (all among type I DM patients) and were managed successfully in ICU. Out of 77 cases of newly diagnosed DM, 14 patients died shortly (1–19 days after diagnosis) from COVID-19 sequelae. Survived diabetic patients (n = 63) were followed for three months with repeated testing of FBS.

3.3. Study Endpoint (Glycemic Control after 3 Months)

Hyperglycemia and the need for anti-diabetic treatment (insulin therapy or oral drugs) persisted in 73% of surviving diabetic patients (46/63), whereas anti-diabetic treatment could be stopped in 17 patients (27%). Hyperglycemia persisted in all survived patients with pre-existing DM (n = 9). In survived subjects with new-onset DM types I and II (n = 54), hyperglycemia persisted in 37 patients (68.5%), including all four patients with DM type I and 66% of patients with DM type II (33/50).

4. Discussion

The COVID-19 outbreak is increasing rapidly throughout the world. The new virus responsible for this epidemic was named as SARS-CoV-2, which has now turned into a global catastrophe [12]. COVID-19 causes a novel pathophysiological alteration in glucose homeostasis (a combination of severe insulin resistance and insulin insufficiency), making COVID-19-related diabetes management difficult [13].

The purpose of this cross-sectional study was to determine the frequency of newly diagnosed DM and its different types among COVID-19 patients and to explore the infection outcome and glycemic control of newly diagnosed diabetic patients during the study.

In the first phase of this biphasic cross-sectional study, newly diagnosed diabetes (FPG > 126) was defined in 77 patients (13.5%). This agreed with several studies. Wang et al. reported that 29.1% (176/605) of COVID-19 patients with no previous diagnosis of DM had FPG ≥ 126 mg/dL [14]. Smith et al. reported that COVID-19 is associated with increased FPG and 15.8% of patients developed new-onset DM [15]. Guan et al. stated that DM was discovered in 7.4% of a cohort of COVID-19 hospitalized patients and appeared to be a risk factor for the severity of illness [16]. Finally, a meta-analysis of eight studies with more than 3700 patients showed a pooled proportion of 14.4% for newly diagnosed diabetes in COVID-19 hospitalized patients [17].

HbA1c was performed for all newly diagnosed diabetic patients to differentiate between new-onset and pre-existing DM; fasting insulin and C-peptide were also performed to differentiate between new-onset type 1 DM and new-onset type 2 DM. Accordingly, out of 77 newly diagnosed diabetic patients, newly discovered pre-existing DM was defined in 12 patients (2.1%), new-onset type 1 DM developed in 7 patients (1.2%), and 58 patients (10.2%) had new-onset type 2 DM. However, in some studies, HbA1c was not performed for all participants, so it was not possible to differentiate between new-onset and previously undiagnosed diabetes [14,18].

In the present study, as compared to non-diabetic patients, the newly diagnosed diabetic patients had significantly older age (57.7 $\pm$ 11.4, vs. 46.4 $\pm$ 10, $p < 0.001$), higher BMI (32 $\pm$ 9 vs. 25 $\pm$ 4.5, $p < 0.001$), and positive family history of diabetes (44.2% vs. 4.5%, $p < 0.001$). This was in agreement with Li H et al., who reported that COVID-19 patients with newly diagnosed DM and hyperglycemia were slightly older and obese [19].

In the current work, four patients (all with new-onset type 1 DM) presented with diabetic ketoacidosis (DKA) on admission. This was in agreement with Reddy et al., who stated that COVID-19 may accelerate DKA in those with new-onset or pre-existing DM [20].

Our study also revealed that patients with newly diagnosed DM had more severe infection symptoms such as fever, dyspnea, and cough, as well as elevated levels of inflammatory markers such as CRP, LDH, and ferritin than non-diabetic patients. Our results were in concordance with Li H et al., who stated that patients with newly diagnosed diabetes and hyperglycemia often had more severe symptoms as well as higher levels of inflammatory markers [19]. Infection with COVID-19 decreases ACE2 expression, resulting in hyperinflammation, cellular damage, and respiratory failure [21].

The results of the current study revealed that positive chest CT findings (89% vs. 46%, $p < 0.001$) and D-dimer (1.5 $\pm$ 2 vs. 0.9 $\pm$ 1.2, $p < 0.001$) were higher in diabetic group as compared to non-diabetic group.

Mortality within the COVID-19 patients of our study was significantly higher among newly diagnosed diabetic than non-diabetic patients (18.2% vs. 9.7%, $p = 0.046$). Likewise, one study from the United States found that COVID-19 patients who are diabetics had a markedly higher mortality than patients without diabetes (28.8% vs. 6.2%) [22]. Furthermore, Li H et al. reported that in patients with COVID-19, newly diagnosed DM is connected to increased mortality when compared to known DM and normal glucose levels [19]. Chronic hyperglycemia was linked to decreased immunity, and hyperglycemia was found to be an independent predictor of lower respiratory tract infection and poor prognosis [4].

Our logistic regression analysis showed that older age, higher BMI, elevated CRP, and elevated ferritin were the significant predictors of newly diagnosed DM among COVID-19 patients ($p < 0.001$).

The results of the current study revealed that increasing age, hypertension, IHD, and high levels of D-dimer were reported as important predictors of mortality among COVID-19 patients. This agreed with Zhou et al., who confirmed that the death rate was higher in elderly patients with COVID-19 [23]. Rodelo et al. stated that increased levels of D-dimer have been linked to 28-day mortality in patients with severe infection or sepsis in intensive care units [24]. A pooled analysis stated that hypertension is associated with a 2.5-fold increased risk of both severity and mortality in COVID-19 patients [25]. Moreover, Bonow et al. found that patients with underlying cardiovascular disease are more likely to have serious COVID-19 outcomes, including death, as we discovered in our study [26].

Out of the 77 patients with DM, 14 (18.2%) patients died shortly (1–19 days) due to COVID-19 sequelae. The remaining 63 patients were followed for three months. Hyperglycemia and the need for anti-diabetic treatment persisted in 46 (73%) patients, while 17 (27%) patients became euglycemic and did not need anti-diabetic treatment after recovery from the acute illness, indicating that they had stress-induced hyperglycemia, an adaptive immune-neurohormonal response to physiological stress.

To the best of our knowledge, this is the first study to assess the different types of newly diagnosed DM among COVID-19 patients and to explore the persistence of hyperglycemia over the study duration, as assessed by laboratory measurements and follow-up. As a contribution of this study, it raises the hypothesis for the development of a large-scale multinational study to assess the development and prevention of DM in COVID-19 patients. The relatively short follow-up duration was a limitation to this study.

5. Conclusions

A significant proportion of COVID-19 patients (13.5%) experienced the appearance of new-onset DM and expression of pre-existing DM during disease course, both being frequent with more severe infection. The newly diagnosed DM persisted for three months in about two-thirds of affected subjects. COVID-19 patients with newly diagnosed diabetes had high risk of mortality compared with COVID-19 patients without diabetes. Increasing age, hypertension, IHD, and high levels of D-dimer were reported as important predictors of mortality among COVID-19 patients. We recommend that a patient with COVID-19 infection have their blood glucose levels constantly checked for the emergence of full-blown diabetes. Newly diagnosed diabetes should be handled early and effectively.

Author Contributions: A.A.F. and K.E. selected the idea, designed the study, and completed the final revision of the data; H.M.H., H.H.S., and E.S.A.e. helped with the data collection and analysis; A.S. and A.M.S. carried out the laboratory work. All authors have read and agreed to the published version of the manuscript.

Funding: This work has not received any funding.

Institutional Review Board Statement: The study was carried out in a manner consistent with the ethical principles of the Declaration of Helsinki, and it was approved by the Institutional Review Board (IRB) of the Faculty of Medicine, Zagazig University, Zagazig, Egypt (approval no. 6790).

Informed Consent Statement: Written informed consent was received from all subjects involved in the study.

Data Availability Statement: Not applicable.

Acknowledgments: The authors thank all patients who participated in the study and all resident physicians and nursing staff who helped to complete this study.

Conflicts of Interest: The authors declare no conflict of interest.

References

1. Wang, Y.; Wang, Y.; Chen, Y.; Qin, Q. Unique epidemiological and clinical features of the emerging 2019 novel coronavirus pneumonia (COVID-19) implicate special control measures. *J. Med. Virol.* **2020**, *92*, 568–576. [CrossRef]
2. Lu, R.; Zhao, X.; Li, J.; Niu, P.; Yang, B.; Wu, H.; Wang, W.; Song, H.; Huang, B.; Zhu, N.; et al. Genomic characterisation and epidemiology of 2019 novel coronavirus: Implications for virus origins and receptor binding. *Lancet* **2020**, *395*, 565–574. [CrossRef]
3. WHO. Coronavirus (COVID-19) Dashboard I WHO Coronavirus (COVID-19) Dashboard with Vaccination Data. Available online: https://covid19.who.int/ (accessed on 7 July 2021).
4. Pearson-Stuttard, J.; Blundell, S.; Harris, T.; Cook, D.G.; Critchley, J. Diabetes and infection: Assessing the association with glycaemic control in population-based studies. *Lancet Diabetes Endocrinol.* **2016**, *4*, 148–158. [CrossRef]
5. Gentile, S.; Strollo, F.; Mambro, A.; Ceriello, A. COVID-19, ketoacidosis and new-onset diabetes: Are there possible cause and effect relationships among them? *Diabetes Obes. Metab.* **2020**, *22*, 2507–2508. [CrossRef]
6. Apicella, M.; Campopiano, M.C.; Mantuano, M.; Mazoni, L.; Coppelli, A.; Del Prato, S. COVID-19 in people with diabetes: Understanding the reasons for worse outcomes. *Lancet Diabetes Endocrinol.* **2020**, *8*, 782–792. [CrossRef]
7. Li, J.; Wang, X.; Chen, J.; Zuo, X.; Zhang, H.; Deng, A. COVID-19 infection may cause ketosis and ketoacidosis. *Diabetes Obes. Metab.* **2020**, *22*, 1935–1941. [CrossRef]
8. Maddaloni, E.; Buzzetti, R. COVID-19 and diabetes mellitus: Unveiling the interaction of two pandemics. *Diabetes/Metab. Res. Rev.* **2020**, *36*, e3321. [CrossRef] [PubMed]
9. Prete, M.; Favoino, E.; Catacchio, G.; Racanelli, V.; Perosa, F. SARS-CoV-2 inflammatory syndrome. Clinical features and rationale for immunological treatment. *Int. J. Mol. Sci.* **2020**, *21*, 3377. [CrossRef]

10. *COVID-19 Diagnosis and Treatment Guideline in China*, 7th ed.; National Health Commission of the People's Republic of China. Available online: http://www.nhc.gov.cn/yzygj/s7653p/202003/46c9294a7dfe4cef80dc7f5912eb1989.shtml (accessed on 17 March 2020).
11. American Diabetes Association. 2. Classification and diagnosis of diabetes: Standards of medical Care in diabetes-2020. *Diabetes Care* **2020**, *43* (Suppl. 1), S14–S31. [CrossRef]
12. Chen, Y.; Gong, X.; Wang, L.; Guo, J. Effects of hypertension, diabetes and coronary heart disease on COVID-19 diseases severity: A systematic review and meta-analysis. *medRxiv* **2020**. [CrossRef]
13. Sathish, T.; Tapp, R.J.; Cooper, M.E.; Zimmet, P. Potential metabolic and inflammatory pathways between COVID-19 and new-onset diabetes. *Diabetes Metab.* **2021**, *47*, 101204. [CrossRef]
14. Wang, S.; Ma, P.; Zhang, S.; Song, S.; Wang, Z.; Ma, Y.; Xu, J.; Wu, F.; Duan, L.; Yin, Z.; et al. Fasting blood glucose at admission is an independent predictor for 28-day mortality in patients with COVID-19 without previous diagnosis of diabetes: A multi-centre retrospective study. *Diabetologia* **2020**, *63*, 2102–2111. [CrossRef]
15. Smith, S.M.; Boppana, A.; Traupman, J.A.; Unson, E.; Maddock, D.A.; Chao, K.; Dobesh, D.P.; Brufsky, A.; Connor, R.I. Impaired glucose metabolism in patients with diabetes, prediabetes, and obesity is associated with severe COVID-19. *J. Med. Virol.* **2021**, *93*, 409–415. [CrossRef]
16. Guan, W.J.; Ni, Z.Y.; Hu, Y.; Liang, W.H.; Ou, C.Q.; He, J.X.; Liu, L.; Shan, H.; Lei, C.L.; Hui, D.S.; et al. Clinical characteristics of corona virus disease 2019 in China. *N. Engl. J. Med.* **2020**, *382*, 1708–1720. [CrossRef]
17. Sathish, T.; Kapoor, N.; Cao, Y.; Tapp, R.J.; Zimmet, P. Proportion of newly diagnosed diabetes in COVID-19 patients: A systematic review and meta-analysis. *Diabetes Obes. Metab.* **2021**, *23*, 870–874. [CrossRef] [PubMed]
18. Fadini, G.P.; Morieri, M.L.; Boscari, F.; Fioretto, P.; Maran, A.; Busetto, L.; Tresso, S.; Cattelan, A.M.; Vettor, R. Newly diagnosed diabetes and admission hyperglycemia predict COVID-19 severity by aggravating respiratory deterioration. *Diabetes Res. Clin. Pract.* **2020**, *168*, 108374. [CrossRef] [PubMed]
19. Li, H.; Tian, S.; Chen, T.; Cui, Z.; Shi, N.; Zhong, X.; Qiu, K.; Zhang, J.; Zeng, T.; Chen, L.; et al. Newly diagnosed diabetes is associated with a higher risk of mortality than known diabetes in hospitalized patients with COVID-19. *Diabetes Obes. Metab.* **2020**, *22*, 1897–1906. [CrossRef] [PubMed]
20. Reddy, P.K.; Kuchay, M.S.; Mehta, Y.; Mishra, S.K. Diabetic ketoacidosis precipitated by COVID-19: A report of two cases and review of literature. *Diabetes Metab. Syndr.* **2020**, *14*, 1459–1462. [CrossRef] [PubMed]
21. Hoffmann, M.; Kleine-Weber, H.; Schroeder, S.; Krüger, N.; Herrler, T.; Erichsen, S.; Schiergens, T.S.; Herrler, G.; Wu, N.H.; Nitsche, A.; et al. SARS-CoV-2 Cell Entry Depends on ACE2 and TMPRSS2 and Is Blocked by a Clinically Proven Protease Inhibitor. *Cell* **2020**, *181*, 271–280. [CrossRef]
22. Bode, B.; Garrett, V.; Messler, J.; McFarland, R.; Crowe, J.; Booth, R.; Klonoff, D.C. Glycemic Characteristics and Clinical Outcomes of COVID-19 Patients Hospitalized in the United States. *J. Diabetes Sci. Technol.* **2020**, *14*, 813–821. [CrossRef]
23. Zhou, F.; Yu, T.; Du, R.; Fan, G.; Liu, Y.; Liu, Z.; Xiang, J.; Wang, Y.; Song, B.; Gu, X.; et al. Clinical course and risk factors for mortality of adult inpatients with COVID-19 in Wuhan, China: A retrospective cohort study. *Lancet* **2020**, *395*, 1054–1062. [CrossRef]
24. Rodelo, J.R.; De la Rosa, G.; Valencia, M.L.; Ospina, S.; Arango, C.M.; Gómez, C.I.; García, A.; Nuñez, E.; Jaimes, F.A. D-dimer is a significant prognostic factor in patients with suspected infection and sepsis. *Am. J. Emerg. Med.* **2012**, *30*, 1991–1999. [CrossRef]
25. Lippi, G.; Wong, J.; Henry, B.M. Hypertension in patients with coronavirus disease 2019 (COVID-19): A pooled analysis. *Pol. Arch. Intern. Med.* **2020**, *130*, 304–309. [PubMed]
26. Bonow, R.O.; Fonarow, G.C.; O'Gara, P.T.; Yancy, C.W. Association of coronavirus disease 2019 (COVID-19) with myocardial injury and mortality. *JAMA Cardiol.* **2020**, *5*, 751–753. [CrossRef] [PubMed]

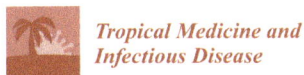

Tropical Medicine and
Infectious Disease

Review

Coagulopathy of Dengue and COVID-19: Clinical Considerations

Amin Islam [1,2,*], Christopher Cockcroft [1], Shereen Elshazly [1,3], Javeed Ahmed [4], Kevin Joyce [1], Huque Mahfuz [5], Tasbirul Islam [6], Harunor Rashid [7,8] and Ismail Laher [9]

1. Department of Haematology, Mid & South Essex University Hospital NHS Foundation Trust, Prittlewell Chase, Westcliff-on-Sea SS0 0RY, UK
2. Department of Haematology, Queen Mary University of London, Mile End Road, London E1 3NS, UK
3. Adult Haemato-Oncology Unit, Faculty of Medicine, Ainshams University, Cairo 11566, Egypt
4. Department of Microbiology and Virology, Mid & South Essex University Hospital NHS Foundation Trust, Westcliff-on-Sea SS0 0RY, UK
5. Department of Haematology and Oncology, Combined Military Hospital, Dhaka 1206, Bangladesh
6. Department of Pulmonology and Critical Care Medicine, Indiana School of Medicine, Lafayette, IN 47907, USA
7. National Centre for Immunisation Research and Surveillance, The Children's Hospital at Westmead, Westmead, NSW 2145, Australia
8. Sydney Institute for Infectious Diseases, The University of Sydney, Westmead, NSW 2145, Australia
9. Department of Anesthesiology, Pharmacology & Therapeutics, Faculty of Medicine, The University of British Colombia, Vancouver, BC V6T 1Z3, Canada
* Correspondence: amin.islam@qmul.ac.uk

Abstract: Thrombocytopenia and platelet dysfunction commonly occur in both dengue and COVID-19 and are related to clinical outcomes. Coagulation and fibrinolytic pathways are activated during an acute dengue infection, and endothelial dysfunction is observed in severe dengue. On the other hand, COVID-19 is characterised by a high prevalence of thrombotic complications, where bleeding is rare and occurs only in advanced stages of critical illness; here thrombin is the central mediator that activates endothelial cells, and elicits a pro-inflammatory reaction followed by platelet aggregation. Serological cross-reactivity may occur between COVID-19 and dengue infection. An important management aspect of COVID-19-induced immunothrombosis associated with thrombocytopenia is anticoagulation with or without aspirin. In contrast, the use of aspirin, nonsteroidal anti-inflammatory drugs and anticoagulants is contraindicated in dengue. Mild to moderate dengue infections are treated with supportive therapy and paracetamol for fever. Severe infection such as dengue haemorrhagic fever and dengue shock syndrome often require escalation to higher levels of support in a critical care facility. The role of therapeutic platelet transfusion is equivocal and should not be routinely used in patients with dengue with thrombocytopaenia and mild bleeding. The use of prophylactic platelet transfusion in dengue fever has strained financial and healthcare systems in endemic areas, together with risks of transfusion-transmitted infections in low- and middle-income countries. There is a clear research gap in the management of dengue with significant bleeding.

Keywords: COVID-19; cross-reactivity; dengue; haemorrhage; thrombocytopenia; thrombosis

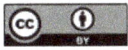

1. Introduction

The exponential spread of COVID-19 that started early in 2020 resulted in one of the worst global pandemics of our lifetime, leading to a gauntlet of clinical challenges, including responding to unique patterns of coagulation anomalies. The COVID-19 outbreak has further added to clinical challenges in tropical and subtropical regions of the world, where dengue fever, caused by dengue virus (DENV) is also endemic. Similarities in clinical manifestations of COVID-19 and dengue fever often create diagnostic dilemmas in dengue-endemic countries with limited resources, often leading to delayed or even incorrect diagnosis. Furthermore, there are growing concerns of cross-reactivity due to pre-existing DENV-antibodies that potentially can enhance COVID-19 antibody-dependent immune responses [1]. Mild to moderate thrombocytopenia are common to both conditions but have different clinico-pathological aetiologies and treatment approaches, making earlier diagnosis key to preventing severe outcomes. Moreover, despite mild to moderate thrombocytopenia in COVID-19 diseases, anticoagulation is an integral part of the treatment protocols of COVID-19 [2]. In contrast, treatment with anticoagulants is contraindicated in dengue infections and non-steroidal anti-inflammatory agents are also avoided merely because of their theoretic risk of aggravated bleeding such as from the gastrointestinal tract [3]. There are concerns about the indiscriminate use of prophylactic platelet transfusions in dengue viral infections, especially in tropical dengue-endemic areas where the availability of safe transfusion services remains a significant challenge due to greater risks of transfusion-transmitted infections and other immunological concerns.

DENVs are the most important human arboviruses worldwide. Transmission of dengue occurs via Aedes mosquitoes, producing four antigenically distinct serotypes (DENV-1 to DENV-4). Clinical presentations range from mild to more severe infections, with significant morbidities and mortalities in endemic areas. It is estimated that there are currently 50–100 million cases of dengue infections worldwide annually, with more than 500,000 reported cases of severe forms of dengue infections such as dengue haemorrhagic fever (DHF) and dengue shock syndrome (DSS) [4]. The immunological cross-reactivity and common pathological processes, such as capillary leakage, thrombocytopenia, and coagulopathy, between SARS-CoV-2 and DENV, make it difficult to distinguish their shared clinical and laboratory characteristics (Table 1) [1]. Patients with dengue fever, including those with positive non-structural protein 1 (NS1) and/or IgM serology results, should be differentiated from those with SARS-CoV-2 infection, and if necessary, dengue IgM/IgG testing should be repeated to identify co-infection or serological overlap [5]. It is necessary to prepare for dengue outbreaks alongside controlling the COVID-19 pandemic, as a resurgence poses a very real threat [6].

Table 1. Comparing dengue and COVID-19, based on data from Henrina et al. [7] and Centers for Disease Control and Prevention guidance [8].

General Features:	Dengue	COVID-19
Virology		
Family	Flaviviridae	Coronaviridae
Diameter	50 nm	65–125 nm
Genetic Material	ssRNA	ssRNA
Presentation		
Incubation	3–10 days	2 to 14 (median 4–5) days
Fever	Saddleback fever (with 2 peaks)	No specific fever patterns. Defervescence after 6 days of illness
Headache	45–95%	6.5–13.6%
Myalgia	12%	15–44%
Cough	21.5%	76%
Dyspnoea	9.5–95.2%	55%
Diarrhoea	6%	2–34%
Abdominal pain	17–25%	2%
Vomiting	30–58%	4–5%

Table 1. *Cont.*

General Features:	Dengue	COVID-19
Cutaneous manifestation	Skin flushing that blanch on pressure, petechiae, and convalescent rash	Erythematous rash, urticaria, chickenpox-like vesicles
Warning signs:	Persistent vomiting, mucosal bleeding, difficulty in breathing, lethargy/restlessness, postural hypotension, liver enlargement and progressive increases in haematocrit	Difficulty in breathing, persistent pain or pressure in the chest, new confusion, inability to wake or stay awake, bluish lips or face
Laboratory Findings		
Thrombocytopenia	69.51–100%	12–36.2%
Leukopenia	20–82.2%	25–29%
Lymphopenia	63%	63%
Raised AST	63–97%	31–35%
Raised ALT	45–97%	24–28%
Raised D-dimer	13–87%	46.4%

2. Virology of DENV

DENV is a single-stranded RNA virus of the Flaviviridae family. Each of the four DENV serotypes vary in their epidemiological patterns, but some countries may have hyperendemicity with more than one serotype actively circulating at the same time [4], as in the Indian subcontinent and South East Asia. There may be different genotypes with minor antigenic changes within the same serotype. Life-long immunity develops after infection with the same serotype, but with only a partial and short-lived immunity to another serotype. The recorded number of confirmed dengue cases may not accurately reflect the true burden of dengue, as many patients are asymptomatic or remain undiagnosed.

The gold standard test to confirm dengue is by reverse transcriptase-PCR (rt-PCR) targeting regions within the genome of DENV. Resource-limited countries rely on detecting DENV IgG and IgM. The serology tests could cross-react with other flaviviruses; hence the mainstay is testing for active viremia by rt-PCR [9]. Antigenic assays have recently been developed that target NS1 which is secreted in infected mammalian cells. A serotype-specific mAb-based NS1 antigen-capture ELISA has reliable serotype specificity [10]. Whilst the cross-reactivity is observed in serological assays of DENV, there is no evidence that an infection with DENV confers cross-infectivity to other viruses such as West Nile virus, Japanese Encephalitis virus, or other arthropod-borne flaviviruses. An exception is cross-reactivity of DENV with yellow fever virus, the underlying cause of which remains unknown.

3. Virology of COVID-19

COVID-19 is caused by SARS-CoV-2, of the order Nidovirales within the family Coronaviridae. It is an enveloped, positive-sense single-stranded RNA (+ssRNA) virus of dimension between 65 and 125 nm [8]. Cell membrane attachment is achieved through a spike protein interaction with cell surface receptor angiotensin-converting enzyme receptor 2 (ACE2), leading to membrane fusion and deposition of the virion's genetic material into the cytoplasm.

New sub-variants of SARS-CoV-2 have emerged with varying clinical significance, including transmission rates and susceptibility to vaccination [11,12]. As a whole, SARS-CoV-2 shows structural similarities to two of its relatives, SARS-CoV (Severe Acute Respiratory Syndrome-Coronavirus) and MERS-CoV (Middle Eastern Respiratory Syndrome-Coronavirus) [11] both of which have caused recent epidemics.

4. Epidemiology of Dengue

Dengue is the second most diagnosed cause of fever after malaria in travelers returning from low- and middle-income countries. The global incidence of dengue continues to grow, even though most cases are asymptomatic or mild and self-managed, suggesting that case numbers are likely under-reported. Many cases are also misdiagnosed as other febrile illnesses [13]. Dengue is endemic in 129 countries with 390 million cases globally per year, of which 96 million manifest clinically, with the majority (70%) of the burden being in Asia [14,15]. Dengue is now spreading to new areas including Europe, with explosive outbreaks also occurring. There were 2000 cases of dengue in the Madeira Islands of Portugal in 2012, with imported cases detected in mainland Portugal and 10 other European countries.

The largest recent outbreak of dengue was in 2019, when all the World Health Organization (WHO) Regions were affected. The Region of the Americas alone reported 3.1 million cases, with more than 25,000 cases classified as severe [16]. Dengue affected several countries in 2020; however, cases drastically reduced by 55–65% with the advent of the COVID-19 wave in the year 2021 across the globe indicating an 'inverse relationship' between the two diseases [17].

Lifestyle changes and globalisation place severe limitations on the control of mosquito vectors to reduce dengue viral infections, in part due to rapid urbanisation in many counties. The increasing use of containers for water storage, such as automobile tyres and plastic containers, creates ideal sites for oviposition and larval habitats for *Aedes aegypti* mosquitoes. Most of the mosquito-control efforts directed at adult mosquitoes in the early 1970s used expensive methods that were largely ineffective. Changing human lifestyles creates more larval habitats, thus facilitating dengue transmission by increasing mosquito populations in areas with crowded human habitation [18].

5. Epidemiology of COVID-19

COVID-19 was first described in Wuhan province (China) in December 2019. It quickly spread throughout the world and was designated a Public Health Emergency of International Concern (PHEIC), the WHO's highest level of alert, on 30 January 2020. The resultant pandemic created dramatic lockdown measures across the globe that affected international and local travel. There were over 541 million confirmed COVID-19 cases and 6.3 million deaths reported to the WHO as of 4 July 2022 [19].

SARS-CoV-2 is believed to have crossed the species barrier to humans from an animal reservoir, most likely from bats [20]. Transmission is believed to occur either through large droplets or aerosols in the form of coughing or sneezing [21]. As such, the infection spreads best in densely packed communities, especially where physical distancing is not practiced, and where cough etiquette is not observed meticulously. There are also rare reports of faeco-oral or vertical transmissions [22].

The incubation period is variably reported to be between 2 and 14 days [22,23]. The period of infectivity extends from a few days before the symptom onset to several days post-symptom resolution [24]. Such a lag before the onset of warning signs and the cessation of infectivity, along with cases of asymptomatic spreading [25], allows COVID-19 to continue to spread even in a population vigilant of the signs and practicing symptomatic isolation.

The spectrum of COVID-19 severity varies from asymptomatic to life-threatening/fatal infection. Risk factors for severe infection include advanced age and presence of comorbidities [22] (Table 2). Vaccinations have become the leading deterrent for severe illness and hospitalisation [26].

Table 2. Risk factors for severe dengue and COVID-19, based on Centers for Disease Control and Prevention guidance [27–29].

	Dengue	COVID-19
Viral characteristics	Viral titer correlates with disease severity. There may be strain and serotype differences in pathogenicity.	Relationship between viral titer and severity poorly understood. Certain variants, (via increased transmission, vaccine resistance etc.).
Host factors	Age (infant) Women, especially pregnant women. Patients with chronic medical conditions, including diabetes, asthma, obesity and heart disease. Patients with secondary DENV infection.	Age (elderly) Pregnant/recently pregnant women. Comorbidities, such as chronic kidney disease, malignancy, chronic lung disease, dementia, cardiovascular disease, diabetes, immunosuppression, multiple comorbidities.

At the time of writing, the global outbreak of COVID-19 is largely receding, with the last peak recorded in January 2022 [19]. The WHO regions with the greatest burden of disease are the Americas, Europe and the Western Pacific region; however, inconsistencies in global surveillance and reporting systems are likely to misrepresent the true magnitude of the pandemic.

6. Severe Dengue in Adults and Infants

The risk of dengue infection in various patient groups is summarised in Table 2.

6.1. Antibody-Dependent Enhancement and Severe Dengue

Severe dengue most commonly occurs in infants and adults with secondary dengue infections (i.e., infection with a DENV type different from a previous DENV infection). The most widely cited hypothesis for this is antibody-dependent enhancement (ADE) of disease, which occurs when non-neutralising anti-DENV antibodies bind to, but do not neutralise, an infecting DENV. This virus-antibody complex allows for enhanced viral entry into host cells (specifically dendritic cells and macrophages) and the virus replicates and generates higher viral titers in blood than when the anti-DENV antibody is not present, resulting in a 'cytokine storm' and exacerbating the disease.

6.2. Severe Dengue among Infants

Infants in dengue-endemic areas have anti-DENV IgG antibodies at birth. Anti-DENV IgG antibodies are passed from a mother to foetus (IgM does not cross placenta). This passively transferred maternal anti-DENV IgG can protect the infant for a few months after birth, which can explain why the occurrence of dengue in infants under 4 months of age is unusual. However, as the maternal anti-DENV IgG titer falls 4–6 months after birth, ADE outweighs neutralisation, and the infant is at higher risk for severe disease even with a primary DENV infection. Children aged one year or more are not at increased risk.

7. General Aspects of Platelets and Haemostasis

Platelets play an integral part in primary haemostasis by forming a thrombus at the site of vascular injury; new platelets are produced daily to maintain a platelet count of $150–400 \times 10^9$ platelets/L blood [30–32]. Activated platelets undergo actin-mediated shape changes (from smooth discoid to spiny spheres) when passing through damaged blood vessels. Various receptors for adhesive and clotting proteins in activated platelets then attract other platelets to form a plug that limits vascular leakage [33].

Platelets activate neutrophils, monocytes and lymphocytes to form platelet-leukocyte aggregates, and thus participate in immune responses. It is possible that platelet surface receptors such as toll-like receptors (TLRs) and glycoprotein V1 play roles in immune responses [34]. A haemostatic envelope which prevents excessive bleeding after vascular injury is formed by exposure to membrane-bound tissue factor (TF) that is constitutively expressed on the cell surfaces of fibroblasts and muscle cells [35]. The conversion of factor X to Xa occurs after catalysis by TF-V11a, which further assembles the prothrombinase complex formed by factor Xa, factor Va, factor II (prothrombin) and Ca^{2+}, resulting in the generation of thrombin [36]. The semipermeable properties of endothelial cells are supported by platelets in a well-recognised process, where platelet activation releases proangiogenic molecules that mediate the migration and proliferation of vascular cells, and vessel organisation and stabilisation [37,38].

8. Coagulopathy in Dengue

Thrombocytopenia remains a potential indicator of clinical severity of dengue infection as per WHO guidelines, with the most recent WHO guidelines (from 2009) describing rapid decreases in platelet count, or a count of less than 150,000 per microliter of blood [39]. Coagulation and fibrinolytic pathways are activated during an acute dengue infection [40]. Thrombocytopenia, coagulopathy and vasculopathy are related to the platelet and endothelial dysfunction observed in severe dengue. A recent study reports that mild to moderate thrombocytopenia occurs 3 to 7 days (significantly on the 4th day) after infection and returns to normal levels on day 8 or 9 of infections in adult patients without shock [41]. There is no clear relationship between the platelet count, disease severity and bleeding manifestations in dengue viral infections in children [42]. A platelet count of 5×10^9/L and haematocrit (HCT) > 50 L/L (normal range 0.40–0.52) is associated with bleeding symptoms in adults, though a study of 245 dengue patients showed there is no clear correlation between clinical bleeding and platelet count, whereas 81 non-bleeding patients had a platelet count of $<20 \times 10^9$/L [43], while another study of 225 patients demonstrated bleeding to be more frequent when the platelet count reached below 20×10^9/L [44].

Most clinical guidelines recommend that platelet transfusions should be given to patients who develop serious haemorrhagic symptoms or when platelet count is below $10–20 \times 10^9$/L without haemorrhage. It is also advised that platelet transfusion should be considered in patients with bleeding manifestations when platelet count is below 50×10^9/L. However, the efficacy of platelet transfusions in dengue viral infection remains a matter of debate. A study involving 106 children with DSS who had thrombocytopenia and coagulopathy indicated no significant differences in bleeding manifestations between children who received platelets or not. Patients who received platelet transfusions had more transfusion-associated pulmonary oedema and longer hospital stays [45].

Severe thrombocytopenia and the secondary effects of hypoxia due to prolonged shock resulting in acidosis can trigger disseminated intravascular coagulation (DIC) and major haemorrhagic manifestations in some patients. Despite less severe bleeding and some minor abnormalities of basic clotting tests, all major pathways of the coagulation cascade are changed in children with DSS. Levels of proteins C, S and antithrombin are reduced secondary to leakage through the vascular endothelium, and correlate with the severity of shock in critical dengue infections. Direct activation of fibrinolysis by DENV may be secondary to raised levels of TF, thrombomodulin and plasminogen activator inhibitor 1 (PAI-1) which can then activate endothelial cells, platelets and monocytes.

The details of the pathogenesis of thrombocytopenia and bleeding are poorly understood, with many hypotheses offered on the pathogenesis, such as that DENV directly or indirectly affects bone marrow progenitor cells by inhibiting their function and reducing proliferative capacities [46], as supported by findings that DENV induces bone marrow hypoplasia during acute phases of the disease [47]. In addition to low platelet counts, functional disruption of platelets is associated with deregulation of the plasma kinin system and the immunopathogenesis of dengue [48]. Dengue viral infection induces platelet consumption due to DIC, platelet destruction due to increased apoptosis, lysis by the complement system and activation of antiplatelet antibodies [49]. Cytokines (e.g., TNF-α), interleukins (IL-2, IL-6, IL-8) and interferons (IFN-α and IFN-γ) also have roles in thrombocytopenia by suppressing haematopoiesis. Levels of these cytokines correlate with the clinical severity of dengue infection [50].

Other comorbidities increase the risk of severity of dengue; for example, allergy or diabetes increase the risk of DHF by 2.5 times, and hepatitis also increases the risk of complications. Increases in viral infections, hyperferritinaemia and the activation of coagulation and fibrinolytic systems occur in children with dengue compared to those without hyperferritinaemia. Other contributing factors to thrombocytopenia include cytokines, coagulation mediators, adhesive molecules and proteins, which encourage inflammatory response promoting cell interactions between platelets, immune cells and the endothelium. In addition, thrombocytopenia resulting from decreased bone marrow production and increased peripheral destruction of platelets, causes immune thrombocytopenia (ITP).

NS1 correlates well with levels of viremia, and is particularly high in patients suffering from DHF. Several mechanisms have been proposed by which NS1 contributes to the coagulopathy seen in DHF, such as proinflammatory cytokine release via activation of macrophages, and activation of complement, whilst expressed on the surface of infected cells and when released into the surrounding plasma, both of which contribute to endothelial damage and increase permeability, leading to DHF [51]. Anti-NS1 (a cross-reactive anti-dengue antibody) and prM (structural precursor-membrane protein), and coronavirus E proteins all target platelets, endothelial cells and coagulation molecules. This process contributes to endothelial damage, macrophage activation and more platelet dysfunction, ultimately leading to further worsening of coagulopathy. Increased vascular fragility and impaired platelet function leads to haemorrhage, which can further contribute to plasma leakage in DHF/DSS [52]. There may also be other more complex mechanisms involved in dengue immunopathogenesis, platelet dysfunction and thrombocytopenia [53].

9. Thrombocytopenia Associated with COVID Vaccines

Thrombotic thrombocytopenia syndrome (TTS), a complication of COVID-19 vaccines, involves thrombosis and thrombocytopenia with infrequent arterial thrombosis. TTS appears to mostly affect females aged between 20 and 50 years old, with no predisposing risk factors conclusively identified so far. Cases are characterised by thrombocytopenia, higher levels of D-dimers than commonly observed in venous thromboembolic events (VTE), inexplicably low fibrinogen levels and worsening thrombosis. Hyper-fibrinolysis associated with bleeding can also occur. Antibodies that bind platelet factor 4, like those associated with heparin-induced thrombocytopenia, have also been identified but in the absence of patient exposure to heparin treatment. TTS is an extremely rare but increasingly recognised serious adverse event related to thromboembolism at unusual sites, such as cerebral venous sinus thrombosis (CVST) or abdominal thromboses (splanchnic, mesenteric or portal vein), all of which are associated with thrombocytopenia. 'CVST with thrombocytopenia' is a rare subtype of cerebrovascular accident, with an incidence of 5.0 per million in those receiving Vaxzevria (manufactured by AstraZeneca) and 4.1 per million in those receiving mRNA-based vaccines, and the prevalence is three times greater in younger to middle aged women (mean age 35). Several countries have suspended the use of adenovirus-vectored vaccines for younger individuals. The prevailing opinion is that the risk of developing COVID-19 disease, including thrombosis, far exceeds the extremely low risk of TTS associated with highly efficacious vaccines. Mass vaccination should continue but with caution. Vaccines that are more likely to cause TTS (e.g., Vaxzevria) should be avoided in younger patients for whom an alternative vaccine is available [54]. The only vaccine currently known to cause ITP is the mumps, measles and rubella (MMR) vaccine, but with low incidence.

10. Coagulopathy of Dengue versus COVID-19

The clinical manifestation and magnitude of coagulopathy varies greatly in patients with dengue due to differences in viral virulence, routes of exposure and host conditions [55]. Minor bleeding, including petechiae, epistaxis and bleeding gums, can occur and help to recognise viral haemorrhagic fever in its early stages [56]. Unlike COVID-19, dengue rarely causes respiratory dysfunction and/or acute lung injury. Vascular injury results in increased permeability, hypovolaemia and circulatory shock in the advanced stages of severe viral hemorrhagic fever.

Shock can also occur in COVID-19. Multisystem inflammatory syndrome in children (MIS-C) and multisystem inflammatory syndrome in adults (MIS-A) are rare post-infectious complications characterised by fever, systemic inflammation, abdominal pain and cardiac involvement. The symptoms usually occur late, while the sudden onset of severe systemic inflammation with shock is reminiscent of toxic shock syndrome in bacterial infections. The aetiology of MIS-C and MIS-A is uncertain, but derangement of the autoimmune reaction is a possibility [57]. Increased vascular permeability in viral hemorrhagic fever also induces coagulation defects that can result in severe bleeding [58].

Systemic viral infection also induces an acute inflammatory and hypercoagulable state, causing DIC that increases the risk of multiorgan failure and death. However, except for Ebola and Marburg, bleeding in haemorrhagic fevers is rarely a direct cause of death [59]. Coagulopathy is common in filovirus diseases and also occurs in dengue. Petechiae, gingival and mucosal bleeding, and sustained bleeding at venipuncture site can occur in these patients. These symptoms usually diminish within a week, but a small proportion of patients develop DHF with worsening of bleeding and shock [60]. In 1997, the WHO characterised typical DHF by four major clinical manifestations: (1) sustained high fever for two to seven days; (2) a haemorrhagic tendency, such as a positive tourniquet test, or clinical bleeding; (3) thrombocytopenia (platelets $\leq 100 \times 10^9$/L); and (4) evidence of plasma leakage manifested by haemoconcentration (>20% increase in hematocrit) or pleural effusion [61].

The clinical features of coagulation disorders are quite different in COVID-19 and dengue (see Table 3). COVID-19 is characterised by a high prevalence of thrombotic complications, with an estimated overall prevalence of VTE of 14.1% [62]. The incidence of VTE in COVID-19 is at least threefold higher than in other viral respiratory infections [63]. In more critically ill patients, the incidence of VTE is 45.6%, while it was 23.0% in non-ICU (intensive care unit) patients [62]. Coagulopathy in COVID-19 is initiated by local lung injury, and following the initial localised thrombo-inflammatory response, systemic hypercoagulability becomes prominent. Coagulation tests including prothrombin time (PT) and activated partial thromboplastin time (aPTT) are usually normal; however, more sensitive viscoelastic testing demonstrates a hypercoagulable pattern mainly due to activated platelets [64]. Since SARS-CoV-2 injures vascular endothelial cells, the loss of anticoagulant activity is another critical factor for prothrombotic changes. Internalisation of ACE2 to increase angiotensin II levels causes vasoconstriction, hyperinflammation, and the release of prothrombotic substances such as von Willebrand factor (VWF), P-selectin, factor VIII and angiopoietin 2 [65]. Bleeding rarely occurs in COVID-19, especially in advanced stages of critical illness. Increased haemorrhage is due to thrombocytopenia, platelet dysfunction and consumptive coagulopathy often complicated by secondary infections [66].

Table 3. Coagulation disorders in COVID-19 and dengue (based on Iba et al. [67]).

General	Dengue	COVID-19
Basic comparisons	Consumptive coagulopathy is common	Consumptive coagulation disorder is seen in limited cases
Bleeding in VHF and thrombosis in COVD-19	Increased permeability in viral haemorrhagic fever also induces coagulation defects that can result in critical bleeding. The systemic viral infection also induces an acute inflammatory and hypercoagulable state causing DIC	COVID-19 is characterised by a high prevalence of thrombotic complications. Infrequently, bleeding can occur, especially in advanced stages of critical illness

Table 3. Cont.

General	Dengue	COVID-19
Pathogenesis	Infected dendritic cells and macrophages lose their ability to regulate type I IFN levels, and lymphocytes undergo cell death. Inappropriate dendritic cell function perturbs the innate immune system and increases vascular permeability. Furthermore, the replicated viruses disseminate throughout the body to systemic reactions such as dysfunction of the visceral parenchymal cells, platelet disability and coagulopathy which lead to DIC resulting in uncontrolled haemorrhage	COVID-19 directly infects macrophages/monocytes, provoking inflammation and thrombosis by releasing proinflammatory cytokines, and expressing TF. Activated neutrophils eject neutrophil extracellular traps and disrupt antithrombogenicity by damaging glycocalyx. Thrombin activates endothelial cells, elicits a proinflammatory reaction, prothrombotic change and activates platelet aggregation. COVID-19 also infects endothelial cells by binding to ACE2 and stimulates the release of factor VIII, VWF and angiopoietin 2, resulting in thrombosis

11. Prior Exposure to DENV and COVID-19 Severity

It is possible that prior exposure to DENV could provide some degree of cross-protection to SARS-CoV-2 infection, rendering it less severe in regions where dengue is endemic, as supported by a report from Singapore where a man and a woman (both aged 57 years) were originally COVID-19 virus-positive and false-positive in serological tests for dengue, including DENV-IgM and IgG [68]. Reports are available which show that sero-diagnostic tests for DENV yield false-positive results for SARS-CoV-2 and vice versa in dengue-endemic regions, thereby indicating potential cross-reactivity between the viruses. A recent study that tested the antigenic similarities of SARS-CoV-2 and DENV using computational docking demonstrated that human DENV antibodies can bind to the receptor binding domain of SARS-CoV-2 spike protein. Some of these interactions can also potentially intercept human ACE2 receptor binding to the receptor-binding motif (RBM). Dengue serum samples predating the COVID-19 outbreak cross-reacted with the SARS-CoV-2 spike protein. Of importance is that the m396 and 80R antibodies (against SARS virus) did not dock with RBM of SARS-CoV-2. It is probable that immunological memory/antibodies to DENV in endemic countries could reduce the severity and spread of COVID-19. It is not known whether SARS-CoV-2 antibodies will hinder DENV infections by binding to DENV particles and reduce dengue incidence in the future, or even facilitate DENV infection by deploying ADE [69].

12. Clinical Manifestations

12.1. Haemorrhagic Manifestations of Dengue

Minor bleeding such as that in the nose, gums and gastrointestinal tract is occasionally observed in children without shock [70]. Mucosal bleeding is more common and of greater severity in adults. However, intracranial haemorrhage is very rare but can be a fatal complication [71]. Patients with profound or prolonged shock complicated by metabolic acidosis and/or DIC typically experience gastrointestinal bleeding. The clinical features of dengue infection are summarised in Figure 1.

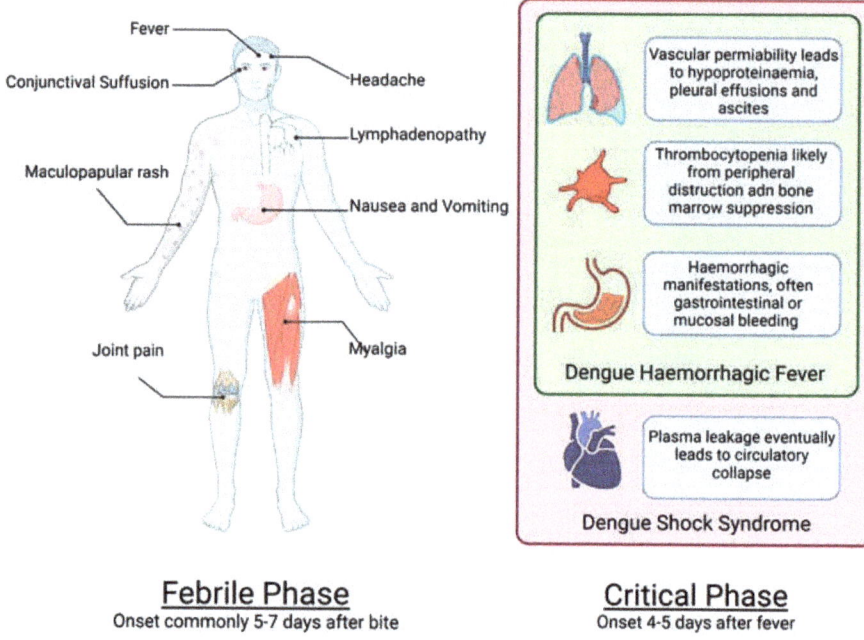

Figure 1. Systemic effects of dengue and time course of infection.

12.2. Thrombosis in COVID-19

Exaggerated inflammatory reactions occur during the advanced stages of COVID-19, including progression to acute respiratory distress syndrome (ARDS) and multi-organ failure, ultimately leading to shock, and the development of DIC [72]. The process is multifactorial but is believed to largely revolve around a disproportionate inflammatory cascade and cytokine storm [73] dysregulating haemostatic failsafe mechanisms. Figure 2 summarises the stages and clinical features of classical COVID-19 infections.

Several coexisting factors predisposing to increased thrombosis are observed throughout the progression of a COVID-19 infection and may manifest as thrombotic events such as myocardial infarction, pulmonary embolism or cerebrovascular disorders, with the highest rates reported among severe cases, particularly those needing ICU admission [22]. However, there are reports of thrombosis in otherwise asymptomatic individuals and occurring weeks after symptom resolution [72]. Mechanisms of coagulopathy include viral interaction with the renin angiotensin system (RAS) via its binding to ACE2 receptors in the lungs, leading to an upregulation of the prothrombotic angiotensin-II, a cytokine storm and complement activation, endothelial dysfunction and sepsis-driven and hypoxia-driven coagulopathy [72,74,75]. Severe COVID-19 has further been associated with the shutdown of normal fibrinolysis, an essential failsafe in thrombotic homeostasis [76]. This is believed to be due to increased release of antifibrinolytic agents, most notably plasminogen activator inhibitor 1 (PAI-1) from activated platelets and damaged endothelium [77]. Thus, clots not only form more easily, but are broken down less efficiently once formed. Not all these mechanisms are confined to the severely ill patients, but new mechanisms will exacerbate disease progression. Thus, the risk of thrombosis persists throughout a COVID-19 infection, with the risk of thrombosis being greater in more severely affected patients [78].

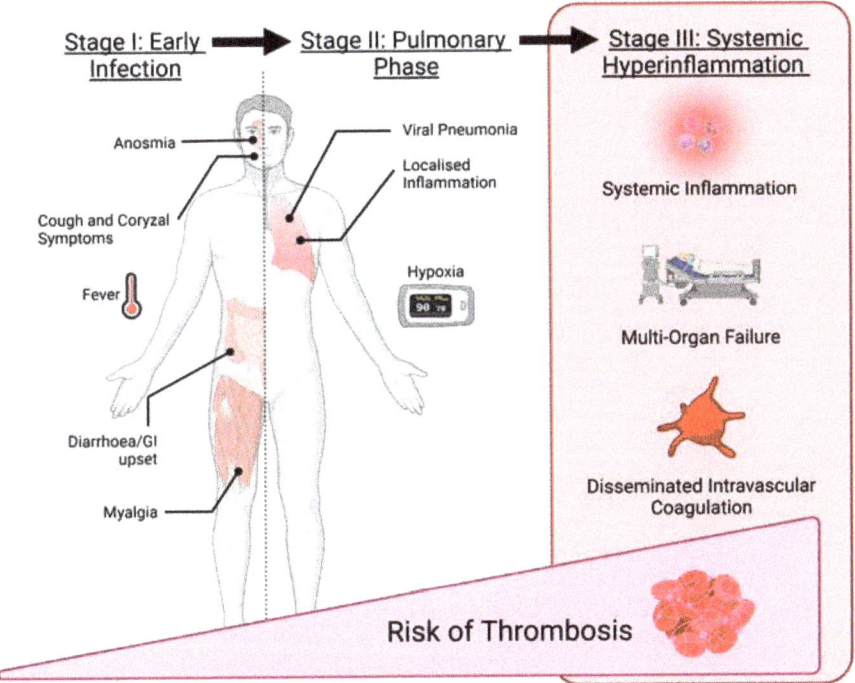

Figure 2. Typical stages of a COVID-19 infection and their clinical features.

13. Serological Cross-Reactivity between Dengue and COVID-19

It is often difficult to distinguish between COVID-19 and dengue owing to their shared clinical and laboratory features, including possible cross-reactivity. Failing to consider COVID-19 due to false-positive dengue serology can have serious implications and vice versa. In a report published from Israel using clinical data and serum samples from 55 individuals with COVID-19, dengue-specific antibodies were detected by lateral-flow rapid tests and enzyme-linked immunosorbent assay (ELISA) in 12 (21.8%) COVID-19 patients compared to zero positive cases in a control group of 70 healthy individuals ($p < 0.001$). Of the 12 positive cases, nine had IgM positivity, two had IgG IgM positivity and one had both IgM and IgG IgM positivity. ELISA testing for dengue was positive in two additional subjects using envelope protein-directed antibodies but negative by lateral flow rapid testing. Out of 95 samples obtained from patients diagnosed with dengue before September 2019, SARS-CoV-2 serology targeting the S protein was positive/equivocal in 21 (22%) (16 IgA, 5 IgG) versus 4 positives/equivocal in 102 controls (4%) ($p < 0.001$). Subsequent in silico analysis revealed possible similarities between SARS-CoV-2 epitopes in the HR2 domain of the spike protein and the dengue envelope protein. This finding supports possible cross-reactivity between DENV and SARS-CoV-2, which can lead to false-positive dengue serology among COVID-19 patients and vice versa—which has important therapeutic and public health implications [79].

14. Management Recommendations for COVID-19 Coagulopathy

The best practice management of coagulopathy in the context of a COVID-19 infection continues to evolve as new evidence emerges, and no guidance can adequately cover every possible situation. However, some recommendations can be made regarding approaches to mitigate and treat coagulopathy in these patients. The scope of this paper does not cover all eventualities such as management of specific thrombotic syndromes (e.g., acute coronary syndrome) in COVID-19, but instead lays out recommendations for general prophylactic management.

14.1. Mild COVID-19 Infection

Anticoagulation should not be commenced routinely in patients with mild, early symptoms, as the risk of coagulation disorders is the lowest in these patients who can be treated at home [75]. Appropriate counselling should be offered, including increased risk of coagulopathy, warning signs of clotting and basic measures for prevention (e.g., staying well hydrated, staying mobile).

A risk–benefit analysis should be conducted for patients with other co-morbidities that can increase coagulation risk. Anticoagulation should be continued in those already on anticoagulant therapy (for instance, a patient with pre-existing atrial fibrillation treated with a direct-acting oral anticoagulant). However, there are specific considerations concerning the suitability of treatment in light of their current infection status, such as safe access to international normalised ratio (INR) clinics if a patient's warfarin dosing is unstable, in which case an alternative anticoagulant may be more appropriate.

14.2. Moderate to Severe COVID-19 Infection

In patients with a COVID-19 syndrome severe enough to be admitted to hospital, management of thrombotic risk requires a more proactive approach. Close monitoring is recommended for signs of either developing a VTE or coagulation abnormality and anticoagulation is recommended in the first instance, with or without mechanical prophylaxis.

Specific agents and dosing will differ, and these should be sought from local or national guidelines related to the place of treatment, and at the discretion of the clinician treating the patient. For instance, the National Institute of Clinical Excellence in the UK currently recommends that prophylactic low molecular weight heparin be offered to all COVID-positive patients without contraindications, unless already receiving a suitable prophylaxis agent, with several considerations for escalating to a short-term therapeutic dosing regimen [80]; however, the optimal dosing in patients without evidence of current VTE remains unclear [75].

Monitoring of biochemical markers is recommended for inpatients, not only for disease progression, but for signs of coagulopathy. Raised D-dimer levels are associated with increased morbidity and mortality [72,78] and should be monitored at 2–3 day intervals [75]. Though it is not generally recommended to dose anticoagulation treatment based on D-dimers [80], this can be used to identify a deteriorating patient, or the presence of thrombus development.

Severe COVID-19, as with many other critical conditions, represents an increased risk of developing DIC [72]. Close clinical and biochemical monitoring of signs of DIC is recommended in the form of platelet counts and coagulation panels, including fibrinogen levels and D-dimers. Decisions on the anticoagulation should be on a patient-to-patient basis, with considerations balanced between the risks of thrombosis and bleeding. It is generally recommended that prophylactic anticoagulation be continued in the absence of overt bleeding [75], and most reports suggest that incidence of life-threatening bleeding is less than that of major thrombosis [72]. Consultation with a local haematologist is advised to optimise care in such cases.

15. Management Recommendations in Dengue

General Aspects of Management of Dengue

There are three phases of clinical presentations of dengue infections: febrile, critical (leakage) and convalescence (Figure 1). The convalescent phase can be divided into early (24–36 h after shock or 48–60 h after leakage) and a later convalescence phase (36 h after shock or 60 h after leakage). Disease manifestations are DHF (grades I and II) and DSS (grades III and IV). Expanded dengue syndrome is considered the most severe because this can lead to complications and death if not managed in a timely manner. Patients with DHF and DSS have different clinical presentations from other patients infected with dengue. Plasma leaks occur during the critical phases of DHF and DSS [81]. Most patients with dengue present with an undifferentiated febrile illness, but DHF/DSS occurs in only a small number of patients. Early diagnosis of DHF/DSS is important to initiate management promptly to prevent shock, severe illness and death. Symptomatic and supportive treatment is only needed during the early febrile phase. Dengue patients usually have high persistent fevers for 4–5 (range 2–7) days. Common signs and symptoms are severe headache, retro-orbital pain, myalgia, arthralgia and minor haemorrhagic manifestations such as petechial rash, epistaxis, gum bleeding and coffee-ground vomiting. Haematemesis and melena are both common symptoms. Haemoglobinuria is common on urine testing of haemolytic anaemias, especially in cases of thalassemia, other haemoglobinopathy and G-6-PD deficiency. Erythematous or maculopapular or petechial rash is especially common in adults. Nausea and vomiting along with poor appetite and malaise are common but nonspecific symptoms [82].

The use of an early tourniquet when diagnosing DHF and DSS is very helpful, where blood pressure is measured using an appropriately sized cuff. Cuff pressure is increased to a value that is mid-way between systolic and diastolic pressure for 5 min, and the cuff is then released. Results can be obtained after 1 min, or once normal skin circulation is noted. The test is regarded as positive if there are $\geq$310 petechiae/mm^3 [83]. Paracetamol is the only recommended antipyretic to treat fever, both in children and in adults; non-steroidal anti-inflammatory drugs and aspirin are contraindicated. Anti-emetics are allowed for patients with nausea and vomiting. Other supportive and symptomatic medicines may be provided at the physician's discretion, depending on clinical signs and symptoms. Some examples include anticonvulsants, anti-histamines and gastro protectives such as proton pump inhibitors. Antibiotics are not indicated unless superimposed secondary bacterial infections are suspected.

Shock or impending shock should be suspected in dengue patients with narrow pulse pressure ($\leq$20 mmHg), hypotension, those with clinical signs of shock (rapid and weak pulse, mottled, cold and calmy skin, delayed capillary refill time (>3 s)), thrombocytopenia and raised haematocrit (320%), leukopenia, which can be related to a poor appetite, clinical deterioration or significant bleeding during defervescence. Any patient with shock or impending shock needs urgent hospitalisation for intensive monitoring of vital signs and prompt management [84].

16. Management of Haemorrhage in Dengue

The risk of clinically significant bleeding in dengue is unpredictable and often contributes to adverse outcomes. A large systematic review of 11 studies on prophylactic and therapeutic interventions for bleeding in dengue failed to identify any effective intervention in preventing or treating clinically significant bleeding in dengue [85].

A retrospective study evaluated 256 patients with dengue infection who developed thrombocytopenia (platelet count, <20 $\times$ 10^3 platelets/μL) without prior bleeding, of which 188 received platelet transfusions. Subsequent bleeding, platelet increases, and platelet recovery times were similar between patients either receiving or not receiving platelet transfusions. Prophylactic platelet transfusion did not prevent bleeding in adult patients with dengue infection [86]. Another multicentre, open-label, randomised controlled trial (RCT) assigned 372 patients to transfusion (n = 188) or control (n = 184) groups. The intention-to-treat analysis shows clinical bleeding by day 7 or at hospital discharge occurred in 40 (21%) patients in the transfusion group and 48 (26%) patients in the control group (risk difference $-$4.98% (95% confidence interval (CI) $-$15.08 to 5.34); relative risk 0.81 (95% CI 0.56 to 1.17); p = 0.16); however, significantly more adverse events occurred in the transfusion group (5.81% (95% CI $-$4.42 to 16.01) versus 6.26% (95% CI 1.43 to 27.34); p < 0.01). No deaths were reported. The authors concluded that prophylactic platelet transfusion was not superior to supportive care in preventing bleeding in adult patients with dengue and thrombocytopenia, and could be associated with adverse events [87].

Some treatment recommendations are outlined below [85]:
1. Prophylactic platelet transfusion should not be routinely prescribed based on low platelet counts in patients with dengue and no bleeding.
2. Therapeutic platelet transfusion should not be routinely prescribed in patients with dengue with thrombocytopaenia and mild bleeding.
3. There is insufficient evidence to support or refute the use of platelet transfusion in patients with severe bleeding in dengue.
4. There is a need for further, well-designed RCTs to evaluate the role of platelets and plasma transfusion in patients in both the prevention of bleeding and in the setting of clinically significant bleeding in dengue infection.
5. There is currently insufficient evidence regarding the role of rFVIIa, anti-D globulin, Ig or tranexamic acid in the prevention or treatment of bleeding in dengue infection and there is a need for further research on these therapeutic agents.

17. Conclusions

Significant coagulation abnormalities, including thrombocytopenia, are common in both dengue and COVID-19 infections. This review discusses their common pathogenesis, clinical features including potential serological false positivity, and diagnostic challenges especially in dengue-endemic areas. We also review the importance of not transfusing platelets routinely as this can further stress already stretched services globally.

There are multiple complex mechanisms responsible for coagulation disturbances, thrombocytopenia and platelet dysfunction in dengue and paradoxical thromboembolism in COVID-19. The important aspects of treating COVID-19-induced immunothrombosis associated with thrombocytopenia are anticoagulation with or without aspirin. However, aspirin, nonsteroidal anti-inflammatory agents and anticoagulants are contraindicated in dengue infections.

The importance of recognising the similar clinical presentations of both diseases and excluding COVID-19 in the differential diagnoses in the setting of a dengue pandemic is paramount in preventing potential serious consequences in the current management of DENV-induced thrombocytopenia. While both dengue fever and COVID-19 infections can result in thrombocytopenia and coagulopathy, their clinical manifestations and management are quite different. Prevention and control strategies combined with vaccinations are key to controlling disease burden. While successful vaccinations for dengue currently remain largely ineffective, COVID 19 vaccinations have largely been successful.

Author Contributions: Conceptualisation, A.I.; resources, A.I., S.E., K.J., I.L. and C.C.; writing—A.I., I.L, S.E., J.A. and C.C.; review—writing and editing, A.I., S.E., J.A., T.I., H.R., H.M., C.C. and I.L.; supervision, A.I. and I.L.; Figure 1 was original crafted by K.J., Figure 2 was original crafted by C.C. All authors have read and agreed to the published version of the manuscript.

Funding: This work received no external funding.

Institutional Review Board Statement: Not applicable.

Informed Consent Statement: Not applicable.

Data Availability Statement: No new data was created or analysed in this study. Data sharing is not applicable to this article.

Acknowledgments: Figures 1 and 2 were created with BioRender.com (accessed on 30 June 2022), with license to publish.

Conflicts of Interest: The authors declare no conflict of interest.

References

1. Harapan, H.; Ryan, M.; Yohan, B.; Abidin, R.S.; Nainu, F.; Rakib, A.; Jahan, I.; Emran, T.B.; Ullah, I.; Panta, K.; et al. COVID-19 and Dengue: Double Punches for Dengue-Endemic Countries in Asia. *Rev. Med. Virol.* **2021**, *31*, e2161. [CrossRef] [PubMed]
2. Gao, Y.; Li, T.; Han, M.; Li, X.; Wu, D.; Xu, Y.; Zhu, Y.; Liu, Y.; Wang, X.; Wang, L. Diagnostic Utility of Clinical Laboratory Data Determinations for Patients with the Severe COVID-19. *J. Med. Virol.* **2020**, *92*, 791–796. [CrossRef]
3. Kellstein, D.; Fernandes, L. Symptomatic treatment of dengue: Should the NSAID contraindication be reconsidered? *Postgrad. Med.* **2019**, *131*, 109–116. [CrossRef]
4. Simmons, C.P.; Farrar, J.J.; van Vinh Chau, N.; Wills, B. Dengue. *N. Engl. J. Med.* **2012**, *366*, 1423–1432. [CrossRef] [PubMed]
5. Kembuan, G.J. Dengue Serology in Indonesian COVID-19 Patients: Coinfection or Serological Overlap? *IDCases* **2020**, *22*, e00927. [CrossRef]
6. Wilder-Smith, A.; Tissera, H.; Ooi, E.E.; Coloma, J.; Scott, T.W.; Gubler, D.J. Preventing Dengue Epidemics during theCOVID-19 Pandemic. *Am. J. Trop. Med. Hyg.* **2020**, *103*, 570–571. [CrossRef]
7. Henrina, J.; Putra, I.C.S.; Lawrensia, S.; Handoyono, Q.F.; Cahyadi, A. Coronavirus Disease of 2019: A Mimicker of Dengue Infection? *SN Compr. Clin. Med.* **2020**, *2*, 1109–1119. [CrossRef]
8. Centers for Disease Control and Prevention (CDC). Is It Dengue or Is It COVID-19? Available online: https://www.cdc.gov/dengue/healthcare-providers/dengue-or-covid.html (accessed on 18 August 2022).
9. Vaughn, D.W.; Green, S.; Kalayanarooj, S.; Innis, B.L.; Nimmannitya, S.; Suntayakorn, S.; Endy, T.P.; Raengsakulrach, B.; Rothman, A.L.; Ennis, F.A.; et al. Dengue Viremia Titer, Antibody Response Pattern, and Virus Serotype Correlate with Disease Severity. *J. Infect. Dis.* **2000**, *181*, 2–9. [CrossRef]
10. Peeling, R.W.; Artsob, H.; Pelegrino, J.L.; Buchy, P.; Cardosa, M.J.; Devi, S.; Enria, D.A.; Farrar, J.; Gubler, D.J.; Guz-man, M.G.; et al. Evaluation of Diagnostic Tests: Dengue. *Nat. Rev. Microbiol.* **2010**, *8*, S30–S37. [CrossRef]
11. Mohamadian, M.; Chiti, H.; Shoghli, A.; Biglari, S.; Parsamanesh, N.; Esmaeilzadeh, A. COVID-19: Virology, biology and novel laboratory diagnosis. *J. Gene. Med.* **2021**, *23*, e3303. [CrossRef]
12. Rowe, B.; Canosa, A.; Meslem, A.; Rowe, F. Increased airborne transmission of COVID-19 with new variants, implications for health policies. *Build. Environ.* **2022**, *219*, 109132. [CrossRef]
13. Waggoner, J.J.; Gresh, L.; Vargas, M.J.; Ballesteros, G.; Tellez, Y.; Soda, K.J.; Sahoo, M.K.; Nuñez, A.; Balmaseda, A.; Harris, E.; et al. Viremia and Clinical Presentation in Nicaraguan Patients Infected with Zika Virus, Chikungunya Virus, and Dengue Virus. *Clin. Infect. Dis.* **2016**, *63*, 1584–1590. [CrossRef]
14. Bhatt, S.; Gething, P.W.; Brady, O.J.; Messina, J.P.; Farlow, A.W.; Moyes, C.L.; Drake, J.M.; Brownstein, J.S.; Hoen, A.G.; Sankoh, O.; et al. The Global Distribution and Burden of Dengue. *Nature* **2013**, *496*, 504–507. [CrossRef] [PubMed]
15. Brady, O.J.; Gething, P.W.; Bhatt, S.; Messina, J.P.; Brownstein, J.S.; Hoen, A.G.; Moyes, C.L.; Farlow, A.W.; Scott, T.W.; Hay, S.I. Refining the Global Spatial Limits of Dengue Virus Transmission by Evidence-Based Consensus. *PLoS Negl. Trop. Dis.* **2012**, *6*, e1760. [CrossRef] [PubMed]
16. World Health Organization (WHO). Dengue and Severe Dengue. Available online: https://www.who.int/news-room/fact-sheets/detail/dengue-and-severe-dengue (accessed on 18 August 2022).
17. Sharma, H.; Ilyas, A.; Chowdhury, A.; Poddar, N.K.; Chaudhary, A.A.; Shilbayeh, S.A.R.; Ibrahim, A.A.; Khan, S. Does COVID-19 lockdowns have impacted on global dengue burden? A special focus to India. *BMC Public Health* **2022**, *22*, 1402. [CrossRef] [PubMed]
18. Banerjee, S.; Aditya, G.; Saha, G.K. Household Wastes as Larval Habitats of Dengue Vectors: Comparison between Urban and Rural Areas of Kolkata, India. *PLoS ONE* **2015**, *10*, e0138082. [CrossRef]
19. World Health Organization (WHO). Weekly Epidemiological Update on COVID-19-29 June 2022. Available online: https://www.who.int/publications/m/item/weekly-epidemiological-update-on-covid-19---29-june-2022 (accessed on 18 August 2022).
20. Rehman, S.; Shafique, L.; Ihsan, A.; Liu, Q. Evolutionary Trajectory for the Emergence of Novel Coronavirus SARS-CoV-2. *Pathogens* **2020**, *9*, 240. [CrossRef]
21. Centres of Disease Control and Prevention (CDC). COVID-19 Overview and Infection Prevention and Control Priorities in Non-U.S. Healthcare Settings. Available online: https://www.cdc.gov/coronavirus/2019-ncov/hcp/non-us-settings/overview (accessed on 18 August 2022).
22. Bulut, C.; Kato, Y. Epidemiology of COVID-19. *Turk. J. Med. Sci.* **2020**, *50*, 563–570. [CrossRef]
23. Tsai, P.; Lai, W.; Lin, Y.; Luo, Y.; Lin, Y.; Chen, H.; Chen, Y.M.; Lai, Y.C.; Kuo, L.C.; Chen, S.D.; et al. Clinical manifestation and disease progression in COVID-19 infection. *J. Chin. Med. Assoc.* **2021**, *84*, 3–8. [CrossRef]
24. Siordia, J. Epidemiology and clinical features of COVID-19: A review of current literature. *J. Clin. Virol.* **2020**, *127*, 104357. [CrossRef]
25. Hu, Z.; Song, C.; Xu, C.; Jin, G.; Chen, Y.; Xu, X.; Ma, H.; Chen, W.; Lin, Y.; Zheng, Y.; et al. Clinical characteristics of 24 asymptomatic infections with COVID-19 screened among close contacts in Nanjing, China. *Sci. China Life Sci.* **2020**, *63*, 706–711. [CrossRef] [PubMed]
26. Lopez Bernal, J.; Andrews, N.; Gower, C.; Robertson, C.; Stowe, J.; Tessier, E.; Simmons, R.; Cottrell, S.; Roberts, R.; O'Doherty, M.; et al. Effectiveness of the Pfizer-BioNTech and Oxford-AstraZeneca vaccines on COVID-19 related symptoms, hospital admissions, and mortality in older adults in England: Test negative case-control study. *BMJ* **2021**, *373*, n1088. [CrossRef] [PubMed]

27. Centers for Disease Control and Prevention (CDC). Dengue Clinical Case Management Course. Available online: https://www.cdc.gov/dengue/training/cme.html (accessed on 18 August 2022).
28. Centers for Disease Control and Prevention (CDC). COVID-19 Information for Specific Groups of People. Available online: https://www.cdc.gov/coronavirus/2019-ncov/need-extra-precautions/index.html (accessed on 18 August 2022).
29. Centers for Disease Control and Prevention (CDC). Serology Testing for COVID-19 at CDC. Available online: https://www.cdc.gov/coronavirus/2019-ncov/lab/serology-testing.html (accessed on 18 August 2022).
30. Coller, B.S.; Shattil, S.J. The GPIIb/IIIa (Integrin AlphaIIbbeta3) Odyssey: A Technology-Driven Saga of a Receptor with Twists, Turns, and Even a Bend. *Blood* **2008**, *112*, 3011–3025. [CrossRef] [PubMed]
31. Gawaz, M.; Langer, H.; May, A.E. Platelets in Inflammation and Atherogenesis. *J. Clin. Investig.* **2005**, *115*, 3378–3384. [CrossRef]
32. Kaushansky, K. Lineage-Specific Hematopoietic Growth Factors. *N. Engl. J. Med.* **2006**, *354*, 2034–2045. [CrossRef]
33. Semple, J.W.; Italiano, J.E.; Freedman, J. Platelets and the Immune Continuum. *Nat. Rev. Immunol.* **2011**, *11*, 264–274. [CrossRef]
34. Trzeciak-Ryczek, A.; Tokarz-Deptuła, B.; Deptuła, W. Platelets-an Important Element of the Immune System. *Pol. J. Vet. Sci.* **2013**, *16*, 407–413. [CrossRef]
35. Kasthuri, R.S.; Glover, S.L.; Boles, J.; Mackman, N. Tissue Factor and Tissue Factor Pathway Inhibitor as Key Regulators of Global Hemostasis: Measurement of Their Levels in Coagulation Assays. *Semin. Thromb. Hemost.* **2010**, *36*, 764–771. [CrossRef]
36. Daubie, V.; Pochet, R.; Houard, S.; Philippart, P. Tissue Factor: A Mini-Review. *J. Tissue Eng. Regen. Med.* **2007**, *1*, 161–169. [CrossRef]
37. Danielli, J.F. Capillary Permeability and Oedema in the Perfused Frog. *J. Physiol.* **1940**, *98*, 109–129. [CrossRef]
38. Andia, I.; Abate, M. Platelet-Rich Plasma: Underlying Biology and Clinical Correlates. *Regen. Med.* **2013**, *8*, 645–658. [CrossRef] [PubMed]
39. World Health Organization (WHO). Dengue Guidelines for Diagnosis, Treatment, Prevention and Control: New Edition. Available online: https://apps.who.int/iris/handle/10665/44188 (accessed on 18 August 2022).
40. Rothman, A.L.; Ennis, F.A. Immunopathogenesis of Dengue Hemorrhagic Fever. *Virology* **1999**, *257*, 1–6. [CrossRef] [PubMed]
41. Mitrakul, C. Bleeding Problem in Dengue Haemorrhagic Fever: Platelets and Coagulation Changes. *Southeast Asian J. Trop. Med. Public Health* **1987**, *18*, 407–412.
42. Malavige, G.N.; Ranatunga, P.K.; Velathanthiri, V.G.N.S.; Fernando, S.; Karunatilaka, D.H.; Aaskov, J.; Seneviratne, S.L. Patterns of Disease in Sri Lankan Dengue Patients. *Arch. Dis. Child.* **2006**, *91*, 396–400. [CrossRef]
43. Chaudhary, R.; Khetan, D.; Sinha, S.; Sinha, P.; Sonkar, A.; Pandey, P.; Das, S.; Agarwal, P.; Ray, V. Transfusion Support to Dengue Patients in a Hospital Based Blood Transfusion Service in North India. *Transf. Apheresis Sci.* **2007**, *35*, 239–244. [CrossRef]
44. Makroo, R.N.; Raina, V.; Kumar, P.; Kanth, R.K. Role of Platelet Transfusion in the Management of Dengue Patients in a Tertiary Care Hospital. *Asian J. Transf. Sci.* **2007**, *1*, 4. [CrossRef]
45. Lum, L.C.S.; Abdel-Latif, M.E.-A.; Goh, A.Y.T.; Chan, P.W.K.; Lam, S.K. Preventive Transfusion in Dengue Shock Syndrome-Is It Necessary? *J. Pediatr.* **2003**, *143*, 682–684. [CrossRef]
46. Murgue, B.; Cassar, O.; Guigon, M.; Chungue, E. Dengue Virus Inhibits Human Hematopoietic Progenitor Growth in Vitro. *J. Infect. Dis.* **1997**, *175*, 1497–1501. [CrossRef]
47. Nakao, S.; Lai, C.J.; Young, N.S. Dengue Virus, a Flavivirus, Propagates in Human Bone Marrow Progenitors and Hematopoietic Cell Lines. *Blood* **1989**, *74*, 1235–1240. [CrossRef]
48. Edelman, R.; Nimmannitya, S.; Colman, R.W.; Talamo, R.C.; Top, F.H. Evaluation of the Plasma Kinin System in Dengue Hemorrhagic Fever. *J. Lab. Clin. Med.* **1975**, *86*, 410–421.
49. Hottz, E.D.; Oliveira, M.F.; Nunes, P.C.G.; Nogueira, R.M.R.; Valls-de-Souza, R.; Da Poian, A.T.; Weyrich, A.S.; Zimmerman, G.A.; Bozza, P.T.; Bozza, F.A. Dengue Induces Platelet Activation, Mitochondrial Dysfunction and Cell Death through Mechanisms That Involve DC-SIGN and Caspases. *J. Thromb. Haemost.* **2013**, *11*, 951–962. [CrossRef] [PubMed]
50. Laur, F.; Murgue, B.; Deparis, X.; Roche, C.; Cassar, O.; Chungue, E. Plasma Levels of Tumour Necrosis Factor Alpha and Transforming Growth Factor Beta-1 in Children with Dengue 2 Virus Infection in French Polynesia. *Trans. R. Soc. Trop. Med. Hyg.* **1998**, *92*, 654–656. [CrossRef]
51. Pang, X.; Zhang, R.; Cheng, G. Progress towards understanding the pathogenesis of dengue hemorrhagic fever. *Virol. Sin.* **2017**, *32*, 16–22. [CrossRef] [PubMed]
52. Dejnirattisai, W.; Jumnainsong, A.; Onsirisakul, N.; Fitton, P.; Vasanawathana, S.; Limpitikul, W.; Puttikhunt, C.; Edwards, C.; Duangchinda, T.; Supasa, S. Cross-Reacting Antibodies Enhance Dengue Virus Infection in Hu-mans. *Science* **2010**, *328*, 745–748. [CrossRef] [PubMed]
53. De Azeredo, E.L.; Monteiro, R.Q.; de-Oliveira Pinto, L.M. Thrombocytopenia in Dengue: Interrelationship between Virus and the Imbalance between Coagulation and Fibrinolysis and Inflammatory Mediators. *Mediat. Inflamm.* **2015**, *2015*, 313842. [CrossRef]
54. Islam, A.; Bashir, M.S.; Joyce, K.; Rashid, H.; Laher, I.; Elshazly, S. An Update on COVID-19 Vaccine Induced Thrombotic Thrombocytopenia Syndrome and Some Management Recommendations. *Molecules* **2021**, *26*, 5004. [CrossRef]
55. Geisbert, T.W.; Jahrling, P.B. Exotic Emerging Viral Diseases: Progress and Challenges. *Nat. Med.* **2004**, *10*, 110–121. [CrossRef]
56. Hidalgo, J.; Richards, G.A.; Jiménez, J.I.S.; Baker, T.; Amin, P. Viral Hemorrhagic Fever in the Tropics: Report from the Task Force on Tropical Diseases by the World Federation of Societies of Intensive and Critical Care Medicine. *J. Crit. Care.* **2017**, *42*, 366–372. [CrossRef]

57. Buonsenso, D.; Riitano, F.; Valentini, P. Pediatric Inflammatory Multisystem Syndrome Temporally Related with SARS-CoV-2: Immunological Similarities with Acute Rheumatic Fever and Toxic Shock Syndrome. *Front. Pediatr.* **2020**, *8*, 574. [CrossRef]
58. Schnittler, H.-J.; Feldmann, H. Viral Hemorrhagic Fever–a Vascular Disease? *Thromb. Haemost.* **2003**, *89*, 967–972. [CrossRef]
59. Zapata, J.C.; Cox, D.; Salvato, M.S. The Role of Platelets in the Pathogenesis of Viral Hemorrhagic Fevers. *PLoS Negl. Trop. Dis.* **2014**, *8*, e2858. [CrossRef] [PubMed]
60. Kularatne, S.A.M. Dengue Fever. *BMJ* **2015**, *351*, h4661. [CrossRef] [PubMed]
61. World Health Organization (WHO). *Dengue Haemorrhagic Fever: Diagnosis, Treatment, Prevention, and Control*, 2nd ed.; World Health Organization: Geneva, Switzerland, 1997; ISBN 978-92-4-154500-6. Available online: https://apps.who.int/iris/handle/10665/41988 (accessed on 18 August 2022).
62. Nopp, S.; Moik, F.; Jilma, B.; Pabinger, I.; Ay, C. Risk of Venous Thromboembolism in Patients with COVID-19: A Systematic Review and Meta-Analysis. *Res. Pract. Thromb. Haemost.* **2020**, *4*, 1178–1191. [CrossRef] [PubMed]
63. Smilowitz, N.R.; Subashchandran, V.; Yuriditsky, E.; Horowitz, J.M.; Reynolds, H.R.; Hochman, J.S.; Berger, J.S. Thrombosis in Hospitalized Patients with Viral Respiratory Infections versus COVID-19. *Am. Heart J.* **2021**, *231*, 93–95. [CrossRef]
64. Katz, D.; Maher, P.; Getrajdman, C.; Hamburger, J.; Zhao, S.; Madek, J.; Bhatt, H.; Levin, M.; Görlinger, K. Monitoring of COVID-19-Associated Coagulopathy and Anticoagulation with Thromboelastometry. *Transfus. Med. Hemother.* **2021**, *48*, 168–172. [CrossRef]
65. Wibowo, A.; Pranata, R.; Lim, M.A.; Akbar, M.R.; Martha, J.W. Endotheliopathy Marked by High von Willebrand Factor (VWF) Antigen in COVID-19 Is Associated with Poor Outcome: A Systematic Review and Meta-Analysis. *Int. J. Infect. Dis.* **2021**, *117*, 267–273. [CrossRef]
66. Al-Samkari, H.; Karp Leaf, R.S.; Dzik, W.H.; Carlson, J.C.T.; Fogerty, A.E.; Waheed, A.; Goodarzi, K.; Bendapudi, P.K.; Bornikova, L.; Gupta, S.; et al. COVID-19 and Coagulation: Bleeding and Thrombotic Manifestations of SARS-CoV-2 Infection. *Blood* **2020**, *136*, 489–500. [CrossRef]
67. Iba, T.; Levy, J.H.; Levi, M. Viral-Induced Inflammatory Coagulation Disorders: Preparing for Another Epidemic. *Thromb. Haemost.* **2021**, *122*, 8–19. [CrossRef]
68. Nath, H.; Mallick, A.; Roy, S.; Sukla, S.; Basu, K.; De, A.; Biswas, S. 2021 Archived Dengue Serum Samples Produced False-Positive Results in SARS-CoV-2 Lateral Flow-Based Rapid Antibody Tests. *J. Med. Microbiol.* **2021**, *70*, 001369. [CrossRef]
69. Nath, H.; Mallick, A.; Roy, S.; Sukla, S.; Biswas, S. Computational Modelling Supports That Dengue Virus Envelope Antibodies Can Bind to SARS-CoV-2 Receptor Binding Sites: Is Pre-Exposure to Dengue Virus Protective against COVID-19 Severity? *Comput. Struct. Biotechnol. J.* **2021**, *19*, 459–466. [CrossRef]
70. Carlos, C.C.; Oishi, K.; Cinco, M.T.D.D.; Mapua, C.A.; Inoue, S.; Cruz, D.J.M.; Pancho, M.A.M.; Tanig, C.Z.; Matias, R.R.; Morita, K.; et al. Comparison of Clinical Features and Hematologic Abnormalities between Dengue Fever and Dengue Hemorrhagic Fever among Children in the Philippines. *Am. J. Trop. Med. Hyg.* **2005**, *73*, 435–440. [CrossRef] [PubMed]
71. Wani, A.M.; Mejally, M.A.A.; Hussain, W.M.; Maimani, W.A.; Hanif, S.; Khoujah, A.M.; Siddiqi, A.; Akhtar, M.; Bafaraj, M.G.; Fareed, K. Skin Rash, Headache and Abnormal Behaviour: Unusual Presentation of Intracranial Haemorrhage in Dengue Fever. *BMJ Case Rep.* **2010**, *2010*, bcr0620091949. [CrossRef] [PubMed]
72. Hanff, T.; Mohareb, A.; Giri, J.; Cohen, J.; Chirinos, J. Thrombosis in COVID-19. *Am. J. Hematol.* **2020**, *95*, 1578–1589. [CrossRef] [PubMed]
73. England, J.T.; Abdulla, A.; Biggs, C.M.; Lee, A.Y.Y.; Hay, K.A.; Hoiland, R.L.; Wellington, C.L.; Sekhon, M.; James, S.; Shojania, K.; et al. Weathering the COVID-19 storm: Lessons from hematologic cytokine syndromes. *Blood Rev.* **2021**, *45*, 100707. [CrossRef]
74. Gomez-Mesa, J.; Galindo-Coral, S.; Montes, M.; Martin, M. Thrombosis and Coagulopathy in COVID-19. *Curr. Prob. Cardiol.* **2021**, *46*, 100742. [CrossRef]
75. Karim, S.; Islam, A.; Rafiq, S.; Laher, I. The COVID-19 Pandemic: Disproportionate Thrombotic Tendency and Management Recommendations. *Trop. Med. Infect. Dis.* **2021**, *6*, 26. [CrossRef]
76. Tsantes, A.E.; Frantzeskaki, F.; Tsantes, A.G.; Rapti, E.; Rizos, M.; Kokoris, S.I.; Paramythiotou, E.; Katsadiotis, G.; Karali, V.; Flevari, A.; et al. The haemostatic profile in critically ill COVID-19 patients receiving therapeutic anticoagulant therapy: An observational study. *Medicine* **2020**, *99*, e23365. [CrossRef]
77. Meizoso, J.; Moore, H.; Moore, E. Fibrinolysis Shutdown in COVID-19: Clinical Manifestations, Molecular Mechanisms, and Therapeutic Implications. *J. Am. Coll. Surg.* **2021**, *232*, 995–1003. [CrossRef]
78. De Brune, S.; Bos, L.; van Roon, M.; Tuip-de Boer, A.; Schuurman, A.; Koel-Simmelink, M.; Bogaard, H.J.; Tuinman, P.R.; van Agtmael, M.A.; Hamann, J.; et al. Clinical features and prognostic factors in COVID-19: A prospective cohort study. *EBioMedicine* **2021**, *67*, 103378. [CrossRef]
79. Lustig, Y.; Keler, S.; Kolodny, R.; Ben-Tal, N.; Atias-Varon, D.; Shlush, E.; Gerlic, M.; Munitz, A.; Doolman, R.; Asraf, K.; et al. Potential Antigenic Cross-Reactivity Between Severe Acute Respiratory Syndrome Coronavirus 2 (SARS-CoV-2) and Dengue Viruses. *Clin. Infect. Dis.* **2021**, *73*, 2444–2449. [CrossRef] [PubMed]
80. National Institute of Clinical Excellence (NICE). COVID-19 Rapid Guidelines: Managing COVID-19; Section 8.3: Venous Thromboembolism (VTE) Prophylaxis. Available online: https://app.magicapp.org/#/guideline/L4Qb5n/rec/LwomXL (accessed on 18 August 2022).
81. Halstead, S.B.; Lum, L.C. Assessing the Prognosis of Dengue-Infected Patients. *F1000 Med. Rep.* **2009**, *1*, 73. [CrossRef] [PubMed]

82. Vaughn, D.W.; Green, S.; Kalayanarooj, S.; Innis, B.L.; Nimmannitya, S.; Suntayakorn, S.; Rothman, A.L.; Ennis, F.A.; Nisalak, A. Dengue in the Early Febrile Phase: Viremia and Antibody Responses. *J. Infect. Dis.* **1997**, *176*, 322–330. [CrossRef] [PubMed]
83. Gubler, D.J. Dengue and Dengue Hemorrhagic Fever. *Clin. Microbiol. Rev.* **1998**, *11*, 480–496. [CrossRef]
84. Kalayanarooj, S. Dengue Classification: Current WHO vs. the Newly Suggested Classification for Better Clinical Application? *J. Med. Assoc. Thai* **2011**, *94*, 74–84.
85. Rajapakse, S.; de Silva, N.L.; Weeratunga, P.; Rodrigo, C.; Fernando, S.D. Prophylactic and Therapeutic Interventions for Bleeding in Dengue: A Systematic Review. *Trans. R. Soc. Trop. Med. Hyg.* **2017**, *111*, 433–439. [CrossRef] [PubMed]
86. Lye, D.C.; Lee, V.J.; Sun, Y.; Leo, Y.S. Lack of Efficacy of Prophylactic Platelet Transfusion for Severe Thrombocytopenia in Adults with Acute Uncomplicated Dengue Infection. *Clin. Infect. Dis.* **2009**, *48*, 1262–1265. [CrossRef]
87. Lye, D.C.; Archuleta, S.; Syed-Omar, S.F.; Low, J.G.; Oh, H.M.; Wei, Y.; Fisher, D.; Ponnampalavanar, S.S.L.; Wijaya, L.; Lee, L.K.; et al. Prophylactic Platelet Transfusion plus Supportive Care versus Supportive Care Alone in Adults with Dengue and Thrombocytopenia: A Multicentre, Open-Label, Randomised, Superiority Trial. *Lancet* **2017**, *389*, 1611–1618. [CrossRef]

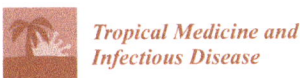

Tropical Medicine and
Infectious Disease

Review

COVID-19: Current Status in Gastrointestinal, Hepatic, and Pancreatic Diseases—A Concise Review

Jorge Aquino-Matus, Misael Uribe and Norberto Chavez-Tapia *

Digestive Diseases and Obesity Clinic, Medica Sur Clinic & Foundation, Mexico City 14070, Mexico
* Correspondence: nchavezt@medicasur.org.mx

Abstract: The gastrointestinal tract plays an important role in the pathogenesis of COVID-19. The angiotensin-converting enzyme 2 receptor and the transmembrane protease serine 2 receptor bind and activate SARS-CoV-2 and are present in high concentrations throughout the gastrointestinal tract. Most patients present with gastrointestinal symptoms and/or abnormal liver function tests, both of which have been associated with adverse outcomes. The mechanisms of liver damage are currently under investigation, but the damage is usually transient and nonsevere. Liver transplantation is the only definitive treatment for acute liver failure and end-stage liver disease, and unfortunately, because of the need for ventilators during the COVID-19 pandemic, most liver transplant programs have been suspended. Patients with gastrointestinal autoimmune diseases require close follow-up and may need modification in immunosuppression. Acute pancreatitis is a rare manifestation of COVID-19, but it must be considered in patients with abdominal pain. The gastrointestinal tract, including the liver and the pancreas, has an intimate relationship with COVID-19 that is currently under active investigation.

Keywords: COVID-19; SARS-CoV-2; diarrhea; liver; pancreas; inflammatory bowel diseases; liver transplantation

1. Introduction

The new coronavirus SARS-CoV-2 infection (COVID-19) reported in Wuhan, China, in December 2019, and by 11 March 2020, the World Health Organization declared it a global pandemic [1]. Time has passed, many people have succumbed to the infection, and a global effort has been carried out to study the virus, both to develop an effective vaccine and to prevent further complications among survivors. Coronaviruses are 65–125 nm diameter (26–32 kb genome) positive monocatenary RNA viruses from the family *Coronaviridae* and subfamily *Orthocoronavirinae*, which are subdivided into *Alphacoronavirus*, *Betacoronavirus*, *Gammacoronavirus*, and *Deltacoronavirus* [2]. The two previous *Betacoronavirus* pandemics were SARS-CoV in 2003 and MERS-CoV in 2012, with mortality of 10% and 37%, respectively [3]. Interestingly, the new coronavirus SARS-CoV-2 genome shows 96.2% homology with the RaTG13 virus in bats (Bat-RaTG13 and Bat-SL-CoVZXC21) [4].

Coronaviruses are known to cause severe acute respiratory distress syndrome and death, and the gastrointestinal tract has been described as playing a key role in the route of infection, clinical manifestations, and disease outcomes. In addition, many gastrointestinal diseases (e.g., autoimmune hepatitis, Crohn's disease) require immunosuppressive treatment and whether the clinical course or risk of complications may be halted by treatment for COVID-19 infection is still under investigation. Moreover, liver transplant as the only intervention for terminal liver disease has also been affected by the pandemic. Specifically, most transplant programs in the world have been halted, which will result in longer waiting lists, liver decompensation, and death in the short term for many such patients.

The objective of the current review is to describe the intimate relationship between the gastrointestinal tract, including the liver and pancreas, and the pathogenesis, clinical course, and outcomes of the COVID-19 pandemic.

Citation: Aquino-Matus, J.; Uribe, M.; Chavez-Tapia, N. COVID-19: Current Status in Gastrointestinal, Hepatic, and Pancreatic Diseases—A Concise Review. *Trop. Med. Infect. Dis.* **2022**, *7*, 187. https://doi.org/10.3390/tropicalmed7080187

Academic Editors: Peter A. Leggat, John Frean and Lucille Blumberg

Received: 1 July 2022
Accepted: 9 August 2022
Published: 16 August 2022

Publisher's Note: MDPI stays neutral with regard to jurisdictional claims in published maps and institutional affiliations.

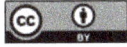

Copyright: © 2022 by the authors. Licensee MDPI, Basel, Switzerland. This article is an open access article distributed under the terms and conditions of the Creative Commons Attribution (CC BY) license (https://creativecommons.org/licenses/by/4.0/).

2. The Gastrointestinal Tract in the Pathogenesis of COVID-19

Coronaviruses express four structural proteins: spike (S), membrane (M), envelope (E), and nucleocapsid (N). The S protein receptor-binding domain shares 75% of the amino acid sequence of the SARS-CoV virus [2]. The conformational change of protein S, which binds with the angiotensin-converting enzyme 2 (ACE2) receptor and transmembrane protease serine 2 receptor (TMPRSS2) of the host cell, allows fusion of the viral envelope with the cell membrane and internalization of the virus [5]. Interferon upregulates the expression of ACE2 and TMPRSS2 receptors in the nasal secretory cells, type II pneumocytes, and enterocytes. Thus, the tropism of the virus is determined by the tissue distribution of ACE2 and TMPRSS2 receptors [6,7]. The affinity of SARS-CoV-2 for the ACE2 receptor in the gastrointestinal tract is 10–20 times greater than that of SARS-CoV [8].

Although fecal isolates of SARS-CoV-2 are capable of infecting cells cultured in vitro, fecal–oral transmission, though possible, has not been demonstrated [9]. In a retrospective study, a positive fecal real-time polymerase chain reaction (RT-PCR) was detected two to five days after a positive sputum RT-PCR with fecal excretion of the virus for up to 11 days [10].

Interestingly, SARS-CoV-2 RNA was identified in the sewage water of hospitals in Beijing and when seeded, could remain infectious for 14 days at 4 °C and 2 days at 20 °C [11]. Evidence for gastrointestinal infection of SARS-CoV-2 is controversial. For example, a 78-year-old man with COVID-19 developed gastrointestinal bleeding during hospitalization, with a hematoxylin and eosin (H&E) stain of endoscopic samples showing damage with infiltrating lymphocytes in the esophageal epithelium and plasma cells with interstitial edema in the stomach, duodenum, and rectum [12].

Gut microbiota could play a potential role as a diagnostic or prognostic biomarker in patients with COVID-19, as reported in a comprehensive systematic review including 1668 studies [13]. Patients with COVID-19 develop gut microbiota dysbiosis with depletion of *Ruminococcus*, *Alistipes*, *Eubacterium*, *Bifidobacterium*, *Faecalibacterium*, *Roseburia*, *Fusicathenibacter*, and *Blautia*, and enrichment of *Eggerthella*, *Bacteroides*, *Actinomyces*, *Clostridium*, *Streptococcus*, *Rothia*, and *Collinsella*. A dysregulated gut environment could increase the expression of ACE2 in the gut and favor more severe disease [14]. Table 1 summarizes examples of basic and translational implications of COVID-19.

Table 1. Basic and translational implications of COVID-19.

Study	Hypothesis	Design	Results	Implications
Jiao [15]	The gastrointestinal tract could play a central role in the pathogenesis of COVID-19	Infection of Rhesus monkeys with an intragastric or intranasal challenge with SARS-CoV-2	Both intranasal and intragastric inoculation caused pneumonia and gastrointestinal dysfunction	Possible connections through inflammatory cytokines
Wang [16]	SARS-CoV-2 could be potentially transmitted other than through the respiratory tract	Biodistribution of SARS-CoV-2 among different tissues of inpatients	SARS-CoV-2 detected in respiratory tissue, feces, and blood but not in urine	Transmission of the virus through extra-respiratory routes (feces) could explain the rapid spread
Irham [17]	Individual expression of TMPRSS2 may influence SARS-CoV-2 susceptibility	Multiple large genome databases (GTEx portal, SNP nexus, Ensembl genome project)	Four variants (rs464397, rs469390, rs2070788, and rs383510) affect expression of TMPRSS2 in lung tissue	Higher frequency of upregulating variants in European and American populations
Cao [18]	ACE2 variants could reduce the binding of S protein in SARS-CoV-2	Analysis of variants of ACE2 gene and allele frequencies in ChinaMAP and 1 KgP databases	Singleton truncating variant of ACE2 (Gln300X) and higher allele frequency in China of the SNP rs2285666	Lack of natural resistant mutations for coronavirus S protein binding

3. COVID-19 and Gastrointestinal Symptoms

Most patients with COVID-19 report nonspecific symptoms, including fever, headache, fatigue, arthralgias, myalgias, and general malaise. Because SARS-CoV-2 targets primarily the respiratory tract, additional symptoms such as cough, dyspnea, and anosmia are also reported [19]. Furthermore, in most published studies the prevalence of gastrointestinal symptoms varies between 5% and up to 50% of cases, and include diarrhea, nausea, vomiting, anorexia, and abdominal pain. In about 5% of patients, gastrointestinal symptoms may occur prior to respiratory symptoms [20]. A meta-analysis of 1577 patients reported that among gastrointestinal symptoms, diarrhea was the most prevalent with 33.9%, followed by nausea with 12.5%, and vomiting with 11.5%. In this study, the presence of gastrointestinal symptoms was not associated with COVID-19 severity (Odds Ratio (OR) 1.16; 95% Confidence Interval (CI) 0.89–1.52), and only abdominal pain was associated with a more severe disease (OR 2.83; 95% CI 1.34–6.01; $p = 0.007$) [21]. By comparison, in another meta-analysis that included 6686 patients, the presence of gastrointestinal symptoms was associated with a higher risk of acute respiratory distress syndrome (OR 2.85, 95% CI 1.17–7.48), and abdominal pain was associated with greater disease severity (OR 7.10; 95% CI 1.93–26.07) [22].

A systematic review and meta-analysis involving 4682 patients reported that the most significant gastrointestinal symptoms were anorexia (17%; 95% CI 0.06–0.27) and diarrhea (0.08; 95% CI 0.06–0.11), and patients with severe disease were more likely to have diarrhea, anorexia, and abdominal pain [23]. Although the clinical effect of gastrointestinal symptoms on COVID-19 outcomes is mixed, a prospective study in 244 patients reported that diarrhea was not associated with mortality (0% vs. 7.7%, $p = 0.036$) and overall gastrointestinal symptoms were negatively associated with moderate to severe disease ($p = 0.004$) [24].

In a study evaluating the dynamics of fecal RNA shedding in 113 patients, fecal SARS-CoV-2 RNA was detected in 49.2% (95% CI 38.2–60.3%) of patients within the first seven days after diagnosis, and 3.8% (95% CI 2.0–7.3%) of individuals shed for up to seven months [25]. Although it has been postulated that shedding of the virus correlates with gastrointestinal and nongastrointestinal symptoms, no association with long COVID-19 symptoms has been found [26].

Complex gastrointestinal complications of COVID-19 have been reported in severe disease, including ileus, hepatic necrosis, acalculous cholecystitis, and bowel ischemia. A systematic review that included 22 studies reported that 29% of patients presented with arterial mesenteric thromboembolism and 19.3% with portal venous thrombosis, requiring laparotomy and bowel resection in 64.5% with an overall mortality of 38.7% [27]. Although rare, ischemic gastrointestinal complications of COVID-19 can be fatal. Figure 1 highlights the relationship between COVID-19 and gastrointestinal manifestations and complications.

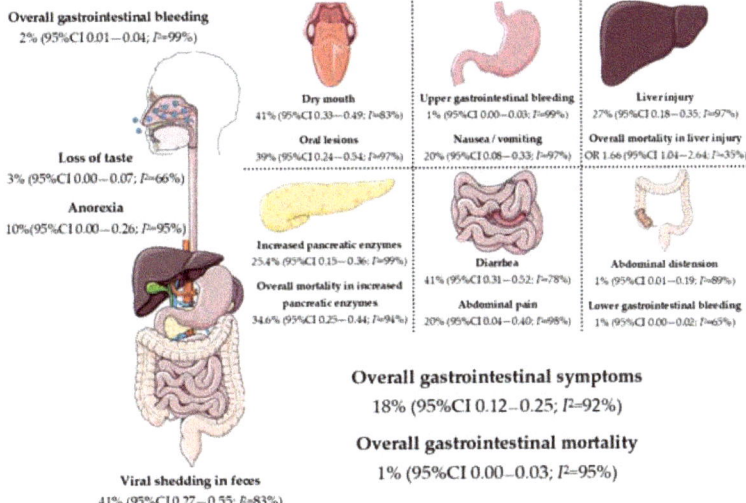

Figure 1. Overview of COVID-19 gastrointestinal, hepatic, and pancreatic manifestations (Adapted from references [14,28–30]).

4. COVID-19 and the Liver

At the beginning of the pandemic, the behavior of COVID-19 was expected to be similar to that of the SARS pandemic of 2003, where liver damage was reported in up to 60% of patients [31]. Early publications reported aberrations in liver tests, suggesting a possible mechanism of liver damage different from that in SARS-CoV-2. Abnormal liver function tests are frequently observed, with a prevalence as high as 76.3% and associated with more severe disease with abnormal alanine aminotransferase (ALT) (OR 1.89; 95% CI 1.30–2.76; p = 0.009) and abnormal aspartate aminotransferase (AST) (OR 3.08; 95% CI 2.14–4.42; p < 0.0001) [22].

The pattern of liver damage has been associated with greater severity of the disease with an OR of 2.73 (95% CI 1.19–6.3) for hepatocellular damage and an OR of 4.44 (95% CI 1.93–10.23) for mixed damage [32]. A meta-analysis that included 12,882 patients reported AST elevation in 41.1% and ALT elevation in 29.1% of cases; acute liver damage was reported in 26.5% of cases, which was associated with worse outcome (OR 1.68; 95% CI 1.04–2.70; p = 0.03) [33]. Abnormal liver tests in COVID-19 may be independent of the presence of pre-existing liver disease [34], which suggests a direct effect of the virus on the liver, among other mechanisms that are discussed below. In most cases, these alterations are transient and nonsignificant [19].

4.1. Proposed Mechanisms of Liver Injury

The liver is the only organ with double blood supply (arterial and portal) and harvests the largest reserve of macrophages, playing a crucial role in the immune response to SARS-CoV-2 through hepatic stellar cells. In addition, endothelial cells in liver sinusoids register and activate the immune response through Toll-like receptors [35].

The interaction between SARS-CoV-2 and the liver is under active investigation because ACE2 receptors are not expressed in Kupffer cells, hepatocytes, or endothelium of the hepatic sinusoids [7]. By contrast, ACE2 receptors are expressed in vascular endothelium and in cholangiocytes, almost in the same proportion as in the type II pneumocytes [31]. The endothelium of bile ducts is more susceptible to SARS-CoV-2, therefore the upregulation of ACE2 receptors favors internalization of the virus and results in liver damage due to compensatory proliferation of hepatocytes [19]. Interestingly, the expression of ACE2 receptors has been reported in fatty liver animal models [36] and in regeneration nodules in liver cirrhosis [35], giving rise to the possibility of greater susceptibility to liver damage in such patients.

Currently, there is no consensus on the exact mechanism of liver damage in COVID-19. However, several hypotheses have been postulated: (1) direct cytopathic damage, (2) systemic inflammatory response with immune-mediated collateral damage, (3) hypoxia and liver ischemia, as in hypoxic hepatitis, (4) acute-on-chronic liver failure, and (5) drug-induced and/or herbal-induced liver injury [37].

Direct cytopathic damage has not been demonstrated and in a study of postmortem liver biopsies, only moderate lymphocytic lobular infiltrate and centrilobular sinusoidal dilatation were reported, findings that the authors attributed to the patient's previous comorbidities [38]. In another postmortem study, no viral inclusions were found in the liver parenchyma [39].

The terms "cytokine release syndrome" and "cytokine storm" have been described in the medical literature since 1992 and refer to the role of a devastating effect of immune dysregulation, characterized by constitutional symptoms, systemic inflammation, and multiorgan dysfunction that can lead to multiorgan failure and death [40]. The cytokine storm in COVID-19 is characterized by high circulating levels of interleukin-1β, interferon-γ, and monocyte chemoattractant protein-1 [35], which upregulates the expression of ACE2 and TMPRSS2 receptors [6].

Hypoxic hepatitis refers to the massive, rapid rise in serum aminotransferases as a result of reduced oxygen delivery to the liver, which most common in cardiac failure, septic shock, and respiratory failure, but may occur in the absence of hypotension or a shock state in about 50% of cases [41]. In COVID-19, hypoxic hepatitis may be secondary to septic shock, COVID-related myocarditis (as cardiogenic shock), and ventilator complications [42]. In a series of 40 patients who died of complications of COVID-19, congestion and centrilobular ischemic necrosis were found in 78% and 40% of cases, respectively [43]. Hypoxic hepatitis may be considered among the differential diagnoses of liver injury in patients with COVID-19.

Acute-on-chronic liver failure (ACLF) refers to an acute decompensation in patients with chronic liver disease that is associated with a high risk of short-term mortality [44]. This syndrome is characterized by intense systemic inflammation, a close precipitating event, and single or multiple organ failure [45]. The mortality burden of ACLF in wait-listed patients is high, with prompt liver transplantation required in survivors. It has been hypothesized that patients with cirrhosis and ACLF have an increased risk of developing severe COVID-19 because of immune dysregulation (or immune paralysis). In cirrhosis, immune dysregulation is responsible for 30% of the mortality and is characterized by increases in anti-inflammatory cytokines, suppression of proinflammatory cytokines, increased gut permeability, reduced intestinal transit, and altered intestinal microbiota, which increases the risk of bacterial translocation and endotoxemia [46]. In a study that included 2460 patients, 35% met the definition of ACLF from the European Association for the Study of the Liver (EASL)-Chronic Liver Failure Consortium and exhibited prolonged hospital stay (14.7 ± 17.3 days vs. 5.4 ± 5.3 days, $p = 0.004$), severe COVID-19 (25% vs. 3%, $p = 0.03$), need for intensive care unit (45% vs. 11%, $p = 0.003$), and higher mortality (30% vs. 5%, $p = 0.01$) than patients without ACLF [47].

Drug-induced liver injury (DILI) and herb-induced liver injury (HILI) are defined as liver dysfunction and/or abnormalities in liver function tests secondary to the use of medications, herbs, or xenobiotics within the reasonable exclusion of other etiologies [48]. Many drugs have been used to treat patients with COVID-19, including antiviral agents (e.g., lopinavir, ritonavir, remdesivir, darunavir, umifenovir, and favipiravir), antibiotics (e.g., azithromycin), antimalarials (e.g., chloroquine and hydroxychloroquine), monoclonal antibodies (e.g., tocilizumab), JAK inhibitors (e.g., baricitinib), tyrosin kinase inhibitors (e.g., imatinib) [49,50], complementary alternative medicine (e.g., chlorine dioxide and Ayurvedic Kadha), and home remedies (*Allium sativum*) [51], many of which have been associated with hepatotoxicity alone or in combination as compassionate treatment. In this context, the Réseau d'Étude Francophone de l'Hépatotoxicité des Produits de Santé, a European study network focused on DILI, reported four cases of lopinavir/ritonavir suspected hepatotoxicity [52]. In clinical practice, polypharmacy is not uncommon, and physicians must be aware of DILI and HILI as potential causes of liver injury in patients with COVID-19. The same work-up and recommendations for patients without COVID-19 should be started upon suspicion of polypharmacy and DILI, especially discontinuation of the offending drug.

The exact mechanism of liver damage in COVID-19 is complex, challenging, and multifactorial in nature.

4.2. Implications in Fatty Liver Disease

Information concerning the association of hepatic steatosis and fibrosis with COVID-19 outcomes is limited. A more severe illness and worse outcomes are expected because a higher expression of ACE2 receptors has been found in hepatocytes of animal models of fatty liver [36].

A retrospective study that included 202 patients with fatty liver assessed by a hepatic steatosis index (HSI) > 36 points and/or confirmation by liver ultrasound reported a higher risk of progression of COVID-19 (6.6% vs. 44.7%, $p < 0.00001$) and longer shedding time (17.5 days vs. 12.1 days, $p < 0.00001$) in comparison with patients without fatty liver disease [53].

Obesity and metabolic syndrome are common risk factors for metabolic associated fatty liver disease (MAFLD) and in many cases coexist with COVID-19 in an alarming way. A prospective study of 214 patients with COVID-19 reported a 30.8% prevalence of MAFLD, of whom 68.2% had obesity associated with greater severity of disease (OR 6.32; 95% CI 1.16–34.54, p = 0.033) [54].

Establishing the risk of MAFLD through noninvasive predictive models at the time of hospitalization for COVID-19 may result in an overestimation of the prevalence of MAFLD because biomarkers (e.g., transaminases) used in the models (e.g., HSI, NAFLD-FS) may be altered by COVID-19. In addition, imaging techniques such as ultrasound have an overall sensitivity of 84.8% (95% CI 79.5–88.9) and a specificity of 93.6% (95% CI 87.2–97.0) for the detection of moderate to severe fatty liver [55], which could be considered as a reliable bedside diagnostic tool for fatty liver and for excluding other causes of abnormal liver tests.

In a systematic review and meta-analysis including 16 observational studies and 1746 MAFLD patients, the prevalence of COVID-19 was 29% (95% CI 0.19–0.40, p = 0.04) and was associated with increased severity (OR 3.07; 95% CI 2.30–4.09) and risk of ICU admission (OR 1.46; 95% CI 1.12–1.91, p = 0.28) but not associated with mortality (OR 1.45; 95% CI 0.74–2.87, p > 0.05) [56]. Patients with MAFLD seem to be at higher risk of developing complications related to COVID-19, but further research is needed.

4.3. Implications in Liver Cirrhosis

Liver cirrhosis is estimated to affect 4.5–9% of the world's population [57], and a high proportion of patients with cirrhosis are expected to be infected with COVID-19. A multicenter study of 160 patients reported a prevalence of advanced fibrosis of 28.1% assessed with FIB-4 $\geq$ 2.67, which was associated with a higher risk for requiring intensive care (OR 3.41; 95% CI 1.30–8.92) [58].

The two most important international registries of patients with chronic liver disease and COVID-19 are COVID-Hep.net (University of Oxford and EASL) and SECURE-Cirrhosis Registry (University of North Carolina at Chapel Hill). In the first report, which included 745 patients (386 with cirrhosis and 359 controls), a mortality of 32% was found in patients with cirrhosis, which increased according to liver disease severity to 35% (OR 4.14; 95% CI 1.03–3.52) in Child–Pugh B and 51% (OR 9.32; 95% CI 4.80–18.08) in Child–Pugh C. Acute decompensation was observed in 46% of cases, of which 21% had no respiratory symptoms and 50% presented as ACLF [59].

An additional concern during the COVID-19 pandemic is the role of immunosuppression in patients with autoimmune liver diseases due to the increased risk of respiratory tract infections. However, a greater severity of infection has not yet been demonstrated in this group of patients. In this regard, recommendations for the approach to this group of patients are summarized in Table 2 [60].

Table 2. Recommendations for patients with autoimmune liver disease and COVID-19 (adapted from Lleo [60]).

Summary of Recommendations
• Organize independent access to health services to avoid contact with COVID-19-positive patients. • Limit invasive screening procedures to only emergency interventions (e.g., endoscopy). • Initiate immunosuppressive treatment at standard doses for the treatment of exacerbation of autoimmune hepatitis. • Coordinate care with the transplant committee in case of acute liver failure. • Reduce immunosuppression in case of infection, especially antimetabolites in patients with lymphopenia.

4.4. Implications in Liver Transplantation

Since 1980, transplant programs around the world have responded to the pandemics of HIV, SARS-CoV, East Nile Virus, Influenza A/H1N1, Zika, and Ebola, maintaining their operation with the evaluation of the transmission to the donor, the severity of the disease in the recipient, and the risk of transmission to health personnel [61]. Unlike other solid organ transplant programs where alternatives or bridging therapies exist, such as hemodialysis, cardiac assist devices, and extracorporeal membrane oxygenation, in the case of patients with acute liver failure or end-stage liver disease, liver transplantation is the only treatment alternative. Currently, liver transplantation programs are among the most vulnerable around the world.

During the COVID-19 pandemic, the availability of intensive care beds has been vital, and this need is shared by transplant programs whose patients require specialized postoperative care. Therefore, a staggered-phase approach has been proposed with a decrease in the activity of transplant programs according to the tolerance of transplant risk, hospital capacity, and pandemic activity in the locality [61]. In a health system completely overwhelmed by the care of COVID-19 patients, the transplant program must be reduced by 100%.

Early experience at the beginning of the COVID-19 pandemic has been reported in a prospective nationwide study containing 111 liver transplant patients with COVID-19. At a median of 23 days, up to 86.5% of patients were hospitalized, 19.8% required intubation, 10.88% were admitted to the intensive care unit, and 18% died [62]. Currently, there is no consensus regarding the time of liver transplant in patients with COVID-19. Even so, successful liver transplants have been reported in patients with asymptomatic COVID-19 [63].

Recently, a study involving 792 patients from the EASL-COVID-Hep network and 283 patients from the UK OCTAVE study were compared with 93 healthy controls from the UK PITCH consortium. The study reported that liver transplant recipients had reduced anti-S Ig titer following two doses of BNT162b2 or ChAdOx1 vaccines [64]. It is still unknown why liver transplant patients failed to generate a response following vaccination.

4.5. COVID-19 and Inflammatory Bowel Disease

Patients with inflammatory bowel disease (IBD) share a similar inflammatory cytokine profile with acute exacerbation and "cytokine storm", and such patients could benefit from treatment with interleukin-1 or interleukin-6 antagonists [65].

Two forms of the ACE2 receptor have been described, a soluble one that lacks a transmembrane domain and circulates in small amounts in the bloodstream and a complete one made up of an extracellular domain and a transmembrane domain and is responsible for the internalization of the virus into the host cell [66]. The soluble ACE2 receptor is upregulated in patients with IBD, and in vitro studies have shown that it can prevent virus binding to the transmembrane ACE2 receptor by acting as a competitive inhibitor [65].

In a multicenter study from the SECURE-IBD database (University of North Carolina at Chapel Hill), 232 patients with IBD (101 with Crohn's disease, 93 with ulcerative colitis, and 38 with indeterminate colitis) were compared with 19,776 controls, and although there was no difference between the groups regarding the severity of the infection, the risk of severe COVID-19 was higher in patients under treatment with steroids (OR 1.60, 95% CI 1.01–2.57; p = 0.04) [67]. From this database, 209 patients under 18 years of age were analyzed and hospitalization was required in 7% with 1% requiring mechanical ventilation; no mortality was reported. Interestingly, patients receiving anti-TNF monotherapy had a lower rate of hospitalization (7% vs. 51%, p < 0.01) [68].

A meta-analysis containing 24 studies reported a pooled incidence rate of COVID-19 of 4.02 per 1000 persons with IBD (95% CI 1.44–11.17, I^2 = 98%) with a pooled relative risk of acquiring COVID-19 no different from the general population (0.47; 95% CI 0.18–1.26, I^2 = 89%) nor type of IBD (1.03, 95% CI 0.62–1.71, I^2 = 0); pooled mortality was 4.27% [69]. As reported in previous studies, the relative risk of hospitalization, intensive care unit admission, and mortality was lower for patients on biologics but higher for those taking steroids or 5-aminosalicylates. In a prospective study including 5457 patients with IBD (I-CARE project), 4.3% reported COVID-19 with 0.2% severe cases and no COVID-19-related mortality [70]. Currently, there is no evidence that IBD is associated with a higher risk of COVID-19 infection or worse outcomes.

Similar to autoimmune liver diseases, IBD relapse may occur with inappropriate discontinuation of corticosteroids, antimetabolites, immunomodulators, and/or biologics [71]. Therefore, discussion with IBD experts is warranted in the treatment and follow-up of these patients.

4.6. COVID-19 and the Pancreas

Because COVID-19 manifests as a multisystemic disease, pancreatic involvement is expected, although limited evidence is available. Multiple viruses affect the pancreas, including hepatotropic viruses (hepatitis A, B, and E, Epstein–Barr, Coxsackie, Cytomegalovirus, and herpes zoster), as well as HIV, mumps, measles, and varicella zoster [72].

Higher levels of ACE2 messenger RNA have been found in the pancreas than in the lungs, a finding that could explain the pancreatic damage with infection [73]. In addition, obesity increases visceral adipose tissue, including intrapancreatic fat, in which the content of unsaturated fatty acids from triglycerides in adipocytes is released by hydrolysis and perpetuates fat necrosis in cases of acute pancreatitis that ultimately results in a "cytokine storm" and multi-organ failure, a similar scenario to that observed in COVID-19 [72].

Although the presence of SARS-CoV-2 in the pancreas has not been demonstrated in necropsy studies of patients with COVID-19, in 2004 SARS-CoV was detected by murine monoclonal antibodies in four patients with SARS [74]. Because of the similarity in viral structure and pathogenesis of SARS-CoV with SARS-CoV-2, a similar distribution can be expected in tissues and organs between the two viruses.

Abnormal pancreatic enzyme levels have been described in 8.5% to 17.3% of COVID-19 cases. Nonetheless, only 0.76% of cases met the Atlanta criteria for acute pancreatitis [72]. In a multicenter retrospective study of 71 hospitalized patients with COVID-19, only 12.1% presented with hyperlipasemia and 2.8% had a report of serum lipase levels at least three times the upper limit of normal, which was not associated with worse outcomes and no patient met the criteria for acute pancreatitis [75]. In patients with severe COVID-19, a higher prevalence of elevated pancreatic enzymes has been reported, and in a retrospective study of 1003 patients, 16.8% presented with lipase more than three times the upper limit of normal, which was associated with a higher rate of admission to intensive care (OR 8.93; 95% CI 2.43–38.5, $p < 0.002$) and intubation (OR 12.5; 95% CI 2.95–68.4, $p < 0.002$) when reported in the range of 81 to 701 IU/L [76].

Most cases of acute pancreatitis have been documented in patients with severe COVID-19, even without respiratory symptoms at the onset of the disease [72]. In a multicenter retrospective study of 48,012 hospitalized patients, only 0.39% met acute pancreatitis criteria, of whom 17% had COVID-19, and this combination was associated with a higher rate of intubation (OR 5.65; 95% CI 1.49–21.52, $p = 0.01$) and length of hospital stay (OR 3.22; 95% CI 1.34–7.75, $p = 0.009$) compared with patients without COVID-19 [77].

Finally, treatments used for COVID-19 can precipitate acute pancreatitis both directly (e.g., steroids and baricitinib) and indirectly (e.g., hypertriglyceridemia from tocilizumab and lopinavir/ritonavir) [72]. Therefore, although acute pancreatitis is not the most frequent manifestation of COVID-19, it should be considered within the differential diagnosis of patients with gastrointestinal symptoms, specifically abdominal pain.

As expected, in a study comparing admissions for acute pancreatitis (baseline group) with admissions during the same period in 2020 (pandemic group), patients in the pandemic group were more likely to present with systemic inflammatory response syndrome (40% vs. 25%, $p < 0.01$) and pancreatic necrosis (14% vs. 10%, $p = 0.03$), reflecting an avoidance of hospitalization for milder cases [78].

5. Conclusions

The role of the gastrointestinal tract in terms of presentation, progression, and outcomes in COVID-19 infection is becoming increasingly more important. Gastrointestinal symptoms and liver damage are common and can be associated with worse outcomes. Patients with cirrhosis are at increased risk of severe COVID-19. Patients with IBD are not at higher risk of complications, except for those on steroids. Immunosuppressive treatment should be continued and adjusted according to the clinical scenario of each individual case. Evidence of pancreatic involvement in patients with COVID-19 is still scarce.

Author Contributions: Conceptualization, J.A.-M., M.U. and N.C.-T.; methodology, J.A.-M. and N.C.-T.; investigation, J.A.-M.; writing—original draft preparation, J.A.-M. and N.C.-T.; writing—review and editing, J.A.-M. and N.C.-T.; visualization, J.A.-M.; supervision, M.U. and N.C.-T.; funding acquisition, M.U. All authors have read and agreed to the published version of the manuscript.

Funding: This research was partially funded by Medica Sur Clinic & Foundation.

Institutional Review Board Statement: Not applicable.

Informed Consent Statement: Not applicable.

Data Availability Statement: Not applicable.

Acknowledgments: The authors acknowledge the use of Servier Medical Art, provided by Servier, licensed under a Creative Commons Attribution 3.0 unported license, for partially generating Figure 1.

Conflicts of Interest: All authors declare no conflict of interest.

References

1. WHO Director-General's Opening Remarks at the Media Briefing on COVID-19—11 March 2020. Available online: https://www.who.int/dg/speeches/detail/who-director-general-s-opening-remarks-at-the-media-briefing-on-covid-19---11-march-2020 (accessed on 17 October 2020).
2. Shereen, M.A.; Khan, S.; Kazmi, A.; Bashir, N.; Siddique, R. COVID-19 Infection: Origin, Transmission, and Characteristics of Human Coronaviruses. *J. Adv. Res.* **2020**, *24*, 91–98. [CrossRef] [PubMed]
3. Huang, C.; Wang, Y.; Li, X.; Ren, L.; Zhao, J.; Hu, Y.; Zhang, L.; Fan, G.; Xu, J.; Gu, X.; et al. Clinical Features of Patients Infected with 2019 Novel Coronavirus in Wuhan, China. *Lancet* **2020**, *395*, 497–506. [CrossRef]
4. Amoroso, L.; Simonato, L.E.; Ramos, R.R. Phylogeny and Pathogenesis of SARS-CoV-2: A Systematic Study. *J. Mod. Med. Chem.* **2020**, *8*, 49–55.
5. Wu, F.; Zhao, S.; Yu, B.; Chen, Y.M.; Wang, W.; Song, Z.G.; Hu, Y.; Tao, Z.W.; Tian, J.H.; Pei, Y.Y.; et al. A New Coronavirus Associated with Human Respiratory Disease in China. *Nature* **2020**, *579*, 265–269. [CrossRef] [PubMed]
6. Ziegler, C.G.K.; Allon, S.J.; Nyquist, S.K.; Mbano, I.M.; Miao, V.N.; Tzouanas, C.N.; Cao, Y.; Yousif, A.S.; Bals, J.; Hauser, B.M.; et al. SARS-CoV-2 Receptor ACE2 Is an Interferon-Stimulated Gene in Human Airway Epithelial Cells and Is Detected in Specific Cell Subsets across Tissues. *Cell* **2020**, *181*, 1016–1035.e19. [CrossRef] [PubMed]
7. Hamming, I.; Timens, W.; Bulthuis, M.L.C.; Lely, A.T.; Navis, G.J.; van Goor, H. Tissue Distribution of ACE2 Protein, the Functional Receptor for SARS Coronavirus. A First Step in Understanding SARS Pathogenesis. *J. Pathol.* **2004**, *203*, 631–637. [CrossRef]
8. D'Amico, F.; Baumgart, D.C.; Danese, S.; Peyrin-Biroulet, L. Diarrhea during COVID-19 Infection: Pathogenesis, Epidemiology, Prevention and Management. *Clin. Gastroenterol. Hepatol.* **2020**, *18*, 1663–1672. [CrossRef]
9. Hindson, J. COVID-19: Faecal–Oral Transmission? *Nat. Rev. Gastroenterol. Hepatol.* **2020**, *17*, 259. [CrossRef]
10. Tian, Y.; Rong, L.; Nian, W.; He, Y. Review Article: Gastrointestinal Features in COVID-19 and the Possibility of Faecal Transmission. *Aliment. Pharmacol. Ther.* **2020**, *51*, 843–851. [CrossRef]
11. Yeo, C.; Kaushal, S.; Yeo, D. Enteric Involvement of Coronaviruses: Is Faecal–Oral Transmission of SARS-CoV-2 Possible? *Lancet Gastroenterol. Hepatol.* **2020**, *5*, 335–337. [CrossRef]
12. Xiao, F.; Tang, M.; Zheng, X.; Liu, Y.; Li, X.; Shan, H. Evidence for Gastrointestinal Infection of SARS-CoV-2 Fei. *Gastroenterology* **2020**, *158*, 1831–1833. [CrossRef] [PubMed]
13. Farsi, Y.; Tahvildari, A.; Arbabi, M.; Vazife, F.; Sechi, L.A.; Shahidi Bonjar, A.H.; Jamshidi, P.; Nasiri, M.J.; Mirsaeidi, M. Diagnostic, Prognostic, and Therapeutic Roles of Gut Microbiota in COVID-19: A Comprehensive Systematic Review. *Front. Cell. Infect. Microbiol.* **2022**, *12*, 804644. [CrossRef] [PubMed]
14. Chen, T.; Hsu, M.; Lee, M.; Chou, C. Gastrointestinal Involvement in SARS-CoV-2 Infection. *Viruses* **2022**, *14*, 1188–1205. [CrossRef] [PubMed]
15. Jiao, L.; Li, H.; Xu, J.; Yang, M.; Ma, C.; Li, J.; Zhao, S.; Wang, H.; Yang, Y.; Yu, W.; et al. The Gastrointestinal Tract Is an Alternative Route for SARS-CoV-2 Infection in a Nonhuman Primate Model. *Gastroenterology* **2021**, *160*, 1647–1661. [CrossRef]
16. Wang, W.; Xu, Y.; Gao, R.; Han, K.; Wu, G.; Tan, W. Detection of SARS-CoV-2 in Different Types of Clinical Specimens. *JAMA* **2020**, *323*, 1843–1844. [CrossRef] [PubMed]
17. Irham, L.M.; Chou, W.H.; Calkins, M.J.; Adikusuma, W.; Hsieh, S.L.; Chang, W.C. Genetic Variants That Influence SARS-CoV-2 Receptor TMPRSS2 Expression among Population Cohorts from Multiple Continents. *Biochem. Biophys. Res. Commun.* **2020**, *529*, 263–269. [CrossRef]

18. Cao, Y.; Li, L.; Feng, Z.; Wan, S.; Huang, P.; Sun, X.; Wen, F.; Huang, X.; Ning, G.; Wang, W. Comparative Genetic Analysis of the Novel Coronavirus (2019-NCoV/SARS-CoV-2) Receptor ACE2 in Different Populations. *Cell Discov.* **2020**, *6*, 11. [CrossRef]
19. Patel, K.P.; Patel, P.A.; Vunnam, R.R.; Hewlett, A.T.; Jain, R.; Jing, R.; Vunnam, S.R. Gastrointestinal, Hepatobiliary, and Pancreatic Manifestations of COVID-19. *J. Clin. Virol.* **2020**, *128*, 104386. [CrossRef]
20. Schmulson, M.; Dávalos, M.F.; Berumen, J. Beware: Gastrointestinal Symptoms Can Be a Manifestation of COVID-19. *Rev. Gastroenterol. Mex.* **2020**, *85*, 282–287. [CrossRef]
21. Deidda, S.; Tora, L.; Firinu, D.; Del Giacco, S.; Campagna, M.; Meloni, F.; Orrù, G.; Chessa, L.; Carta, M.G.; Melis, A.; et al. Gastrointestinal Coronavirus Disease 2019: Epidemiology, Clinical Features, Pathogenesis, Prevention, and Management. *Expert Rev. Gastroenterol. Hepatol.* **2021**, *15*, 41–50. [CrossRef]
22. Mao, R.; Qiu, Y.; He, J.S.; Tan, J.Y.; Li, X.H.; Liang, J.; Shen, J.; Zhu, L.R.; Chen, Y.; Iacucci, M.; et al. Manifestations and Prognosis of Gastrointestinal and Liver Involvement in Patients with COVID-19: A Systematic Review and Meta-Analysis. *Lancet Gastroenterol. Hepatol.* **2020**, *5*, 667–678. [CrossRef]
23. Dong, Z.Y.; Xiang, B.J.; Jiang, M.; Sun, M.J.; Dai, C. The Prevalence of Gastrointestinal Symptoms, Abnormal Liver Function, Digestive System Disease and Liver Disease in COVID-19 Infection. *J. Clin. Gastroenterol* **2021**, *55*, 67–76. [CrossRef] [PubMed]
24. Singh, S.; Samanta, J.; Suri, V.; Bhalla, A.; Puri, G.D.; Sehgal, R.; Kochhar, R. Presence of Diarrhea Associated with Better Outcomes in Patients with COVID-19—A Prospective Evaluation. *Indian J. Med. Microbiol.* **2022**. in press. [CrossRef] [PubMed]
25. Natarajan, A.; Zlitni, S.; Brooks, E.F.; Vance, S.E.; Dahlen, A.; Hedlin, H.; Park, R.M.; Han, A.; Schmidtke, D.T.; Verma, R.; et al. Gastrointestinal Symptoms and Fecal Shedding of SARS-CoV-2 RNA Suggest Prolonged Gastrointestinal Infection. *Med. (N. Y.)* **2022**, *3*, 371–387.e9. [CrossRef]
26. Sneller, M.C.; Liang, C.J.; Marques, A.R.; Chung, J.Y.; Shanbhag, S.M.; Fontana, J.R.; Raza, H.; Okeke, O.; Dewar, R.L.; Higgins, B.P.; et al. A Longitudinal Study of COVID-19 Sequelae and Immunity: Baseline Findings. *Ann. Intern. Med.* **2022**, *175*, 969–979. [CrossRef] [PubMed]
27. Keshavarz, P.; Rafiee, F.; Kavandi, H.; Goudarzi, S.; Heidari, F.; Gholamrezanezhad, A. Ischemic Gastrointestinal Complications of COVID-19: A Systematic Review on Imaging Presentation. *Clin. Imaging* **2021**, *73*, 86–95. [CrossRef]
28. Qi, X.; Northridge, M.E.; Hu, M.; Wu, B. Oral Health Conditions and COVID-19: A Systematic Review and Meta-Analysis of the Current Evidence. *Aging Health Res.* **2022**, *2*, 100064. [CrossRef]
29. Yadav, D.K.; Singh, A.; Zhang, Q.; Bai, X.; Zhang, W.; Yadav, R.K.; Singh, A.; Zhiwei, L.; Adhikari, V.P.; Liang, T. Involvement of Liver in COVID-19: Systematic Review and Meta-Analysis. *Gut* **2021**, *70*, 807–809. [CrossRef]
30. Yang, F.; Xu, Y.; Dong, Y.; Huang, Y.; Fu, Y.; Li, T.; Sun, C.; Pandanaboyana, S.; Windsor, J.A.; Fu, D. Prevalence and Prognosis of Increased Pancreatic Enzymes in Patients with COVID-19: A Systematic Review and Meta-Analysis. *Pancreatology* **2022**, *22*, 539–546. [CrossRef]
31. Jothimani, D.; Venugopal, R.; Abedin, M.F.; Kaliamoorthy, I.; Rela, M. COVID-19 and the Liver. *J. Hepatol.* **2020**, *73*, 1231–1240. [CrossRef]
32. Cai, Q.; Huang, D.; Yu, H.; Zhu, Z.; Xia, Z.; Su, Y.; Li, Z.; Zhou, G.; Gou, J.; Qu, J.; et al. COVID-19: Abnormal Liver Function Tests. *J. Hepatol.* **2020**, *73*, 566–574. [CrossRef] [PubMed]
33. Sharma, A.; Jaiswal, P.; Kerakhan, Y.; Saravanan, L.; Murtaza, Z.; Zergham, A.; Honganur, N.-S.; Akbar, A.; Deol, A.; Francis, B.; et al. Liver Disease and Outcomes among COVID-19 Hospitalized Patients—A Systematic Review and Meta-Analysis. *Ann. Hepatol.* **2021**, *21*, 100273. [CrossRef] [PubMed]
34. Zhang, C.; Shi, L.; Wang, F.S. Liver Injury in COVID-19: Management and Challenges. *Lancet Gastroenterol. Hepatol.* **2020**, *5*, 428–430. [CrossRef]
35. Lizardo-Thiebaud, M.J.; Cervantes-Alvarez, E.; Limon-de la Rosa, N.; Tejeda-Dominguez, F.; Palacios-Jimenez, M.; Méndez-Guerrero, O.; Delaye-Martinez, M.; Rodriguez-Alvarez, F.; Romero-Morales, B.; Liu, W.-H.; et al. Direct or Collateral Liver Damage in SARS-CoV-2-Infected Patients. *Semin. Liver Dis.* **2020**, *40*, 321–330. [CrossRef]
36. Zhang, W.; Li, C.; Liu, B.; Wu, R.; Zou, N.; Xu, Y.Z.; Yang, Y.Y.; Zhang, F.; Zhou, H.M.; Wan, K.Q.; et al. Pioglitazone Upregulates Hepatic Angiotensin Converting Enzyme 2 Expression in Rats with Steatohepatitis. *Ann. Hepatol.* **2013**, *12*, 892–900. [CrossRef]
37. Méndez-Sánchez, N.; Valencia-Rodríguez, A.; Qi, X.; Yoshida, E.M.; Romero-Gómez, M.; George, J.; Eslam, M.; Abenavoli, L.; Xie, W.; Teschke, R.; et al. What Has the COVID-19 Pandemic Taught Us so Far? Addressing the Problem from a Hepatologist's Perspective. *J. Clin. Transl. Hepatol.* **2020**, *8*, 109–112. [CrossRef]
38. Tian, S.; Xiong, Y.; Liu, H.; Niu, L.; Guo, J.; Liao, M.; Xiao, S.Y. Pathological Study of the 2019 Novel Coronavirus Disease (COVID-19) through Postmortem Core Biopsies. *Mod. Pathol.* **2020**, *33*, 1007–1014. [CrossRef]
39. Barton, L.M.; Duval, E.J.; Stroberg, E.; Ghosh, S.; Mukhopadhyay, S. COVID-19 Autopsies, Oklahoma, USA. *Am. J. Clin. Pathol.* **2020**, *153*, 725–733. [CrossRef]
40. Fajgenbaum, D.C.; June, C.H. Cytokine Storm. *N. Engl. J. Med.* **2020**, *383*, 2255–2273. [CrossRef]
41. Waseem, N.; Chen, P.H. Hypoxic Hepatitis: A Review and Clinical Update. *J. Clin. Transl. Hepatol.* **2016**, *4*, 263–268.
42. Hamid, S.; Alvares Da Silva, M.R.; Burak, K.W.; Chen, T.; Drenth, J.P.H.; Esmat, G.; Gaspar, R.; Labrecque, D.; Lee, A.; Macedo, G.; et al. WGO Guidance for the Care of Patients with COVID-19 and Liver Disease. *J. Clin. Gastroenterol.* **2021**, *55*, 1–11. [CrossRef] [PubMed]

43. Lagana, S.M.; Kudose, S.; Iuga, A.C.; Lee, M.J.; Fazlollahi, L.; Remotti, H.E.; Del Portillo, A.; De Michele, S.; de Gonzalez, A.K.; Saqi, A.; et al. Hepatic Pathology in Patients Dying of COVID-19: A Series of 40 Cases Including Clinical, Histologic, and Virologic Data. *Mod. Pathol.* **2020**, *33*, 2147–2155. [CrossRef] [PubMed]
44. Arroyo, V.; Moreau, R.; Jalan, R. Acute-on-Chronic Liver Failure. *N. Engl. J. Med.* **2020**, *382*, 2137–2145. [CrossRef] [PubMed]
45. Asrani, S.K.; O'Leary, J.G. Acute-On-Chronic Liver Failure. *Clin. Liver Dis.* **2014**, *18*, 561–574. [CrossRef]
46. Noor, M.T.; Manoria, P. Immune Dysfunction in Cirrhosis. *J. Clin. Transl. Hepatol.* **2017**, *5*, 50–58. [CrossRef]
47. Kumar, P.; Sharma, M.; Sulthana, S.F.; Kulkarni, A.; Rao, P.N.; Reddy, D.N. SARS-CoV-2 Related Acute on Chronic Liver Failure (S-ACLF). *J. Clin. Exp. Hepatol.* **2021**, *11*, 404–406. [CrossRef]
48. Suk, K.T.; Kim, D.J. Drug-Induced Liver Injury: Present and Future. *Clin. Mol. Hepatol.* **2012**, *18*, 249–257. [CrossRef]
49. Alqahtani, S.A.; Schattenberg, J.M. Liver Injury in COVID-19: The Current Evidence. *United Eur. Gastroenterol. J.* **2020**, *8*, 509–519. [CrossRef]
50. Boeckmans, J.; Rodrigues, R.M.; Demuyser, T.; Piérard, D.; Vanhaecke, T.; Rogiers, V. COVID-19 and Drug-Induced Liver Injury: A Problem of Plenty or a Petty Point? *Arch. Toxicol.* **2020**, *94*, 1367–1369. [CrossRef]
51. Charan, J.; Bhardwaj, P.; Dutta, S.; Kaur, R.; Bist, S.K.; Detha, M.D.; Kanchan, T.; Yadav, D.; Mitra, P.; Sharma, P. Use of Complementary and Alternative Medicine (CAM) and Home Remedies by COVID-19 Patients: A Telephonic Survey. *Indian J. Clin. Biochem.* **2020**, *36*, 108–111. [CrossRef]
52. Olry, A.; Meunier, L.; Délire, B.; Larrey, D.; Horsmans, Y.; Le Louët, H. Drug-Induced Liver Injury and COVID-19 Infection: The Rules Remain the Same. *Drug Saf.* **2020**, *43*, 615–617. [CrossRef] [PubMed]
53. Ji, D.; Qin, E.; Xu, J.; Zhang, D.; Cheng, G.; Wang, Y.; Lau, G. Non-Alcoholic Fatty Liver Diseases in Patients with COVID-19: A Retrospective Study. *J. Hepatol.* **2020**, *73*, 451–453. [CrossRef] [PubMed]
54. Zheng, K.I.; Gao, F.; Wang, X.B.; Sun, Q.F.; Pan, K.H.; Wang, T.Y.; Ma, H.L.; Liu, W.Y.; George, J.; Zheng, M.H. Letter to the Editor: Obesity as a Risk Factor for Greater Severity of COVID-19 in Patients with Metabolic Associated Fatty Liver Disease. *Metabolism* **2020**, *108*, 154244. [CrossRef]
55. Hernaez, R.; Lazo, M.; Bonekamp, S.; Kamel, I.; Brancati, F.L.; Guallar, E.; Clark, J.M. Diagnostic Accuracy and Reliability of Ultrasonography for the Detection of Fatty Liver: A Meta-Analysis. *Hepatology* **2011**, *54*, 1082–1090. [CrossRef] [PubMed]
56. Hayat, U.; Ashfaq, M.Z.; Johnson, L.; Ford, R.; Wuthnow, C.; Kadado, K.; El Jurdi, K.; Okut, H.; Kilgore, W.R.; Assi, M.; et al. The Association of Metabolic-Associated Fatty Liver Disease with Clinical Outcomes of COVID-19: A Systematic Review and Meta-Analysis. *Kansas J. Med.* **2022**, *15*, 241–246. [CrossRef] [PubMed]
57. Méndez-Sánchez, N.; Zamarripa-Dorsey, F.; Panduro, A.; Purón-González, E.; Coronado-Alejandro, E.U.; Cortez-Hernández, C.A.; de la Tijera, F.H.; Pérez-Hernández, J.L.; Cerda-Reyes, E.; Rodríguez-Hernández, H.; et al. Current Trends of Liver Cirrhosis in Mexico: Similitudes and Differences with Other World Regions. *World J. Clin. Cases* **2018**, *6*, 922–930. [CrossRef]
58. Ibáñez-Samaniego, L.; Bighelli, F.; Usón, C.; Caravaca, C.; Carrillo, C.F.; Romero, M.; Barreales, M.; Perelló, C.; Madejón, A.; Marcos, A.C.; et al. Elevation of Liver Fibrosis Index FIB-4 Is Associated With Poor Clinical Outcomes in Patients With COVID-19. *J. Infect. Dis.* **2020**, *222*, 726–733. [CrossRef]
59. Marjot, T.; Moon, A.M.; Cook, J.A.; Abd-Elsalam, S.; Aloman, C.; Armstrong, M.J.; Brenner, E.J.; Cargill, T. Outcomes Following SARS-CoV-2 Infection in Patients with Chronic Liver Disease: An International Registry Study. *J. Hepatol.* **2021**, *74*, 567–577. [CrossRef]
60. Lleo, A.; Invernizzi, P.; Lohse, A.W.; Aghemo, A.; Carbone, M. Management of Patients with Autoimmune Liver Disease during COVID-19 Pandemic. *J. Hepatol.* **2020**, *73*, 453–455. [CrossRef]
61. Kumar, D.; Manuel, O.; Natori, Y.; Egawa, H.; Grossi, P.; Han, S.H.; Fernández-Ruiz, M.; Humar, A. COVID-19: A Global Transplant Perspective on Successfully Navigating a Pandemic. *Am. J. Transplant.* **2020**, *20*, 1773–1779. [CrossRef]
62. Colmenero, J.; Rodríguez-Perálvarez, M.; Salcedo, M.; Arias-Milla, A.; Muñoz-Serrano, A.; Graus, J.; Nuño, J.; Gastaca, M.; Bustamante-Schneider, J.; Cachero, A.; et al. Epidemiological Pattern, Incidence, and Outcomes of COVID-19 in Liver Transplant Patients. *J. Hepatol.* **2021**, *74*, 148–155. [CrossRef] [PubMed]
63. Mouch, C.A.; Alexopoulos, S.P.; LaRue, R.W.; Kim, H.P. Successful Liver Transplantation in Patients with Active 2 Infection. *Am. J. Transpl.* **2022**. *online ahead of print*. [CrossRef]
64. Burba, K. Liver Transplantation Linked to Lower Antibody, T-Cell Response to COVID-19 Vaccine. Healio Gastroenterology. Available online: https://www.healio.com/news/gastroenterology/20220628/liver-transplantation-linked-to-lower-antibody-tcell-response-to-covid19-vaccine (accessed on 20 June 2022).
65. Monteleone, G.; Ardizzone, S. Are Patients with Inflammatory Bowel Disease at Increased Risk for Covid-19 Infection? *J. Crohns. Colitis* **2020**, *14*, 1334–1336. [CrossRef] [PubMed]
66. Du, L.; He, Y.; Zhou, Y.; Liu, S.; Zheng, B.J.; Jiang, S. The Spike Protein of SARS-CoV-A Target for Vaccine and Therapeutic Development. *Nat. Rev. Microbiol.* **2009**, *7*, 226–236. [CrossRef] [PubMed]
67. Singh, S.; Khan, A.; Chowdhry, M.; Bilal, M.; Kochhar, G.S.; Clarke, K. Risk of Severe Coronavirus Disease 2019 in Patients with Inflammatory Bowel Disease in the United States: A Multicenter Research Network Study. *Gastroenterology* **2020**, *159*, 1575–1578.e4. [CrossRef] [PubMed]
68. Brenner, E.J.; Pigneur, B.; Focht, G.; Zhang, X.; Ungaro, R.C.; Colombel, J.-F.; Turner, D.; Kappelman, M.D.; Ruemmele, F.M. Benign Evolution of SARS-CoV-2 Infections in Children with Inflammatory Bowel Disease: Results from Two International Databases. *Clin. Gastroenterol. Hepatol.* **2020**, *19*, 394–396.e5. [CrossRef] [PubMed]

69. Singh, A.K.; Jena, A.; Kumar-M, P.; Sharma, V.; Sebastian, S. Risk and Outcomes of Coronavirus Disease (COVID-19) in Patients with Inflammatory Bowel Disease: A Systematic Review and Meta-Analysis. *United Eur. Gastroenterol. J.* **2021**, *9*, 159–176. [CrossRef]
70. Amiot, A.; Rahier, J.-F.; Baert, F.; Nahon, S.; Hart, A.; Viazis, N.; Biancone, L.; Domenech, E.; Reenears, C.; Peyrin-Biroulet, L.; et al. The Impact of COVID-19 on Patients with IBD in a Prospective European Cohort Study. *J. Crohn's Colitis*, 2022. *online ahead of print*. [CrossRef]
71. Al-Ani, A.H.; Prentice, R.E.; Rentsch, C.A.; Johnson, D.; Ardalan, Z.; Heerasing, N.; Garg, M.; Campbell, S.; Sasadeusz, J.; Macrae, F.A.; et al. Review Article: Prevention, Diagnosis and Management of COVID-19 in the IBD Patient. *Aliment. Pharmacol. Ther.* **2020**, *52*, 54–72. [CrossRef]
72. Samanta, J.; Gupta, R.; Singh, M.P.; Patnaik, I.; Kumar, A.; Kochhar, R. Coronavirus Disease 2019 and the Pancreas. *Pancreatology* **2020**, *20*, 1567–1575. [CrossRef]
73. Liu, F.; Long, X.; Zhang, B.; Zhang, W.; Chen, X.; Zhang, Z. ACE2 Expression in Pancreas May Cause Pancreatic Damage After SARS-CoV-2 Infection. *Clin. Gastroenterol. Hepatol.* **2020**, *18*, 2128–2130.e2. [CrossRef]
74. Ding, Y.; He, L.; Zhang, Q.; Huang, Z.; Che, X.; Hou, J.; Wang, H.; Shen, H.; Qiu, L.; Li, Z.; et al. Organ Distribution of Severe Acute Respiratory Syndrome (SARS) Associated Coronavirus (SARS-CoV) in SARS Patients: Implications for Pathogenesis and Virus Transmission Pathways. *J. Pathol.* **2004**, *203*, 622–630. [CrossRef]
75. McNabb-Baltar, J.; Jin, D.X.; Grover, A.S.; Redd, W.D.; Zhou, J.C.; Hathorn, K.E.; McCarty, T.R.; Bazarbashi, A.N.; Shen, L.; Chan, W.W. Lipase Elevation in Patients With COVID-19. *Am. J. Gastroenterol.* **2020**, *115*, 1286–1288. [CrossRef] [PubMed]
76. Barlass, U.; Wiliams, B.; Dhana, K.; Adnan, D.; Khan, S.R.; Mahdavinia, M.; Bishehsari, F. Marked Elevation of Lipase in COVID-19 Disease: A Cohort Study. *Clin. Transl. Gastroenterol.* **2020**, *11*, e00215. [CrossRef] [PubMed]
77. Inamdar, S.; Benias, P.C.; Liu, Y.; Sejpal, D.V.; Satapathy, S.K.; Trindade, A.J. Prevalence, Risk Factors, and Outcomes of Hospitalized Patients with COVID-19 Presenting as Acute Pancreatitis. *Gastroenterology* **2020**, *159*, 2226–2228.e2. [CrossRef] [PubMed]
78. Ramsey, M.L.; Patel, A.; Sobotka, L.A.; Lim, W.; Kirkpatrick, R.B.; Han, S.; Hart, P.A.; Krishna, S.G.; Papachristou, G.I. Hospital Trends of Acute Pancreatitis During the Coronavirus Disease 2019 Pandemic. *Pancreas*, 2022. *online ahead of print*. [CrossRef]

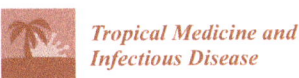

Opinion

Overlapping of Pulmonary Fibrosis of Postacute COVID-19 Syndrome and Tuberculosis in the Helminth Coinfection Setting in Sub-Saharan Africa

Luis Fonte [1,*], Armando Acosta [2], María E. Sarmiento [2], Mohd Nor Norazmi [2], María Ginori [3], Yaxsier de Armas [4,5] and Enrique J. Calderón [6,7,8,*]

1. Department of Parasitology, Institute of Tropical Medicine "Pedro Kourí", Havana 11400, Cuba
2. School of Health Sciences, Universiti Sains Malaysia, Kubang Kerian 16150, Kelantan, Malaysia; ducmar13@gmail.com (A.A.); mariesarmientogarcia@gmail.com (M.E.S.); norazmimn@usm.my (M.N.N.)
3. Department of Teaching, Polyclinic "Plaza de la Revolución", Havana 11300, Cuba; maginorig@infomed.sld.cu
4. Department of Clinical Microbiology Diagnostic, Hospital Center of Institute of Tropical Medicine "Pedro Kourí", Havana 11400, Cuba; yaxsier2017@gmail.com
5. Department of Pathology, Hospital Center of Institute of Tropical Medicine "Pedro Kourí", Havana 11400, Cuba
6. Instituto de Biomedicina de Sevilla, Hospital Universitario Virgen del Rocío, Consejo Superior de Investigaciones Científicas, Universidad de Sevilla, 41013 Sevilla, Spain
7. Centro de Investigación Biomédica en Red de Epidemiología y Salud Pública (CIBERESP), 28029 Madrid, Spain
8. Depatamento de Medicina, Facultad de Medicina, Universidad de Sevilla, 41009 Sevilla, Spain
* Correspondence: luisfonte@infomed.sld.cu (L.F.); ecalderon@us.es (E.J.C.)

Abstract: There is an increasing attention to the emerging health problem represented by the clinical and functional long-term consequences of SARS-CoV-2 infection, referred to as postacute COVID-19 syndrome. Clinical, radiographic, and autopsy findings have shown that a high rate of fibrosis and restriction of lung function are present in patients who have recovered from COVID-19. Patients with active TB, or those who have recovered from it, have fibrotic scarred lungs and, consequently, some degree of impaired respiratory function. Helminth infections trigger predominantly type 2 immune responses and the release of regulatory and fibrogenic cytokines, such as TGF-β. Here, we analyze the possible consequences of the overlapping of pulmonary fibrosis secondary to COVID-19 and tuberculosis in the setting of sub-Saharan Africa, the region of the world with the highest prevalence of helminth infection.

Keywords: pulmonary fibrosis; postacute COVID-19 syndrome; tuberculosis; helminth coinfection; sub-Saharan Africa

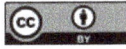

1. Introduction

Reports on the development of fibrotic lesions secondary to coronavirus infection are not new. Clinical, chest computed tomography (CT), and postmortem findings of pulmonary fibrosis (PF) were observed in people who suffered from severe acute respiratory syndrome (SARS) and Middle East respiratory syndrome (MERS), the previous two coronavirus pandemics in the current century [1]. However, the high lethality and the short duration of these pandemics did not allow comprehensive studies to be performed on patients who survived the acute forms of these viral infections.

Even at the beginning of the current pandemic, Paolo Spagnolo et al. [2] predicted that in COVID-19 convalescents, despite the removal of the cause for lung damage, the possibility for the development of progressive and irreversible PF, especially for those with pre-existing pulmonary conditions, may be real. Two years later, the overlapping of PF secondary to COVID-19 with the fibrotic sequelae of other diseases was demonstrated [1,3–5]. Here, we analyze the possible consequences of the overlapping of PF secondary to COVID-19 and tuberculosis (TB) in the setting of sub-Saharan Africa (SSA), the region of the world with the highest prevalence of helminth infection.

2. Pulmonary Fibrosis (PF) of Postacute COVID-19 Syndrome (PACS)

The natural evolution of SARS-CoV-2 infection can be asymptomatic, evolve with mild symptoms or progress to severe clinical forms. This wide spectrum is a result of triggering host immune responses which, in children and healthy adults, generally contain viral replication at the higher portions of the respiratory system and lead to recovery and, in elderly and patients with comorbidities, can generate an intense pulmonary inflammatory reaction, additional clinical complications, and death [6]. Due to the severe clinical forms of the acute phase of COVID-19, 5,993,901 people had died worldwide as of 8 March 2022 [7].

Although the development and implementation of more effective tools to reduce the incidence and the severity of COVID-19 continues to be a priority, there is an increasing attention to the emerging health problem represented by the unfavorable long-term consequences of that infectious disease. Those adverse consequences include a myriad of clinical manifestations corresponding to injuries in almost all organs, referred to as postacute COVID-19 syndrome (PACS) [8,9].

One important manifestation of PACS is PF, which is a long-lasting and progressive lung disorder caused by excessive deposition of collagen and other extracellular matrix (ECM) components in the organ parenchyma. PF, left to its natural course, can severely impair respiratory function and lead to the development of fatal disability [10,11]. Among the main morphological features of that disorder are the following: (i) an incorrect reestablishment of the injured alveolar epithelium, (ii) fibroblast persistence, (iii) a disproportionate accumulation of ECM components such as collagen, and (iv) the disappearance of regular pulmonary structure [12].

Clinical, chest CT, and postmortem findings have shown that fibrosis and restriction of pulmonary function are frequently present in patients who have recovered from COVID-19: (i) more than a third of the patients with severe forms of COVID-19 may show limited lung function after hospital discharge [12,13], (ii) PF on chest CT have been reported in patients who had recovered from severe or critical disease [12–14], and (iii) in an autopsy study involving patients with acute respiratory distress syndrome (ARDS), the finding of PF was more frequent as more time had elapsed since the onset of clinical manifestations of COVID-19 [15]. PF is already recognized among the most important sequelae of SARS-CoV-2 infection [16].

The processes involved in the progress to PF in persons who suffered from acute COVID-19 are complex and, in general, not clearly understood. Several mechanisms, some of them interconnected, have been suggested to explain its development. Of those, three are noteworthy: (i) the downregulation (endocytosis upon virus binding) of the angiotensin-converting enzyme 2 (ACE2) reduces the anti-inflammatory and antifibrotic components of the renin–angiotensin system, leading first to more inflammation and afterwards to fibrosis [17]; (ii) the involvement of type 2 immune cytokines, mainly interleukin-4 (IL-4) and IL-13, each one exhibiting profibrotic activity by promoting the recruitment, activation, and proliferation of the corresponding cellular types [1,10]; and (iii) the increased secretion of transforming growth factor-β (TGF-β), which is a characteristic event in lung fibrotic process [18]. SARS-CoV-2 upregulates TGF-β expression and both TGF-β mRNA as TGF-β protein levels in fibrotic pulmonary tissue are increased [19]. TGF-β can trigger PF by inducing myofibroblast expansion, a key effector event in lung fibrogenesis, and promoting the production and deposition of ECM proteins [20,21].

3. Overlapping of Pulmonary Fibrosis (PF) of Postacute COVID-19 Syndrome (PACS) and Tuberculosis (TB)

TB is a chronic and debilitating disease caused by organisms of the *Mycobacterium tuberculosis* (Mtb) complex [22,23]. Although Mtb is primarily a lung pathogen, it can affect practically any organ or tissue. During the last decades, the estimated global TB incidence rate has decreased; nevertheless, TB continues to be an important sanitary problem, mainly in low- and middle-income countries of Africa and Asia, where factors such as poverty, HIV infection, and multidrug resistant TB are fueling the pandemic [23,24].

Depending on the host immune competence, the Mtb infection can evolve from containment, in which the bacteria are isolated within granulomas in latent TB infection (LTBI), to a contagious state, in which the patient will show symptoms that can include cough, fever, night sweats, and weight loss, among others (active TB) [22]. Protection against Mtb requires a distinctly defined type 1 response, mediated by interferon-gamma (IFNγ), IL-2, and tumor necrosis factor-alpha (TNFα), which may clear the infection or restrain it into an immune-mediated containment, also known as latency [23,25]. Active TB is characterized by unlimited mycobacterial multiplication, considerable collagen deposition, and fibrosis [26]. Even though tissue repair during fibrosis is a healing process, large fibrosis with scar formation damages pulmonary function [27].

Early in the pandemic, the World Health Organization (WHO) predicted that patients coinfected with both TB and COVID-19 may have unfavorable clinical evolution [28]. While some studies have not found a significant association of coinfection and disease severity [29,30], others have described a notable higher frequency of undesirable clinical progression among patients with TB and COVID-19 coinfection [31,32].

A recent systematic review and meta-analysis of previous data on the association of COVID-19 and active TB included studies performed almost exclusively in high-TB-burden countries [3]. The overall pooled incidence and lethality found were 1.07% (43 studies) and 1.5% (17 studies), respectively. In agreement with the prediction of WHO, COVID-19 patients with TB had a higher risk of severity (relative risk/risk ratio (RR) 1.46, 95% confidence interval (CI) 1.05–2.02); and mortality (RR 1.93, 95% CI 1.56–2.39), from 20 and 17 studies, respectively, compared to COVID-19 patients without TB.

More recently, another systematic review and meta-analysis performed on data obtained exclusively from high-TB-burden countries of SSA showed that the overall incidence and lethality due to COVID-19/TB coinfection were 2% (20 studies) and 10% (9 studies), respectively [4]. Although the data included in this review corresponded both to people with previous TB and to patients with active infection, the incidence and case-fatality rates of the association were higher than those previously reported [3].

As mentioned above, active TB patients, or those who have recovered from it, are left with fibrotic scarred lungs and, consequently, with some degree of impaired respiratory function. It has been estimated that more than half of all TB survivors have some form of persistent pulmonary dysfunction despite microbiological cure, leaving patients potentially more susceptible to other infectious diseases, included COVID-19 [5]. On the other hand, post-COVID fibrosis may also exacerbate the fibrotic sequelae of pulmonary TB causing a more profound and prolonged disability [3].

4. Pulmonary Fibrosis (PF) in the Helminth Coinfection Setting in Sub-Saharan Africa (SSA)

Africa, in particular SSA region, is the continent with the highest prevalence of helminth infections [33]. It is estimated that more than half of SSA's population is affected by one or more helminth infections, especially by soil-transmitted helminths and schistosomes [23]. Millions of years of host–helminth coevolution have resulted in the development of defensive responses by the hosts and sophisticated immune regulatory mechanisms by the helminths. For more complexity, the immune responses against those parasites, which are relatively large and multicellular organisms, include injury repair processes, necessary to lessen the tissue damage that those pathogens may cause as they move through host organs.

To control helminth infection, the human host typically develops type 2 immune responses (increase of Th2 cells and release of cytokines, primarily IL-4, IL-5, and IL-13) [34,35]. To persist in their host, helminths induce an important immunomodulatory, anti-inflammatory, and fibrogenic pathway: the expansion of FOXP3+ T regulatory cells, B regulatory cells, and M2 macrophages, which together cause the secretion of regulatory cytokines, mainly TGF-β [36]. In relation with this regulatory scenery, it has recently been demonstrated that helminth extracellular vesicles (small membrane-bound vesicles secreted by helminths which contain functional proteins, carbohydrates, lipids, mRNA, and noncoding RNAs) can trigger several events that modulate host–parasite interactions [37,38].

The expanded population of T regulatory cells resulting from the host–helminth interaction can downmodulate both Th1 and Th2 inflammatory responses and interfere with other effector T-cell functions [20,34–36]. A prolonged exposure to parasitic helminth infection has been associated with generalized immune hyporesponsiveness [35]. Th2, Tregs, and the immunoregulatory cytokines they produce (such IL-4, IL-5, IL-13, IL-10, and TGF-β) may act as potent inhibitors of the Th1 responses which are required, as it was commented above, for immunity against Mtb infection [23]. Interestingly, some of those cytokines, mainly TGF-β, can trigger PF by promoting the production and deposition of ECM proteins [20,21]. It may be a way for the exacerbation of fibrotic sequelae of pulmonary TB in helminth infection settings.

Despite the underdeveloped economies and limited health care infrastructures of the majority of SSA nations, the lethality of COVID-19 in that region apparently was lower than in the rest of the world during the first part of the pandemic (the time before the massive administration of COVID-19 vaccines in Europe and the Unites States of America).

Some reasons, or combinations of them, have been alluded to explain that unexpected evolution: nonextensive diagnostic testing, age and genetic background of the population, under-reporting of COVID-19 mortality, mutational variations of SARS-CoV-2, environmental temperature and humidity nonfavorable for viral replication, Bacillus Calmette–Guérin (BCG) vaccination policies, composition of the microbiome, endemicity of other infections, and anti-inflammatory component of the helminth immune modulation, among others [39–43].

At times, the prevalence of helminth infections in SSA has been very high [33]. For surviving, helminths modulate the immune responses of their hosts [34–36]. The helminths' immune modulation is highly anti-inflammatory, to the point that allergic and autoimmune events in SSA are relatively rare [35]. The COVID-19 lethality is mainly due to inflammatory phenomena [44]. Some authors have related the relatively low lethality of COVID-19 in SSA with the modulation of immune responses by helminths [41,42,45–49]. Woldey et al. demonstrated that parasite coinfection was associated with a reduced risk of severe COVID-19 in African patients, supporting the hypothesis that parasite coinfection may silence the hyperinflammation associated with severe COVID-19 [49] (Figure 1).

Nevertheless, the long-term outcomes of COVID-19 in SSA may not be as benevolent as the acute phase of the disease as observed in that region. The adverse consequences of the overlapping of fibrotic sequelae of COVID-19 and TB may be amplified by the cytokine profile elicited by helminth coinfection in that setting. As commented above, data obtained from SSA, where the prevalence of helminth infection is very high, showed that the overall incidence and lethality due to COVID-19/TB coinfection were higher there than those reported in other parts of the world [3,4]. The overlapping of post-COVID fibrosis and the fibrotic sequelae of pulmonary TB in a setting of helminth immune modulation (with a predominant type 2 immunity and an increased release of regulatory and fibrogenic cytokines, such as TGF-β), as observed in SSA, may result in more fibrosis and, consequently, a greater disruption of the organ's architecture (Figure 1).

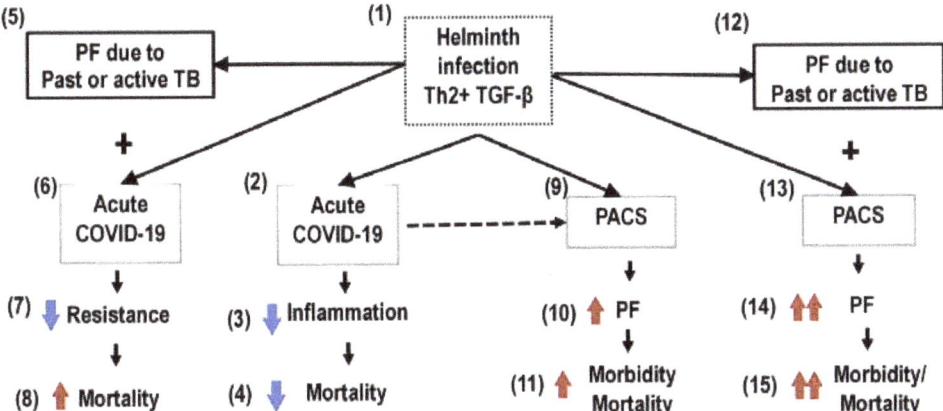

Figure 1. Overlapping of acute COVID-19 and postacute COVID-19 syndrome (PACS) and tuberculosis (TB) in the helminth coinfection setting in sub-Saharan Africa (SSA) population. (1) Helminth coinfection inhibits inflammation and amplifies pulmonary fibrosis (PF) processes; (2–4) helminth coinfection inhibits COVID-19 lung inflammation and decreases mortality; (5–8) infection by *Mycobacterium tuberculosis* and PF due to past or active TB limit resistance to COVID-19 and increase mortality; (9–11) PACS, amplified by helminth infection, increases morbidity and mortality; (12–15) the overlapping of PF due to past or active TB with PF due to PACS, amplified by helminth infection, increases morbidity and mortality.

5. Conclusions

Clinical, chest CT, and postmortem findings have shown that a high rate of fibrosis and restriction of lung function are present in patients recovered from COVID-19. Patients with active TB, or those who have recovered from it, have fibrotic scarred lungs and, consequently, some degree of impaired respiratory function. Helminth infections trigger predominantly type 2 immune responses and the release of regulatory and fibrogenic cytokines, such as TGF-β. The overlapping of post-COVID fibrosis and fibrotic sequelae of pulmonary TB, and its adverse clinical consequences, may be amplified by the cytokine profile elicited by helminth coinfection in SSA, the region of the world with the highest prevalence of helminth infection.

Recent findings indicate that the risks of COVID-19 associated with previous and/or current TB may be underestimated in SSA, as this coinfection is under-reported due to logistical constraints [4]. Nevertheless, in spite of the scarcity of accurate data about that association, its fatality rate has been estimated as high [3,4]. For that reason, professionals dealing with TB or COVID-19 patients, mainly in high-burden TB regions, should take into consideration the potential adverse consequences of the association of the fibrotic sequelae of those diseases. The convergence of lung disease after TB and lung disease after COVID-19 necessitates the follow-up of patients with post-TB lung disease who had COVID-19 pneumonia and the prioritization of their linkage to respiratory services for optimal care [50].

At the epidemiological level, the long-term consequences of PF secondary to COVID-19 and TB and their potential amplification by helminth coinfection require more research. Therefore, prospective studies on COVID-19 survivors of SSA populations are necessary to institute better strategies to reduce further disabilities and death in that impoverished region, and possibly in other settings [50].

The administration of effective COVID-19 and TB vaccines may help to decrease the potential burden associated with the COVID-19 and TB PF overlapping in SSA. However, in the development and distribution of vaccines against both pathogens it must be taken into account that helminth infections can impair human immune responses to immuno-gens prepared to control other infectious diseases [51]. Thus, as long as time and resources allow, clinical trials of COVID-19 and TB vaccines to be used in SSA must include the corresponding helminth-infected groups.

In the short-term, and also taking into consideration the global necessity for reducing the number of persons at risk, efforts should be made to speed up the administration of appropriate COVID-19 vaccines in SSA, where, as of March 2022, only 15% of its populations had received a complete schedule of immunization against SARS-CoV-2 infection [7].

Author Contributions: All authors listed have made a substantial, direct, and intellectual contribution to the work, and approved it for publication. All authors have read and agreed to the published version of the manuscript.

Funding: This research received no external funding.

Institutional Review Board Statement: Not applicable.

Informed Consent Statement: Not applicable.

Data Availability Statement: Not applicable.

Conflicts of Interest: The authors declare no conflict of interest.

References

1. Vianello, A.; Guarnieri, G.; Braccioni, F.; Lococo, S.; Molena, B.; Cecchetto, A.; Giraudo, C.; De Marchi, L.B.; Caminati, M.; Senna, G. The pathogenesis, epidemiology and biomarkers of susceptibility of pulmonary fibrosis in COVID-19 survivors. *Clin. Chem. Lab. Med.* **2022**, *60*, 307–316. [CrossRef] [PubMed]
2. Spagnolo, P.; Balestro, E.; Aliberti, S.; Cocconcelli, E.; Biondini, D.; Della Casa, G.; Sverzellati, N.; Maher, T.M. Pulmonary fibrosis secondary to COVID-19: A call to arms? *Lancet* **2020**, *8*, 750–752. [CrossRef]
3. Aggarwal, A.N.; Agarwal, R.; Dhooria, S.; Prasad, K.T.; Sehgal, I.S.; Muthu, V. Active pulmonary tuberculosis and coronavirus disease 2019: A systematic review and meta-analysis. *PLoS ONE* **2021**, *16*, e0259006. [CrossRef] [PubMed]
4. Tamuzi, J.L.; Lulendo, G.; Mbuesse, P. The incidence and mortality of COVID-19 related TB infection in Sub-Saharan Africa: A systematic review and meta-analysis. *Int. Clin. Img. Med. Rev.* **2022**, *1*, 1036. Available online: https://ijcimr.org/articles/IJCIMR-V1-1036.pdf (accessed on 18 May 2022).
5. Udwadia, Z.F.; Vora, A.; Tripathi, A.R.; Malu, K.N.; Lange, C.; Raju, R.S. COVID-19 -Tuberculosis interactions: When dark forces collide. *Indian J. Tuberc.* **2020**, *67*, S155–S162. [CrossRef]
6. Wang, Y.; Wang, Y.; Chen, Y.; Qin, Q. Unique epidemiological and clinical features of the emerging 2019 novel coronavirus pneumonia (COVID-19) implicate special control measures. *J. Med. Virol.* **2020**, *92*, 568–576. [CrossRef]
7. World Health Organization. *Coronavirus Disease 2019 (COVID-19): Weekly Epidemiological Update, 8 March 2022*; WHO: Geneva, Switzerland, 2022; Available online: https://www.who.int/publications/m/item/weekly-epidemiological-update-on-covid-19---8-march-2022 (accessed on 10 March 2022).
8. Nalbandian, A.; Sehgal, K.; Gupta, A.; Madhavan, M.V.; McGroder, C.; Stevens, J.S.; Cook, J.R.; Nordvig, A.S.; Shalev, D.; Sehrawat, T.S.; et al. Post-acute COVID-19 syndrome. *Nat. Med.* **2021**, *27*, 601–615. [CrossRef]
9. Datta, S.D.; Talwar, A.; Lee, J.T. A Proposed Framework and Timeline of the Spectrum of Disease Due to SARS-CoV-2 Infection: Illness beyond acute infection and public health implications. *JAMA* **2020**, *324*, 2251–2252. [CrossRef] [PubMed]
10. Wilson, M.S.; A Wynn, T. Pulmonary fibrosis: Pathogenesis, etiology and regulation. *Mucosal. Immunol.* **2009**, *2*, 103–121. [CrossRef]
11. Gause, W.C.; Wynn, T.A.; Allen, J.E. Type 2 immunity and wound healing: Evolutionary refinement of adaptive immunity by helminths. *Nat. Rev. Immunol.* **2013**, *13*, 607–614. [CrossRef]
12. Tanni, S.E.; Fabro, A.T.; de Albuquerque, A.; Ferreira, E.V.M.; Verrastro, C.G.Y.; Sawamura, M.V.Y.; Ribeiro, S.M.; Baldi, B.G. Pulmonary fibrosis secondary to COVID-19: A narrative review. *Expert Rev. Respir. Med.* **2021**, *15*, 791–803. [CrossRef]
13. Liang, J.; Liu, G.; Yu, Y.; Yang, Y.; Li, Y.; Tian, H.; Chen, Z.; Gong, W. Dynamic Changes in Chest CT Images Over 167 Days in 11 Patients with COVID-19: A Case Series and Literature Review. *Zoonoses* **2021**, *1*, 1–11. [CrossRef]
14. Safont, B.; Tarraso, J.; Rodriguez-Borja, E.; Fernández-Fabrellas, E.; Sancho-Chust, J.N.; Molina, V.; Lopez-Ramirez, C.; Lope-Martinez, A.; Cabanes, L.; Andreu, A.L.; et al. Lung Function, Radiological Findings and Biomarkers of Fibrogenesis in a Cohort of COVID-19 Patients Six Months After Hospital Discharge. *Arch. Bronconeumol.* **2021**, *58*, 142–149. [CrossRef] [PubMed]
15. Thille, A.W.; Esteban, A.; Fernández-Segoviano, P.; Rodriguez, J.-M.; Aramburu, J.-A.; Vargas-Errázuriz, P.; Martín-Pellicer, A.; Lorente, J.A.; Frutos-Vivar, F. Chronology of histological lesions in acute respiratory distress syndrome with diffuse alveolar damage: A prospective cohort study of clinical autopsies. *Lancet Respir. Med.* **2013**, *1*, 395–401. [CrossRef]
16. Hu, Z.-J.; Xu, J.; Yin, J.-M.; Li, L.; Hou, W.; Zhang, L.-L.; Zhou, Z.; Yu, Y.-Z.; Li, H.-J.; Feng, Y.-M.; et al. Lower Circulating Interferon-Gamma Is a Risk Factor for Lung Fibrosis in COVID-19 Patients. *Front. Immunol.* **2020**, *11*, 585647. [CrossRef]

17. Furuhashi, M.; Moniwa, N.; Takizawa, H.; Ura, N.; Shimamoto, K. Potential differential effects of renin-angiotensin system inhibitors on SARS-CoV-2 infection and lung injury in COVID-19. *Hypertens. Res.* **2020**, *43*, 837–840. [CrossRef] [PubMed]
18. Zuo, W.; Zhao, X.; Chen, Y.-G. SARS Coronavirus and Lung Fibrosis. In *Molecular Biology of the SARS-Coronavirus*; Lal, S.K., Ed.; Springer: Berlin/Heidelberg, Gremany, 2010. [CrossRef]
19. Rübe, C.E.; Uthe, D.; Schmid, K.W.; Richter, K.D.; Wessel, J.; Schuck, A.; Willich, N.; Rübe, C. Dose-dependent induction of transforming growth factor β (TGF-β) in the lung tissue of fibrosis-prone mice after thoracic irradiation. *Int. J. Radiat. Oncol. Biol. Phys.* **2000**, *47*, 1033–1042. [CrossRef]
20. Liu, F.; Matsuura, I. Inhibition of Smad Antiproliferative Function by CDK Phosphorylation. *Cell Cycle* **2005**, *4*, 63–66. [CrossRef]
21. Derynck, R.; Akhurst, R. Differentiation plasticity regulated by TGF-β family proteins in development and disease. *Nat. Cell Biol.* **2007**, *9*, 1000–1004. [CrossRef]
22. Barry, C.E., III; Boshoff, H.I.; Dartois, V.; Dick, T.; Ehrt, S.; Flynn, J.; Schnappinger, D.; Wilkinson, R.; Young, D. The spectrum of latent tuberculosis: Rethinking the biology and intervention strategies. *Nat. Rev. Microbiol.* **2009**, *7*, 845–855. [CrossRef]
23. Cadmus, S.I.; Akinseye, V.O.; Taiwo, B.O.; Pinelli, E.O.; van Soolingen, D.; Rhodes, S.G. Interactions between helminths and tuberculosis infections: Implications for tuberculosis diagnosis and vaccination in Africa. *PLOS Neglected Trop. Dis.* **2020**, *14*, e0008069. [CrossRef] [PubMed]
24. Global Tuberculosis Report 2021. Available online: https://www.who.int/publications/digital/global-tuberculosis-report-2021/tb-disease-burden/incidence (accessed on 28 March 2022).
25. Chen, Q.; Ghilardi, N.; Wang, H.; Baker, T.; Xie, M.-H.; Gurney, A.; Grewal, I.; De Sauvage, F.J. Development of Th1-type immune responses requires the type I cytokine receptor TCCR. *Nature* **2000**, *407*, 916–920. [CrossRef] [PubMed]
26. Hunter, R.L. Pathology of post primary tuberculosis of the lung: An illustrated critical review. *Tuberculosis* **2011**, *91*, 497–509. [CrossRef] [PubMed]
27. Tsenova, L.; Singhal, A. Effects of host-directed therapies on the pathology of tuberculosis. *J. Pathol.* **2020**, *250*, 636–646. [CrossRef] [PubMed]
28. World Health Organization. Information Note: Tuberculosis and COVID-19. 12 May 2020. Available online: https://www.who.int/docs/default-source/documents/tuberculosis/infonote-tb-covid-19.pdf (accessed on 8 March 2022).
29. Gao, Y.; Liu, M.; Chen, Y.; Shi, S.; Geng, J.; Tian, J. Association between tuberculosis and COVID-19 severity and mortality: A rapid systematic review and meta-analysis. *J. Med. Virol.* **2020**, *93*, 194–196. [CrossRef] [PubMed]
30. Oh, T.K.; Song, I.-A. Impact of coronavirus disease-2019 on chronic respiratory disease in South Korea: An NHIS COVID-19 database cohort study. *BMC Pulm. Med.* **2021**, *21*, 12. [CrossRef]
31. Tadolini, M.; Codecasa, L.; García-García, J.-M.; Blanc, F.-X.; Borisov, S.; Alffenaar, J.-W.; Andréjak, C.; Bachez, P.; Bart, P.-A.; Belilovski, E.; et al. Active tuberculosis, sequelae and COVID-19 co-infection: First cohort of 49 cases. *Eur. Respir. J.* **2020**, *56*, 2001398. [CrossRef]
32. Kumar, M.S.; Surendran, D.; Manu, M.S.; Rakesh, P.S.; Balakrishnan, S. Mortality due to TB-COVID-19 coinfection in India. *Int. J. Tuberc. Lung Dis.* **2021**, *25*, 250–251. [CrossRef] [PubMed]
33. Hotez, P.J.; Kamath, A. Neglected Tropical Diseases in Sub-Saharan Africa: Review of Their Prevalence, Distribution, and Disease Burden. *PLOS Negl. Trop. Dis.* **2009**, *3*, e412. [CrossRef]
34. Harris, N.L.; Loke, P. Recent Advances in Type-2-Cell-Mediated Immunity: Insights from Helminth Infection. *Immunity* **2017**, *47*, 1024–1036. [CrossRef] [PubMed]
35. Maizels, R.M. Regulation of immunity and allergy by helminth parasites. *Allergy* **2020**, *75*, 524–534. [CrossRef] [PubMed]
36. Turner, J.; Jackson, J.A.; Faulkner, H.; Behnke, J.; Else, K.; Kamgno, J.; Boussinesq, M.; Bradley, J.E. Intensity of Intestinal Infection with Multiple Worm Species Is Related to Regulatory Cytokine Output and Immune Hyporesponsiveness. *J. Infect. Dis.* **2008**, *197*, 1204–1212. [CrossRef] [PubMed]
37. Yang, Y.; Liu, L.; Liu, X.; Zhang, Y.; Shi, H.; Jia, W.; Zhu, H.; Jia, H.; Liu, M.; Bai, X. Extracellular Vesicles Derived From Trichinella spiralis Muscle Larvae Ameliorate TNBS-Induced Colitis in Mice. *Front. Immunol.* **2020**, *11*, 1174. [CrossRef]
38. Ryan, S.; Shiels, J.; Taggart, C.C.; Dalton, J.P.; Weldon, S. Fasciola hepatica-Derived Molecules as Regulators of the Host Immune Response. *Front. Immunol.* **2020**, *11*, 2182. [CrossRef] [PubMed]
39. Napoli, P.E.; Nioi, M. Global Spread of Coronavirus Disease 2019 and Malaria: An Epidemiological Paradox in the Early Stage of A Pandemic. *J. Clin. Med.* **2020**, *9*, 1138. [CrossRef] [PubMed]
40. Gursel, M.; Gursel, I. Is global BCG vaccination coverage relevant to the progression of SARS-CoV-2 pandemic? *Allergy* **2020**, *75*, 1815–1819. [CrossRef] [PubMed]
41. Hays, R.; Pierce, D.; Giacomin, P.; Loukas, A.; Bourke, P.; McDermott, R. Helminth coinfection and COVID-19: An alternate hypothesis. *PLOS Neglected Trop. Dis.* **2020**, *14*, e0008628. [CrossRef]
42. Fonte, L.; Acosta, A.; Sarmiento, M.E.; Ginori, M.; García, G.; Norazmi, M.N. COVID-19 Lethality in Sub-Saharan Africa and Helminth Immune Modulation. *Front. Immunol.* **2020**, *11*, 574910. [CrossRef]
43. Acosta, A.; Fonte, L.; Sarmiento, M.E.; Norazmi, M.N. Does our Mycobacteriome Influence COVID-19 Morbidity and Lethality? *Front. Microbiol.* **2021**, *12*, 589165. [CrossRef]
44. Zhou, Y.; Fu, B.; Zheng, X.; Wang, D.; Zhao, C.; Qi, Y.; Sun, R.; Tian, Z.; Xu, X.; Wei, H. Pathogenic T-cells and inflammatory monocytes incite inflammatory storms in severe COVID-19 patients. *Natl. Sci. Rev.* **2020**, *7*, nwaa041. [CrossRef]

45. Tcheutchoua, D.N.; Tankeu, A.T.; Angong, D.L.W.; Agoons, B.B.; Nguemnang, N.Y.Y.; Djeunga, H.C.N.; Kamgno, J. Unexpected low burden of coronavirus disease 2019 (COVID-19) in sub-Saharan Africa region despite disastrous predictions: Reasons and perspectives. *Pan Afr. Med. J.* **2020**, *37*, 352. [CrossRef] [PubMed]
46. Abdoli, A. Helminths and COVID-19 Co-Infections: A Neglected Critical Challenge. *ACS Pharmacol. Transl. Sci.* **2020**, *3*, 1039–1041. [CrossRef] [PubMed]
47. Cepon-Robins, T.J.; Gildner, T.E. Old friends meet a new foe. *Evol. Med. Public Health* **2020**, *2020*, 234–248. [CrossRef] [PubMed]
48. Parker, W.; Sarafian, J.T.; A Broverman, S.; Laman, J.D. Between a hygiene rock and a hygienic hard place. *Evol. Med. Public Health* **2021**, *9*, 120–130. [CrossRef] [PubMed]
49. Wolday, D.; Gebrecherkos, T.; Arefaine, Z.G.; Kiros, Y.K.; Gebreegzabher, A.; Tasew, G.; Abdulkader, M.; Abraha, H.E.; Desta, A.A.; Hailu, A.; et al. Effect of co-infection with intestinal parasites on COVID-19 severity: A prospective observational cohort study. *eClinicalMedicine* **2021**, *39*, 101054. [CrossRef] [PubMed]
50. Dheda, K.; Perumal, T.; Moultrie, H.; Perumal, R.; Esmail, A.; Scott, A.J.; Udwadia, Z.; Chang, K.C.; Peter, J.; Pooran, A.; et al. The intersecting pandemics of tuberculosis and COVID-19: Population-level and patient-level impact, clinical presentation, and corrective interventions. *Lancet Respir. Med.* **2022**, *10*, 603–622. [CrossRef]
51. Wait, L.F.; Dobson, A.P.; Graham, A.L. Do parasite infections interfere with immunisation? A review and meta-analysis. *Vaccine* **2020**, *38*, 5582–5590. [CrossRef] [PubMed]

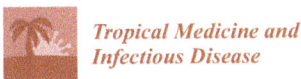 *Tropical Medicine and Infectious Disease*

Commentary

Commentary on COVID-19 Vaccine Hesitancy in sub-Saharan Africa

Severin Kabakama [1,*], Eveline T. Konje [2], Jerome Nyhalah Dinga [3,4], Colman Kishamawe [5], Imran Morhason-Bello [6], Peter Hayombe [7], Olufela Adeyemi [8], Ernest Chimuka [9], Ivan Lumu [10], John Amuasi [11], Theophilus Acheampong [12] and Tafadzwa Dzinamarira [13]

1. Humanitarian and Public Health Consultant, Mwanza P.O. Box 511, Tanzania
2. Department of Biostatistics, Epidemiology and Behavioral Sciences, School of Public Health, Catholic University of Health and Allied Sciences, Mwanza P.O. Box 1464, Tanzania; ekonje28@bugando.ac.tz
3. Michael Gahnyam Gbeugvat Foundation, Buea P.O. Box 63, Cameroon; djnyhalah@yahoo.com
4. Biotechnology Unit, University of Buea, Buea P.O. Box 63, Cameroon
5. National Institute for Medical Research, Mwanza P.O. Box 1462, Tanzania; kishamawe@yahoo.com
6. Department of Obstetrics & Gynaecology, Faculty of Clinical Sciences, Institute for Advanced Medical Research and Training (IAMRAT), College of Medicine, University of Ibadan, Ibadan 200132, Nigeria; iomorhason-bello@com.ui.edu.ng
7. Khasto Consultants, Nairobi P.O. Box 18690-00100, Kenya; pkhayombe@khastoconsultants.org
8. Ascendant & Company Ltd., 515 Freetown Highway, Sima Town, Western Area, Waterloo, Sierra Leone; olufela.adeyemi@asendantandcompny.com
9. Apolowil Consultants, 113A Fife Avenue, Harare, Zimbabwe; ernest@apolowilconsultants.com
10. Global Health Security Department, Infectious Diseases Institute, Makerere University College of Health Sciences, Kampala P.O. Box 22418, Uganda; ilumu@idi.co.ug
11. Kwame Nkrumah University of Science and Technology (KNUST), Kumasi, Ghana; amuasi@kccr.de
12. iRIS Research Consortium, 6 Ashur Suites, North Legon, Accra, Ghana; theo.acheampong@gmail.com
13. Faculty of Health Sciences, 31 Bophelo Road, Gezina, University of Pretoria, Pretoria 0084, South Africa; td2581@cumc.columbia.edu
* Correspondence: skabaka@yahoo.com

Abstract: Rates of vaccination against COVID-19 remain lower in sub-Saharan Africa than in other low and middle-income regions. This is, in part, attributed to vaccine hesitancy, mainly due to misinformation about vaccine origin, efficacy and safety. From August to December 2021, we gathered the latest experiences and opinions on four vaccine hesitancy-related areas (policies, perceived risk religious beliefs, and misinformation) from 12 sub-Saharan African researchers, four of whom have published about COVID-19 vaccine hesitancy. The authors included two political and business experts, six public health specialists, five epidemiologists, and four biostatisticians from ten sub-Saharan African countries(Cameroon, Ghana, Kenya, Liberia, Nigeria, Sierra Leone, South Africa, Tanzania, Uganda, and Zimbabwe). The authors' overarching opinions were that political influences, religious beliefs and low perceived risk exists in sub-Saharan Africa, and they collectively contribute to COVID-19 vaccine hesitancy. Communication strategies should target populations initially thought by policy makers to be at low risk, use multiple communication avenues and address major concerns in the population.

Keywords: COVID-19; vaccine hesitancy; sub-Saharan Africa

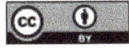

1. Introduction

Globally, there had been 522 million COVID-19 cases and six million COVID-19-related deaths by the third week of May 2022 [1]. The African region has reported over nine million cumulative COVID-19 cases and 172,308 deaths since the pandemic started. COVID-19 vaccines have proved to be an effective solution to preventing morbidity and mortality. These are complemented by other non-pharmaceutical interventions such as mask-wearing, social distancing, and hand washing.

Public health experts in the African region are increasingly concerned about the low vaccination uptake in sub-Saharan Africa, with eight in ten African countries unlikely to have attained the mid-2022 target of 70% vaccination rate [2]. This is despite the commendable efforts from global initiatives such as COVAX and the African Vaccine Acquisition Trust (AVAT) to attain equitable COVID-19 vaccine access. Such low levels of uptake are in part attributed to the high vaccine hesitancy, varying from 33% of the population in Mali [3], 50% of the people in Zimbabwe [4] and Ghana [5], and 85% reported in Cameroon [6].

Vaccine mistrust issues, vaccine safety, and the lack of reliable information are observed barriers to the uptake of COVID-19 vaccines [4–6]. The higher rate of observed COVID-19 vaccine hesitancy in some sub-Saharan African countries compared to high-income countries has been attributed to perceptions of low vaccine effectiveness, perceived low risk of contracting SARS CoV-2, misinformation and a fear of side effects [7].

The intent to vaccinate against COVID-19 was higher in some countries such as Ghana [5]. However, the context changed after the vaccine was introduced, due to mistrust of the vaccine-manufacturing companies or countries [5], doubts about vaccine efficacy [6,7], and fear of severe adverse effects following vaccination [7]. In sub-Saharan Africa, misinformation is widespread [4,6], hence driving hesitancy [6].

The purpose of this commentary is to highlight the barriers to COVID-19 vaccination and propose some solutions to accelerate the attainment of COVID-19 vaccination targets in the sub-Saharan African region.

2. Methods

Three authors (SK, EK, CK) from Tanzania drafted the commentary concept note and methods. They also requested, via email, expert opinions and experiences from nine other experts from nine sub-Saharan African countries, including Cameroon, Ghana, Kenya, Liberia, Nigeria, Sierra Leone South Africa, Uganda, and Zimbabwe. Four of the selected authors have published about COVID-19 vaccine hesitancy. The authors included two political and business experts, six public health specialists, five epidemiologists and four biostatisticians. Seven of the authors were affiliated with consultancies, two with research organisations, and seven with university faculties. All authors provided input on hesitancy-related thematic areas from their countries about: health policies related to COVID-19 vaccines, religious beliefs, perceived risks of COVID-19 infection, and influences of social media. Three authors (SK, EK, and CK) consolidated the inputs into a final commentary and synthesized the information according to theme and country into a final manuscript, which all authors reviewed.

3. Results

Policies promoting vaccine hesitancy: One of the strategies to increase equitable vaccine access for low-and middle-income countries has been the COVAX free vaccine program. Whereas 74% (34/46) of sub-Saharan countries, including Kenya, Uganda, and Zimbabwe, had started vaccinating their populations in January 2021, other countries, including Tanzania, had neither joined COVAX nor commenced vaccination against COVID-19 as of June 2021 [8]. The initial denial of COVID-19 existence and the "eradication of COVID-19" by divine powers and an antivaccine sentiments from key government officials delayed the COVID-19 vaccination program rollout in Tanzania [8]. As a result, after the vaccine was introduced in August 2021, dispelling the rumours became difficult despite government efforts, including hosting a national-level launch of the COVID-19 vaccination campaign.

At the beginning of the vaccination programs, some countries did not wish to be accountable for the vaccine related adverse effects; they insisted the program was optional and voluntary. For example, in Uganda and Tanzania, the official communication from the relevant health ministries and directorates did not distinguish voluntary from necessary vaccination. Requiring written consent before vaccination exonerated the government from any blame for any adverse effects but increased fear and suspicion in the population. However, realizing the hesitancies of policymakers, affluent groups, for instance the rich and diplomats began the importation of vaccines ahead of the government (Kenya and Tanzania). This led to an assortment of vaccine brands in these countries, making the provision of the desirable vaccination schedule and regulatory oversight practically impossible.

Initially, the vaccine was reserved for at-risk group such as the elderly, and provided at limited distribution points. However, these distribution points were few compared to the target population. Also, turnout at the designated health facilities remained low. As a result, governments lifted the limitations and more distribution points opened (Cameroon, Ghana, Kenya, Nigeria, Sierra Leone, Tanzania, Uganda and Zimbabwe). For instance, in Cameroon, Kenya and Tanzania all, hospitals at regional and district levels were providing the vaccine. In Uganda, as of November 2021, several private facilities and small health centres were permitted to vaccinate.

Religious beliefs: In some countries in sub-Saharan Africa, faith-based groups, which make up a significant section of the population, resist health care, including vaccines [9]. Religious leaders are trusted sources of information; however, as the COVID-19 pandemic entered its second wave, religious leaders became divided on the decision to vaccinate. Some religious leaders openly got vaccinated on national TV while others used religious gatherings to advance antivaccine campaigns (Ghana, Kenya, South Africa, Tanzania, and Zimbabwe). Meanwhile, despite some sects having beliefs against vaccination in Uganda, they did not publicly express antivaccine sentiments for fear of prosecution by the government. In Zimbabwe, apostolic sects have a history of resistance to vaccination programs and vaccine acceptance for most of these sects remains low [10]. However, when sect leaders realized the seriousness of the pandemic at the peak of the second wave, many churches decided to opened their doors only to those vaccinated against COVID-19 (Zimbabwe).

Perceived low risk and complacency: In the early phase of the pandemic, some scholars believed that sub-Saharan Africans were less vulnerable to COVID-19, which might have contributed to poor vaccine uptake [6,11].

The targeted vaccination program caused the rest of the population to think that the vaccine was not for them, as the messages delivered prioritised at-risk groups such as health care workers, persons over 50 years, security officers, teachers and those with chronic ailments or comorbidities (Cameroon, Uganda, Tanzania, Ghana and Kenya). Those left out were considered by policy makers to be at low risk; hence many did not see the importance of vaccination (Cameroon, Nigeria, Sierra Leone and Uganda). Some countries even embraced herbal medicine and steam inhalations as both protective and curative for COVID-19. Hence, the populations did not think that taking the vaccine was important as the herbal medicine (Cameroon, Uganda, Sierra Leone and Tanzania).

Social media and misinformation: Vaccine myths, misconceptions, and the spread of misinformation via social media platforms [12], led to the rapid growth of anti-COVID-19 vaccine campaigns. This was enabled by challenges in COVID-19 health communication, such as the lack of access to accurate information and protracted lockdowns that subjected people to unreliable social media channels as the only source of information.

Several circulating myths, misconceptions and rumours regarding the origins of SARS-CoV-2 and the dangers of the vaccines in the population have circulated widely on various social media platforms (Cameroon, Ghana, South Africa and Zimbabwe) despite stricter media laws prohibiting the circulation of misinformation through social media (Cameroon, Sierra Leone, Tanzania). Predominantly, the misinformation was associated with misinterpretation of scientific information (Cameroon, Ghana, and Kenya). In specific cases, the misinformation was directed to certain brands of vaccines as being ineffective (Cameroon, Uganda).

4. Suggested Solutions for Vaccine Hesitancy

We highlight below some high-level interventions that could address COVID-19 Vaccine hesitancy and improve vaccine uptakes in sub-Saharan Africa.

1. Governments, policymakers and health workers at all levels should be conversant with the scientific basis of the COVID-19 interventions. They should be able to explicitly counter rumours and adequately explain the facts. This includes, for example, addressing concerns about why the development of COVID-19 vaccines was hastened and reassuring the public about the effectiveness and safety of the vaccine.
2. Countries should strive to resolve the mistrust of COVID-19 vaccines by advocating and lobbying for technology transfer to foster local vaccine production. South Africa is already producing some vaccines, and the government of Kenya has commissioned the production of COVID-19 vaccines through local research institutes.
3. Countries should initiate a context-tailored approach to COVID-19 vaccine awareness initiatives and integrate them in existing structures and programs, including involving religious leaders. Additionally, ethnographic research is required to identify multifaceted community engagement interventions which could include a cocktail of approaches to health communications appropriate for specific age groups within the population.
4. Public health experts in sub-Saharan Africa should counter misinformation, targeting younger people who are not only the majority but also the heaviest social media users.
5. Health workers should proactively guide the community on seeking credible information about the COVID-19 vaccines from trustworthy sources.

Funding: This research was funded in part by the Bill and Melinda Gates Foundation (Grant number: OPP1075938-PEARL Program Support) awarded to Jerome Nyhalah Dinga.

Conflicts of Interest: The authors declare no conflict of interest.

References

1. World Health Organization. *COVID-19 Weekly Epidemiological Update (25 May 2022)*; WHO: Geneva, Switzerland, 2022; pp. 1–33. Available online: https://www.who.int/publications/m/item/covid-19-weekly-epidemiological-update (accessed on 15 June 2022).
2. WHO Africa. Eight in 10 African Countries to Miss Crucial COVID-19 Vaccination Goal. 2021, p. 2021. Available online: https://www.afro.who.int/news/eight-10-african-countries-miss-crucial-covid-19-vaccination-goal (accessed on 20 September 2021).
3. Kanyanda, S.; Markhof, Y.; Wollburg, P.; Zezza, A. Acceptance of COVID-19 vaccines in sub-Saharan Africa: Evidence from six national phone surveys. *BMJ Open* **2021**, *11*, e055159. [CrossRef] [PubMed]
4. Mundagowa, P.T.; Tozivepi, S.N.; Chiyaka, E.T.; Mukora-Mutseyekwa, F.; Makurumidze, R. Assessment of COVID-19 vaccine hesitancy among Zimbabweans: A rapid national survey. *PLoS ONE* **2021**, *17*, e0266724. [CrossRef] [PubMed]
5. Acheampong, T.; Akorsikumah, E.A.; Osae-kwapong, J.; Khalid, M.; Appiah, A.; Amuasi, J.H. Examining Vaccine Hesitancy in sub-Saharan Africa: A Survey of the Knowledge and Attitudes among Adults to Receive COVID-19 Vaccines in Ghana. *Vaccines* **2021**, *9*, 814. [CrossRef] [PubMed]
6. Dinga, J.N.; Sinda, L.K.; Titanji, V.P.K. Assessment of Vaccine Hesitancy to a COVID-19 Vaccine in Cameroonian Adults and Its Global Implication. *Vaccines* **2021**, *9*, 175. [CrossRef] [PubMed]
7. Solís Arce, J.S.; Warren, S.S.; Meriggi, N.F.; Scacco, A.; McMurry, N.; Voors, M.; Syunyaev, G.; Malik, A.A.; Aboutajdine, S.; Adeojo, O.; et al. COVID-19 vaccine acceptance and hesitancy in low- and middle-income countries. *Nat. Med.* **2021**, *27*, 1385–1394. [CrossRef] [PubMed]
8. Jerving, S. Tanzania Rethinks Its Approach to COVID-19. Devex. 2021. Available online: https://www.devex.com/news/tanzania-finally-joins-covax-100172 (accessed on 20 August 2021).
9. Dzinamarira, T.; Nachipo, B.; Phiri, B.; Musuka, G. COVID-19 Vaccine Roll-Out in South Africa and Zimbabwe: Urgent Need to Address Community Preparedness, Fears and Hesitancy. *Vaccines* **2021**, *9*, 250. [CrossRef] [PubMed]
10. McAbee, L.; Tapera, O.; Kanyangarara, M. Factors Associated with COVID-19 Vaccine Intentions in Eastern Zimbabwe: A Cross-Sectional Study. *Vaccines* **2021**, *9*, 1109. [CrossRef] [PubMed]
11. Musa, H.H.; Musa, T.H.; Musa, I.H.; Musa, I.H.; Ranciaro, A.; Campbell, M.C. Addressing Africa's pandemic puzzle: Perspectives on COVID-19 transmission and mortality in sub-Saharan Africa. *Int. J. Infect. Dis.* **2021**, *102*, 483–488. [CrossRef]
12. UNICEF. Countering Online Misinformation Resource Pack. 2020. Available online: https://www.unicef.org/eca/media/13636/file (accessed on 15 June 2022).

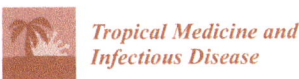

Systematic Review

Characteristics of COVID-19 Breakthrough Infections among Vaccinated Individuals and Associated Risk Factors: A Systematic Review

Shilpa Gopinath [1,*], Angela Ishak [2], Naveen Dhawan [3,4,5], Sujan Poudel [2], Prakriti Singh Shrestha [2], Prabhjeet Singh [6], Emily Xie [7], Peggy Tahir [8], Sima Marzaban [2], Jack Michel [2] and George Michel [9]

1. Department of Internal Medicine, Division of Infectious Disease, Johns Hopkins University, Baltimore, MD 21205, USA
2. Division of Research and Academic Affairs, Larkin Community Hospital, South Miami, FL 33143, USA; aishak@larkinhospital.com (A.I.); spoudel@larkinhospital.com (S.P.); prakritisingh@hotmail.com (P.S.S.); smarzban@larkinhospital.com (S.M.); jmichel@larkinhospital.com (J.M.)
3. Department of Bioengineering and Therapeutic Sciences, University of California San Francisco (UCSF), San Francisco, CA 94158, USA; naveen.dhawan@ucsf.edu
4. Department of Bioengineering, University of California Berkeley, Berkeley, CA 94704, USA
5. Krieger School of Arts and Sciences, Johns Hopkins University, Baltimore, MD 21218, USA
6. Bloomberg School of Public Health, Johns Hopkins University, Baltimore, MD 21205, USA; psingh40@jh.edu
7. Department of Plant and Microbial Biology, University of California, Berkeley, CA 94720, USA; emily.x@berkeley.edu
8. University of California San Francisco (UCSF) Library, San Francisco, CA 94143, USA; peggy.tahir@ucsf.edu
9. Department of Internal Medicine, Larkin Community Hospital, South Miami, FL 33143, USA; gmichel@larkinhospital.com

* Correspondence: sgopina2@jh.edu; Tel.: +1-443-927-3219

Abstract: We sought to assess breakthrough SARS-CoV-2 infections in vaccinated individuals by variant distribution and to identify the common risk associations. The PubMed, Web of Science, ProQuest, and Embase databases were searched from 2019 to 30 January 2022. The outcome of interest was breakthrough infections (BTIs) in individuals who had completed a primary COVID-19 vaccination series. Thirty-three papers were included in the review. BTIs were more common among variants of concern (VOC) of which Delta accounted for the largest number of BTIs (96%), followed by Alpha (0.94%). In addition, 90% of patients with BTIs recovered, 11.6% were hospitalized with mechanical ventilation, and 0.6% resulted in mortality. BTIs were more common in healthcare workers (HCWs) and immunodeficient individuals with a small percentage found in fully vaccinated healthy individuals. VOC mutations were the primary cause of BTIs. Continued mitigation approaches (e.g., wearing masks and social distancing) are warranted even in fully vaccinated individuals to prevent transmission. Further studies utilizing genomic surveillance and heterologous vaccine regimens to boost the immune response are needed to better understand and control BTIs.

Keywords: COVID-19; SARS-CoV-2; variants; reinfections; breakthrough infections; vaccination

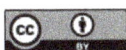

1. Introduction

The severe acute respiratory syndrome coronavirus type 2 (SARS-CoV-2) that emerged in December 2019 in Wuhan, China, and was the cause of coronavirus 2019 disease (COVID-19), continues to cause morbidity as part of the ongoing pandemic. As of 4 March 2022, 440,807,756 confirmed cases of COVID-19, including 5,978,096 deaths have been reported [1]. Mortality due to COVID-19 has substantially decreased since the introduction of vaccines and mass vaccination efforts worldwide. As of 27 February 2022, a total of 10,585,766,316 vaccine doses have been administered around the world [1].

However, emerging variants of SARS-CoV-2 and waning immunity in vaccinated individuals continue to hinder efforts to control the disease. Breakthrough infections (BTIs)

are defined by the United States (U.S.) Centers for Disease Control and Prevention (CDC) as a positive COVID-19 test by a reverse transcription-polymerase chain reaction (RT-PCR) or rapid antigen test > 14 days following the final dose of the recommended vaccination regimen [2]. In the U.S. as of 22 January 2022, the rate of BTIs was 846.73 per 100,000 in individuals who had completed a primary series of vaccination and 642.19 per 100,000 in those who had completed a primary series and a booster dose [3]. The death rate was 0.96 per 100,000 individuals vaccinated with a primary series and 9.68 in unvaccinated people [3].

The CDC and SARS-CoV-2 Interagency Group (SIG) variant classification define four classes of SARS-CoV-2 variants: variants being monitored (VBM), variants of interest (VOI), variants of concern (VOC), and variants of high consequence (VHC) [4]. VBM includes variants that were associated with an increased rate of transmission but are no longer detected and do not pose a threat to public health in the U.S. These currently include Alpha (B.1.1.7 and Q lineages), Beta (B.1.351, descendent lineages), Gamma (P.1, descendent lineages), Epsilon (B.1.427, B.1.429), Eta (B.1.525), Iota (B.1.526), Kappa (B.1.617.1), 1.617.3, Mu (B.1.621, B.1.621.1), and Zeta (P.2). VOI are associated with increased transmissibility and higher levels of infection. Iota (B.1.526) and B.1.525, identified in the United States, and Zeta (P. 2), first detected in Brazil, belong to this class [4]. Increased transmissibility and disease severity is seen in VOC. These include Alpha (B.1.1.7), first detected in the United Kingdom; Gamma (P.1), first detected in Brazil; Beta (B.1.351) from South Africa; and Epsilon (B.1.427 and B.1.429), detected in the United States [4]. Among all the variants, the Delta (B.1.617.2) variant was reported to have the most transmissibility and severity based on the hospitalization rate until the advent of Omicron (B.1.1.529), which was detected for the first time in South Africa on 24 November 2021 [5,6]. Recent reports suggest that certain VOC might result in a less robust immune response, among other factors, following vaccination against COVID-19, especially in patients with immunosuppression [7,8].

On a mass scale, BTIs pose a serious challenge in tackling the pandemic as these patients may serve as a source of viral spread [9]. With the emergence of VOC such as Omicron and its variants and waning immunity in certain populations after vaccination, a better understanding of BTIs and their attributes, particularly with variant profiles, is essential. These data can help guide public health efforts in determining specific populations that could benefit the most from booster doses of COVID-19 vaccines and help to assess vaccine effectiveness against specific variants.

We explored the current literature on BTIs of SARS-CoV-2 among vaccinated individuals, with a particular focus on the type of vaccine, the SARS-CoV-2 variant involved, common etiology, and immune parameters. This study aimed to identify any associated risk factors and to determine the extent to which BTIs are due to an immune evasion by VOCs as opposed to the failure of vaccines to elicit a satisfactory immune response.

2. Materials and Methods

2.1. Search Strategy and Selection Criteria

This systematic review was performed in accordance with the standards of the Preferred Reporting Items for Systematic Review and Meta-Analysis (PRISMA) Statement [10]. Approval from the Institutional Review Board was not needed. PubMed, Web of Science, ProQuest, and Embase databases were systematically searched from 2019 until 30 January 2022. A medical subject headings (MeSH) term and keyword search of each database was performed using the Boolean operators OR and AND. Keywords used included: SARS-CoV-2, SARS-CoV-2 variants, and breakthrough infections. The full search strategy for each database is provided in the Supplementary Materials.

Studies were included if they:

- Were conducted on adult patients with confirmed COVID-19 diagnosis.
- Reported COVID-19 breakthrough infections.
- Were written in the English language.
- Were peer-reviewed.

- Were either clinical trials, observational studies consisting of prospective cohort, retrospective cohort, case-control studies, case reports, or case series.
- Studies were excluded if they:
- Contained incomplete data.
- Were animal studies.
- Presented outcomes of no interest.

2.2. Data Extraction and Analysis

Two authors (A.I. and S.G.) independently performed the title and abstract screening. Relevant articles were then retrieved for full-text screening which was performed by two independent authors (P.S.S. and S.G.). All conflicts were resolved by a third author (A.I.). The references of the included articles were also reviewed to identify any articles missed by electronic database search.

The primary outcome of this systematic review was BTIs in vaccinated individuals; the variants causing these BTIs were also noted. The secondary outcomes were clinical and symptom severity in the vaccinated BTIs.

3. Results

Our initial search generated 848 studies; 139 duplicates were removed; 528 studies were excluded by title and abstract screening; and 181 studies were screened for full text. We then identified 33 eligible studies describing infection with COVID-19 in those with prior vaccination (Table 1). Figure 1 depicts in detail the flow of the article selection following the PRISMA guidelines.

The total number of participants in the review who were vaccinated with two doses of vaccine was 651,595. Among these, 25,743 (3.95%) presented with BTIs. The age of the patients ranged from <15 to >83 years with a mean age of 52 years. Out of the 25,743 patients with BTIs, 11,648 (44.24%) were male and 14,068 (54.65%) were female patients. The gender of three patients was reported as "others" and the gender of 18 patients (0.07%) was unknown. BTIs presented from <4 to 185 days with a mean of 52.33 days after full vaccination (defined as completing a primary series of vaccination as recommended for the vaccine type excluding the booster).

Table 1. Included studies and patient characteristics of reinfection in vaccinated individuals.

Study	Type of Study	Number of Fully Vaccinated Individuals (Breakthrough Infections)	Country	Gender	Age (Years)	Number of Days since Vaccination	Vaccine Received	Symptoms	Comorbidities	Variants [Reported Mutations]	Ct (Cycle Threshold) Value	Complications & Outcome
Bergwerk et al., 2021 [11]	Case control	11,453 (39)	Israel	Females: 25; Males: 14	Mean: 42	Median: 39 (Range: 11–102)	BNT162b2 (Pfizer-BioNTech)	Upper respiratory congestion (36%), myalgia (28%), loss of smell or taste (28%); fever or rigors (21%); Asymptomatic (33%)	Immunosuppressed (1), CLL*(1), ITP*(1), metabolic syndrome (6), thyroid disorder (3), other (migraines, fibromyalgia, osteoporosis, PCOS*) (4)	Alpha (B.1.1.7): 85% of samples	<30 (74%); >30 (26%)	Recovery
Estofolete et al., 2021 [12]	Case Report	2 (2)	Brazil	Male	60	106	Corona Vac (Sinovac)	Anosmia, malaise, myalgia, dyspnea	Type 2 diabetes mellitus, hypertension, obesity degree I (BMI*: 32.3 kg/m²)	Gamma (P.1) [K417T, E484K, N501Y]	Unknown	Hospitalization with supplemental oxygen → Recovery
				Male	55	122		Sore throat, headache, malaise, chills, coryza, sneezing, dyspnea, hypoxia	None			
Fabiani et al., 2021 [13]	Case Report	1 (1)	Italy	Male	83	23	BNT162b2 (Pfizer-BioNTech)	Slight headache, mild cold	None	Gamma (P.1) [K417T, E484K, N501Y, D614G]	13	Recovery
Philomina et al., 2021 [14]	Retrospective cohort	6 (6)	India	Female	25	35	AZD1222/Covishield (SII)	Influenza-like illness	Unknown	B.1.1.306 [E484K]	16.45	Recovery
				Male	50	30		Fever, malaise, anosmia, headache			20	
					53	28		Rhinitis			21	
				Female	25	26		Fever, loose stools, abdominal pain, dry cough, myalgia, rhinitis, anosmia		Alpha (B.1.1.7) [N501Y]	24	
					32	25		Mild nasal congestion, headache			26	
					33	17		Loss of smell, loose stools, rhinitis		B.1.1 B.1.560 [S477N]	14	

Table 1. Cont.

Study	Type of Study	Number of Fully Vaccinated Individuals (Breakthrough Infections)	Country	Gender	Age (Years)	Number of Days since Vaccination	Vaccine Received	Symptoms	Comorbidities	Variants [Reported Mutations]	Ct (Cycle Threshold) Value	Complications & Outcome
Hacisuleyman et al., 2021 [15]	Prospective cohort	417 (2)	USA		51	19	mRNA-1273 (Moderna)	Sore throat, congestion, headache, anosmia		Alpha (B.1.1.7) [E484K D614G T95I, del142-144]	24.2	Recovery
				Female	65	36	BNT162b2 (Pfizer-BioNTech)	Fatigue, sinus congestion, headache	None	Alpha (B.1.1.7) [S477N T95I, del142-144 R190T F2201 R237K R246T D614G]	33.3	Recovery
Kroidl et al., 2021 [16]	Case report	1 (1)	Germany	Unknown	Early 60s	26	BNT162b2 (Pfizer-BioNTech)	Headache, congested nose	None	Beta (B.1.351)	Unknown	Recovery
Almaghrabi et al., 2022 [17]	Case series	4 (4)	Saudi Arabia		68	73		Fever, chills, vomiting	Liver transplant, diabetes mellitus, hypertension, immunosuppressive medication	Alpha (B.1.1.7) [E484K]	25	Severe pneumonia →Mechanical ventilation →Death
				Male	69	150	BNT162b2 (Pfizer-BioNTech)	Shortness of breath, hypoxia	Renal transplant, diabetes mellitus, hypertension, immunosuppressive medication	Alpha (B.1.1.7)	30	Pneumonia → Mechanical ventilation, septic shock →Death
					41	39		Mild coughs, shortness of breath	Renal transplant, immunosuppressive medications	Beta (B.1.351)	29	ICU* admission with HFNC*→ Recovery
				Female	48	21	ChAdOx1 nCoV-19 vaccine (AstraZeneca)	Fever, hypoxia	Renal transplant, post-transplant lymphoma, immunosuppressive medications	Delta (B.1.617.2)	19	Hospital acquired infection, HFNC*→ Recovery

Table 1. Cont.

Study	Type of Study	Number of Fully Vaccinated Individuals (Breakthrough Infections)	Country	Gender	Age (Years)	Number of Days since Vaccination	Vaccine Received	Symptoms	Comorbidities	Variants [Reported Mutations]	Ct (Cycle Threshold) Value	Complications & Outcome
Baj et al., 2021 [18]	Retrospective cohort Study	4 (4)	Italy	Female	80	77	mRNA-1273 (Moderna)	Fatigue, headache, myalgia, dyspnea	Unknown	Delta (B.1.617.2)[E484K]	22	Recovery
				Male	77	67	Pfizer-BioNTech (BNT162b2)	Fever			19	
				Female	83	87	BNT162b2 (Pfizer-BioNTech)	Fever, fatigue, ageusia, anosmia			18	
				Female	81	45	mRNA-1273 (Moderna)	Dyspnea, fever, myalgia, fatigue			21	Hospital admission → Recovery
Bignardi et al., 2022 [19]	Case report	1 (1)	Italy	Male	61	120	mRNA vaccine -type not specified	Dyspnea, cough, fever	Hypertension, obesity	Delta (B.1.617.2)	Unknown	Pneumonia → Death
Chau et al., 2021 [20]	Cohort	866 (62) [a]	Vietnam	Females: 29 Males:33	Median: 41.5 (IQR: 32–50)	49–56 (97%)	Oxford-AstraZeneca	Fever (27%), cough (37%), sore throat (34%), runny nose (36%), loss of smell (39%), loss of taste (8%), muscle pain (27%), headache (19%), chest pain (3%), nausea (8%), shortness of breath (4%), pneumonia (5%), asymptomatic (21%)	Overweight (6), obesity (3), hypertension (3), hepatitis B (3), diabetes mellitus (2), pregnancy (1)	Delta (B.1.617.2)	31.9 (IQR: 23.3–34.9)	Recovery
Connor et al., 2021 [21]	Case report	2 (2)	USA	Male	63	60	BNT162b2 (Pfizer-BioNTech)	Nasal congestion, headache, dry cough	Hypertension, benign prostatic hypertrophy, overweight	B.1.617.2 B.1.619 [35 mutations detected, including 9 in the spike protein]	31.3	Recovery
				Male	25	90		Upper respiratory symptoms, headaches	None	B.1.617.2 [7/12 shared S-gene mutations]	25.2	Recovery

Table 1. Cont.

Study	Type of Study	Number of Fully Vaccinated Individuals (Breakthrough Infections)	Country	Gender	Age (Years)	Number of Days since Vaccination	Vaccine Received	Symptoms	Comorbidities	Variants [Reported Mutations]	Ct (Cycle Threshold) Value	Complications & Outcome
Gharpure et al., 2022 [22]	Cohort	1128 (918)	USA	Females: 90 Males: 822	19–49 (66%), 50–64 (30%), 65–74 (4%), >75 (0.4%)	>14	BNT162b2 (Pfizer-BioNTech): 504 mRNA-1273 (Moderna): 293 Johnson & Johnson: 121	Abdominal pain (6%), chills (35%), congestion (58%), cough (73%), diarrhea (20%), shortness of breath (10%), fatigue (41%), fever (43%), headache (47%), loss of appetite (16%), loss of smell or taste (50%), muscle pain (39%), sore throat (42%), vomiting (3%)	Active cancer (3), autoimmune disease (11), cardiovascular disease (36), chronic kidney disease (3), chronic lung disease (22), pregnancy (3), diabetes mellitus (21), HIV* infection (6), solid organ transplant (1), other immunosuppressive conditions (41)	Delta (B.1.617.2): 98% Delta (AY3 sublineage: 0.3%, Delta (AY4 sublineage): 0.8% Gamma (P1): 0.8%	Unknown	Hospitalized (7), ICU* (2) → Recovery
Galan Huerta et al., 2022 [23]	Case-control	53 (53)	Mexico	Females: 28; Males: 25	Mean: 59.7 (50–70)	7	AstraZeneca/Oxford: 8 (15%) BNT162b2 (Pfizer/BioNTech): 8 (15%) Convidecia (CanSino): 24 (45%) CoronoVac (Sinovac): 10 (19%) Unspecified: 3	Mostly mild or asymptomatic	Hospitalized: hypertension (11), Type 2 diabetes mellitus (13), obesity (1), smoking (4); Ambulatory: hypertension (5), Type 2 diabetes mellitus (5), obesity (2), smoking (1)	Delta (B.1.617.2) (AY.1, AY.2, AY.3, AY4 lineage): 67.92% Gamma (P.1, P.1.1, P.1.2): 7.55% Mu (B.1.621): 7.55% Alpha (B.1.1.7): 5.66%	Hospitalized: 19.58 (17.19–22.49); Ambulatory: 18.81 (15.72–21.24)	Hospitalized: High-flow O2 (14), intubation (10), ICU* admission (1), death (4); Ambulatory: all recovered (30)

Table 1. Cont.

Study	Type of Study	Number of Fully Vaccinated Individuals (Breakthrough Infections)	Country	Gender	Age (Years)	Number of Days since Vaccination	Vaccine Received	Symptoms	Comorbidities	Variants [Reported Mutations]	Ct (Cycle Threshold) Value	Complications & Outcome
				Female	60			Rhinorrhea	None	Alpha 20I/S: 501Y.V1	18.8	
				Male	58		BNT162b2 (Pfizer-BioNTech)	Chill, subjective fever	None	Alpha (20I/S: 501Y.V1)	19.1	
					48			Weakness, congestion loss of taste/smell, fatigue	Smoker	Alpha (20I/S: 501Y.V1)	20.9	Recovery
					51		mRNA vaccine type not provided	Headache, cough, rhinorrhea ageusia, anosmia	Immunosuppressive medication, non-alcoholic steatohepatitis	Gamma (20J/S: 501Y.V3)	17.1	
				Female	37		mRNA-1273 (Moderna)	Asymptomatic	None	20G	19.5	
					50		BNT162b2 (Pfizer-BioNTech)	Asymptomatic	None	Unknown	34.2	
					81		Johnson & Johnson	Shortness of breath, cough	Heart disease, cerebrovascular disease	Alpha (20I/S: 501Y.V1)	18.8	Hospitalization → recovery
Deng et al., 2021 [24]	Case control	14 (14)	USA		65	Range: (14–109)		Diarrhea, myalgia, chills, fever	Immunosuppressive medication, kidney and heart transplant	Alpha (20I/S: 501Y.V1)	20.1	Pneumonia → recovery
				Male	55		BNT162b2 (Pfizer-BioNTech)	Cough, acute hypoxic respiratory failure, sepsis	Immunosuppressive medication, kidney transplant	Alpha (20I/S: 501Y.V1)	22.3	Intensive Care Unit (ICU) → Death
					70			Cough, weakness, fever, dyspnea	Immunosuppressive medication, liver transplant	Gamma (20J/S: 501Y.V3)	19.6	Hospitalization → recovery
					68		mRNA-1273 (Moderna)	Acute hypoxia, acute pneumonia, hemoptysis	Immunosuppressive medication, lung transplant	Gamma (20J/S: 501Y.V3)	21.4	
				Female	60			Shortness of breath, fever, chills, body aches, hypoxia	Immunosuppressive medication, lung transplant	Gamma (20J/S: 501Y.V3)	15.7	Intensive Care Unit (ICU) → Recovery
				Male	65		BNT162b2 (Pfizer-BioNTech)	Diarrhea, nausea, weakness cough, dyspnea	Immunosuppressive medication, liver transplant	Epsilon (CAL.20C)	22.1	Hospitalization → Recovery
				Female	76			Fever, chills, acute respiratory failure	None	20G	18.3	Intensive Care Unit (ICU) → Recovery

Table 1. Cont.

Study	Type of Study	Number of Fully Vaccinated Individuals (Breakthrough Infections)	Country	Gender	Age (Years)	Number of Days since Vaccination	Vaccine Received	Symptoms	Comorbidities	Variants [Reported Mutations]	Ct (Cycle Threshold) Value	Complications & Outcome
De Souza et al., 2021 [25]	Case control	42 (22)	Brazil	Females: 17 Males: 5	77 (IQR: 51–87)	5–27	CoronaVac (SinoVac)	Asymptomatic (75%) Mild COVID-19 symptoms (25%)	Unknown	Alpha (B.1.1.7)	Unknown	Death: 1% Recovery: 99%
Gupta et al., 2021 [26]	Case control	592 (592)	India	Females: 207; Males: 385	Mean 44 (31–56)	39 (19–58)	Covaxin: 71 (10.5%/Covishield (AstraZeneca): 604 (89.2%) Covilo (Sinopharm): 2 (0.3%)	Symptomatic (71%) with one or more symptoms, fever (69%), body ache, headache and nausea (56%), cough (45%), sore throat (37%), loss of smell and taste (22%), diarrhea (6%), breathlessness (6%), ocular irritation, redness (1%); Asymptomatic (29%)	Type 2 diabetes mellitus, hypertension, obesity, chronic cardiac, renal, and pulmonary diseases	Delta (B.1.617.2): 384 Alpha (B.1.1.7): 28 Kappa (B.1.617.1): 22 B.1.617.3: 2 B.1.36: 2 B.1.1.294: 1 B.1.36.16: 1 B.1.1.306: 1 Delta (AY.2): 2	<30	Fully vaccinated: hospitalized (53), Recovered (589), Death (3)
Kale et al., 2021 [27]	Cohort	1639 (156)	India	Female: 86 Males: 70	Median: 34 (IQR 21–67)	>14	ChAdOx1 nCoV-19/Covishield (SII)	Fever, muscle aches	Unknown	Delta (B.1.617.2): 32 Kappa (B.1.617.1):11 Alpha (B.1.1.7): 1	23.2 (IQR 0.0–33.1)	Recovery; Hospitalization (0.22%)
Schulte et al., 2021 [28]	Case report	1 (1)	Germany	Male	42	49	BNT162b2 (Pfizer-BioNTech)	Asymptomatic	None	B.1.525	9.44	Recovery
Malhotra et al., 2022 [29]	Retrospective cohort	1079 (17)	India	Unknown 660 (60.6%); ≥25–44: 357 (32.8%)	<25:72 (6.6%);	>15	BBV152/Covaxin (Bharat Biotech)	Symptomatic:–Fever, rhinorrhea, sore throat, cough, chest pain, wheezing, difficulty breathing, shortness of breath, anosmia, dysgeusia, fatigue, myalgia, headache, abdominal pain, nausea, diarrhea. Asymptomatic: 3	Hypertension; chronic heart, lung, or kidney disease; cancer; hypothyroidism	Gamma (B.1.617.2)	Unknown	Recovery
Shastri et al., 2021 [30]	Case report	1(1) [b]	India	Female	61	28	ChAdOx1 nCoV-19(Covishield)	1st infection episode: Abdominal pain, fever, myalgia, fatigue 2nd infection episode: Body ache, fatigue, headache, cough, breathlessness, fever, rhinorrhea, vomiting	Prediabetes, bronchial asthma, hypertension	Alpha (B.1.1.7);1st Delta (B.1.617.2);2nd	1st infection: 35.2 2nd infection: 20.4	Recovery

Table 1. *Cont.*

Study	Type of Study	Country	Number of Fully Vaccinated Individuals (Breakthrough Infections)	Gender	Age (Years)	Number of Days since Vaccination	Vaccine Received	Symptoms	Comorbidities	Variants [Reported Mutations]	Ct (Cycle Threshold) Value	Complications & Outcome
Rovida et al., 2021 [31]	Cohort	Italy	3702 (33)	Females:26 Males: 7	Unknown	47 (Range 7–90)	BNT162b2 (Pfizer-BioNTech)	Asymptomatic (48%), fever (6%), asthenia (6%), headache (6%), arthralgia (9%), pharyngodynia (3%), rhinitis (27%), cough (9%), anosmia (9%), ageusia (3%), nausea (9%), diarrhea (10%)	Unknown	Alpha (B.1.1.7)	Unknown	Recovery
Rumke et al., 2022 [32]	Cohort	Netherlands	14 (14)		45	43	BNT162b2 (Pfizer-BioNTech)	Anosmia, arthralgia, fever, headache, myalgia, peripheral neuropathy, rhinosinusitis	None	Alpha (B.1.1.7)	18.5	Recovery
					62	78		Anosmia, rhinosinusitis	None	Alpha (B.1.1.7)	23.7	
				Female	27	64		Rhinitis	None	Alpha (B.1.1.7) [A771V]	23.5	
					52	61		Cough, dyspnea, fever	Asthma	Alpha (B.1.1.7)	19.6	
					35	74		Anosmia, cough, rhinitis	None	Alpha (B.1.1.7) [H245Y]	21.5	
					35	80		Anosmia, rhinosinusitis	None	Alpha (B.1.1.7) [S494P]	24.7	
				Male	58	80		Asymptomatic	None	Alpha (B.1.1.7)	31.9	
					26	111		Fever, rhinitis	None	Alpha (B.1.1.7) [V382L]	19.8	
					38	38		Cough, fever, pharyngitis, rhinosinusitis	None	Alpha (B.1.1.7) [D88V]	18.9	
					57	37	Ad26.COV2.S (Johnson & Johnson)	Cough, dyspnea	None	Alpha (B.1.1.7) [V483I, A706V]	21.5	
				Female	50	20		Asymptomatic	None	Alpha (B.1.1.7) [S12F; D905N]	23.6	
					54	45		Cough, fever, headache, myalgia, otitis	Atopic dermatitis	Delta (B.617.2)	31.3	
					38	18		Asymptomatic	Hashimoto thyroiditis	Alpha (B.1.1.7)	29.0	
					48	52		Anosmia, fever, headache, myalgia, sinusitis	None	Delta (B.617.2) [G142D]	29.2	

Table 1. *Cont.*

Study	Type of Study	Country	Number of Fully Vaccinated Individuals (Breakthrough Infections)	Gender	Age (Years)	Number of Days since Vaccination	Vaccine Received	Symptoms	Comorbidities	Variants [Reported Mutations]	Ct (Cycle Threshold) Value	Complications & Outcome
Yi et al., 2022 [33]	Cohort	South Korea	24 (24)	Females:18	78.9 (Range 34–99)	Mean: 40 (Range, 80–117)	BNT162b2 (Pfizer-BioNTech)	Asymptomatic (48%) Symptomatic (48%)	Unknown	Delta (B.1.617.2):13	18.1 (symptomatic); 20 (asymptomatic)	Recovery (96%), Death (4%)
Robilotti et al., 2021 [34]	Cohort	USA	12,046 (80: pre-Delta)	Females: 60 Males: 20	Median:37 (Range:22–65)	Median: 56 (Range:1–100)	BNT162b2 (Pfizer-BioNTech): 91% mRNA-1273 (Moderna): 9%	Asymptomatic (20%) Headache (55%) Fatigue (45%) Body aches (28%) Fever (including subjective) (19%) Loss of smell/taste (28%) Chills (20%) Sore throat (21%) Rhinorrhea, nasal congestion, sneezing (53%) GI symptoms (nausea, vomiting, diarrhea or abdominal pain) (18%) Cough (31%) Shortness of breath (8%)	Unknown	Alpha (B.1.1.7) [E484K K417T/N S477N N501Y]	Unknown	Recovery
			(179: post-Delta)	Females: 127 Males: 52	Median 33 (Range 21–63)	Median: 185 (Range 8–235)	BNT162b2 (Pfizer-BioNTech): 79% mRNA-1273 (Moderna): 21%	Asymptomatic (8%) Headache (45%) Fatigue (55%) Body aches (37%) Fever (including subjective) (32%) Loss of smell/taste (28%) Chills (27%) Sore throat (44%) Rhinorrhea, nasal congestion, sneezing (52%) GI symptoms (nausea, vomiting, diarrhea or abdominal pain) (17%) Cough (53%) Shortness of breath (9%)	Unknown	Delta (B.1.617.2) [L452R T478K E484Q]	Unknown	Recovery
Vignier et al., 2021 [35]	Cohort	French Guiana	25 (15)	Males: 15	Median: 53.3	>14	BNT162b2 (Pfizer-BioNTech): 56.8%	Symptomatic: Fever, dyspnea (87%)	Hypertension, diabetes mellitus, obesity, cardiac insufficiency	Gamma (P.1)	18–35	Recovery

Table 1. Cont.

Study	Type of Study	Country	Number of Fully Vaccinated Individuals (Breakthrough Infections)	Gender	Age (Years)	Number of Days since Vaccination	Vaccine Received	Symptoms	Comorbidities	Variants [Reported Mutations]	Ct (Cycle Threshold) Value	Complications & Outcome
Tober-lau et al., 2021 [36]	Longitudinal	Germany	20 (16)	Females: 12 Males: 4	>65 years	4–5	BNT162b2 (Pfizer-BioNTech)	Asymptomatic mostly. Diarrhea, fatigue, cough or shortness of breath (31.25%)	Hypertension, Type 2 diabetes mellitus, chronic kidney disease dementia	Alpha (B.1.1.7)	Unknown	Hospitalization (31.25%) Supplemental oxygen (6.3%) Death (12.5%)
Servellita et al., 2022 [37]	Cohort	USA	1373 (125) [c]	Females: 68 Males: 57	Mean: 49 (Range 22–97)	Median: 73.5 (range 15–140)	BNT162b2 (Pfizer-BioNTech): 51% mRNA-1273 (Moderna): 31% Johnson & Johnson: 10%	Asymptomatic (26%) COVID-19 pneumonia (15.4%)	Immunocompromised (23%)	Delta (B.1.617.2:31%, Alpha (B.1.1.7): 18.3%, Gamma (P.1): 15.6%, Iota (B.1.526): 11.9%, Epsilon (B.1.427/B.1.429): 6.4%, Beta (B.1.351): 3.7%, Other: 12.8% [L452R/Q, E484K/Q and/or F490S]	23.1	Recovery (100%) ICU (2.6%), Hospitalizations (15.4%)
Singer et al., 2021 [38]	Prospective cohort	Israel	343 (31)	Females: 17 Males: 14	Median: 58 (21–87)	>7	BNT162b2 (Pfizer-BioNTech)	Asymptomatic (05%)	Unknown	Beta (B.1.351)	Unknown	Recovery
Thangaraj et al., 2022 [39]	Prospective cohort	India	113 (113)	Females: 44 Males:66 Others:3	Median:54 (42–64)	>14	Covaxin: 27.4% Covishield: 70.8% Unknown: 1.8%	Symptomatic (88.5%)	Unspecified comorbidities (46%)	Delta (B.1.617.2):74.3% B.1.617.1: 0.9% AY.1: 0.9% Alpha (B.1.1.7): 0.9% Beta (B.1.351): 0.9%	<30	Recovery
Olsen et al., 2021 [40]	Cohort	USA	12,476 (207)	Females: 53% Males: 47% [d]	Median: 52.5 [d]	>14	BNT162b2 (Pfizer-BioNTech): 87% mRNA-1273 (Moderna): 13%	Unknown	BMI > 30 (42.7%)	Alpha (B.1.1.7): 126; Gamma (P.1): 5 Epsilon (B.1.429): 3 B.1526: 1 B.1526.1.1 Eta (B.1.525): 1 non-VOC: 70	23.9	Hospitalization (34.8%)
Singh et al., 2022 [41]	Cohort	India	63 (36)	Females: 13 Male: 23	Median: 37 (21–92)	Unknown	AZD1222/Covishield (SII): 15.87% BBV152/Covaxin: 84.13%	High-grade unremitting fever, shortness of breath, headache	None	Delta (B.1.617.2): 63.9% B.1.617.1: 11.1% Alpha (B.1.1.7) 2.8%	Range: 11.3–31	Recovery

Table 1. *Cont.*

Study	Type of Study	Number of Fully Vaccinated Individuals (Breakthrough Infections)	Country	Gender	Age (Years)	Number of Days since Vaccination	Vaccine Received	Symptoms	Comorbidities	Variants [Reported Mutations]	Ct (Cycle Threshold) Value	Complications & Outcome
Tay et al., 2022 [42]	Prospective case-control	55 (55)	Singapore	Females: 19 Males: 36	Median: 46 (IQR 36.5–59.5)	82 (IQR 51.5–99)	BNT162b2 (Pfizer-BioNTech)	Asymptomatic (21.8%) Mild symptoms (78.2%)	Chronic venous, asthma, other chronic lung diseases, rheumatologic disease, chronic liver disease, diabetes mellitus, chronic kidney disease, malignancies, or HIV (6)	Delta (B.1.617.2): 87.3% Unknown: 7.3% Non-Delta:5.5%	Unknown	Recovery
Sun et al., 2021 [43]	Retrospective cohort	604,035 (22,917)	USA	Females: 13,040 Males: 9877	Median: 51 (IQR 34–66)	138 (85–178)	BNT162b2 (Pfizer-BioNTech) mRNA-1273 (Moderna)	Unknown	Immunocompromised (1451).	Delta (B.1.617.2)	Unknown	Recovery (93.5%); Hospitalization: 11.5% Severe outcomes (0.65%)

* Abbreviations: CLL—Chronic Lung Disease; ITP—Idiopathic thrombocytopenic purpura; PCOS—Polycystic ovarian syndrome; BMI—Body mass index; HIV: Human Immunodeficiency Virus; ICU: Intensive Care Unit; HFNC: High flow nasal cannula. [a] Only 62 participants included in the study; [b] Patient had 2 breakthrough infections; [c] Variant breakdown provided for 109 patients; [d] Patient data corresponds to total number of patients.

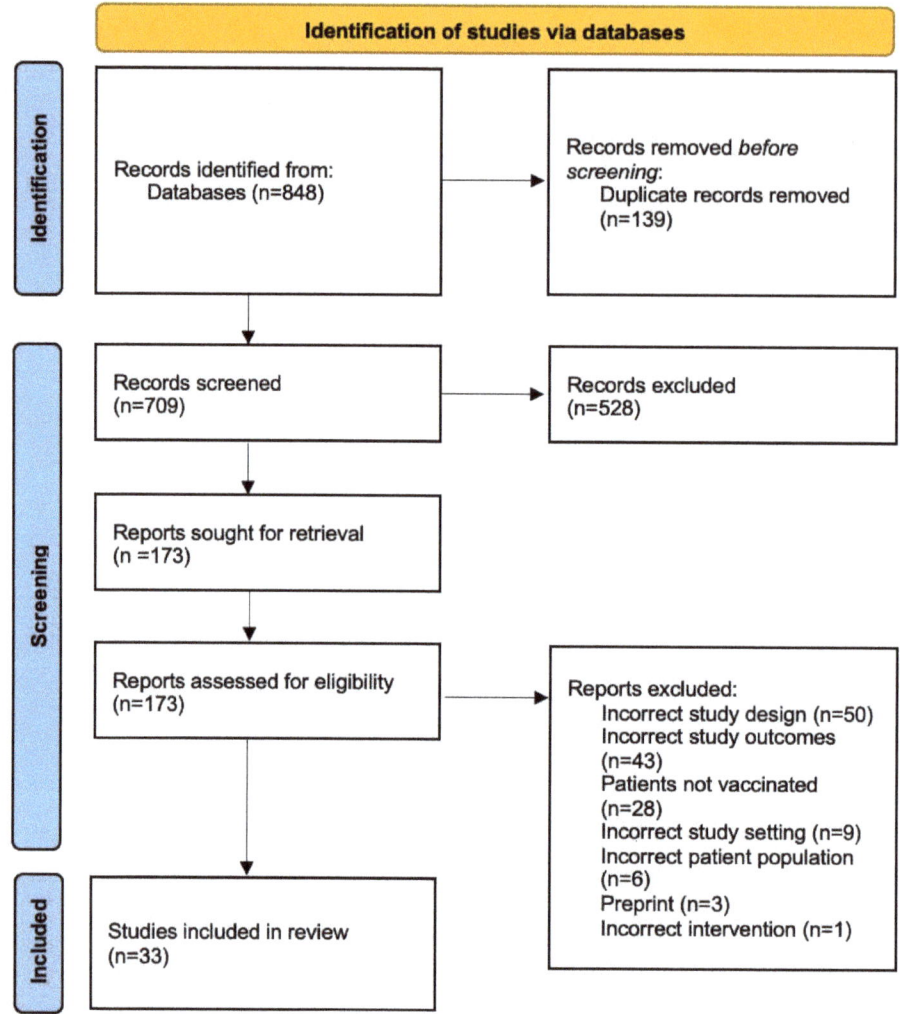

Figure 1. Study selection and screening following the PRISMA 2020 guidelines.

Study Type and Geographical Distribution

All 33 studies were observational; 19 were cohort studies, 7 were case reports, 6 were case-control studies, 1 was a longitudinal study, and 1 was a case series. The majority of the studies were conducted in the United States of America (USA) (9), followed by India (7), Italy (4), Germany (3), Israel (2), Brazil (2), Saudi Arabia, Vietnam, Mexico, Netherlands, South Korea, French Guiana, and Singapore.

Most individuals received the mRNA COVID-19 vaccinations Pfizer/BioNTech (23 studies) and Moderna (9 studies). Other vaccinations included were Covishield/AstraZeneca (10 studies), Johnson & Johnson/Janssen vaccine (4 studies), Covaxin (4 studies), Sinovac (3 studies), CanSino, and Sinopharm. Two studies did not specify which mRNA vaccine the patients received.

Among the reviewed studies, 96% of BTIs occurred with the Delta variant (B.1.617.2) and 0.94% of BTIs were due to the Alpha variant (B.1.1.7). Other variants included Gamma-P.1 (0.21%), Beta-B.1.351 (0.15%), and Kappa-B.1.617.1 (0.14%). In addition, 70 patients

(0.27%) had BTIs due to non-VOCs; 19 patients were reported as other; and 17 had BTIs due to the Iota (B.1.526) variant. The serum samples of nine patients with BTIs revealed the Epsilon (B.1.427 and B.1.429) variant and four patients with the Mu (B.1.621) variant. The B.1.1.306, B.1.617.3, and 20G variants were seen in two patients each, whereas the Eta (B.1.525) and B.1.560 variants were seen in one patient each. The variant distribution for four patients was reported as unknown. Among the reported mutations, the most commonly identified were the N501Y, E484K, and the L452R mutations. Of interest, the AY.1 lineage of the Delta variant was also identified in a subset of BTIs.

A total of 8.4% of patients had pre-existing comorbidities, which included chronic bronchitis, smoking, obesity, dyslipidemia, type 2 diabetes mellitus, and immunosuppressive conditions. Moreover, 591 (2.3%) of the reported BTIs occurred in healthcare workers (HCW). The symptoms in the BTIs ranged from asymptomatic to severe pneumonia as well as intensive care unit (ICU) admission with mechanical ventilation. The majority of patients recovered without any complications. However, 11.6% of patients were hospitalized requiring oxygen supplementation, intubation, or ECMO, and 0.6% died.

4. Discussion

This systematic review aimed to assess the existing evidence on BTIs of SARS-CoV-2. The results shed light on the distribution of variant type, clinical outcomes, and symptom severity in BTIs, and the associative factors. SARS-CoV-2 structure and function. An understanding of BTIs begins with consideration of the characteristics of SARS-CoV-2, which comprises two groups of proteins: structural proteins (SP) and non-structural proteins (NSP). SPs are encoded by four genes, including E (envelope), M (membrane), S (spike), and N (nucleocapsid) genes [44]. NSPs are mostly enzymes or functional proteins that play a role in viral replication and methylation and may induce host responses to infection [44]. These genes are encoded in several groups, namely ORF1a (NSP1–11), ORF1b (NSP12–16), ORF3a, ORF6, ORF7a, ORF7b, ORF8, and ORF10 [44]. Importantly, not all genetic mutations lead to an increase in viral infectivity. VOCs mostly carry mutations in the spike gene, and the ORF1a frame is the critical region for mutations in the E, M, and S genes [44]. As of February 2022, over 8,600,000 sequences and eight variants of interest or concern have been identified in the global SARS-CoV-2 sequence database operated by the Global Initiative on Sharing Avian Influenza Data (GISAID) [45].

SARS-CoV-2 viral entry into the cells is facilitated by the spike protein, which attaches to the angiotensin-converting enzyme 2 (ACE2) receptor on the cell's surface. The spike protein is split into two subunits, S1 and S2. Mutations in the S1 region, which is the receptor-binding domain (RBD) site, lower the affinity to neutralizing antibodies and show increased affinity to ACE2 receptors [46,47]. These include the N501Y (N asparagine replaced with Y tyrosine), K417N (lysine K replaced with asparagine N), and E484K (glutamic acid E replaced with lysine K) mutations in the Alpha variant. In the Beta variant, in addition to the N501Y mutation, the E484K mutations were seen, whereas both the E484K and K417T mutations were seen in the Gamma variant. The Delta and Kappa variants share the E484Q (glutamic acid E replaced with glutamine Q) and L452R (leucine L altered by arginine R) mutations. Another mutation unique to the Delta variant is T478K (threonine T replaced by lysine K) [48–50]. In addition to the above, mutations at the non-receptor binding site, D614G, increase the density of the spike proteins, thus leading to more functional spikes and increased replication and infectivity [51–53].

4.1. COVID-19 Vaccines and Efficacy

As of February 2022, the vaccines recommended by the World Health Organization (WHO) as part of its emergency use listing include the Comirnaty vaccine by Pfizer/BioNTech, the ChAdOx1-S nCov-19 vaccines by AstraZeneca, the Janssen/Ad26.COV 2.S vaccine by Johnson & Johnson, mRNA 1273 by Moderna, Sinopharm COVID-19 vaccine, the CoronaVac vaccine by Sinovac, BBV152 Covaxin by Bharat Biotech, Covishield (ChAdOx1-S [recombinant]) and the Covovax (NVX–CoV2373) vaccine by the Serum Institute of India, the Nuvaxovid (NVX–CoV2373) vaccine by Novavax, and the Inactivated COVID-19 Vaccine (Vero Cell) by the Beijing Institute of Biological Products [54]. The United States Food and Drug Administration (FDA) has approved three different vaccinations against SARS-CoV-2: BNT162b2 (Pfizer-BioNTech), mRNA-1273 (Moderna), and Ad26.COV2. S (Janssen) [55]. The final list of studies included these vaccines, in addition to Ad5-nCoV by CanSino, which was not yet approved for emergency use by WHO or FDA [54].

The Pfizer–BioNTech vaccine is estimated to be 90% effective after the second dose in individuals aged 80 years or older and at least 97% effective in preventing symptomatic COVID-19 cases, hospitalizations, and deaths [56]. The mRNA-1273 vaccine by Moderna is highly effective against SARS-CoV-2 after six months and has an efficacy of 94.1% against COVID-19 14 days after the first dose [57]. The Pfizer-BioNTech and Moderna vaccines contain synthetic nucleoside-modified mRNA encapsulated in lipid nanoparticles (LNP). The mRNA is translated in the cytoplasm of the cells by ribosomes into viral spike proteins activating the host immune response [58]. The AstraZeneca vaccine has a 76% efficacy in preventing symptomatic SARS-CoV-2 infection, specifically during the 15 days after the second dose (with a 29-day interval between the two doses). The vaccine utilizes an inactivated adenovirus DNA as a vector that carries the SARS-CoV-2 spike protein gene, which is then transcribed into mRNA, ultimately activating the immune system and antibody production in a manner similar to the Pfizer-BioNTech and Moderna vaccines [59]. The Sinopharm vaccine is an inactivated vaccine that stimulates the host's immune system. It has an efficacy of 79% against symptomatic SARS-CoV-2 infection 14 days or more after the second dose (with a 21-day interval between the two doses). The Ad5-nCoV by CanSino is an adenovirus-based viral vector vaccine with an efficacy rate of 57.5% against symptomatic COVID-19 infection [60]. Ad.26.COV2.S or JNJ-78436725 Janssen vaccine is known to elicit a durable immune response for a minimum of eight months post-vaccination with minimal reductions in antibody levels [61]. The vaccine efficacy is 85.4% against critical illness and 93.1 % against hospitalization [62]. This recombinant vaccine contains an adenovirus serotype 26 (Ad26) vector that expresses a SARS-CoV-2 spike protein, which is then translated into mRNA that stimulates cellular immune responses and antibody formation against the S antigen [63]. The Sinovac vaccine is an inactivated virus vaccine, which is 51% efficacious against symptomatic SARS-CoV-2 infection, and Covaxin is an inactivated vaccine that induces a robust immune response using an adjuvant called Alhydroxiquim-II [64]. It has an efficacy of 78% against severe COVID-19 disease [64].

4.2. SARS-CoV-2 Variants and Breakthrough Infections

However, despite the above vaccine efficacy rates, BTIs occur. Most BTIs in our review were due to the Delta variant. This confirms the results of other studies in the literature where lowered effectiveness of the vaccines has been due to the highly transmissible Delta variant (which is 60% more transmissible than the Alpha variant) [7,64,65]. B.1.617.1 also partially impairs neutralizing antibodies elicited by BNT162b2 and ChAdOx1 nCoV-19 (Covishield) vaccines [20]. The T478K mutation in the Delta variant may also facilitate an escape by antibodies generated by vaccines or natural infection [45,66]. The AY.4 lineage of the Delta variant was seen predominantly in hospitalized patients vaccinated by the CanSino vaccine where around 67% of vaccinated individuals developed milder symptoms of COVID-19 [23]. Despite the asymptomatic or mild disease, the BTIs were associated with low levels of neutralizing antibodies, high viral load, and prolonged positivity on PCR tests, thus potentially contributing to ongoing transmission from fully vaccinated individuals [66]. Another study that analyzed the viral loads of over 16,000 infections during the predominantly Delta wave in Israel, found lower viral loads in BTIs in fully vaccinated individuals compared to infections in the unvaccinated. However, this effect started to decline after 2 months [23].

Moderate reductions in vaccine efficacy with the E484K, L452R, S477N, and N501Y mutations during the Delta variant surge were also observed in New York City between November 2020 and August 2021 [34]. However, the immune escape mutations in the spike protein gene were evenly distributed among the partially and fully vaccinated cases [34]. BTIs in which Delta was the predominant variant also revealed lowered humoral and cell-mediated immunity with Eotaxin, SCF, SDF-1a, and PIGF-1; low memory B cell cytokines (IL-1b, TNF, IFNc) and chemokines (Eotaxin, SCF, SDF-1a, PIGF-1); increased levels of plasmablast cells; and a higher frequency of CD4+ and IL-2 cells after vaccination with the BNT162b2 vaccine [42]. Compared to plasma antibodies, memory B cells were found to have a higher neutralizing effect against VOCs potentially implying that the lowered memory B cells with the Delta variant may have led to BTIs [67]. Data also shows that there is a 3-fold and 16-fold reduction in neutralization against the Delta and Beta variants as compared with the Alpha variant with BNT162b2 vaccinated sera, and a 5-fold and 9-fold reduction against the same with ChAdOx1 nCoV-19 [68].

The N501Y mutation predominantly seen in the studies yielded by our review also lowers the neutralization capacity of the vaccines [25,69]. Infections with the N501Y mutation in the Alpha variant led to low neutralizing antibodies against the AZD1222 vaccine compared to non-Alpha variants [14].

Similarly, both the E484K and S477 mutations, found in P.1 and P.6 respectively, are reported to escape neutralization by a range of mAbs [70]. E484K is also associated with a decrease in the neutralizing activity of convalescent and post-vaccination (BNT162b2) sera [71–73]. E484K causes resistance to many class 2 RBD-directed antibodies, including bamlanivimab [74,75]. The most potent mRNA vaccine-elicited monoclonal antibodies were over 10-fold less effective against pseudotyped viruses carrying the E484K mutation [18]. In the study by Olsen et al., BTIs in fully vaccinated patients due to the E484K variant mutations in the Alpha variant had a significantly lower cycle threshold (a proxy for higher virus load) and significantly higher hospitalization rate [40]. Other variants (e.g., B.1.429 and B.1.427, P.1, P.2 (Zeta), and R.1) also increased rapidly, although the magnitude was less than that in Alpha [40]. Additionally, patients infected with the B.1.617.1 or B.1.617.2 variants also had a high rate of hospitalization despite vaccination[51]. In addition to the above, the L452R mutation, where Leucine-452 that is located at the point of interaction with the ACE2 receptor in the RBD receptor is replaced by arginine, also causes greater receptor affinity and escape from neutralizing antibodies [20,24,76].

Although most BTIs reported in the final 33 studies occurred before full vaccine-induced immunity, a few reinfections were also reported despite the presence of neutralizing antibodies [28]. Schulte et al. reported the case of an HCW who developed infection with the Eta (B.1.525) variant despite the presence of neutralizing antibodies seven weeks after vaccination [77]. The authors hypothesized that this could be attributed to the absence of an N-specific antibody and spike-based neutralization post-vaccination, which prevents antibody responses to the nucleocapsid, thus demonstrating the need for protective measures such as masks even after full vaccination [78]. As per their study, neutralization assays demonstrated differences against variants by a factor of 4. Variant B.1.525 is the best at neutralizing, followed by the B.3 and B.1.1.7 variants. The B.1.351 variant neutralizes the least. The study concluded that differences in spike proteins play a crucial role in neutralization [78]. Another study showed similar results, with higher neutralization against B.1.525 and B.1.1.7 and weaker neutralization against B.1.351 compared to B.1 [79].

4.3. Breakthrough Infections in at-Risk Populations

4.3.1. Immunosuppression

Laboratory and clinical investigations among the final 33 studies showed that post-vaccine antibody responses against SARS-CoV-2 variants are less than antibody responses against wild SARS-CoV-2 but are still protective against severe disease and death [80,81]. This phenomenon is applicable for immunocompetent patients who are mounting high antibody responses that can overcome the mutations in the spike protein but inadequate for solid organ transplant recipients and those with immunosuppression who mount a suboptimal antibody response against wild SARS-CoV-2 [82]. In patients with solid organ transplantation, lower antibody response and waning immunity render those patients at higher risk of BTIs after vaccination. In addition, immunosuppressive medications such as calcineurin inhibitors, mycophenolic acid, and antiproliferative drugs were reported to increase the risk of SARS-CoV-2 BTIs by lowering the immunogenicity of vaccines and in developing an adequate immune response [17,83].

In a study by Deng et al., BTIs occurred in fully vaccinated individuals over four weeks of follow-up [76]. Fourteen patients were identified and 42.8% were solid organ transplant (SOT) recipients. Another study by Almaghrabi et al. demonstrated that BTIs after COVID-19 mRNA vaccination were highest in immunocompromised patients with primary immunodeficiencies, active malignancies, and transplantation [84]. In one study, patients with cancer undergoing chemotherapy had lower levels of antibodies compared to healthy controls following the second dose of the BNT162b2 vaccine [43]. Sun et al. demonstrated that full vaccination was associated with a reduced rate of BTIs regardless of the immune status [85]. However, even among these, the rate of BTIs was still higher in the immunocompromised group thus necessitating the need for alternate strategies such as monoclonal antibodies and non-pharmaceutical personal protective measures such as masks, social distancing, and avoiding large gatherings [85]. Immunosuppressed individuals also had a higher risk factor for BTIs when controlled for age, gender, and comorbidities [85]. To combat this, the third dose of the vaccine was initially recommended for immunocompromised patients [86]. However, studies still revealed a substantially lower immune response compared to the general population, thus paving the way for treatment with monoclonal antibodies [87,88].

4.3.2. Aging

Our study revealed that the aging of the immune system or immunosenescence, which decreases the number of naive T & B cells, can also lead to reduced vaccine efficacy, particularly in older individuals, thus predisposing them to BTIs [84,89]. A recent study that described humoral and cell-mediated responses after two doses of mRNA vaccination against SARS-CoV-2 VOCs in relation to different age groups showed that patients above eighty years old had lower cell-mediated responses compared to younger patients [90]. Another multicenter study in the USA that examined the factors affecting COVID-19 immunity in individuals who were administered two doses of the BNT162b2 vaccine, found that antibody titers were negatively correlated with increasing age [11]. Sun et al. who analyzed the risk of BTIs in immunocompromised patients, found that although full vaccination was associated with a 28% reduced risk of BTIs, older individuals still had a higher rate of BTIs [85].

4.3.3. Occupational Risk

Lastly, the results showed that reinfections were seen due to prolonged exposure, predominantly in healthcare workers despite vaccination [16,20,29,31,41,69,91]. Although occupational exposure other than healthcare settings was not reported in the studies in our review, prolonged exposure to COVID-19 has also been known to occur in retail workers, meat and poultry workers, shelter staff, call center staff, and transit operators [92]. As per the WHO prior to the availability of COVID-19 vaccines, HCWs accounted for 14% of COVID-19 cases [93]. Several studies have also reported milder infection in HCWs, and this could be due to the availability of frequent testing and detection [94]. Although our review reported no comorbidities among HCWs, around 6% of HCWs in previous studies who presented with severe infection had comorbidities such as obesity [94]. The risk of BTIs among HCWs is said to have declined after the introduction of COVID-19 vaccinations, with a greater proportion of infections from community exposure. Despite this, BTIs due to waning immunity and the emergence of variants still present a risk to patients and coworkers, highlighting the need for ongoing screening and testing in this population [95].

4.3.4. Ct (Cycle Threshold) Values & Viral Loads

The Ct (cycle threshold) value is the number of cycles it takes for the RT-PCR test to detect the virus. Ct levels are inversely proportional to the amount of target nucleic acid in the sample. The higher the amount of the viral nucleic acid in the sample, the lower the Ct value. An important issue for controlling the spread of variants is to determine if the BTI is associated with high viral loads that may result in a secondary spread. Previous studies reported that low viral loads and a high Ct value were detected following vaccination [23,96]. In contrast, a study by Deng et al. detected relatively high viral loads (median Ct of 19.6) even in non-immunosuppressed vaccinated subjects exhibiting asymptomatic or mild infection [28]. This finding is consistent with other studies that reported that individuals with BTIs with the Alpha variant had a significantly lower Ct value compared to non-Alpha patients [40]. Although this could be viewed as an enhanced transmissibility potential of Alpha, no clear correlation between Ct values and transmission rates has been confirmed.

4.3.5. Heterogenous Vaccination Regimens

Numerous studies have shown a stronger immune response where mix and match vaccine regimens are used [19,97,98]. Individuals who receive different types of COVID-19 vaccines for their first, second, and subsequent booster doses show more potent immune responses. One study in our review described the transmission of infection from a fully vaccinated spouse, thus hypothesizing that this was due to a lack of immune response against the nucleocapsid protein, against which the mRNA vaccines are not effective. A study by Nordstrom et al., found that those who received a mixed vaccine regimen were 68% less likely to develop an infection compared to unvaccinated people, whereas those who received two doses of the same vaccine (Astra Zeneca) were 50% less likely to do so [82]. Another study also showed similar results where the vaccine efficacy against SARS-CoV-2 infection was 88% when ChAdOx1 and an mRNA vaccine were combined [83]. Additionally, there is some evidence that heterologous vaccination may also confer greater protection, with combined cellular and humoral immunity in immunocompromised individuals [84].

5. Limitations

Importantly, our study has several notable limitations. Given the nature of surveillance, testing, and reporting, oftentimes not all cases are documented. There may also have been some overlap in status (e.g., some individuals who had been vaccinated may have been previously infected at some point). We describe the cases that have been documented in the scientific literature. Additionally, we must consider the possibility of asymptomatic viral transmission among vaccinated individuals; these numbers are not reflected in these studies. Thus, it could be possible that the extent of SARS-CoV-2 transmissibility among vaccinated individuals is greater than expected as per our current understanding. Data reported from hospital settings where exposure to infection is higher, may not reflect the infection rates in the general population. Also, data in several studies were collected from electronic medical records and hence may be prone to error. Similarly, the history of exposure in those with BTIs may not always be accurate and the source of infection is not always known. Among the data from the immunocompromised patients, there were no specific mentions of which condition may have had a greater contribution towards the lowered immunity.

6. Conclusions

BTIs remain a critical challenge in controlling the epidemic. Whether individuals with BTIs contribute substantially to the onward transmission of SARS-CoV-2 in the population currently remains unclear. In our review, we found that BTIs do not reflect selection towards specific immunity-evading variants, rather, they reflect the most prevalent variant in the community at that time. Hence a standardized surveillance reporting protocol for suspected BTIs is necessary to better assess the nature and extent of the burden of reinfections in vaccinated individuals. Studies on BTIs could be helpful to understand the neutralizing response to SARS-CoV-2 infection and the corresponding immunity. However, the absence of systematic genomic sequencing of positive cases worldwide impedes advances in public health surveillance to manage the pandemic at the individual and collective levels. Further investigations, including a genetic comparison of SARS-CoV-2 strains, would be beneficial to understanding the frequency and pathophysiology of SARS-CoV-2 reinfections. Although COVID-19 vaccines have proven to be highly effective, the possibility of BTIs remains a reality, particularly in the context of emerging variants of concern. Many factors contribute to BTIs including the transmission dynamics of SARS-CoV-2 variants and their biological capacity to survive, behavioral characteristics of individuals, and vaccination status. Future studies should explore the role of combining different types of vaccines, post-exposure prophylaxis, and close monitoring for disease progression including disease progression and transmission in high-risk individuals such as HCWs or immunocompromised patients.

Supplementary Materials: The following are available online at https://www.mdpi.com/article/10.3390/tropicalmed7050081/s1, The full search strategy for each database.

Author Contributions: Conceptualization, S.G. and N.D.; Methodology, P.T., S.G. and N.D.; Formal Analysis, S.G., A.I., S.P. and P.S.S.; Data Curation, S.G., A.I., S.P., P.S.S., P.S. and E.X.; Writing—Original Draft Preparation: S.G., A.I., N.D., S.P. and P.S.S.; Writing—Review and Editing: S.G., A.I. and N.D.; Supervision, S.G., S.M., J.M. and G.M.; Project Administration, S.G., S.M., J.M. and G.M. All authors have read and agreed to the published version of the manuscript.

Funding: This research received no external funding.

Institutional Review Board Statement: Not Applicable.

Informed Consent Statement: Not Applicable.

Conflicts of Interest: The authors declare no conflict of interest.

References

1. World Health Organization. WHO Coronavirus (COVID-19) Dashboard. 2022. Available online: https://covid19.who.int/ (accessed on 4 February 2022).
2. CDC COVID-19 Vaccine Breakthrough Case Investigations Team. COVID-19 Vaccine Breakthrough Infections Reported to CDC—United States, 1 January—30 April 2021. *MMWR Morb. Mortal. Wkly. Rep.* **2021**, *70*, 792–793. [CrossRef] [PubMed]
3. Centers for Disease Control and Prevention. Rates of COVID-19 Cases and Deaths by Vaccination Status. 2022. Available online: https://covid.cdc.gov/covid-data-tracker/#rates-by-vaccine-status (accessed on 4 March 2022).
4. Centers for Disease Control and Prevention. Investigative Criteria for Suspected Cases of SARS-CoV-2 Reinfection (ICR). 2020. Available online: https://www.cdc.gov/coronavirus/2019-ncov/php/invest-criteria.html (accessed on 9 January 2022).
5. Krause, P.R.; Fleming, T.R.; Longini, I.M.; Peto, R.; Briand, S.; Heymann, D.L.; Beral, V.; Snape, M.D.; Rees, H.; Ropero, A.M.; et al. SARS-CoV-2 Variants and Vaccines. *N. Engl. J. Med.* **2021**, *385*, 179–186. [CrossRef] [PubMed]
6. World Health Organization. Classification of Omicron (B.1.1.529): SARS-CoV-2 Variant of Concern. 2021. Available online: https://www.who.int/news/item/26-11-2021-classification-of-omicron-(b.1.1.529)-SARS-CoV-2-variant-of-concern (accessed on 27 November 2021).
7. Lopez Bernal, J.; Andrews, N.; Gower, C.; Gallagher, E.; Simmons, R.; Thelwall, S.; Stowe, J.; Tessier, E.; Groves, N.; Dabrera, G.; et al. Effectiveness of COVID-19 Vaccines against the B.1.617.2 (Delta) Variant. *N. Engl. J. Med.* **2021**, *385*, 585–594. [CrossRef] [PubMed]
8. Fendler, A.; Shepherd, S.; Au, L.; Wilkinson, K.; Wu, M.; Byrne, F.; Cerrone, M.; Schmitt, A.M.; Joharatnam-Hogan, N.; Shum, B.; et al. Adaptive immunity and neutralizing antibodies against SARS-CoV-2 variants following vaccination in patients with cancer: The Capture study. *Nat. Cancer* **2021**, *2*, 1321–1337. [CrossRef] [PubMed]
9. Seyed Alinaghi, S.; Oliaei, S.; Kianzad, S.; Afsahi, A.M.; MohsseniPour, M.; Barzegary, A.; Barzegary, A.; Mirzapour, P.; Behnezhad, F.; Noori, T.; et al. Reinfection risk of novel coronavirus (COVID-19): A systematic review of current evidence. *World J. Virol.* **2020**, *9*, 79–90. [CrossRef]
10. Page, M.J.; McKenzie, J.E.; Bossuyt, P.M.; Boutron, I.; Hoffmann, T.C.; Mulrow, C.D.; Shamseer, L.; Tetzlaff, J.M.; Akl, E.A.; Brennan, S.E.; et al. The PRISMA 2020 statement: An updated guideline for reporting systematic reviews. *Syst. Rev.* **2021**, *10*, 89. [CrossRef]
11. Bergwerk, M.; Gonen, T.; Lustig, Y.; Amit, S.; Lipsitch, M.; Cohen, C.; Mandelboim, M.; Levin, E.G.; Rubin, C.; Indenbaum, V.; et al. COVID-19 Breakthrough Infections in Vaccinated Health Care Workers. *N. Engl. J. Med.* **2021**, *385*, 1474–1484. [CrossRef]

12. Estofolete, C.F.; Banho, C.A.; Campos, G.R.F.; Marques, B.C.; Sacchetto, L.; Ullmann, L.S.; Possebon, F.S.; Machado, L.F.; Syrio, J.D.; Araújo Junior, J.P.; et al. Case Study of Two Post Vaccination SARS-CoV-2 Infections with P1 Variants in CoronaVac Vaccinees in Brazil. *Viruses* **2021**, *13*, 1237. [CrossRef]
13. Fabiani, M.; Margiotti, K.; Viola, A.; Mesoraca, A.; Giorlandino, C. Mild Symptomatic SARS-CoV-2 P.1 (B.1.1.28) Infection in a Fully Vaccinated 83-Year-Old Man. *Pathogens* **2021**, *10*, 614. [CrossRef]
14. Philomina, J.B.; Jolly, B.; John, N.; Bhoyar, R.C.; Majeed, N.; Senthivel, V.; Cp, F.; Rophina, M.; Vasudevan, B.; Imran, M.; et al. Genomic survey of SARS-CoV-2 vaccine breakthrough infections in healthcare workers from Kerala, India. *J. Infect.* **2021**, *83*, 237–279. [CrossRef]
15. Hacisuleyman, E.; Hale, C.; Saito, Y.; Blachere, N.E.; Bergh, M.; Conlon, E.G.; Schaefer-Babajew, D.J.; DaSilva, J.; Muecksch, F.; Gaebler, C.; et al. Vaccine Breakthrough Infections with SARS-CoV-2 Variants. *N. Engl. J. Med.* **2021**, *384*, 2212–2218. [CrossRef] [PubMed]
16. Kroidl, I.; Mecklenburg, I.; Schneiderat, P.; Müller, K.; Girl, P.; Wölfel, R.; Sing, A.; Dangel, A.; Wieser, A.; Hoelscher, M. Vaccine breakthrough infection and onward transmission of SARS-CoV-2 Beta (B.1.351) variant, Bavaria, Germany, February to March 2021. *Eurosurveillance* **2021**, *26*, 2100673. [CrossRef] [PubMed]
17. Almaghrabi, R.S.; Alhamlan, F.S.; Dada, A.; Al-Tawfiq, J.A.; Al Hroub, M.K.; Saeedi, M.F.; Alamri, M.; Alhothaly, B.; Alqasabi, A.; Al-Qahtani, A.A.; et al. Outcome of SARS-CoV-2 variant breakthrough infection in fully immunized solid organ transplant recipients. *J. Infect. Public Health* **2022**, *15*, 51–55. [CrossRef] [PubMed]
18. Olsen, R.J.; Christensen, P.A.; Long, S.W.; Subedi, S.; Hodjat, P.; Olson, R.; Nguyen, M.; Davis, J.J.; Yerramilli, P.; Saavedra, M.O.; et al. Trajectory of Growth of Severe Acute Respiratory Syndrome Coronavirus 2 (SARS-CoV-2) Variants in Houston, Texas, January through May 2021, Based on 12,476 Genome Sequences. *Am. J. Pathol.* **2021**, *191*, 1754–1773. [CrossRef]
19. Schmidt, T.; Klemis, V.; Schub, D.; Schneitler, S.; Reichert, M.C.; Wilkens, H.; Sester, U.; Sester, M.; Mihm, J. Cellular immunity predominates over humoral immunity after homologous and heterologous mRNA and vector-based COVID-19 vaccine regimens in solid organ transplant recipients. *Am. J. Transplant.* **2021**, *21*, 3990–4002. [CrossRef]
20. Chau, N.V.V.; Ngoc, N.M.; Nguyet, L.A.; Quang, V.M.; Ny, N.T.H.; Khoa, D.B.; Phong, N.T.; Toan, L.M.; Hong, N.T.; Tuyen, N.T.K.; et al. An observational study of breakthrough SARS-CoV-2 Delta variant infections among vaccinated healthcare workers in Vietnam. *EClinicalMedicine* **2021**, *41*, 101143. [CrossRef]
21. Connor, B.A.; Couto-Rodriguez, M.; Barrows, J.E.; Gardner, M.; Rogova, M.; O'Hara, N.B.; Nagy-Szakal, D. Monoclonal Antibody Therapy in a Vaccine Breakthrough SARS-CoV-2 Hospitalized Delta (B1.617.2) Variant Case. *Int. J. Infect. Dis.* **2021**, *110*, 232–234. [CrossRef]
22. Gharpure, R.; Sami, S.; Vostok, J.; Johnson, H.; Hall, N.; Foreman, A.; Sabo, R.T.; Schubert, P.L.; Shephard, H.; Brown, V.R.; et al. Multistate Outbreak of SARS-CoV-2 Infections, Including Vaccine Breakthrough Infections, Associated with Large Public Gatherings, United States. *Emerg. Infect. Dis.* **2022**, *28*, 35–43. [CrossRef]
23. Galán-Huerta, K.A.; Flores-Treviño, S.; Salas-Treviño, D.; Bocanegra-Ibarias, P.; Rivas-Estilla, A.M.; Pérez-Alba, E.; Lozano-Sepúlveda, S.A.; Arellanos-Soto, D.; Camacho-Ortiz, A. Prevalence of SARS-CoV-2 Variants of Concern and Variants of Interest in COVID-19 Breakthrough Infections in a Hospital in Monterrey, Mexico. *Viruses* **2022**, *14*, 154. [CrossRef]
24. Deng, X.; Evdokimova, M.; O'Brien, A.; Rowe, C.L.; Clark, N.M.; Harrington, A.; Reid, G.E.; Uprichard, S.L.; Baker, S.C. Breakthrough Infections with Multiple Lineages of SARS-CoV-2 Variants Reveals Continued Risk of Severe Disease in Immunosuppressed Patients. *Viruses* **2021**, *13*, 1743. [CrossRef]
25. De Souza, W.M.; Muraro, S.P.; Souza, G.F.; Amorim, M.R.; Sesti-Costa, R.; Mofatto, L.S.; Forato, J.; Barbosa, P.P.; Toledo-Teixeira, D.A.; Bispo-Dos-Santos, K.; et al. Clusters of SARS-CoV-2 Lineage B.1.1.7 Infection after Vaccination with Adenovirus-Vectored and Inactivated Vaccines. *Viruses* **2021**, *13*, 2127. [CrossRef] [PubMed]
26. Gupta, N.; Kaur, H.; Yadav, P.D.; Mukhopadhyay, L.; Sahay, R.R.; Kumar, A.; Nyayanit, D.A.; Shete, A.M.; Patil, S.; Majumdar, T.; et al. Clinical Characterization and Genomic Analysis of Samples from COVID-19 Breakthrough Infections during the Second Wave among the Various States of India. *Viruses* **2021**, *13*, 1782. [CrossRef] [PubMed]
27. Kale, P.; Gupta, E.; Bihari, C.; Patel, N.; Rooge, S.; Pandey, A.; Bajpai, M.; Khillan, V.; Chattopadhyay, P.; Devi, P.; et al. Vaccine Breakthrough Infections by SARS-CoV-2 Variants after ChAdOx1 nCoV-19 Vaccination in Healthcare Workers. *Vaccines* **2021**, *10*, 54. [CrossRef]
28. Schulte, B.; Marx, B.; Korencak, M.; Emmert, D.; Aldabbagh, S.; Eis-Hübinger, A.M.; Streeck, H. Case Report: Infection With SARS-CoV-2 in the Presence of High Levels of Vaccine-Induced Neutralizing Antibody Responses. *Front. Med.* **2021**, *8*, 704719. [CrossRef] [PubMed]
29. Malhotra, S.; Mani, K.; Lodha, R.; Bakhshi, S.; Mathur, V.P.; Gupta, P.; Kedia, S.; Sankar, J.; Kumar, P.; Kumar, A.; et al. SARS-CoV-2 Reinfection Rate and Estimated Effectiveness of the Inactivated Whole Virion Vaccine BBV152 Against Reinfection Among Health Care Workers in New Delhi, India. *JAMA Netw. Open* **2022**, *5*, e2142210. [CrossRef]
30. Shastri, J.; Parikh, S.; Aggarwal, V.; Agrawal, S.; Chatterjee, N.; Shah, R.; Devi, P.; Mehta, P.; Pandey, R. Severe SARS-CoV-2 Breakthrough Reinfection with Delta Variant After Recovery from Breakthrough Infection by Alpha Variant in a Fully Vaccinated Health Worker. *Front. Med.* **2021**, *8*, 737007. [CrossRef] [PubMed]
31. Rovida, F.; Cassaniti, I.; Paolucci, S.; Percivalle, E.; Sarasini, A.; Piralla, A.; Giardina, F.; Sammartino, J.C.; Ferrari, A.; Bergami, F.; et al. SARS-CoV-2 vaccine breakthrough infections with the alpha variant are asymptomatic or mildly symptomatic among health care workers. *Nat. Commun.* **2021**, *12*, 6032. [CrossRef]

32. Rümke, L.W.; Groenveld, F.C.; van Os, Y.M.G.; Praest, P.; Tanja, A.A.N.; de Jong, D.T.C.M.; Symons, J.; Schuurman, R.; Reinders, T.; Hofstra, L.M.; et al. In-depth Characterization of Vaccine Breakthrough Infections With SARS-CoV-2 Among Health Care Workers in a Dutch Academic Medical Center. *Open Forum Infect. Dis.* **2021**, *9*, ofab553. [CrossRef]
33. Yi, S.; Kim, J.M.; Choe, Y.J.; Hong, S.; Choi, S.; Ahn, S.B.; Kim, M.; Park, Y.J. SARS-CoV-2 Delta Variant Breakthrough Infection and Onward Secondary Transmission in Household. *J. Korean Med. Sci.* **2022**, *37*, e12. [CrossRef]
34. Robilotti, E.V.; Whiting, K.; Lucca, A.; Poon, C.; Guest, R.; McMillen, T.; Jani, K.; Solovyov, A.; Kelson, S.; Browne, K.; et al. Clinical and Genomic Characterization of SARS-CoV-2 infections in mRNA Vaccinated Health Care Personnel in New York City. *Clin. Infect. Dis.* **2021**, ciab886. [CrossRef]
35. Vignier, N.; Bérot, V.; Bonnave, N.; Peugny, S.; Ballet, M.; Jacoud, E.; Michaud, C.; Gaillet, M.; Djossou, F.; Blanchet, D.; et al. Breakthrough Infections of SARS-CoV-2 Gamma Variant in Fully Vaccinated Gold Miners, French Guiana, 2021. *Emerg. Infect. Dis.* **2021**, *27*, 2673–2676. [CrossRef] [PubMed]
36. Tober-Lau, P.; Schwarz, T.; Hillus, D.; Spieckermann, J.; Helbig, E.T.; Lippert, L.J.; Thibeault, C.; Koch, W.; Bergfeld, L.; Niemeyer, D.; et al. Outbreak of SARS-CoV-2 B.1.1.7 Lineage after Vaccination in Long-Term Care Facility, Germany, February–March 2021. *Emerg. Infect. Dis.* **2021**, *27*, 2169–2173. [CrossRef] [PubMed]
37. Servellita, V.; Morris, M.K.; Sotomayor-Gonzalez, A.; Gliwa, A.S.; Torres, E.; Brazer, N.; Zhou, A.; Hernandez, K.T.; Sankaran, M.; Wang, B.; et al. Predominance of antibody-resistant SARS-CoV-2 variants in vaccine breakthrough cases from the San Francisco Bay Area, California. *Nat. Microbiol.* **2022**, *7*, 277–288. [CrossRef] [PubMed]
38. Singer, S.R.; Angulo, F.J.; Swerdlow, D.L.; McLaughlin, J.M.; Hazan, I.; Ginish, N.; Anis, E.; Mendelson, E.; Mor, O.; Zuckerman, N.S.; et al. Effectiveness of BNT162b2 mRNA COVID-19 vaccine against SARS-CoV-2 variant Beta (B.1.351) among persons identified through contact tracing in Israel: A prospective cohort study. *EClinicalMedicine* **2021**, *42*, 101190. [CrossRef] [PubMed]
39. Thangaraj, J.W.V.; Yadav, P.; Kumar, C.G.; Shete, A.; Nyayanit, D.A.; Rani, D.S.; Kumar, A.; Kumar, M.S.; Sabarinathan, R.; Saravana Kumar, V.; et al. Predominance of delta variant among the COVID-19 vaccinated and unvaccinated individuals, India, May 2021. *J. Infect.* **2022**, *84*, 94–118. [CrossRef] [PubMed]
40. Motozono, C.; Toyoda, M.; Zahradnik, J.; Saito, A.; Nasser, H.; Tan, T.S.; Ngare, I.; Kimura, I.; Uriu, K.; Kosugi, Y.; et al. SARS-CoV-2 spike L452R variant evades cellular immunity and increases infectivity. *Cell Host Microbe* **2021**, *29*, 1124–1136. [CrossRef]
41. Singh, U.B.; Rophina, M.; Chaudhry, R.; Senthivel, V.; Bala, K.; Bhoyar, R.C.; Jolly, B.; Jamshed, N.; Imran, M.; Gupta, R.; et al. Variants of concern responsible for SARS-CoV-2 vaccine breakthrough infections from India. *J. Med. Virol.* **2022**, *94*, 1696–1700. [CrossRef]
42. Tay, M.Z.; Rouers, A.; Fong, S.W.; Goh, Y.S.; Chan, Y.H.; Chang, Z.W.; Xu, W.; Tan, C.W.; Chia, W.N.; Torres-Ruesta, A.; et al. Decreased memory B cell frequencies in COVID-19 delta variant vaccine breakthrough infection. *EMBO Mol. Med.* **2022**, *14*, e15227. [CrossRef]
43. Sun, J.; Zheng, Q.; Madhira, V.; Olex, A.L.; Anzalone, A.J.; Vinson, A.; Singh, J.A.; French, E.; Abraham, A.G.; Mathew, J.; et al. Association Between Immune Dysfunction and COVID-19 Breakthrough Infection After SARS-CoV-2 Vaccination in the US. *JAMA Intern. Med.* **2022**, *182*, 153–162. [CrossRef]
44. Wu, F.; Zhao, S.; Yu, B.; Chen, Y.M.; Wang, W.; Song, Z.G.; Hu, Y.; Tao, Z.W.; Tian, J.H.; Pei, Y.Y.; et al. A new coronavirus associated with human respiratory disease in China. *Nature* **2020**, *579*, 265–269. [CrossRef]
45. GISAID. Tracking of Variants. 2022. Available online: https://www.gisaid.org/hcov19-variants (accessed on 5 March 2022).
46. Piccoli, L.; Park, Y.J.; Tortorici, M.A.; Czudnochowski, N.; Walls, A.C.; Beltramello, M.; Silacci-Fregni, C.; Pinto, D.; Rosen, L.E.; Bowen, J.E.; et al. Mapping Neutralizing and Immunodominant Sites on the SARS-CoV-2 Spike Receptor-Binding Domain by Structure-Guided High-Resolution Serology. *Cell* **2020**, *183*, 1024–1042.e21. [CrossRef] [PubMed]
47. Starr, T.N.; Greaney, A.J.; Addetia, A.; Hannon, W.W.; Choudhary, M.C.; Dingens, A.S.; Li, J.Z.; Bloom, J.D. Prospective mapping of viral mutations that escape antibodies used to treat COVID-19. *Science* **2021**, *371*, 850–854. [CrossRef] [PubMed]
48. Zhou, D.; Dejnirattisai, W.; Supasa, P.; Liu, C.; Mentzer, A.J.; Ginn, H.M.; Zhao, Y.; Duyvesteyn, H.M.E.; Tuekprakhon, A.; Nutalai, R.; et al. Evidence of escape of SARS-CoV-2 variant B.1.351 from natural and vaccine-induced sera. *Cell* **2021**, *184*, 2348–2361.e6. [CrossRef] [PubMed]
49. Cele, S.; Gazy, I.; Jackson, L.; Hwa, S.; Tegally, H.; Lustig, G.; Giandhari, J.; Pillay, S.; Wilkinson, E.; Naidoo, Y.; et al. Escape of SARS-CoV-2 501Y.V2 from neutralization by convalescent plasma. *Nature* **2021**, *593*, 142–146. [CrossRef]
50. Wang, P.; Casner, R.G.; Nair, M.S.; Wang, M.; Yu, J.; Cerutti, G.; Liu, L.; Kwong, P.D.; Huang, Y.; Shapiro, L.; et al. Increased resistance of SARS-CoV-2 variant P.1 to antibody neutralization. *Cell Host Microbe* **2021**, *29*, 747–751.e4. [CrossRef]
51. Starr, T.N.; Greaney, A.J.; Hilton, S.K.; Ellis, D.; Crawford, K.H.D.; Dingens, A.S.; Navarro, M.J.; Bowen, J.E.; Tortorici, M.A.; Walls, A.C.; et al. Deep Mutational Scanning of SARS-CoV-2 Receptor Binding Domain Reveals Constraints on Folding and ACE2 Binding. *Cell* **2020**, *182*, 1295–1310.e20. [CrossRef]
52. Zhang, L.; Jackson, C.B.; Mou, H.; Ojha, A.; Peng, H.; Quinlan, B.D.; Rangarajan, E.S.; Pan, A.; Vanderheiden, A.; Suthar, M.S.; et al. SARS-CoV-2 spike-protein D614G mutation increases virion spike density and infectivity. *Nat. Commun.* **2020**, *11*, 6013. [CrossRef]
53. Hou, Y.J.; Chiba, S.; Halfmann, P.; Ehre, C.; Kuroda, M.; Dinnon, K.H., 3rd; Leist, S.R.; Schäfer, A.; Nakajima, N.; Takahashi, K.; et al. SARS-CoV-2 D614G variant exhibits efficient replication ex vivo and transmission in vivo. *Science* **2020**, *370*, 1464–1468. [CrossRef]

54. World Health Organization. Coronavirus Disease (COVID-19): Vaccines. 2022. Available online: https://www.who.int/news-room/questions-and-answers/item/coronavirus-disease-(covid-19)-vaccines (accessed on 4 March 2022).
55. Lythgoe, M.P.; Middleton, P. Comparison of COVID-19 Vaccine Approvals at the US Food and Drug Administration, European Medicines Agency, and Health Canada. *JAMA Netw. Open.* **2021**, *4*, e2114531. [CrossRef]
56. Lopez Bernal, J.; Andrews, N.; Gower, C.; Robertson, C.; Stowe, J.; Tessier, E.; Simmons, R.; Cottrell, S.; Roberts, R.; O'Doherty, M.; et al. Effectiveness of the Pfizer-BioNTech and Oxford-AstraZeneca vaccines on COVID-19 related symptoms, hospital admissions, and mortality in older adults in England: Test negative case-control study. *BMJ* **2021**, *373*, n1088. [CrossRef]
57. Doria-Rose, N.; Suthar, M.S.; Makowski, M.; O'Connell, S.; McDermott, A.B.; Flach, B.; Ledgerwood, J.E.; Mascola, J.R.; Graham, B.S.; Lin, B.C.; et al. mRNA-1273 Study Group. Antibody Persistence through 6 Months after the Second Dose of mRNA-1273 Vaccine for COVID-19. *N. Engl. J. Med.* **2021**, *384*, 2259–2261. [CrossRef] [PubMed]
58. Zhou, X.; Jiang, X.; Qu, M.; Aninwene, G.E.; Jucaud, V.; Moon, J.J.; Gu, Z.; Sun, W.; Khademhosseini, A. Engineering Antiviral Vaccines. *ACS Nano* **2020**, *14*, 12370–12389. [CrossRef] [PubMed]
59. Mascellino, M.T.; Di Timoteo, F.; De Angelis, M.; Oliva, A. Overview of the Main Anti-SARS-CoV-2 Vaccines: Mechanism of Action, Efficacy and Safety. *Infect. Drug Resist.* **2021**, *14*, 3459–3476. [CrossRef] [PubMed]
60. Halperin, S.A.; Ye, L.; MacKinnon-Cameron, D.; Smith, B.; Cahn, P.E.; Ruiz-Palacios, G.M.; Ikram, A.; Lanas, F.; Guerrero, M.L.; Navarro, S.R.M.; et al. CanSino COVID-19 Global Efficacy Study Group. Final efficacy analysis, interim safety analysis, and immunogenicity of a single dose of recombinant novel coronavirus vaccine (adenovirus type 5 vector) in adults 18 years and older: An international, multicentre, randomised, double-blinded, placebo-controlled phase 3 trial. *Lancet* **2022**, *399*, 237–248. [CrossRef]
61. Barouch, D.H.; Stephenson, K.E.; Sadoff, J.; Yu, J.; Chang, A.; Gebre, M.; McMahan, K.; Liu, J.; Chandrashekar, A.; Patel, S.; et al. Durable Humoral and Cellular Immune Responses 8 Months after Ad26.COV2.S Vaccination. *N. Engl. J. Med.* **2021**, *385*, 951–953. [CrossRef]
62. World Health Organization. The Janssen Ad26.COV2.S COVID-19 Vaccine: What You Need to Know. 2021. Available online: https://www.who.int/news-room/feature-stories/detail/the-j-j-covid-19-vaccine-what-you-need-to-know (accessed on 4 March 2022).
63. Grifoni, A.; Weiskopf, D.; Ramirez, S.I.; Mateus, J.; Dan, J.M.; Moderbacher, C.R.; Rawlings, S.A.; Sutherland, A.; Premkumar, L.; Jadi, R.S.; et al. Targets of T Cell Responses to SARS-CoV-2 Coronavirus in Humans with COVID-19 Disease and Unexposed Individuals. *Cell* **2020**, *181*, 1489–1501.e15. [CrossRef]
64. National Institute of Health. Adjuvant Developed with NIH Funding Enhances Efficacy of India's COVID-19 Vaccine. 2021. Available online: https://www.nih.gov/news-events/news-releases/adjuvant-developed-nih-funding-enhances-efficacy-indias-covid-19-vaccine (accessed on 4 March 2022).
65. Liu, Y.; Rocklöv, J. The reproductive number of the Delta variant of SARS-CoV-2 is far higher compared to the ancestral SARS-CoV-2 virus. *J. Travel Med.* **2021**, *28*, taab124. [CrossRef]
66. Levine-Tiefenbrun, M.; Yelin, I.; Alapi, H.; Katz, R.; Herzel, E.; Kuint, J.; Chodick, G.; Gazit, S.; Patalon, T.; Kishony, R.; et al. Viral loads of Delta-variant SARS-CoV-2 breakthrough infections after vaccination and booster with BNT162b2. *Nat. Med.* **2021**, *27*, 2108–2110. [CrossRef]
67. Sokal, A.; Barba-Spaeth, G.; Fernández, I.; Broketa, M.; Azzaoui, I.; de La Selle, A.; Vandenberghe, A.; Fourati, S.; Roeser, A.; Meola, A.; et al. mRNA vaccination of naive and COVID-19-recovered individuals elicits potent memory B cells that recognize SARS-CoV-2 variants. *Immunity* **2021**, *54*, 2893–2907.e5. [CrossRef]
68. Abdool Karim, S.S.; de Oliveira, T. New SARS-CoV-2 Variants—Clinical, Public Health, and Vaccine Implications. *N. Engl. J. Med.* **2021**, *384*, 1866–1868. [CrossRef]
69. Emary, K.R.W.; Golubchik, T.; Aley, P.K. Efficacy of ChAdOx1 nCoV-19 (AZD1222) vaccine against SARS-CoV-2 variant of concern 202012/01 (B.1.1.7): An exploratory analysis of a randomized controlled trial. *Lancet* **2021**, *397*, 1351–1362. [CrossRef]
70. Liu, Z.; VanBlargan, L.A.; Bloyet, L.M.; Rothlauf, P.W.; Chen, R.E.; Stumpf, S.; Zhao, H.; Errico, J.M.; Theel, E.S.; Liebeskind, M.J.; et al. Identification of SARS-CoV-2 spike mutations that attenuate monoclonal and serum antibody neutralization. *Cell Host Microbe* **2021**, *29*, 477–488.e4. [CrossRef] [PubMed]
71. Jangra, S.; Ye, C.; Rathnasinghe, R.; Stadlbauer, D.; Personalized Virology Initiative Study Group; Krammer, F.; Simon, V.; Martinez-Sobrido, L.; García-Sastre, A.; Schotsaert, M.; et al. SARS-CoV-2 spike E484K mutation reduces antibody neutralisation. *Lancet Microbe* **2021**, *2*, e283–e284. [CrossRef]
72. Li, Q.; Nie, J.; Wu, J.; Zhang, L.; Ding, R.; Wang, H.; Zhang, Y.; Li, T.; Liu, S.; Zhang, M.; et al. SARS-CoV-2 501Y.V2 variants lack higher infectivity but do have immune escape. *Cell* **2021**, *184*, 2362–2371.e9. [CrossRef]
73. Greaney, A.J.; Starr, T.N.; Barnes, C.O.; Weisblum, Y.; Schmidt, F.; Caskey, M.; Gaebler, C.; Cho, A.; Agudelo, M.; Finkin, S.; et al. Mapping mutations to the SARS-CoV-2 RBD that escape binding by different classes of antibodies. *Nat. Commun.* **2021**, *12*, 4196. [CrossRef] [PubMed]
74. Starr, T.N.; Greaney, A.J.; Dingens, A.S.; Bloom, J.D. Complete map of SARS-CoV-2 RBD mutations that escape the monoclonal antibody LY-CoV555 and its cocktail with LY-CoV016. *Cell Rep. Med.* **2021**, *2*, 100255. [CrossRef] [PubMed]
75. Baj, A.; Novazzi, F.; Pasciuta, R.; Genoni, A.; Ferrante, F.D.; Valli, M.; Partenope, M.; Tripiciano, R.; Ciserchia, A.; Catanoso, G.; et al. Breakthrough Infections of E484K-Harboring SARS-CoV-2 Delta Variant, Lombardy, Italy. *Emerg. Infect. Dis.* **2021**, *27*, 3180–3182. [CrossRef]

76. García, L.F. Immune Response, Inflammation, and the Clinical Spectrum of COVID-19. *Front. Immunol.* **2020**, *11*, 1441. [CrossRef]
77. Zani, A.; Caccuri, F.; Messali, S.; Bonfanti, C.; Caruso, A. Serosurvey in BNT162b2 vaccine-elicited neutralizing antibodies against authentic B.1, B.1.1.7, B.1.351, B.1.525 and P.1 SARS-CoV-2 variants. *Emerg. Microbes Infect.* **2021**, *10*, 1241–1243. [CrossRef]
78. Edridge, A.W.D.; Kaczorowska, J.; Hoste, A.C.R.; Bakker, M.; Klein, M.; Loens, K.; Jebbink, M.F.; Matser, A.; Kinsella, C.M.; Rueda, P.; et al. Seasonal coronavirus protective immunity is short-lasting. *Nat. Med.* **2020**, *26*, 1691–1693. [CrossRef]
79. Becker, M.; Dulovic, A.; Junker, D.; Ruetalo, N.; Kaiser, P.D.; Pinilla, Y.T.; Heinzel, C.; Haering, J.; Traenkle, B.; Wagner, T.R.; et al. Immune response to SARS-CoV-2 variants of concern in vaccinated individuals. *Nat. Commun.* **2021**, *12*, 3109. [CrossRef] [PubMed]
80. Wang, Z.; Schmidt, F.; Weisblum, Y.; Muecksch, F.; Barnes, C.O.; Finkin, S.; Schaefer-Babajew, D.; Cipolla, M.; Gaebler, C.; Lieberman, J.A.; et al. mRNA vaccine-elicited antibodies to SARS-CoV-2 and circulating variants. *Nature* **2021**, *592*, 616–622. [CrossRef] [PubMed]
81. Hall, V.G.; Ferreira, V.H.; Ierullo, M.; Ku, T.; Marinelli, T.; Majchrzak-Kita, B.; Yousuf, A.; Kulasingam, V.; Humar, A.; Kumar, D.; et al. Humoral and cellular immune response and safety of two-dose SARS-CoV-2 mRNA-1273 vaccine in solid organ transplant recipients. *Am. J. Transplant.* **2021**, *21*, 3980–3989. [CrossRef] [PubMed]
82. Holden, I.K.; Bistrup, C.; Nilsson, A.C.; Hansen, J.F.; Abazi, R.; Davidsen, J.R.; Poulsen, M.K.; Lindvig, S.O.; Justesen, U.S.; Johansen, I.S.; et al. Immunogenicity of SARS-CoV-2 mRNA vaccine in solid organ transplant recipients. *J. Intern. Med.* **2021**, *290*, 1264–1267. [CrossRef] [PubMed]
83. Chavarot, N.; Morel, A.; Leruez-Ville, M.; Vilain, E.; Divard, G.; Burger, C.; Serris, A.; Sberro-Soussan, R.; Martinez, F.; Amrouche, L.; et al. Weak antibody response to three doses of mRNA vaccine in kidney transplant recipients treated with belatacept. *Am. J. Transplant.* **2021**, *21*, 4043–4051. [CrossRef]
84. Shroff, R.T.; Chalasani, P.; Wei, R.; Pennington, D.; Quirk, G.; Schoenle, M.V.; Peyton, K.L.; Uhrlaub, J.L.; Ripperger, T.J.; Jergović, M.; et al. Immune responses to two and three doses of the BNT162b2 mRNA vaccine in adults with solid tumors. *Nat. Med.* **2021**, *27*, 2002–2011. [CrossRef] [PubMed]
85. Kamar, N.; Abravanel, F.; Marion, O.; Couat, C.; Izopet, J.; Del Bello, A. Three doses of an mRNA COVID-19 vaccine in solid-organ transplant recipients. *N. Engl. J. Med.* **2021**, *385*, 661–662. [CrossRef]
86. Food and Drug Administration. Coronavirus (COVID-19) Update: FDA Authorizes New Long-Acting Monoclonal Antibodies for Pre-exposure Prevention of COVID-19 in Certain Individuals. 2021. Available online: https://www.fda.gov/news-events/press-announcements/coronavirus-covid-19-update-fda-authorizes-new-long-acting-monoclonal-antibodies-pre-exposure (accessed on 4 March 2022).
87. O'Brien, M.P.; Forleo-Neto, E.; Musser, B.J.; Isa, F.; Chan, K.C.; Sarkar, N.; Bar, K.J.; Barnabas, R.V.; Barouch, D.H.; Cohen, M.S.; et al. Subcutaneous REGEN-COV Antibody Combination to Prevent COVID-19. *N. Engl. J. Med.* **2021**, *385*, 1184–1195. [CrossRef]
88. Chen, R.E.; Zhang, X.; Case, J.B.; Winkler, E.S.; Liu, Y.; VanBlargan, L.A.; Liu, J.; Errico, J.M.; Xie, X.; Suryadevara, N.; et al. Resistance of SARS-CoV-2 variants to neutralization by monoclonal and serum-derived polyclonal antibodies. *Nat. Med.* **2021**, *27*, 717–726. [CrossRef]
89. Richman, D.D. COVID-19 vaccines: Implementation, limitations, and opportunities. *Glob. Health Med.* **2021**, *3*, 1–5. [CrossRef]
90. Nomura, Y.; Sawahata, M.; Nakamura, Y.; Kurihara, M.; Koike, R.; Katsube, O.; Hagiwara, K.; Niho, S.; Masuda, N.; Tanaka, T.; et al. Age and Smoking Predict Antibody Titres at 3 Months after the Second Dose of the BNT162b2 COVID-19 Vaccine. *Vaccines* **2021**, *9*, 1042. [CrossRef] [PubMed]
91. De Gier, B.; de Oliveira Bressane Lima, P.; van Gaalen, R.D.; de Boer, P.T.; Alblas, J.; Ruijten, M.; van Gageldonk-Lafeber, A.B.; Waegemaekers, T.; Schreijer, A.; van den Hof, S.; et al. Occupation- and age-associated risk of SARS-CoV-2 test positivity, the Netherlands, June to October 2020. *Eurosurveillance* **2020**, *25*, 2001884. [CrossRef] [PubMed]
92. World Health Organization. Prevention, Identification, and Management of Health Worker Infection in the Context of COVID-19. 2020. Available online: https://www.who.int/publications/i/item/10665-336265 (accessed on 4 March 2022).
93. Chou, R.; Dana, T.; Buckley, D.I.; Selph, S.; Fu, R.; Totten, A.M. Epidemiology of and Risk Factors for Coronavirus Infection in Health Care Workers: A Living Rapid Review. *Ann. Intern. Med.* **2020**, *173*, 120. [CrossRef] [PubMed]
94. Goldberg, L.; Levinsky, Y.; Marcus, N.; Hoffer, V.; Gafner, M.; Hadas, S.; Kraus, S.; Mor, M.; Scheuerman, O. SARS-CoV-2 Infection among Health Care Workers Despite the Use of Surgical Masks and Physical Distancing-the Role of Airborne Transmission. *Open Forum Infect. Dis.* **2021**, *8*, ofab036. [CrossRef]
95. Teran, R.A.; Walblay, K.A.; Shane, E.L.; Xydis, S.; Gretsch, S.; Gagner, A.; Samala, U.; Choi, H.; Zelinski, C.; Black, S.R.; et al. Postvaccination SARS-CoV-2 infections among skilled nursing facility residents and staff members—Chicago, Illinois, December 2020–March 2021. *Am. J. Transplant.* **2021**, *21*, 2290–2297. [CrossRef]
96. Nordström, P.; Ballin, M.; Nordström, A. Effectiveness of heterologous ChAdOx1 nCoV-19 and mRNA prime-boost vaccination against symptomatic COVID-19 infection in Sweden: A nationwide cohort study. *Lancet Reg. Health Eur.* **2021**, *11*, 100249. [CrossRef]

97. Gram, M.A.; Nielsen, J.; Schelde, A.B.; Nielsen, K.F.; Moustsen-Helms, I.R.; Sørensen, A.K.B.; Valentiner-Branth, P.; Emborg, H.D. Vaccine effectiveness against SARS-CoV-2 infection, hospitalization, and death when combining a first dose ChAdOx1 vaccine with a subsequent mRNA vaccine in Denmark: A nationwide population-based cohort study. *PLoS Med.* **2021**, *18*, e1003874. [CrossRef]
98. Bignardi, E.; Brogna, C.; Capasso, C.; Brogna, B. A fatal case of COVID-19 breakthrough infection due to the delta variant. *Clin. Case Rep.* **2022**, *10*, e05232. [CrossRef]

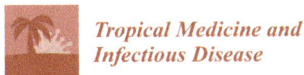

Systematic Review

Global and Regional Prevalence and Outcomes of COVID-19 in People Living with HIV: A Systematic Review and Meta-Analysis

Tope Oyelade [1,*], Jaber S. Alqahtani [2], Ahmed M. Hjazi [3], Amy Li [4], Ami Kamila [5] and Reynie Purnama Raya [5,6]

1. Institute for Liver and Digestive Health, Division of Medicine, University College London, London NW3 2PF, UK
2. Department of Respiratory Care, Prince Sultan Military College of Health Sciences, Dammam 34313, Saudi Arabia; jaber.alqahtani.18@alumni.ucl.ac.uk
3. Centre for Haematology, Department of Inflammatory and Inflammation, College of Medicine, Imperial College London, London W12 0NN, UK; a.hjazi18@imperial.ac.uk
4. Division of Surgery and Interventional Science, University College London, London NW3 2PS, UK; yutong.a.li@ucl.ac.uk
5. Faculty of Science, Universitas 'Aisyiyah Bandung, Bandung 40264, Indonesia; amikamila.unisabdg@gmail.com (A.K.); reynie.raya.18@ucl.ac.uk (R.P.R.)
6. Institute for Global Health, Faculty of Population Health Sciences, University College London, London NW3 2PF, UK
* Correspondence: t.oyelade@ucl.ac.uk; Tel.: +44(0)-20-7679-5203

Abstract: Background: The relationship between HIV (human immunodeficiency virus) and COVID-19 clinical outcome is uncertain, with conflicting data and hypotheses. We aimed to assess the prevalence of people living with HIV (PLWH) among COVID-19 cases and whether HIV infection affects the risk of severe COVID-19 or related death at the global and continental level. Methods: Electronic databases were systematically searched in July 2021. In total, 966 studies were screened following the Preferred Reporting Items for Systematic Reviews and Meta-Analyses guidelines. Narratives were synthesised and data pooled for the global and continental prevalence of HIV–SARS-CoV-2 coinfection. The relative risks of severity and mortality in HIV-infected COVID-19 patients were computed using a random-effect model. Risk of bias was assessed using the Newcastle–Ottawa score and Egger's test, and presented as funnel plots. Results: In total, 43 studies were included involving 692,032 COVID-19 cases, of whom 9097 (1.3%) were PLWH. The global prevalence of PLWH among COVID-19 cases was 2% (95% CI = 1.7–2.3%), with the highest prevalence observed in sub-Saharan Africa. The relative risk (RR) of severe COVID-19 in PLWH was significant only in Africa (RR = 1.14, 95% CI = 1.05–1.24), while the relative risk of mortality was 1.5 (95% CI = 1.45–2.03) globally. The calculated global risk showed that HIV infection may be linked with increased COVID-19 death. The between-study heterogeneity was significantly high, while the risk of publication bias was not significant. Conclusions: Although there is a low prevalence of PLWH among COVID-19 cases, HIV infection may increase the severity of COVID-19 in Africa and increase the risk of death globally.

Keywords: COVID-19; HIV; public health; pandemic; infectious disease

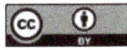

1. Introduction

The 2019 coronavirus (COVID-19) pandemic caused by SARS-CoV-2 remains a global public health challenge that has affected over 186 million people and caused over 4 million deaths globally [1]. While most cases of COVID-19 are clinically mild or asymptomatic, older age and certain underlying illness, such as cardiovascular, respiratory, and digestive diseases, have been reported to increase the risk of severe COVID-19 cases or death [2–4]. Such comorbidities are associated with an increased fatality rate and present a challenge for intensive care management of COVID-19 patients [5,6].

Human immunodeficiency virus (HIV) belongs to a genus of zoonotic lentiviruses that causes acute immune deficiency syndrome (AIDS) [7]. Data from the Joint United Nations Programme on HIV/AIDS (UNAIDS) puts the number of people living with HIV (PLWH) at 38 million globally, with 1.5 million new infections in 2020 and about 6 million people unaware of their HIV infection status [8]. Accordingly, the number of PLWH is projected to increase due to treatment availability and the associated reduction in AIDS-related deaths [9].

HIV is associated with dysregulation of the immune system, which predisposes patients to opportunistic infectious diseases [10]. Indeed, most HIV-related deaths have been linked to secondary infections and abnormal inflammatory response resulting from AIDS [11]. This is especially so in patients with uncontrolled HIV replication, a high viral load and a low CD4/CD8 count. Giving the immune-compromised state of most PLWH and the increased possibility of secondary dysfunctions, an increased risk of infection, severity and death due to COVID-19 may be expected. However, an attenuated immune response may also protect against the cytokine release storm and the corresponding acute respiratory distress syndrome (ARDS) linked with severe SARS-CoV-2 infection or the associated mortality [12]. Indeed, various ARTs (antiretroviral therapies) used for HIV treatment were also proposed as candidates for the treatment of SARS-CoV-2 infection in the early stage of the COVID-19 pandemic, and there have been initial hypotheses that HIV patients undergoing ART or pre-exposure prophylaxis (PrEP) may have collateral immunity to COVID-19. However, most findings showed no significant positive effect of ART on COVID-19 infection or outcomes compared with standard care [13–15]. Further, a study by Ayerdi et al. assessing whether ART or PrEP usage had a preventative effect on the seroprevalence and clinical course of COVID-19 among men who have sex with men and transgender women found no significant positive effect [16].

To understand the relationship between COVID-19 and HIV infection, previous systematic reviews and meta-analysis have been published, including the studies by Mellor et al. and Hariyanto et al., which both found increased risks of severe COVID-19 and mortality in PLWH compared with HIV-negative COVID-19 cases [17,18]. Moreover, a systematic review by Ssentongo et al., involving 22 reports from Africa, Asia, Europe and North America, showed an increased risk of mortality from COVID-19 in PLWH [19]. On the contrary, the study by Gao et al., reported no significant increase in the risk of severe COVID-19 or related death due to HIV infection [20]. This was corroborated by the study by Lee et al. involving 643,018 PLWH, which reported no significant increase in the risk of adverse outcomes of COVID-19 in PLWH [21]. Hence, the association between HIV infection and COVID-19 outcomes remain unclear, with sparse and conflicting reports.

Aside from the heterogeneity from the established difference in the epidemiology of HIV between countries and continents, variability also exists in the treatment and management of HIV infection, as well as the behaviour of PLWH in various regions of the world. These, amongst other factors, determine the rate of spread, as well as the availability and uptake of preventative and treatment measures for HIV [22]. The disruption to clinical care of various chronic diseases due to the diversion of medical resources to manage the increasing COVID-19 cases around the world at the peak of the COVID-19 pandemic further contributes to the increased global variability in the clinical course of COVID-19 in PLWH [23]. This review aimed to provide an updated insight into the global and continental prevalence of PLWH among COVID-19 cases and the potential risk of severe COVID-19 and death associated with HIV infection by conducting a meta-analysis of HIV-positive and HIV-negative COVID-19 patients grouped by continents.

2. Methods

The protocol of this systematic review was registered prospectively to PROSPERO (CRD42021264151). Following the Preferred Reporting in Systematic Reviews and Meta-Analyses (PRISMA) guidelines [24], the Medline and Embase databases were searched on 2 July 2021 using keywords and MeSH terms (Figure S1). Further, a search of preprint databases (www.medrxiv.org and www.preprint.org, accessed on 2 July 2021) was also performed on the 2nd of July 2021 because of the rapidly developing nature of the topic. The search of preprint databases did not follow a systemic search strategy because concatenation was not feasible. However, the MeSH terms for HIV and COVID-19 as described in the supplemental figure (Figure S1) were combined consecutively and the resulting studies' titles were screened. Studies retrieved from the databases were imported into EndNote software, and duplicate records were removed. The resulting duplicate-free studies were then uploaded to Rayyan software, and title, abstract and whole-text screening was carried out (RPR, AK). Reference screening of the included studies and relevant peer-reviewed previously published reports was also performed to retrieve studies that were not covered by the search strategy. The reference search did not include any search strategy and involved identifying references that were cited within published studies that that were published on the topic.

2.1. Inclusion and Exclusion Criteria

The inclusion/exclusion of studies followed the PECO (Population, Exposure, Comparison and Outcome) model [25]. We included only studies that presented the clinical characteristics and/or composite endpoints of COVID-19 patients and reported the proportion of these patients with a pre-existing HIV infection. Studies that included both hospitalized and community-based COVID-19 patients were also included to understand the overall prevalence of HIV infection as a comorbidity in COVID-19 cases, irrespective of the hospitalization status. However, only studies with clinically confirmed outcomes of COVID-19 cases were included in the meta-analysis for the risk of severity and mortality associated with HIV comorbidity. Studies that combined HIV and other immunosuppressive diseases and conditions (cancer, congenital, or medically induced), non-English language publications, reviews, case reports, qualitative studies, editorials, and studies including only patients that died from COVID-19 were excluded. Studies that also focused on only HIV patients coinfected with SARS-CoV-2 were included in the systematic review but not in the meta-analysis. This is because most of these studies focused only on HIV patient recruitment and did not provide a comparative analysis of risk in patients without HIV. Moreover, studies focused on HIV patients alone may introduce bias in recruitment, which may target PLWH more. For studies in which suspected and confirmed COVID-19 cases were reported [26], we only synthesised the number of confirmed cases. In addition, studies including the same (duplicate) population of patients were identified and included in the systematic review [27,28]. However, only the latest study was included in the meta-analysis [27].

2.2. Data Collection

Two authors (RPR, AK) independently screened the titles and abstracts of potentially eligible studies, and conflicts were resolved through mediation by a third reviewer (TO). The full text of potential studies that were included from the abstract screening stage were fully read and assessed against the inclusion/exclusion criteria.

2.3. Data Extraction and Analysis

The authors and year of publication, the study design and period, the country of study, the sample size of COVID-19 cases and the proportion that had HIV as a comorbidity, as well as the clinical outcomes of both groups (PLWH and non-HIV COVID-19 patients) were extracted into a table. Clinical outcomes identified were the severity of the COVID-19 and death linked to infection with the SARS-CoV-2 virus. Severe COVID-19 was defined as a prolonged hospital stay, ICU admission and/or need for mechanical ventilation (MV) as a result of reduced oxygen saturation (<90% of room air), and a respiratory rate of >30 breaths/minute and signs of severe respiratory distress according to the WHO recommendations [29]. Analysis was performed using Stata/MP 17; prevalence was calculated by the "metaprop" procedure using the random effect model. Forest plots were used to present the pooled prevalence of PLWH in COVID-19 cases grouped by the continent of study. Continent-grouped effect sizes (95% confidence intervals, CIs) and the test results of between-study heterogeneity (I^2 statistic, p-value) were also computed using the random effect model. The "metan" procedure was used to assess the risk of severity and mortality in PLWH-COVID-19 patients compared with the general population in the included studies, and the risk ratios were grouped by continents to further assess the intercontinental variation in these risks. All meta-analysis was performed using the random effect model, which is more robust to the between-study heterogeneity expected in the pooled studies, which were performed in different regions of the world with different health, socio-economic and research standards.

2.4. Quality Assessment

A modified version of the Newcastle–Ottawa Score (NOS) was used to assess the risk of bias in the included studies [21]. This includes 3 domains and 9 questions scored accordingly with a star. The "selection" domain assessed the randomness and multicentre involvement in the selection of the study population, as well as the sample size. The multicentre recruitment of patients was scored because this design provides better quality data and more generalizable results because more centres better represent the study population than a single centre [30]. A sample size of ≥ 100 was decided on the basis of previous studies' estimates of ~1% prevalence of HIV infection in COVID-19 cases [21,31]. The standard ascertainment of COVID-19 and HIV were also assessed against the WHO guidelines [32,33]. Finally, the follow-up time (≥ 2 weeks), mode of outcome confirmation and whether all patients were accounted for were also assessed (Table S1). Studies with ≥ 5 stars (>50%) were considered unbiased. To further assess publication bias in the studies pooled for prevalence and the risk of severity and mortality in COVID-19-infected PLWH, funnel plots and the Egger test were computed using the "metafunnel" and "metabias" procedures respectively in STATA. Statistical significance was set at 95% ($p < 0.05$).

We also performed a "leave-one-out" sensitivity analysis using the "meta forestplot, leaveoneout" procedure in STATA to assess whether any of the studies included in the computation of the prevalence and risk ratios were producing misleading and exaggerated effect sizes. The procedure usually performs multiple computations by consecutive removal of one study at each analysis and presenting the effect sizes generated in a forest plot.

3. Results

The systematic search of databases including preprints and the reference search generated an initial total of 955 studies, including 245 duplicates, to give a total of 710 studies. Initial title and abstract screening led to the exclusion of 664 studies, followed by full-text review of the 46 potentially eligible studies. Full-text screening resulted in further exclusion of 14 studies, while screening of the references of relevant studies resulted in 11 eligible studies to give a total of 43 studies which satisfied the inclusion/exclusion criteria (Figure 1).

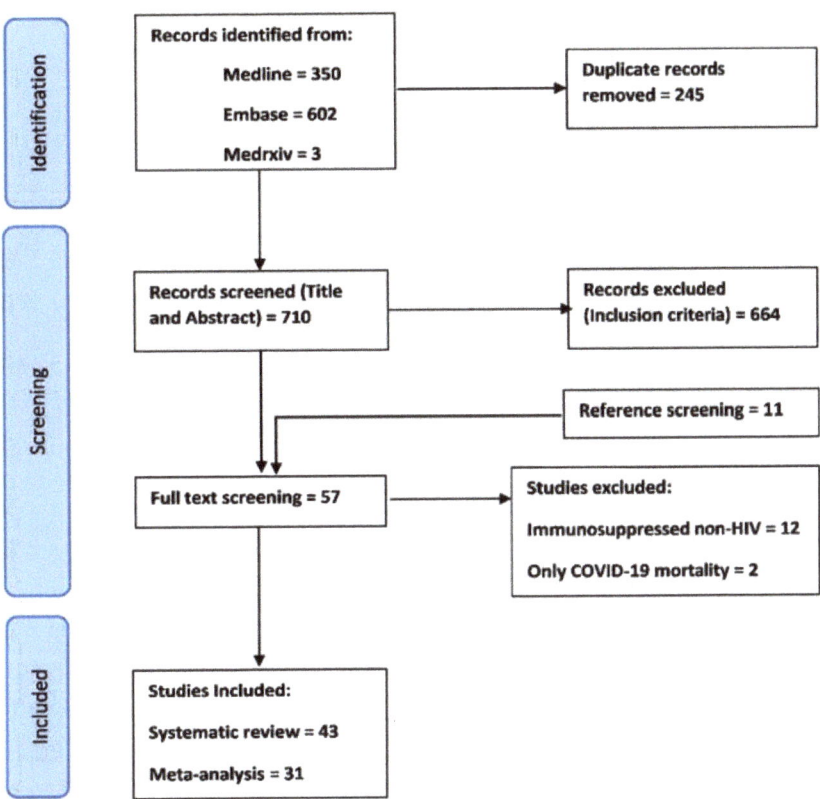

Figure 1. Global and regional prevalence and outcomes of COVID-19 in people living with HIV: A systematic review and meta-analysis according to the Preferred Reporting for Systematic Reviews and Meta-analyses diagram.

3.1. General Description of the Studies Included

The 43 studies in the systematic review included 692,032 COVID-19 cases, of which 9097 (1.3%) were PLWH. The sample sizes of the included studies ranged from 20 to 378,248, with data from 15 countries across five continents. Overall, 27 of the studies were retrospectively performed, with 11 prospective studies, 2 descriptive studies and 3 case series (Table 1). Of the included studies, 10 assessed only PLWH coinfected with SARS-CoV-2 and were excluded from further analysis. Another study was excluded because it involved selective matching of PLWH and non-HIV COVID-19 cases [34], and one study [28] that was conducted on the same cohort of patients was excluded in favour of the more recently published one [27]. The risk of bias assessment showed low bias in the included studies, with 86% (37/43) of the studies below the bias threshold (Table S1).

Table 1. General characteristics of included studies.

Study Name (Year)	Country	Type of Study	Study Participants	Sample Size (M; F; T)	Age (Mean ± SD or Median, Range)	PLWH	PLWH Surviving	PLWH Non-Surviving	PLWH Severe	PLWH Non-Severe
Borobia et al. (2020) [35]	Spain	Retrospective	COVID-19 cases	2226 (M = 1074; F = 1152)	61 (IQR 46–78)	13	9	4	NR	NR
Boulle et al. (2020) [36]	South Africa	Retrospective	COVID-19 cases	22,308 (NR)	(NR)	3978	3863	115	601	3262
Ceballos et al. (2021) [37]	Chile	Prospective	COVID-19 cases	18,321 (M = 10300; F = 8021)	NR	36	31	5	11	25
Collins et al. (2020) [38]	USA	Case series	COVID-19 cases	530 (NR)	NR	20	17	3	3	17
Del Amo et al. (2020) [39]	Spain	Prospective	HIV-SARS-CoV-2 coinfected cases	236 (M = 204; F = 32; all PLWH)	NR	236	216	20	15	221
Di Biagio et al. (2020) [40]	Italy	Prospective	HIV-SARS-CoV-2 coinfected cases	69 (NR; all PLWH)	NR	69	62	7	4	58
Docherty et al. (2020) [28]	UK	Prospective	COVID-19 cases	20,133 (M = 12,068; F = 8065)	73 (IQR 58–62)	83	37	23	NR	NR
Erinoso et al. (2020) [41]	Nigeria	Retrospective	COVID-19 cases	632 (M = 385; F = 247)	40.1 (SD = 13.9)	3	NR	NR	NR	NR
Etienne et al. (2020) [42]	France	Prospective	HIV-SARS-CoV-2 coinfected cases	54 (M = 33; F = 21; all PLWH)	54 (range 47–60)	54	53	1	19	35
Geretti et al. (2020) [27]	UK	Prospective	COVID-19 cases	47,592 (NR)	NR	122	75	30	NR	NR
Gervasoni et al. (2020) [43]	Italy	Retrospective	COVID-19 cases	549 (NR)	51 ± 11	47	45	2	2	34
Getenen et al. (2021) [44]	Ethiopia	Retrospective	COVID-19 cases	372 (M = 279; F = 93)	30 (5–85)	6	5	1	1	5
Gudipati et al. (2020) [45]	USA	Case series	COVID-19 cases	7372 (NR)	NR	14	11	3	2	12
Hadi et al. (2020) [46]	USA	Retrospective	COVID-19 cases	50,167 (NR)	NR	404	384	20	78	326
Harter et al. (2020) [47]	Germany	Retrospective	HIV-SARS-CoV-2 coinfected cases	33 (M = 30; F = 3)	48 (range 26–82)	33	29	3	8	25
Ho et al. (2021) [48]	USA	Retrospective	HIV-SARS-CoV-2 coinfected cases	93 (M = 67; F = 23, T = 3; all PLWH)	58 (range 52–65)	93	74	19	19	74
Huang et al. (2020) [49]	China	Retrospective	COVID-19 cases	50368 (NR)	NR	35	33	2	15	20
Inciarte et al. (2020) [50]	Spain	Prospective	HIV-SARS-CoV-2 coinfected cases	53 (NR)	NR	53	51	2	10	43
Isernia et al. (2020) [51]	France	Case series	COVID-19 cases	390 (NR)	NR	30	24	2	4	24
Izquierdo et al. (2020) [52]	Spain	Retrospective	COVID-19 cases	10504 (M = 5519; F = 4984)	58.2 ± 19.7	34	NR	NR	1	33
Karim et al. (2020) [53]	South Africa	Retrospective	COVID-19 cases	124 (M = 30; F = 94)	45 (IQR, 35.0–57.4)	55	NR	NR	16	39
Kirenga et al. (2020) [54]	Uganda	Prospective	HIV-SARS-CoV-2 coinfected cases	56 (M = 38; F = 18)	34.2 ± 15.5	4	4	0	NR	NR
Liu et al. (2020) [55]	China	Retrospective	HIV-SARS-CoV-2 coinfected cases	20 (M = 5; F = 15)	46.5 (IQR, 39.3–50.5)	20	19	1	3	17
Maggiolo et al. (2021) [56]	Italy	Prospective	HIV-SARS-CoV-2 coinfected cases	55 (M = 44; F = 11)	54 (49–58)	55	51	4	11	44
Migisha et al. (2020) [57]	Uganda	Retrospective	COVID-19 cases	54 (M = 34; F = 20)	NR	2	2	0	0	2
Miyashita and Kuno (2021) [58]	USA	Retrospective	COVID-19 cases	8912 (NR)	NR	161	138	23	36	125
Nachega et al. (2020) [59]	Congo	Retrospective	COVID-19 cases	766 (M = 500; F = 262; unknown = 4)	34 ± 4.5	12	10	2	3	9
Ombajo et al. (2020) [60]	Kenya	Retrospective	COVID-19 cases	787 (M = 505; F = 282)	43 (range 0–109)	53	42	11	NR	NR

Table 1. Cont.

Study Name (Year)	Country	Type of Study	Study Participants	Sample Size (M; F; T)	Age (Mean ± SD or Median, Range)	PLWH	PLWH Surviving	PLWH Non-Surviving	PLWH Severe	PLWH Non-Severe
Parker et al. (2020) [61]	South Africa	Retrospective	COVID-19 cases	113 (M = 44; F = 69)	NR	24	18	6	5	19
Pujari et al. (2021) [62]	India	Retrospective	HIV-SARS-CoV-2 coinfected cases	86 (M = 66; F = 20)	45 ± 52.3	86	80	6	17	69
Rodriguez-Gonzalez et al. (2021) [63]	Spain	Retrospective	COVID-19 cases	1255 (M = 725; F = 530)	65 (range 51–77)	12	9	3	1	11
Rodriguez-Molinero et al. (2020) [64]	Spain	Prospective	COVID-19 cases	418 (M = 238; F = 180)	65.4 ± 16.6	3	2	1	3	0
Shalev et al. (2020) [65]	USA	Retrospective	COVID-19 cases	2159 (NR)	NR	31	23	8	2	29
Shi et al. (2020) [66]	China	Retrospective	COVID-19 cases	134 (M = 65; F = 69)	46 (IQR: 34–58)	1	1	0	0	1
Sigel et al. (2020) [67]	USA	Retrospective	COVID-19 cases	4402 (NR)	NR	88	70	18	18	70
Silver et al. (2020) [60]	USA	Retrospective	COVID-19 cases	249 (M = 110; F = 139)	59.6	6	NR	NR	NR	NR
Stoeckle et al. (2020) [34]	USA	Retrospective (case-control)	COVID-19 cases	120 (M = 96; F = 24)	60.5 (range 56.6–70.0)	30	24	2	4	NR
Tesoriero et al. (2021) [68]	USA	Descriptive	COVID-19 cases	378248 (M = 192,646; F = 183,319)	NR	2988	689	207	896	2092
Virata et al. (2020) [69]	USA	Retrospective	HIV-SARS-CoV-2 coinfected cases	40 (M = 20; F = 20)	NR	40	40	0	4	36
Vizcarra et al. (2020) [26]	Spain	Prospective	COVID-19 cases	61,577 (NR)	NR	51	44	2	6	45
Wang et al. (2020) [70]	China	Descriptive	COVID-19 cases	125 (M = 71; F = 54)	38.76 ± 13.799	1	1	0	NR	NR
Yang et al. (2021) [71]	China	Retrospective	COVID-19 cases	188	NR	3	NR	NR	NR	NR
Yu et al. (2020) [72]	China	Retrospective	COVID-19 cases	142 (M = 81; F = 61)	61.9 ± 12.4	8	NR	NR	NR	NR

M, male; F, female; T, transgender man/woman; SD, standard deviation; IQR, interquartile range; PLWH, people living with HIV; NR, not reported.

3.2. Prevalence of PLWH among COVID-19 Cases

Of the 43 studies included, 10 studied COVID-19 infections in only PLWH, while one study (68) was designed as a case–control study and was excluded from the meta-analysis [39,40,42,47,48,50,55,56,62,69]. Two studies were identified as duplicate data [27,28] and only the most recent version [27] was included. Nine of the studies analysed for prevalence were conducted in Africa, with eight each conducted in Europe and North America. The global pooled prevalence of PLWH among COVID-19 cases was 2% (95% CI = 1.7–2.3%, $p < 0.001$) while at the continental level, the pooled prevalence for Europe and North America was 0.5% and 1.2%, respectively. Moreover, 75% (6/8) of the studies from the USA included in the meta-analysis were conducted in the states (New York and Georgia) with the highest HIV infection rates, according to recent data [73], which may explain the higher prevalence in North America compared with Europe. The pooled prevalence of studies from Africa was expectedly the highest at 11% (95% CI, 4–18%), while that of continental Asia was 1% (95% CI, −0.1–2%). The negative 95% CI in the pooled prevalence of PLWH in COVID-19 shown by studies from Asia may be associated with the random effect model used for intercontinental pooling of studies. However, the prevalence remained the same (1%) and there was no significant between-study heterogeneity when the analysis was performed for studies from Asia separately (Figure S5). Further, 67% (6/9) of the studies from Africa were from East and Southern Africa, the region with over half (55%) of the total global HIV infections according to the 2021 estimate [74]. The variation in the prevalence of HIV infection in this study is illustrative of the current global epidemiology of HIV, whereby more than two-thirds of PLWH are currently in Sub-Saharan Africa [75]. Moreover, the overall between-study heterogeneity was significantly high ($I^2 = 99.7\%$, $p < 0.001$; Figure 2a) and this was expected, due to the variation in global distribution of PLWH. Publication bias in the pooled studies was further assessed by computing a funnel plot and Egger's test, which was significant (T (95% CI) = 2.17 (0.39–12.18), $p = 0.04$; Figure 2b). The sensitivity test showed that there was no significant reduction in heterogeneity following successive omission of studies, as the global pooled prevalence still ranged between 3% and 4% (Figure S2).

3.3. Severity of COVID-19 in PLWH

Thirteen studies presented data on the severity of COVID-19 in PLWH and non-HIV patients, and were analysed to determine the risk of severity in PLWH compared with non-HIV COVID-19 patients [36,37,44,46,53,58,59,61,63,64,66–68]. These studies included a total of 485,540 COVID-19 cases, of whom 7768 (1.6%) were PLWH. Overall, five, four and two of the pooled studies were conducted in Africa, the USA and Europe, respectively. The pooled global risk ratio was not significant and showed that PLWH may not be at risk of developing severe COVID-19 (RR (95% CI) = 1.21 (0.99–1.48); $p = 0.477$; Figure 3a). However, this result was very close to significance, and including more data in the future may provide further insight into the relationship between HIV infection and the severity of COVID-19. Indeed, this lack of significance was true for both Europe and USA, regions associated with better prevention and management of HIV infections. However, the risk for severe COVID-19 among PLWH from Africa was found to increase by 14% (RR (95% CI) = 1.14 (1.05–1.24) compared with non-HIV COVID-19 patients. Moreover, while the overall heterogeneity was significantly high (85%, $p < 0.001$), there was no between-study variation in the studies from Africa ($I^2 = 0\%$, $p = 0.43$). Indeed, the funnel plot showed no publication bias and the Egger's test showed no small study effect (T (95% CI) = −1.32 (−3.02 to 0.75), $p = 0.21$; Figure 3b). The sensitivity test showed that leaving out some studies produced a significant result (Figure S3). However, doing so did not significantly improve the between-study heterogeneity of the results.

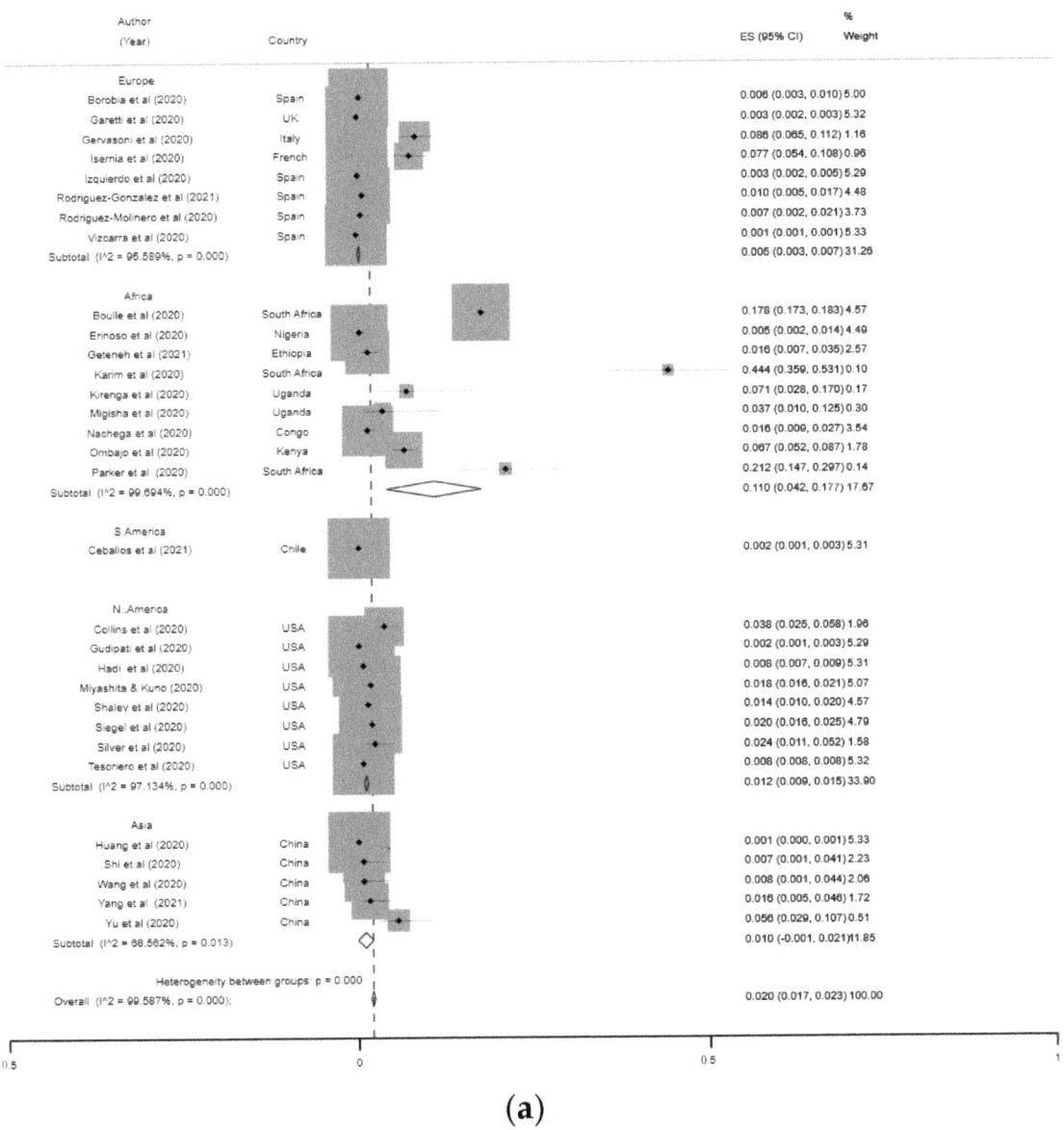

Figure 2. Cont.

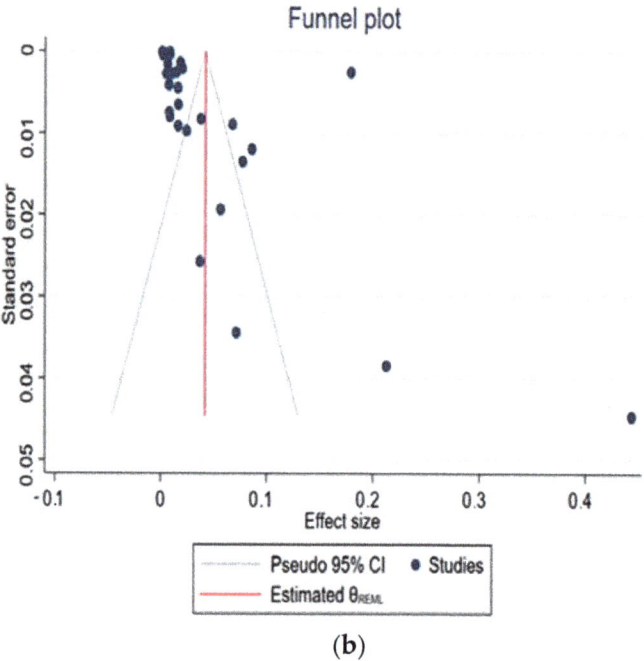

(b)

Figure 2. (**a**) Pooled prevalence of PLWH among COVID-19 cases. The red dotted line represents the overall effect size. The lateral edges of the blue diamonds represent the limits of the 95% confidence intervals (ES: effect size; CI: confidence interval). (**b**) Funnel plot of studies pooled for the prevalence of PLWH among COVID-19 cases (ES: effect size; se: standard error).

3.4. Mortality of PLWH Coinfected with SARS-CoV-2

In total, 17 studies were included in the assessment of the risk of mortality from COVID-19 in PLWH compared with non-HIV COVID-19 patients [27,35–37,43,44,46,49,58–61,63–65,67,68]. The 17 studies had 588,960 COVID-19 cases, including 8013 (1.4%) PLWH. Five each of the analysed studies were conducted in Africa, Europe, and North America. The meta-analysis results showed that HIV infection increased the risk of death from COVID-19 by 2.3-fold globally (RR (95% CI): 2.29 (1.51–3.46); Figure 4a) compared with COVID-19 patients without HIV. On the regional level, there was no significantly increased risk of COVID-19 mortality in PLWH in Africa or Europe. However, a twofold increase in risk of mortality was observed in the USA according to the studies included. Despite this difference in regional risk ratios, the computed funnel plot showed no publication bias (Figure 4b), and Egger's test showed no small study effect in the included studies (T (95% CI) = 1.22 (−1.13 to 4.17)). The sensitivity test showed that the significance was not influenced by the removal of any of the included studies (Figure S4).

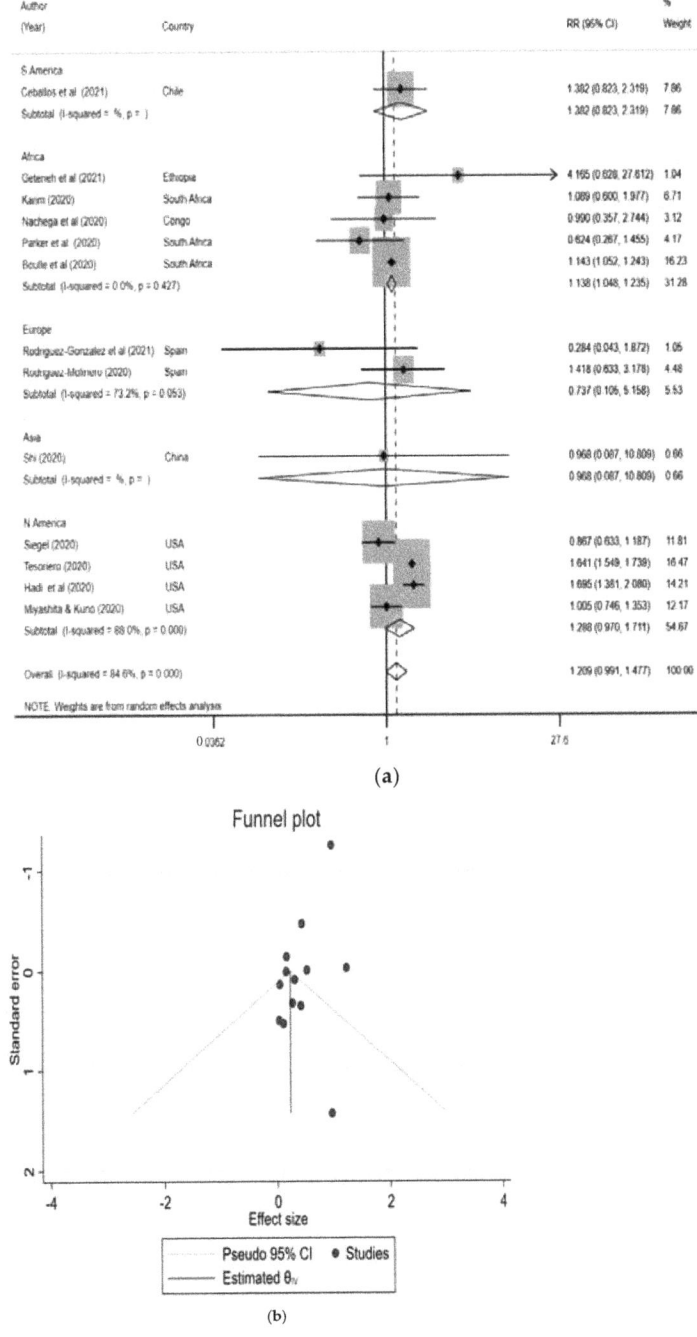

Figure 3. (a) Forest plot of studies pooled for the risk of severe COVID-19 in PLWH. The red dotted line represents the overall effect size/risk ratio. The lateral edges of the blue diamonds represent the limits of the 95% confidence intervals (RR: risk ratio; CI: confidence interval). (b) Funnel plot of studies pooled for the risk of severe COVID-19 in PLWH (CI: confidence interval).

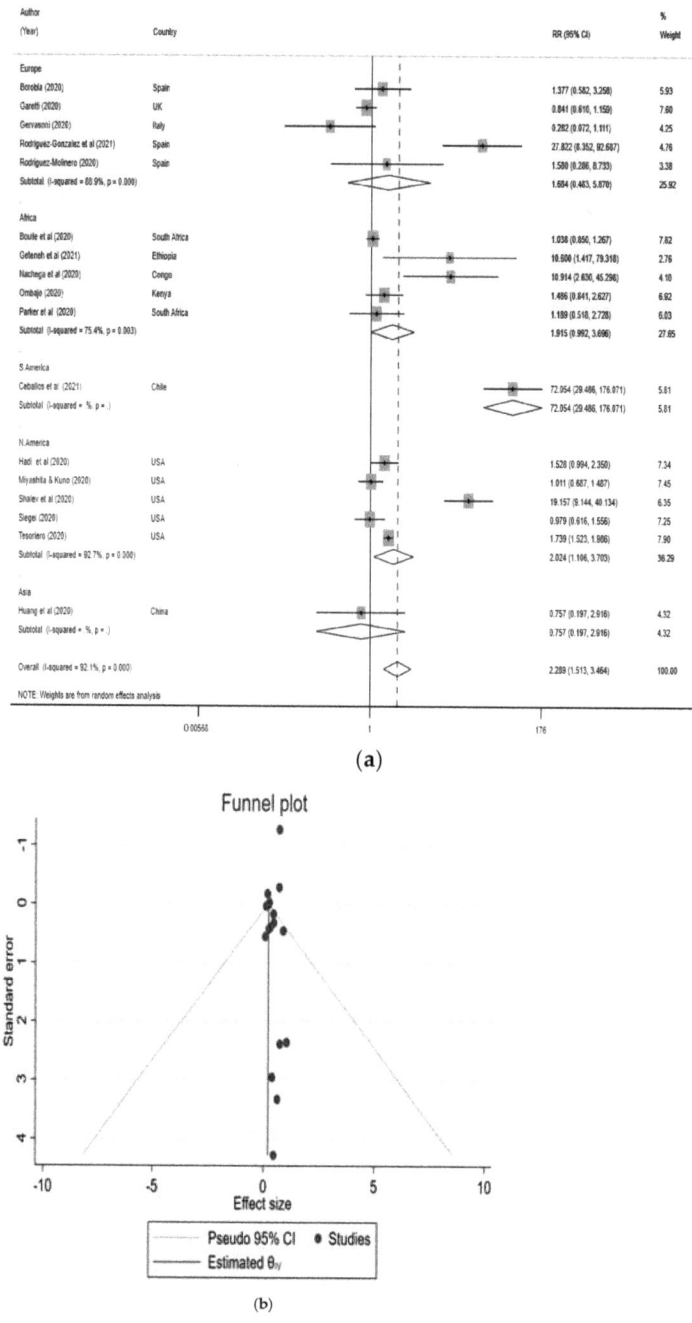

Figure 4. (**a**) Forest plot for COVID-19 mortality in PLWH. The red dotted line represents the overall effect size/risk ratio. The lateral edges of the blue diamonds represent the limits of the 95% confidence intervals (RR: risk ratio; CI: confidence interval). (**b**) Funnel plot of studies pooled for COVID-19 mortality in PLWH (CI: confidence interval).

4. Discussion

This study provides an updated systematic assessment of the prevalence and clinical outcomes of COVID-19 in PLWH compared with the general population. The results were stratified to present the prevalence of PLWH among COVID-19 cases as well as the clinical outcomes at both the global and regional level. To the best of our knowledge, this is the first systematic review and meta-analysis dedicated solely to understanding the clinical outcome of SARS-CoV-2-infected patients who had HIV infection on both the global and continental levels. Our method of analysis considered the regional variation in the prevalence, prevention and management of HIV infection in the included continents. We found a significantly lower global prevalence of PLWH in COVID-19 cases (2%) compared with other comorbidities such as cardiovascular disease and obesity. This is consistent with previous reports which estimated the prevalence of HIV coinfection at 1–2% of COVID-19 patients either admitted to the hospital or in the general population [19,76]. Furthermore, while the proportion was below 2% in Europe, North America and Asia, the prevalence of PLWH in COVID-19 cases was found to be relatively high in Africa (11%). This is reflective of the global epidemiology of HIV, whereby more than half of the global cases are located within continental Africa. Interestingly, 75% of the studies from Africa were performed in the East and Southern Africa region, which accounts for over 54% of the global HIV cases [74]. Our finding is consistent with earlier systematic reviews, which showed a similar prevalence of HIV–SARS-CoV-2 coinfection cases [19,21].

Our result also showed that PLWH may not be at a relatively higher risk of severe COVID-19, defined by admission to intensive care units or the need for mechanical ventilation, at the global level. Interestingly, this lack of an association between HIV infection and COVID-19 severity held true in Europe and the United States, but not in Africa. We found a 15% increase in the risk of severe COVID-19 for PLWH in Africa. Moreover, 60% (3/5) of the studies analysed for the risk of severe COVID-19 in Africa were conducted in South Africa, and all studies originated from sub-Saharan Africa, a region associated with a high HIV infection rate and poorer antiretroviral treatment (ART) availability [74]. Furthermore, we found a twofold increase in the relative risk of death from COVID-19 in PLWH at the global level. However, only the North American (United States) continent showed a significant risk of mortality (twofold) among the regions computed. Moreover, most studies within the USA were conducted in Georgia and New York, both of which are among the top 10 states with the highest HIV infections and that were hardest hit by the COVID-19 pandemic [1,77].

Importantly, our findings corroborate some previous reports on the potential risk of a severe clinical course of COVID-19 in PLWH. Specifically, various meta-analyses were conducted on the difference in risk of severe COVID-19 between HIV-positive and HIV-negative patients with SARS-CoV-2 infection, whereby the risk of severe COVID-19 and mortality were found to be associated with HIV status [17,19]. However, other reports have been conflicting, with no difference in the risk of severe COVID-19 or death between HIV-positive and HIV-negative patients [19,21], with one report proposing a protective effect of HIV infection against COVID-19 [78]. Further, Liang et al. reported that HIV infection was not related to poorer COVID-19 outcomes, and concluded that any risk observed in HIV–SARS-CoV-2 coinfection may be related to the presence of concomitant comorbidities, which may be common in patients with undiagnosed or untreated HIV infection [31]. Lee et al. also reported no relationship between HIV infection and the clinical outcome of COVID-19 following a systematic review of 643,018 PLWH [21]. However, a systematic review by Mellor et al. involving a meta-analysis of five studies showed that PLWH had an increased risk of mortality due to COVID-19 compared with HIV-negative patients [18]. Further, a meta-analysis and meta-regression of PLWH in COVID-19 cases performed by Hariyanto et al. found that an increased risk of mortality was only significant in the studies from Africa and the United States after controlling for age, CD4 cell count or anti-retroviral treatment [16]. The results of this study support our findings regarding the significant increase in the risk of death due to COVID-19 in PLWH from the United States.

However, while the risk of mortality was not significant in Africa, our results were close to statistical significance (0.992–3.696; Figure 4a); more studies may improve this result in future analysis. Notably, most of the previous systematic reviews with or without a meta-analysis were carried out earlier in the COVID-19 pandemic period and included case reports with fewer studies included in the meta-analyses.

The observed increased risk of severe illness (Africa) and death (globally) from COVID-19 in these studies may be attributed to the interplay between several factors. Firstly, the availability of effective HIV management tools in developed countries means that PLWH now live longer in these regions [79]. Increased age is associated with senescence of the natural immune system, which may combine with other immune-dampening features of chronic, untreated HIV infection to increase the risk of severity and death from COVID-19. Moreover, PLWH, especially those with undiagnosed or uncontrolled infections, low CD4 count, opportunistic infections and a high viral load, may present with severe COVID-19 and are at higher risk of death [80]. Aside from CD4 and CD8 T-cell activation, effective and early immunoglobin G (IgG) generation results in effective SARS-CoV-2 clearance and improves clinical outcomes [81]. However, uncontrolled HIV replication may trigger increased CD8 T-cell activation, inflammation, T-cell exhaustion and dysfunction in B-cells' activities [82,83]. The combined breakdown of B- and T-cell functions resulting from natural immune system exhaustion may not only result in poorer COVID-19 outcomes but also compromise the efficacy of vaccines in PLWH. Indeed, the response to and efficacies of various vaccines, including hepatitis B, pneumococcal, influenza vaccines, have been shown to be diminished in PLWH, and repeated or modified vaccine administration has been recommended [84–86]. However, evidence on COVID-19 vaccine efficacy in PLWH is scarce, and vaccination of HIV-positive and -negative people remains similar. Effective ART can attenuate most of the immune dysregulation resulting from uncontrolled HIV infection and replication, and is highly recommended. However, undiagnosed HIV infection and low uptake of ART, both of which are prevalent in Africa, may predispose patients to poorer COVID-19 clinical outcomes [74].

Moreover, the prevention (sensitisation and pre-exposure prophylaxis), diagnosis and management (ART) of HIV and other chronic diseases have been affected by the global shift in medical resources to contain the COVID-19 pandemic [23]. This shift has been suggested to be a contributory factor to the susceptibility of affected groups to severe COVID-19 and death [87–89]. Expectedly, the disruption to healthcare systems, especially HIV clinics, and the downstream effect have been relatively worse in developing countries, possibly resulting in worse outcomes for PLWH coinfected with COVID-19 [90]. However, more data will be needed to establish the extent of these disruptions in regions already behind in the fight against HIV, and the contributory effects of other established confounders that may drive the clinical outcome of COVID-19 in patients with pre-existing HIV infection.

Put together, our result show that while the risk of severity illness and death due to COVID-19 increased respectively in Africa and globally, the mechanistic link between HIV infection and the clinical course of COVID-19 may be more complex than previously thought. Firstly, the regional aggregation performed in this study showed that the prevalence of PLWH in COVID-19 cases is best translated in the context of the current global epidemiology of HIV infections. Indeed, the variability introduced by the differences in regional HIV infection rates made estimation of the global prevalence of HIV–SARS-CoV-2 coinfection less reliable if not controlled for the regional prevalence of HIV. Secondly, there are complex, hardly resolvable confounders when assessing the relationship between HIV infection and COVID-19 outcomes, including age, sex, treatment with ART, race, region, immune state of the patient, number and types of comorbidities and the duration of comorbidities, among other factors, and we recommend further research to clarify this topic in the context of these and other confounders. Indeed, Bhaskaran et al. [91] controlled for age, sex, ethnicity, comorbidities, and time in a population of COVID-19 patients within the United Kingdom. However, the regional differences in prevalence, prevention techniques and clinical management of both HIV and COVID-19, as well as various social-economic factors, mean that their findings may not reflect the situation outside the United Kingdom.

This study has several limitations. Firstly, some of the included studies were case series reporting only PLWH coinfected with SARS-CoV-2. However, such studies were excluded from the prevalence analysis. Moreover, the random effect model was used to reduce the effect of variations in the experimental design on the computed results. Secondly, most studies did not report the distributions of comorbidities, race, age, CD4 and CD8 counts, duration of HIV infection or ART use, among other confounders, in the studied groups. Thus, we could not adjust for these parameters in this study. Moreover, some studies did not report the clinical outcomes (death and severity) of COVID-19 in both PLWH and patients who were HIV-negative, and these could not be included in the relative risk computation. However, Egger's test and the funnel plots showed that there was no publication bias in the analysed records, while the sensitivity analysis also showed no exaggeration of the result due to individual studies. In addition, overlapping data are generally a major limitation in systematic reviews and meta-analyses, which may also limit the interpretation of this study's results [92]. However, records found to be overlapping were excluded in favour of the most recent report. Finally, our database search was restricted to full-text studies alone. Thus, more relevant studies may be available and should be considered for future analyses of this topic.

Our findings have several clinical and research implications. First, it further widens the body of evidence by including more recent and high-quality studies to report that HIV infection may increase the risk of severe COVID-19 and death, and which regions of the world present with more risk to PLWH. Secondly, we show that the risks of severe COVID-19 and death in PLWH varied between continents and may reflect a complex interplay of concomitant contributory factors, which may need to be controlled for to better understand the direct or indirect effects of HIV infection on COVID-19 outcomes. Moreover, the prevalence of HIV–SARS-CoV-2 coinfection is best interpreted in the context of the varied global epidemiology of HIV infection in various regions of the world. Considering the complex effect of HIV infection on the host immune system as well as the dependence of vaccine efficacy on the immune response, future studies should assess the COVID-19 vaccine's pharmacokinetics in HIV-positive patients to decide whether PLWH coinfected with SARS-CoV-2 may benefit from certain types of vaccines, prioritisation, or repeated inoculations.

Supplementary Materials: The following are available online at https://www.mdpi.com/article/10.3390/tropicalmed7020022/s1, Table S1: Quality Assessment; Figure S1: Search Strategy; Figure S2: An influence plot from a "leave-one-out" analysis for the pooled prevalence of PLWH in COVID-19 cases. The red vertical line represents the aggregate effect size when all studies were included in the meta-analysis. The dots represent the aggregate effect size when the study listed next to the dot was removed from the analysis; Figure S3: An influence plot from a "leave-one-out" analysis for the relative risk of severe COVID-19 in PLWH compared to HIV-negative patients. The red vertical line represents the aggregate effect size when all studies were included in the meta-analysis. The dots represent the aggregate effect size when the study listed next to the dot was removed from the analysis; Figure S4: An influence plot from a "leave-one-out" analysis for the relative risk of COVID-19 mortality in PLWH compared to HIV-negative patients. The red vertical line represents the aggregate effect size when all studies were included in the meta-analysis. The dots represent the aggregate effect size when the study listed next to the dot was removed from the analysis; Figure S5: Pooled prevalence of PLWH co-infected with SARS-CoV-2 among COVID-19 cases for Continental Asia alone. The red dotted line represents the overall effect size. The lateral edges of the blue diamond represent the limits of the 95% confidence intervals (ES: Effect size, CI: Confidence Interval).

Author Contributions: Conceptualization, T.O.; methodology, T.O.; software, T.O.; validation, R.P.R., A.K. and T.O., A.M.H.; formal analysis, T.O. and J.S.A.; investigation, T.O., R.P.R., A.K., A.L., J.S.A. and A.M.H.; resources, T.O.; data curation, R.P.R., A.K., T.O. and A.L.; writing—original draft preparation, T.O.; writing—review and editing, T.O., J.S.A. and A.L.; visualization, T.O.; supervision, T.O.; project administration, T.O. All authors have read and agreed to the published version of the manuscript.

Funding: This research received no external funding.

Institutional Review Board Statement: Not applicable.

Informed Consent Statement: Not applicable.

Conflicts of Interest: The authors declare no conflict of interest.

References

1. Worldometer: Coronavirus Update (Live). Available online: https://www.worldometers.info/coronavirus/ (accessed on 25 February 2020).
2. Alqahtani, J.S.; Aldhahir, A.M.; Oyelade, T.; Alghamdi, S.M.; Almamary, A.S. Smoking cessation during COVID-19: The top to-do list. *npj Prim. Care Respir. Med.* **2021**, *31*, 1–3. [CrossRef] [PubMed]
3. Oyelade, T.; Alqahtani, J.; Canciani, G. Prognosis of COVID-19 in Patients with Liver and Kidney Diseases: An Early Systematic Review and Meta-Analysis. *Trop. Med. Infect. Dis.* **2020**, *5*, 80. [CrossRef] [PubMed]
4. Yang, J.; Zheng, Y.; Gou, X.; Pu, K.; Chen, Z.; Guo, Q.; Ji, R.; Wang, H.; Wang, Y.; Zhou, Y. Prevalence of comorbidities in the novel wuhan coronavirus (COVID-19) infection: A systematic review and meta-analysis. *Int. J. Infect. Dis.* **2020**, *94*, 91–95. [CrossRef] [PubMed]
5. Alqahtani, J.S.; Mendes, R.G.; Aldhahir, A.; Rowley, D.; AlAhmari, M.D.; Ntoumenopoulos, G.; Alghamdi, S.M.; Sreedharan, J.K.; Aldabayan, Y.S.; Oyelade, T.; et al. Global Current Practices of Ventilatory Support Management in COVID-19 Patients: An International Survey. *J. Multidiscip. Heal.* **2020**, *13*, 1635–1648. [CrossRef]
6. Guan, W.-J.; Liang, W.-H.; Zhao, Y.; Liang, H.-R.; Chen, Z.-S.; Li, Y.-M.; Liu, X.-Q.; Chen, R.-C.; Tang, C.-L.; Wang, T.; et al. Comorbidity and its impact on 1590 patients with COVID-19 in China: A nationwide analysis. *Eur. Respir. J.* **2020**, *55*, 2000547. [CrossRef]
7. Subgroup 'Assessment of Pathogens Transmissible by Blood' German Advisory Committee Blood (Arbeitskreis Blut) Human Immunodeficiency Virus (HIV). *Transfus. Med. Hemotherapy* **2016**, *43*, 203–222. [CrossRef]
8. Joint United Nations Programme on HIV and AIDS (UNAIDS). FACT SHEET 2021 Preliminary UNAIDS 2021 Epidemiological Estimates, in GLOBAL HIV STATISTICS. 2021. Available online: https://www.unaids.org/en/resources/fact-sheet (accessed on 1 December 2021).
9. Kharsany, A.B.; Karim, Q.A. HIV Infection and AIDS in Sub-Saharan Africa: Current Status, Challenges and Opportunities. *Open AIDS J.* **2016**, *10*, 34–48. [CrossRef]
10. El-Atrouni, W.; Berbari, E.; Temesgen, Z. Hiv-associated opportunistic infections. Bacterial infections. *J. Med. Liban* **2006**, *54*, 80–83.
11. Lewden, C.; Salmon, D.; Morlat, P.; Bévilacqua, S.; Jougla, E.; Bonnet, F.; Héripret, L.; Costagliola, D.; May, T.; Chêne, G. Causes of death among human immunodeficiency virus (HIV)-infected adults in the era of potent antiretroviral therapy: Emerging role of hepatitis and cancers, persistent role of AIDS. *Int. J. Epidemiology* **2004**, *34*, 121–130. [CrossRef]
12. Yazdanpanah, F.; Hamblin, M.R.; Rezaei, N. The immune system and COVID-19: Friend or foe? *Life Sci.* **2020**, *256*, 117900. [CrossRef]
13. Chen, J.; Xia, L.; Liu, L.; Xu, Q.; Ling, Y.; Huang, D.; Huang, W.; Song, S.; Xu, S.; Shen, Y.; et al. Antiviral Activity and Safety of Darunavir/Cobicistat for the Treatment of COVID-19. *Open Forum Infect. Dis.* **2020**, *7*, ofaa241. [CrossRef] [PubMed]
14. De Meyer, S.; Bojkova, D.; Cinatl, J.; Van Damme, E.; Buyck, C.; Van Loock, M.; Woodfall, B.; Ciesek, S. Lack of antiviral activity of darunavir against SARS-CoV-2. *Int. J. Infect. Dis.* **2020**, *97*, 7–10. [CrossRef] [PubMed]
15. Horby, P.W.; Mafham, M.; Bell, J.L.; Linsell, L.; Staplin, N.; Emberson, J.; Palfreeman, A.; Raw, J.; Elmahi, E.; Prudon, B.; et al. Lopinavir–ritonavir in patients admitted to hospital with COVID-19 (recovery): A randomised, controlled, open-label, platform trial. *Lancet* **2020**, *396*, 1345–1352. [CrossRef]
16. Ayerdi, O.; Puerta, T.; Clavo, P.; Vera, M.; Ballesteros, J.; Fuentes, M.E.; Estrada, V.; Rodríguez, C.; Del Romero, J.; Lejarraga, C.; et al. Preventive Efficacy of Tenofovir/Emtricitabine Against Severe Acute Respiratory Syndrome Coronavirus 2 Among Pre-Exposure Prophylaxis Users. *Open Forum Infect. Dis.* **2020**, *7*, ofaa455. [CrossRef]
17. Hariyanto, T.I.; Rosalind, J.; Christian, K.; Kurniawan, A. Human immunodeficiency virus and mortality from coronavirus disease 2019: A systematic review and meta-analysis. *South. Afr. J. HIV Med.* **2021**, *22*, 7. [CrossRef]
18. Mellor, M.M.; Bast, A.C.; Jones, N.R.; Roberts, N.W.; Ordóñez-Mena, J.M.; Reith, A.J.; Butler, C.C.; Matthews, P.C.; Dorward, J. Risk of adverse coronavirus disease 2019 outcomes for people living with HIV. *AIDS* **2021**, *35*, F1–F10. [CrossRef]
19. Ssentongo, P.; Heilbrunn, E.S.; Ssentongo, A.E.; Advani, S.; Chinchilli, V.M.; Nunez, J.J.; Du, P. Epidemiology and outcomes of COVID-19 in HIV-infected individuals: A systematic review and meta-analysis. *Sci. Rep.* **2021**, *11*, 1–12. [CrossRef]
20. Gao, Y.; Chen, Y.; Liu, M.; Shi, S.; Tian, J. Impacts of immunosuppression and immunodeficiency on COVID-19: A systematic review and meta-analysis. *J. Infect.* **2020**, *81*, e93–e95. [CrossRef]
21. Lee, K.; Yap, S.; Ngeow, Y.; Lye, M. COVID-19 in People Living with HIV: A Systematic Review and Meta-Analysis. *Int. J. Environ. Res. Public Heal.* **2021**, *18*, 3554. [CrossRef]

22. Joint United Nations Programme on HIV/AIDS; WHO. *2008 Report on the Global AIDS Epidemic*; WHO: Geneva, Switzerland, 2008. Available online: https://scholar.google.co.uk/scholar?cluster=9760571076381553660&hl=en&as_sdt=0,5&as_vis=1 (accessed on 1 December 2021).
23. Ambrosioni, J.; Blanco, J.L.; Reyes-Urueña, J.M.; Davies, M.-A.; Sued, O.; Marcos, M.A.; Martínez, E.; Bertagnolio, S.; Alcamí, J.; Miro, J.M.; et al. Overview of SARS-CoV-2 infection in adults living with HIV. *Lancet HIV* **2021**, *8*, e294–e305. [CrossRef]
24. Moher, D.; Liberati, A.; Tetzlaff, J.; Altman, D.G.; PRISMA Group. Preferred reporting items for systematic reviews and meta-analyses: The PRISMA statement. *PLoS Med.* **2009**, *6*, e1000097. [CrossRef] [PubMed]
25. Morgan, R.L.; Whaley, P.; Thayer, K.A.; Schünemann, H.J. Identifying the PECO: A framework for formulating good questions to explore the association of environmental and other exposures with health outcomes. *Environ. Int.* **2018**, *121*, 1027–1031. [CrossRef] [PubMed]
26. Vizcarra, P.; Pérez-Elías, M.J.; Quereda, C.; Moreno, A.; Vivancos, M.J.; Dronda, F.; Casado, J.L.; Moreno, S.; Fortún, J.; Navas, E.; et al. Description of COVID-19 in HIV-infected individuals: A single-centre, prospective cohort. *Lancet HIV* **2020**, *7*, e554–e564. [CrossRef]
27. Geretti, A.M.; Stockdale, A.J.; Kelly, S.H.; Cevik, M.; Collins, S.; Waters, L.; Villa, G.; Docherty, A.; Harrison, E.M.; Turtle, L.; et al. Outcomes of Coronavirus Disease 2019 (COVID-19) Related Hospitalization Among People With Human Immunodeficiency Virus (HIV) in the ISARIC World Health Organization (WHO) Clinical Characterization Protocol (UK): A Prospective Observational Study. *Clin. Infect. Dis.* **2020**, *73*, e2095–e2106. [CrossRef] [PubMed]
28. Docherty, A.B.; Harrison, E.M.; Green, C.A.; Hardwick, H.E.; Pius, R.; Norman, L.; Holden, K.A.; Read, J.M.; Dondelinger, F.; Carson, G.; et al. Features of 20 133 UK patients in hospital with COVID-19 using the ISARIC WHO Clinical Characterisation Protocol: Prospective observational cohort study. *BMJ* **2020**, *369*, m1985. [CrossRef]
29. WHO. *COVID-19 Clinical Management: Living Guidance*; WHO: Geneva, Switzerland, 2021.
30. Johnson, J.K.; Barach, P.; Vernooij-Dassen, M.; HANDOVER Research Collaborative. Conducting a multicentre and multinational qualitative study on patient transitions. *BMJ Qual. Saf.* **2012**, *21*, i22–i28. [CrossRef]
31. Liang, M.; Luo, N.; Chen, M.; Chen, C.; Singh, S.; Singh, S.; Tan, S. Prevalence and Mortality due to COVID-19 in HIV Co-Infected Population: A Systematic Review and Meta-Analysis. *Infect. Dis. Ther.* **2021**, *10*, 1267–1285. [CrossRef]
32. WHO. *Laboratory Testing for Coronavirus Disease (COVID-19) in Suspected Human Cases: Interim Guidance*; WHO: Geneva, Switzerland, 2020.
33. WHO. *Consolidated Guidelines on HIV Testing Services: 5Cs: Consent, Confidentiality, Counselling, Correct Results and Connection 2015*; WHO: Geneva, Switzerland, 2015.
34. Stoeckle, K.; Johnston, C.D.; Jannat-Khah, D.P.; Williams, S.C.; Ellman, T.M.; Vogler, M.A.; Gulick, R.M.; Glesby, M.J.; Choi, J.J. COVID-19 in Hospitalized Adults With HIV. *Open Forum Infect. Dis.* **2020**, *7*, ofaa327. [CrossRef]
35. Borobia, A.; Carcas, A.; Arnalich, F.; Álvarez-Sala, R.; Monserrat-Villatoro, J.; Quintana, M.; Figueira, J.; Santos-Olmo, R.T.; García-Rodríguez, J.; Martín-Vega, A.; et al. A Cohort of Patients with COVID-19 in a Major Teaching Hospital in Europe. *J. Clin. Med.* **2020**, *9*, 1733. [CrossRef]
36. Boulle, A.; Davies, M.-A.; Hussey, H.; Ismail, M.; Morden, E.; Vundle, Z.; Zweigenthal, V.; Mahomed, H.; Paleker, M.; Pienaar, D. Risk factors for COVID-19 death in a population cohort study from the Western Cape Province, South Africa. *Clin. Infect. Dis. Off. Publ. Infect. Dis. Soc. Am.* **2020**. [CrossRef]
37. Ceballos, M.E.; Ross, P.; Lasso, M.; Dominguez, I.; Puente, M.; Valenzuela, P.; Enberg, M.; Serri, M.; Muñoz, R.; Pinos, Y.; et al. Clinical characteristics and outcomes of people living with HIV hospitalized with COVID-19: A nationwide experience. *Int. J. STD AIDS* **2021**, *32*, 435–443. [CrossRef] [PubMed]
38. Collins, L.F.; Moran, C.A.; Oliver, N.T.; Moanna, A.; Lahiri, C.D.; Colasanti, J.A.; Kelley, C.F.; Nguyen, M.L.; Marconi, V.C.; Armstrong, W.S.; et al. Clinical characteristics, comorbidities and outcomes among persons with HIV hospitalized with coronavirus disease 2019 in Atlanta, Georgia. *AIDS* **2020**, *34*, 1789–1794. [CrossRef] [PubMed]
39. Del Amo, J.; Polo, R.; Moreno, S.; Diaz-Brito, V.; Martínez, E.; Arribas, J.R.; Jarrín, I.; Hernán, M.A. Incidence and Severity of COVID-19 in HIV-Positive Persons Receiving Antiretroviral Therapy. *Ann. Intern. Med.* **2020**, *173*, 536–541. [CrossRef] [PubMed]
40. Di Biagio, A.; Ricci, E.; Calza, L.; Squillace, N.; Menzaghi, B.; Rusconi, S.; Orofino, G.; Bargiacchi, O.; Molteni, C.; Valsecchi, L.; et al. Factors associated with hospital admission for COVID-19 in HIV patients. *AIDS* **2020**, *34*. [CrossRef]
41. Erinoso, O.A.; Wright, K.O.; Anya, S.; Bowale, A.; Adejumo, O.; Adesola, S.; Osikomaiya, B.; Mutiu, B.; Saka, B.; Falana, A.; et al. Clinical characteristics, predictors of symptomatic coronavirus disease 2019 and duration of hospitalisation in a cohort of 632 Patients in Lagos State, Nigeria. *Niger. Postgrad. Med. J.* **2020**, *27*, 285–292. [CrossRef]
42. Etienne, N.; Karmochkine, M.; Slama, L.; Pavie, J.; Batisse, D.; Usubillaga, R.; Letembet, V.-A.; Brazille, P.; Canouï, E.; Slama, D.; et al. HIV infection and COVID-19: Risk factors for severe disease. *AIDS* **2020**, *34*, 1771–1774. [CrossRef]
43. Gervasoni, C.; Meraviglia, P.; Riva, A.; Giacomelli, A.; Oreni, L.; Minisci, D.; Atzori, C.; Ridolfo, A.; Cattaneo, D. Clinical Features and Outcomes of Patients With Human Immunodeficiency Virus With COVID-19. *Clin. Infect. Dis.* **2020**, *71*, 2276–2278. [CrossRef]
44. Geteneh, A.; Alemnew, B.; Tadesse, S.; Girma, A. Clinical characteristics of patients infected with SARS-CoV-2 in North Wollo Zone, North-East Ethiopia. *Pan Afr. Med. J.* **2021**, *38*. [CrossRef]
45. Gudipati, S.; Brar, I.; Murray, S.; McKinnon, J.E.; Yared, N.; Markowitz, N. Descriptive Analysis of Patients Living With HIV Affected by COVID-19. *JAIDS J. Acquir. Immune Defic. Syndr.* **2020**, *85*, 123–126. [CrossRef]

46. Hadi, Y.B.; Naqvi, S.F.; Kupec, J.T.; Sarwari, A.R. Characteristics and outcomes of COVID-19 in patients with HIV: A multicentre research network study. *AIDS* **2020**, *34*, F3–F8. [CrossRef]
47. Härter, G.; Spinner, C.D.; Roider, J.; Bickel, M.; Krznaric, I.; Grunwald, S.; Schabaz, F.; Gillor, D.; Postel, N.; Mueller, M.C.; et al. COVID-19 in people living with human immunodeficiency virus: A case series of 33 patients. *Infection* **2020**, *48*, 681–686. [CrossRef] [PubMed]
48. Ho, H.-E.; Peluso, M.J.; Margus, C.; Lopes, J.P.M.; He, C.; Gaisa, M.M.; Osorio, G.; Aberg, J.A.; Mullen, M.P. Clinical Outcomes and Immunologic Characteristics of Coronavirus Disease 2019 in People With Human Immunodeficiency Virus. *J. Infect. Dis.* **2020**, *223*, 403–408. [CrossRef] [PubMed]
49. Huang, J.; Xie, N.; Hu, X.; Yan, H.; Ding, J.; Liu, P.; Ma, H.; Ruan, L.; Li, G.; He, N.; et al. Epidemiological, Virological and Serological Features of Coronavirus Disease 2019 (COVID-19) Cases in People Living With Human Immunodeficiency Virus in Wuhan: A Population-based Cohort Study. *Clin. Infect. Dis.* **2020**, *73*, e2086–e2094. [CrossRef] [PubMed]
50. Inciarte, A.; Gonzalez-Cordon, A.; Rojas, J.; Torres, B.; De Lazzari, E.; De La Mora, L.; Martinez-Rebollar, M.; Laguno, M.; Callau, P.; Gonzalez-Navarro, A.; et al. Clinical characteristics, risk factors, and incidence of symptomatic coronavirus disease 2019 in a large cohort of adults living with HIV: A single-center, prospective observational study. *AIDS* **2020**, *34*, 1775–1780. [CrossRef] [PubMed]
51. Isernia, V.; Julia, Z.; Le Gac, S.; Bachelard, A.; Landman, R.; Lariven, S.; Joly, V.; Deconinck, L.; Rioux, C.; Lescure, X.; et al. SARS-COV2 infection in 30 HIV-infected patients followed-up in a French University Hospital. *Int. J. Infect. Dis.* **2020**, *101*, 49–51. [CrossRef] [PubMed]
52. Izquierdo, J.L.; Ancochea, J.; Soriano, J.B. Savana COVID-19 Research Group Clinical Characteristics and Prognostic Factors for Intensive Care Unit Admission of Patients With COVID-19: Retrospective Study Using Machine Learning and Natural Language Processing. *J. Med Internet Res.* **2020**, *22*, e21801. [CrossRef] [PubMed]
53. Karim, F.; Gazy, I.; Cele, S.; Zungu, Y.; Krause, R.; Bernstein, M.; Ganga, Y.; Rodel, H.; Mthabela, N.; Mazibuko, M. Hiv infection alters sars-cov-2 responsive immune parameters but not clinical outcomes in COVID-19 disease. *medRxiv* **2020**. [CrossRef]
54. Kirenga, B.; Muttamba, W.; Kayongo, A.; Nsereko, C.; Siddharthan, T.; Lusiba, J.; Mugenyi, L.; Byanyima, R.K.; Worodria, W.; Nakwagala, F. Characteristics and outcomes of admitted patients infected with sars-cov-2 in uganda. *BMJ Open Respir. Res.* **2020**, *7*, e000646. [CrossRef]
55. Liu, J.; Zeng, W.; Cao, Y.; Cui, Y.; Li, Y.; Yao, S.; Alwalid, O.; Yang, F.; Fan, Y.; Shi, H. Effect of a previous history of antiretroviral treatment on the clinical picture of patients with co-infection of SARS-CoV-2 and hiv: A preliminary study. *Int. J. Infect. Dis.* **2020**, *100*, 141–148. [CrossRef]
56. Maggiolo, F.; Zoboli, F.; Arosio, M.; Valenti, D.; Guarneri, D.; Sangiorgio, L.; Ripamonti, D.; Callegaro, A. SARS-CoV-2 infection in persons living with hiv: A single center prospective cohort. *J. Med. Virol.* **2021**, *93*, 1145–1149. [CrossRef]
57. Migisha, R.; Kwesiga, B.; Mirembe, B.B.; Amanya, G.; Kabwama, S.N.; Kadobera, D.; Bulage, L.; Nsereko, G.; Wadunde, I.; Tindyebwa, T. Early cases of sars-cov-2 infection in uganda: Epidemiology and lessons learned from risk-based testing approaches–march-april 2020. *Glob. Health* **2020**, *16*, 1–9. [CrossRef] [PubMed]
58. Miyashita, H.; Kuno, T. Prognosis of coronavirus disease 2019 (COVID-19) in patients with HIV infection in New York City. *HIV Med.* **2020**, *22*. [CrossRef] [PubMed]
59. Nachega, J.B.; Ishoso, D.K.; Otokoye, J.O.; Hermans, M.P.; Machekano, R.N.; Sam-Agudu, N.A.; Nswe Bongo-Pasi, C.; Mbala-Kingebeni, P.; Ntwan Madinga, J.; Mukendi, S.; et al. Clinical characteristics and outcomes of patients hospitalized for COVID-19 in Africa: Early insights from the Democratic Republic of the Congo. *Am. J. Trop. Med. Hyg.* **2020**, (in press). [CrossRef] [PubMed]
60. Ombajo, L.A.; Mutono, N.; Sudi, P.; Mutua, M.; Sood, M.; Loo, A.M.A.; Juma, P.; Odhiambo, J.; Shah, R.; Wangai, F.; et al. Epidemiological and clinical characteristics of COVID-19 patients in kenya. *medRxiv* **2020**. [CrossRef]
61. Parker, A.; Koegelenberg, C.F.N.; Moolla, M.S.; Louw, E.H.; Mowlana, A.; Nortjé, A.; Ahmed, R.; Brittain, N.; Lalla, U.; Allwood, B.W.; et al. High HIV prevalence in an early cohort of hospital admissions with COVID-19 in Cape Town, South Africa. *S. Afr. Med. J.* **2020**, *110*, 982. [CrossRef]
62. Pujari, S.; Gaikwad, S.; Chitalikar, A.; Dabhade, D.; Joshi, K.; Bele, V. Short Communication: Coronavirus Disease 19 Among People Living with HIV in Western India: An Observational Cohort Study. *AIDS Res. Hum. Retrovir.* **2021**, *37*, 620–623. [CrossRef]
63. Rodriguez-Gonzalez, C.G.; Chamorro-De-Vega, E.; Valerio, M.; Amor-Garcia, M.A.; Tejerina, F.; Sancho-Gonzalez, M.; Narrillos-Moraza, A.; Gimenez-Manzorro, A.; Manrique-Rodriguez, S.; Machado, M.; et al. COVID-19 in hospitalised patients in Spain: A cohort study in Madrid. *Int. J. Antimicrob. Agents* **2020**, *57*, 106249. [CrossRef]
64. Rodríguez-Molinero, A.; Gálvez-Barrón, C.; Miñarro, A.; Macho, O.; López, G.F.; Robles, M.T.; Dapena, M.D.; Martínez, S.; Ràfols, N.M.; Monaco, E.E.; et al. Association between COVID-19 prognosis and disease presentation, comorbidities and chronic treatment of hospitalized patients. *PLoS ONE* **2020**, *15*, e0239571. [CrossRef]
65. Shalev, N.; Scherer, M.; Lasota, E.D.; Antoniou, P.; Yin, M.T.; Zucker, J.; Sobieszczyk, M.E. Clinical Characteristics and Outcomes in People Living With Human Immunodeficiency Virus Hospitalized for Coronavirus Disease 2019. *Clin. Infect. Dis.* **2020**, *71*, 2294–2297. [CrossRef]
66. Shi, P.; Ren, G.; Yang, J.; Li, Z.; Deng, S.; Li, M.; Wang, S.; Xu, X.; Chen, F.; Li, Y.; et al. Clinical characteristics of imported and second-generation coronavirus disease 2019 (COVID-19) cases in shaanxi outside wuhan, china: A multicentre retrospective study. *Epidemiol. Infect.* **2020**, *148*, e238. [CrossRef]

67. Sigel, K.; Swartz, T.; Golden, E.; Paranjpe, I.; Somani, S.; Richter, F.; De Freitas, J.K.; Miotto, R.; Zhao, S.; Polak, P.; et al. Coronavirus 2019 and People Living With Human Immunodeficiency Virus: Outcomes for Hospitalized Patients in New York City. *Clin. Infect. Dis.* **2020**, *71*, 2933–2938. [CrossRef] [PubMed]
68. Tesoriero, J.M.; Swain, C.-A.E.; Pierce, J.L.; Zamboni, L.; Wu, M.; Holtgrave, D.R.; Gonzalez, C.J.; Udo, T.; Morne, J.E.; Hart-Malloy, R.; et al. COVID-19 Outcomes Among Persons Living With or Without Diagnosed HIV Infection in New York State. *JAMA Netw. Open* **2021**, *4*, e2037069. [CrossRef] [PubMed]
69. Virata, M.D.; Shenoi, S.; Ladines-Lim, J.B.; Villanueva, M.; Aoun-Barakat, L. 111. Outcomes Related to COVID-19 Among People Living with HIV: Cohort from a Large Academic Center. *Open Forum Infect. Dis.* **2020**, *7*, S184. [CrossRef]
70. Wang, R.; Pan, M.; Zhang, X.; Han, M.; Fan, X.; Zhao, F.; Miao, M.; Xu, J.; Guan, M.; Deng, X.; et al. Epidemiological and clinical features of 125 Hospitalized Patients with COVID-19 in Fuyang, Anhui, China. *Int. J. Infect. Dis.* **2020**, *95*, 421–428. [CrossRef] [PubMed]
71. Yang, R.; Gui, X.; Zhang, Y.; Xiong, Y.; Gao, S.; Ke, H. Clinical characteristics of COVID-19 patients with HIV coinfection in Wuhan, China. *Expert Rev. Respir. Med.* **2020**, *15*, 403–409. [CrossRef]
72. Yu, Y.; Tu, J.; Lei, B.; Shu, H.; Zou, X.; Li, R.; Huang, C.; Qu, Y.; Shang, Y. Incidence and Risk Factors of Deep Vein Thrombosis in Hospitalized COVID-19 Patients. *Clin. Appl. Thromb.* **2020**, *26*. [CrossRef]
73. Centers for Disease Control and Prevention. *Diagnoses of Hiv Infection in the United States and Dependent Areas, 2014*; HIV Surveillance Report; Centers for Disease Control and Prevention: Atlanta, GA, USA, 2015; Volume 25, pp. 1–82.
74. Joint United Nations Programme on HIV/AIDS (UNAIDS). *Global HIV & AIDS Statistics—Fact Sheet*; UNAIDS: Geneva, Switzerland, 2021.
75. 2020 Global AIDS Update—Seizing the Moment—Tackling Entrenched Inequalities to End Epidemics. Available online: https://www.unaids.org/en/resources/documents/2020/global-aids-report (accessed on 24 August 2021).
76. Blanco, J.L.; Ambrosioni, J.; García, F.; Martínez, E.; Soriano, A.; Mallolas, J.; Miro, J.M. COVID-19 in patients with HIV: Clinical case series. *Lancet HIV* **2020**, *7*, e314–e316. [CrossRef]
77. Centers for Disease Control and Prevention. CDC COVID Data Tracker. Available online: https://covid.cdc.gov/covid-data-tracker/#national-lab (accessed on 24 August 2021).
78. Patel, R.H.; Acharya, A.; Chand, H.S.; Mohan, M.; Byrareddy, S.N. Human Immunodeficiency Virus and Severe Acute Respiratory Syndrome Coronavirus 2 Coinfection: A Systematic Review of the Literature and Challenges. *AIDS Res. Hum. Retroviruses* **2021**, *37*, 266–282. [CrossRef]
79. Pelchen-Matthews, A.; Ryom, L.; Borges, H.; Edwards, S.; Duvivier, C.; Stephan, C.; Sambatakou, H.; Maciejewska, K.; Portu, J.J.; Weber, J.; et al. Aging and the evolution of comorbidities among HIV-positive individuals in a European cohort. *AIDS* **2018**, *32*, 2405–2416. [CrossRef]
80. Zhang, H.; Wu, T. CD4+T, CD8+T counts and severe COVID-19: A meta-analysis. *J. Infect.* **2020**, *81*, e82–e84. [CrossRef]
81. Atyeo, C.; Fischinger, S.; Zohar, T.; Slein, M.D.; Burke, J.; Loos, C.; McCulloch, D.J.; Newman, K.L.; Wolf, C.; Yu, J.; et al. Distinct Early Serological Signatures Track with SARS-CoV-2 Survival. *Immunity* **2020**, *53*, 524–532.e4. [CrossRef] [PubMed]
82. Fenwick, C.; Joo, V.; Jacquier, P.; Noto, A.; Banga, R.; Perreau, M.; Pantaleo, G. T-cell exhaustion in HIV infection. *Immunol. Rev.* **2019**, *292*, 149–163. [CrossRef] [PubMed]
83. Moir, S.; Fauci, A.S. B-cell responses to HIV infection. *Immunol. Rev.* **2017**, *275*, 33–48. [CrossRef] [PubMed]
84. Lee, K.-Y.; Tsai, M.-S.; Kuo, K.-C.; Tsai, J.-C.; Sun, H.-Y.; Cheng, A.C.; Chang, S.-Y.; Lee, C.-H.; Hung, C.-C. Pneumococcal vaccination among HIV-infected adult patients in the era of combination antiretroviral therapy. *Hum. Vaccines Immunother.* **2014**, *10*, 3700–3710. [CrossRef]
85. Ceravolo, A.; Orsi, G.B.; Parodi, V.; Ansaldi, F. Influenza vaccination in HIV-positive subjects: Latest evidence and future perspective. *J. Prev. Med. Hyg.* **2013**, *54*. [CrossRef]
86. Geretti, A.M.; Doyle, T. Immunization for HIV-positive individuals. *Curr. Opin. Infect. Dis.* **2010**, *23*, 32–38. [CrossRef]
87. Hogan, A.B.; Jewell, B.L.; Sherrard-Smith, E.; Vesga, J.F.; Watson, O.J.; Whittaker, C.; Hamlet, A.; Smith, J.A.; Winskill, P.; Verity, R.; et al. Potential impact of the COVID-19 pandemic on HIV, tuberculosis, and malaria in low-income and middle-income countries: A modelling study. *Lancet Glob. Health* **2020**, *8*, e1132–e1141. [CrossRef]
88. Jewell, B.L.; Mudimu, E.; Stover, J.; Ten Brink, D.; Phillips, A.N.; Smith, J.A.; Martin-Hughes, R.; Teng, Y.; Glaubius, R.; Mahiane, S.G.; et al. Potential effects of disruption to HIV programmes in sub-Saharan Africa caused by COVID-19: Results from multiple mathematical models. *Lancet HIV* **2020**, *7*, e629–e640. [CrossRef]
89. Simões, D.; Stengaard, A.R.; Combs, L.; Raben, D. The EuroTEST COVID-19 impact assessment consortium of partners Impact of the COVID-19 pandemic on testing services for HIV, viral hepatitis and sexually transmitted infections in the WHO European Region, March to August 2020. *Eurosurveillance* **2020**, *25*, 2001943. [CrossRef]
90. WHO. *Disruption in HIV, Hepatitis and STI Services Due to COVID-19, in Global HIV, Hepatitis and STI Programmes*; WHO: Geneva, Switzerland, 2020.
91. Bhaskaran, K.; Rentsch, C.T.; MacKenna, B.; Schultze, A.; Mehrkar, A.; Bates, C.J.; Eggo, R.M.; Morton, C.E.; Bacon, S.C.J.; Inglesby, P.; et al. HIV infection and COVID-19 death: A population-based cohort analysis of UK primary care data and linked national death registrations within the OpenSAFELY platform. *Lancet HIV* **2020**, *8*, e24–e32. [CrossRef]
92. Lunny, C.; Pieper, D.; Thabet, P.; Kanji, S. Managing overlap of primary study results across systematic reviews: Practical considerations for authors of overviews of reviews. *BMC Med. Res. Methodol.* **2021**, *21*, 1–14. [CrossRef] [PubMed]

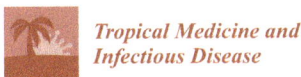

Systematic Review

SARS-CoV-2 mRNA Vaccine Breakthrough Infections in Fully Vaccinated Healthcare Personnel: A Systematic Review

Caterina Ledda [1,*], Claudio Costantino [2], Giuseppe Motta [3], Rosario Cunsolo [4], Patrizia Stracquadanio [5], Giuseppe Liberti [6], Helena C. Maltezou [7] and Venerando Rapisarda [1,5]

1. Occupational Medicine Unit, Department of Clinical and Experimental Medicine, University of Catania, 95123 Catania, Italy; vrapisarda@unict.it
2. Department of Health Promotion, Mother and Child Care, Internal Medicine and Medical Specialties "G. D'Alessandro", University of Palermo, 90133 Palermo, Italy; claudio.costantino01@unipa.it
3. Occupational Medicine Unit, "Garibaldi" Hospital of Catania, 95123 Catania, Italy; giusmotta@gmail.com
4. Hospital Health Management, "G. Rodolico-San Marco" Polyclinic University Hospital, 95123 Catania, Italy; r.cunsolo@ao-ve.it
5. Occupational Medicine Unit, "G. Rodolico-San Marco" University Hospital, 95123 Catania, Italy; patrizia.stracquadanio@ao-ve.it
6. Commissioner Office in Acta for the COVID-19 Emergency, Provincial Health Authority of Catania, 95123 Catania, Italy; commissario.covid@aspct.it
7. Directorate for Research, Studies and Documentation, National Public Health Organization, 15123 Athens, Greece; maltezou.helena@gmail.com
* Correspondence: cledda@unict.it

Citation: Ledda, C.; Costantino, C.; Motta, G.; Cunsolo, R.; Stracquadanio, P.; Liberti, G.; Maltezou, H.C.; Rapisarda, V. SARS-CoV-2 mRNA Vaccine Breakthrough Infections in Fully Vaccinated Healthcare Personnel: A Systematic Review. *Trop. Med. Infect. Dis.* **2022**, *7*, 9. https://doi.org/10.3390/tropicalmed7010009

Academic Editors: Peter A. Leggat, John Frean and Lucille Blumberg

Received: 1 December 2021
Accepted: 10 January 2022
Published: 13 January 2022

Publisher's Note: MDPI stays neutral with regard to jurisdictional claims in published maps and institutional affiliations.

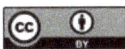

Copyright: © 2022 by the authors. Licensee MDPI, Basel, Switzerland. This article is an open access article distributed under the terms and conditions of the Creative Commons Attribution (CC BY) license (https://creativecommons.org/licenses/by/4.0/).

Abstract: The number of people vaccinated against COVID-19 increases worldwide every day; however, it is important to study the risk of breakthrough infections in vaccinated individuals at high risk of exposure such as healthcare personnel (HCP). A systematic literature review (SLR) applying the PRISMA declaration and the PECOS format using the following entry terms was used: "Health Personnel OR Healthcare Worker OR Healthcare Provider OR Healthcare Personnel AND breakthrough OR infection after vaccine*". The research was carried out utilizing the following databases: SCOPUS, PubMed, Embase, and Web of Sciences. An overall very low incidence of post-vaccination breakthrough infections was found, ranging from 0.011 to 0.001 (per 100 individuals at risk). Our findings further support the published high effectiveness rates of mRNA vaccines in preventing SARS-CoV-2 infections among fully vaccinated HCP. Additional studies are needed to define the duration of the vaccine-induced protection among HCP.

Keywords: mRNA-1273; BNT162b2; TAK-919; COVID-19; SARS-CoV-2; post-vaccination; healthcare personnel; pandemic; vaccination; asymptomatic infection

1. Introduction

Severe acute respiratory syndrome coronavirus 2 (SARS-CoV-2) infections have not been under control in most countries, and the pandemic of coronavirus disease 2019 (COVID-19) continues to be a problem for public health worldwide. As of 10 November 2021, more than 250 million cases and 5 million associated deaths were confirmed [1]. New variants of SARS-CoV-2 strains have emerged, which makes the situation more complex, and new waves recur even in some countries/areas where SARS-CoV-2 infections seemed to be under control [2–4].

Various interventions, including mask-wearing, quarantining, and social distancing, have played a significant role in monitoring and regulating the COVID-19 pandemic [4–7]; nevertheless, vaccination is considered a highly cost-effective intervention to mitigate the pandemic [8,9]. The documented flare-ups and breakthrough cases have been ascribed to three potentials: (1) the circulating variants of SARS-CoV-2 and their effect on vaccine-elicited immunity; (2) the speed of natural decline of antibodies among vaccinated people; and (3) the requirement for booster doses [10,11].

Throughout the past year, COVID-19 vaccines were advanced at an extraordinary speed. As of 10 November 2021, 24 vaccines had been approved by at least one state in the world, 7 vaccines had been authorized for emergency use by the World Health Organization (WHO) [12], and 1 had been fully authorized by the Food and Drug Administration (FDA) [13].

COVID-19 vaccines are created using various technologies: mRNA, protein subunit, inactivated, non-replicating viral vector, and DNA. At first, in December 2020, the United States of America (USA), the United Kingdom, Canada, and the European Union (EU) approved the emergency use of Pfizer-BioNTech's mRNA vaccine (BNT162b2) [12], and in January 2021, the USA and the EU approved the Moderna mRNA-1273 vaccine [12] through the U.S. FDA and European Medicine Agency, respectively. Today, Pfizer-BioNTech's vaccine (BNT162b2) is approved in 103 countries, while Moderna mRNA-1273 in 76 countries, the formulation of the latter has recently been marketed by Takeda (TAK-919) only in Japan [12].

In randomized, placebo-controlled, phase 3 efficacy trials after vaccine rollout, both mRNA vaccines were efficient in inhibiting symptomatic and severe COVID-19 illness [14–17]. Furthermore, a recent study showed that full vaccination of HCP with mRNA vaccine was associated with 66.42% vaccine effectiveness against absenteeism [18]. In clinical trials, the vaccines had 52–95% efficacy for symptomatic disease 14 days later than the first dose and 95% efficacy 7 days later than the second dose [15,16]. Initial observational investigations on mRNA vaccines in healthcare personnel (HCP) indicate 80% effectiveness >14 days following the first dose and 90% >14 days after the second dose [17,19,20]. While the number of vaccinated people increases worldwide, SARS-CoV-2 variants are of interest for their augmented transmissibility, increased disease severity, and immune escaping resulting in the risk of reinfections or breakthrough infections in vaccinated persons [21,22].

Nevertheless, there may be differences in vaccine effectiveness and breakthrough infection rates depending on the timing of testing. Breakthrough infections are mitigated by vaccines and are normally minor in their clinical features [23]. In the first period of vaccination campaigns, institutions had the objective to protect those at the greatest risk of infection because of their high risk of exposure [24]. Therefore, many countries have designated HCP as a main concern group for COVID-19 vaccination [25–27]. Therefore, today, HCP are the oldest, largest, and most at risk of vaccine breakthrough infection group. Moreover, little is known about how many infected vaccinated subjects can spread the infection [28,29].

This systematic literature review (SLR) provides evidence on mRNA reported vaccine breakthrough infections among HCP.

2. Materials and Methods

2.1. Design

An SLR of the records of diverse databases was carried out, subsequent to a pre-set procedure firstly established to minimalize the risk of bias in both choice and publication and safeguarding optimum organization and content. The methodology was to follow the standards specified in the PRISMA declaration [30] and applying the Evidence-Based Health Practice methodology [31], as well as using the Joanna Briggs Inventory (JBI) Checklist for Prevalence Studies tool to evaluate the risk of bias [32]. The instrument was used with the objective of improving consistency in SLR of prevalence records and has been suggested as the most suitable tool for this kind of investigation [33]. The risk of bias was assessed using the nine criteria established by Munn [32]. The level of bias is evaluated by assessing the total sum of criteria with a "yes" reply and transforming this score into a percentage (n/9). Studies obtaining <50% are judged as having high risk of bias, 50–69% medium risk of bias, and ≥70% low risk of bias.

2.2. Literature Search

We searched until 10 November 2021 in SCOPUS, PubMed, Embase, and Web of Sciences. The entry terms used were: "Health Personnel OR Healthcare Worker OR Healthcare Provider OR Healthcare Personnel AND breakthrough OR infection after vaccine*". The examination of the appropriate papers for inclusion in this SLR was also carried out, and the research articles were recovered and reviewed.

2.3. Inclusion and Exclusion Criteria

The following inclusion criterion was used: surveys that assessed SARS-CoV-2 mRNA vaccine breakthrough infections in HCP. The exclusion criteria adopted were: (1) animal studies, (2) abstract and case reports, (3) articles that were not available in English. For replicate studies, the article with more detailed data was integrated.

Moreover, investigations assessed as high risk of bias were excluded from the primary analysis.

2.4. Quality Assessment and Data Extraction

Two reviewers (C.L. and V.R.) studied the manuscripts separately. The title, abstract, and full text of each potentially relevant manuscript were reviewed. Any concerns regarding suitability of the manuscript were defined through consensus. The following data were investigated from all included papers: study design, country, mRNA vaccine, period observed, and breakthrough incidence of fully vaccinated HCP. If incidence was not expressed in the study, it was calculated by the authors. The breakthrough was proven by the detection of SARS-CoV-2 found by Reverse-Transcriptase Polymerase Chain Reaction (RT-PCR) test in swab samples.

3. Results

3.1. Characteristics of Eligible Studies

Following a search of the relevant databases, 121 documents were identified. Of these, 101 were excluded after review of the title and abstract, and 7 studies were excluded after review of the manuscript. After all, nine studies satisfied the inclusion criteria and were included in the SLR [34–42]. A flow-chart depicting the studies selected in the present SLR is shown in Figure 1.

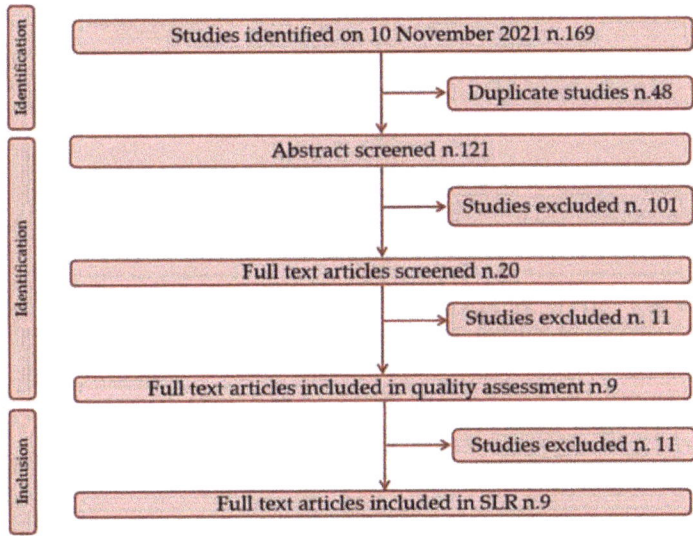

Figure 1. Graph illustrating included and excluded studies in the SLR.

3.2. Results of Eligible Studies

All the studies reviewed investigated COVID-19 infection in HCPs after the emergency vaccination campaign. In detail, seven studies included HCP vaccinated with both the BNT162b2 vaccine and the mRNA-1273 vaccine were conducted in the USA, and only one was conducted in Belgium [17,35–37,39–41]. The other studies were in Israel and Greece using the BNT162b2 vaccine [25,29]. The studies covered a period from 9 December 2020 to 14 August 2021. The breakthrough incidence varied from a minimum of 0.001 to a maximum of 0.011. Table 1 summarizes the features of the studies analyzed.

Table 1. Features of suitable studies.

Reference	JBI Score	Study Design	Country	mRNA Vaccine	Period Observed	Breakthrough Incidence *
Bergwerk et al. [34]	100%	Case-control study	Israel	BNT162b2	20 January 2021–28 April 2021	0.003
Bouton et al. [35]	88%	Prospective cohort study	United States of America	BNT162b2 or mRNA-1273	9 December 2020–23 February 2021	0.003
Fowlkes et al. [36]	88%	Nested cohort study	United States of America	BNT162b2 or mRNA-1273	14 December 2020–14 August 2021	0.011
Geysels et al. [37]	100%	Prospective cohort study	Belgium	BNT162b2 or mRNA-1273	1 March 2021–30 April 2021	0.003
Ioannou et al. [38]	66%	Prospective cohort study	Greece	BNT162b2	4 January 2021–14 April 2021	0.009
Jacobson et al. [39]	100%	Prospective cohort study	United States of America	BNT162b2 or mRNA-1273	18 December 2020–2 April 2021	0.001
North et al. [40]	100%	Prospective cohort study	United States of America	BNT162b2 or mRNA-1273	30 December 2020–2 April 2021	0.001
Teran et al. [41]	100%	Prospective cohort study	United States of America	BNT162b2 or mRNA-1273	28 December 2020–31 March 2021	0.002
Thompson et al. [42]	88%	Prospective cohort study	United States of America	BNT162b2 or mRNA-1273	14 December 2020–10 April 2021	0.001

* = only in fully vaccinated HCP.

Bergwerk et al. [34], to evaluate the effectiveness of the BNT162b2 vaccine, carried out, through a prospective cohort study of 11,453 HCP, a case control investigation among 1497 fully vaccinated HCP. In this study, researchers reported the positivity to SARS-CoV-2 by RT-PCR in 39 fully vaccinated HCP. The mean age of the 39 sick workers was 42 years, and most of them were women (64%). The median period from the second vaccine dose to SARS-CoV-2 finding was 39 days (range, 11 to 102). Only one sick person (3%) was immunosuppressed. Moreover, in 37 cases of breakthrough infection, the suspected source of infection was an unvaccinated person. Of all the HCP with breakthrough infection, 26 (67%) had mild symptoms at various stages, and none needed hospitalization. The residual 13 workers (33% of all cases) were asymptomatic throughout the period of infection. The most frequent symptom that was described was higher respiratory congestion (36% of all cases), subsequent myalgia (28%), and loss of smell or taste (28%); fever or rigors were registered in 21% of participants.

A prospective cohort study was carried out by Bouton and colleagues [35]. They observed a total of 10,590 HCP, but only 5913 had obtained 2 doses of the vaccine (BNT162b2 or mRNA-1273) at that time. In only 17 HCP did post-vaccination cases of SARS-CoV-2 occur. Another prospective cohort study performed in the USA [36] observed 4136 HCP with no earlier laboratory-documented SARS-CoV-2 disease for 35 weeks. Of these, 2976 were fully vaccinated (BNT162b2 or mRNA-1273), and 34 HCP reported the infection of SARS-CoV-2, 80.6% of which were symptomatic.

In Belgium, Geysels et al. [37], in a prospective cohort study of 3491 fully vaccinated (BNT162b2 or mRNA-1273) HCP, 9 workers (0.3%) were positive for SARS-CoV-2 RT-PCR test. Of the nine HCP who were fully vaccinated, five were vaccinated with the BNT162b2 vaccine, and four were vaccinated with the mRNA-1273 vaccine.

Ioannou et al. [38] compared viral load, clinical report at diagnosis, and type of exposure between vaccinated (1800) (with BNT162b2) and non-vaccinated (450) HCP. Among all 55 PCR-positive HCP, 21 were fully vaccinated (diagnosed >2 weeks later than the second dose). Interestingly, the viral load did not differ significantly between vaccinated and non-vaccinated HCP; nevertheless, the kind of symptoms differed significantly. Specifically, rhinorrhea and nasal congestion were significantly more common in vaccinated HCP, while cough and fever were more frequent in non-vaccinated HCP.

A large survey was performed in the USA by Jacobson and colleagues [39] from December 2020 to April 2021 involving 22 271 HCP fully vaccinated with mRNA-based SARS-CoV-2 vaccine. Among these, 26 cases of SARS-CoV-2 occurred in fully vaccinated HCP. The mutation types of breakthrough infections were: 0 (0%) E484K, 10 (55.6%) L452R, N501Y 1 (5.6%), and no mutation 7 (38.9%). Again in the USA, North et al. [40] in a prospective cohort study of 2243 fully vaccinated HCP, observed three infections, among which only one was symptomatic.

Teran [41] reported 22 cases of postvaccination SARS-CoV-2 diseases among skilled nursing facility residents and HCP. Among the 22 individuals with breakthrough infections, 14 (64%) were asymptomatic. Three symptomatic persons had mild, imprecise symptoms; two had mild, certain symptoms; and three had diagnosed pneumonia, one of these, with basic conditions of hypertension, diabetes mellitus, and chronic kidney disease, died.

Lastly, Thompson [42] performed a prospective cohort study including 2686 HCP who received two doses of SARS-CoV-2 mRNA vaccine. SARS-CoV-2 infection was discovered in five fully vaccinated HCP. The authors provided the vaccine effectiveness that was 92% (80–97; 95% CI) among fully vaccinated persons. In particular, the vaccine effectiveness was 94% (82–98; 95% CI) and 84% (31–96: 95% CI) for the BNT162b2 vaccine and the mRNA-1273 vaccine, respectively.

4. Discussion

The present SLR analyzed SARS-CoV-2 breakthrough infections that occurred in HCP fully vaccinated with mRNA SARS-CoV-2 vaccine. Studies included in this systematic review reported a very low incidence (0.001 to 0.011 per 100 individuals at risk) of post-vaccination reinfection among HCP in the first six months following the primary vaccination cycle [25–33]; the death of a single fully vaccinated individual due to COVID-19 breakthrough infection was reported [41]. Vaccine effectiveness on HCP analyzed by this systematic literature review remains high and constant between different countries.

Prior to the kickoff of anti-SARS-CoV-2 vaccination, HCP were the group with the maximum risk of exposure to COVID-19 infection [43,44]. Gholami et al., in a systematic review and meta-analysis, proved that the proportion of HCP who confirmed positive for COVID-19 between 28 surveys was 51.7%, with a 15% rate of hospitalization and a 1.5% death rate [43]. Although breakthrough infections mean that the virus broke through a protective barrier provided by the vaccine, it prevents COVID-19 in more than 90% of beneficiaries [14,15]. Recent investigations carried out among HCP fully vaccinated by mRNA vaccine and continuously examined by routine nasal testing have demonstrated significant decreases, but not a total absence, of SARS-CoV-2-positive tests [17,19,20,34–42]; in detail, almost all of the HCP were asymptomatic and a near absence of hospitalizations was reported, and some case reports just reported the infection among vaccinated HCP [44–49].

Ioannou and colleagues [38] compared the viral loads among vaccinated and unvaccinated HCP and did not find statistically significant differences as regards age, gender, site of acquisition, occurrence of symptoms at diagnosis, and viral loads. His findings, however, are opposite to those found in other studies with stronger enrollment. Thompson et al. [42] showed that among HCP with SARS-CoV-2 infection, the mean viral RNA load was 40% lower (95% CI, 16 to 57) in incompletely or fully vaccinated persons rather than in unvaccinated people. A survey among nursing home residents infected by SARS-CoV-2 and vaccinated with only a single dose of BNT162b2 evidenced that nasopharyngeal viral load was lower in vaccinated people [28].

A comparable outcome was described by Levine-Tiefenbrun et al. [50] in the analysis of a real-world dataset of COVID-19 patients after vaccination by the BNT162b2 mRNA vaccine; they found that the viral load was significantly decreased for infections following 12–37 days after the first dose of vaccine.

Therefore, since the viral load is correlated to transmission [51,52], single-dose mRNA SARS-CoV-2 vaccination might prevent outbreaks. Reduced viral loads indicate a potentially decreased infectiousness, further than reducing vaccine impact on virus spread.

The evaluation of viral loads is critical in the control of breakthrough infections and the management of SARS-CoV-2 variant outbreaks. Jacobson et al. found a high prevalence of breakthrough infection in HCP due to the L452R variant [39]. A study carried out in Israel observed that B117 is associated with higher viral load and observed higher viral load in B117 variant infections when compared to other variants [53]; moreover, higher viral loads in B1351 infections in unvaccinated individuals compared to fully vaccinated persons were reported [54].

An augmented percentage of variants in vaccine breakthrough infections that appears in two distinct windows of period have been reported: The first augmented quantity of B.1.351 was discovered in patients fully vaccinated with BNT162b2, 7–14 days after the second dose, matched to unvaccinated controls. Moreover, an augmented percentage of B.1.1.7 was detected in partially vaccinated persons 14 days after the first dose up to 6 days after the second dose [53].

The behavior of the variants was also studied in in vitro neutralization tests that demonstrated a significant decrease in neutralization against B1351 and a small reduction against B117 in fully vaccinated persons [55–58].

Many seroprevalence studies on SARS-CoV-2 have been conducted. At first, they were carried out to estimate the prevalence among HCP [59–62]. After vaccination, several studies were carried out in order to provide indications on the presence of antibodies after vaccination and the dosages were repeated over time [63–67]. mRNA vaccines stimulate anti-spike IgG in addition to T cell reactions that can be discovered in peripheral blood [68]; however, how long immunity is stimulated by SARS-CoV-2 mRNA vaccine is even under investigation at this phase. Tretyn and colleagues [69] analyzed the components of the immune response in vaccinated persons. After mRNA vaccination, the values of the humoral response were detected in the whole of people enrolled, which verified the effectiveness of the mRNA vaccine in triggering B lymphocytes to release antibodies and T lymphocytes to secrete interferon-γ [69].

Doria-Rose et al. [70] based on ad hoc phase 3 trials of the Moderna mRNA-1273 estimated the half-life of vaccine-binding antibodies and defined the lifetime of the vaccine immune response at 6 months after second dose. Bayart and colleagues [71], in a multicenter prospective study, focused on longer-term kinetics information of the humoral response following the two-dose regimen of BNT162b2 mRNA vaccine and found a significant antibody decrease 6 months post-vaccination. The decrease was highly significant for overall antibodies, IgG, and neutralizing antibodies in both seronegative and seropositive participants. Thus, the clinical implications of serological assays that were not yet clear from a clinical position and the founding of thresholds connected with defense are still needed, but the association between low neutralizing antibody titers and breakthrough infection may not be excluded and might rationalize the request of appropriate vaccination policies, particularly in HCP, frail patients, and their caregivers [34,72–74].

The main limit of the present study could be related to the limited period (less than six months from the completion of primary vaccination cycle) of observation of the studies included in the SLR.

As is well-known, starting from Israel, all European countries, the UK, and the US that began the vaccination campaign among HCP in December 2020–January 2021 have offered the booster doses to HCP since September 2021 (especially those older than 60 years or with at least one comorbidity).

Furthermore, another aspect to underline is the difficulties in the implementation of equitable distribution of anti-SARS-CoV-2 vaccines.

Vaccination has increased slowly worldwide. However, while few high-income countries' governments understand how to vaccinate their whole populations during the pandemic, most low- and middle-income countries have been trusting the COVID-19 Vaccines Global Access (COVAX) facility to acquire vaccines [75]. COVAX aims to require these countries with adequate doses to vaccinate 20% of their people.

Public vaccine improvement efforts should move in the direction of decreasing all characteristics of public health risk instead than favoring its business financial characteristics [76,77].

Future analyses are needed to evaluate the length of the primary vaccination cycle protection among HCP, also standardized for age and at-risk groups.

5. Conclusions

In conclusion, we conducted a systemic review of published evidence on post-vaccination breakthrough SARS-CoV-2 infections among HCP fully vaccinated with mRNA vaccines. An overall very low incidence of post-vaccination breakthrough infections was found, ranging from 0.011 to 0.001 (per 100 individuals at risk). Our findings further support the published high effectiveness rates of mRNA vaccines in stopping SARS-CoV-2 infections including fully vaccinated HCP. Further studies are required to define the duration of the vaccine-induced protection among HCP.

Author Contributions: Conceptualization, C.L., H.C.M. and V.R.; methodology, C.L.; validation, C.C., G.L. and C.L.; formal analysis, P.S., G.M. and R.C.; data curation, C.L.; writing—original draft preparation, C.L.; writing—review and editing, H.C.M. and C.C.; supervision, C.L. All authors have read and agreed to the published version of the manuscript.

Funding: This research received no external funding.

Institutional Review Board Statement: Not applicable.

Informed Consent Statement: Not applicable.

Acknowledgments: The authors thank the Scientific Bureau of the University of Catania for the language support.

Conflicts of Interest: The authors declare no conflict of interest.

References

1. WHO. WHO Coronavirus (COVID-19) Dashboard. Available online: https://covid19.who.int/ (accessed on 23 August 2021).
2. Ramos, A.M.; Vela-Pérez, M.; Ferrández, M.R.; Kubik, A.B.; Ivorra, B. Modeling the Impact of SARS-CoV-2 Variants and Vaccines on the Spread of COVID-19. *Commun. Nonlinear Sci. Numer. Simul.* **2021**, *102*, 105937. [CrossRef] [PubMed]
3. Xiao, Y.; Torok, M.E. Taking the Right Measures to Control COVID-19. *Lancet Infect. Dis.* **2020**, *20*, 523–524. [CrossRef]
4. Arino, J.; Boëlle, P.-Y.; Milliken, E.; Portet, S. Risk of COVID-19 Variant Importation—How Useful Are Travel Control Measures? *Infect. Dis. Model.* **2021**, *6*, 875–897. [CrossRef] [PubMed]
5. Coccia, M. Preparedness of Countries to Face COVID-19 Pandemic Crisis: Strategic Positioning and Factors Supporting Effective Strategies of Prevention of Pandemic Threats. *Environ. Res.* **2022**, *203*, 111678. [CrossRef]
6. Vella, F.; Senia, P.; Ceccarelli, M.; Vitale, E.; Maltezou, H.; Taibi, R.; Lleshi, A.; Venanzi Rullo, E.; Pellicanò, G.F.; Rapisarda, V.; et al. Transmission Mode Associated with Coronavirus Disease 2019: A Review. *Eur. Rev. Med. Pharmacol. Sci.* **2020**, *24*, 7889–7904. [CrossRef]
7. Maniaci, A.; Ferlito, S.; Bubbico, L.; Ledda, C.; Rapisarda, V.; Iannella, G.; La Mantia, I.; Grillo, C.; Vicini, C.; Privitera, E.; et al. Comfort Rules for Face Masks among Healthcare Workers during COVID-19 Spread. *Ann. Ig.* **2021**, *33*, 615–627. [CrossRef] [PubMed]
8. Anderson, R.M.; Heesterbeek, H.; Klinkenberg, D.; Hollingsworth, T.D. How Will Country-Based Mitigation Measures Influence the Course of the COVID-19 Epidemic? *Lancet* **2020**, *395*, 931–934. [CrossRef]

9. Jackson, L.A.; Anderson, E.J.; Rouphael, N.G.; Roberts, P.C.; Makhene, M.; Coler, R.N.; McCullough, M.P.; Chappell, J.D.; Denison, M.R.; Stevens, L.J.; et al. An MRNA Vaccine against SARS-CoV-2—Preliminary Report. *N. Engl. J. Med.* **2020**, *383*, 1920–1931. [CrossRef]
10. Klugar, M.; Riad, A.; Mohanan, L.; Pokorná, A. COVID-19 Vaccine Booster Hesitancy (VBH) of Healthcare Workers in Czechia: National Cross-Sectional Study. *Vaccines* **2021**, *9*, 1437. [CrossRef] [PubMed]
11. Riad, A.; Hocková, B.; Kantorová, L.; Slávik, R.; Spurná, L.; Stebel, A.; Havriľak, M.; Klugar, M. Side Effects of MRNA-Based COVID-19 Vaccine: Nationwide Phase IV Study among Healthcare Workers in Slovakia. *Pharmaceuticals* **2021**, *14*, 873. [CrossRef] [PubMed]
12. McGill University. Interdisciplinary Initiative in Infection and Immunity COVID-19 Vaccine Tracker. Available online: https://covid19.trackvaccines.org/ (accessed on 27 September 2021).
13. FDA. FDA Approves First COVID-19 Vaccine. Available online: https://www.fda.gov/news-events/press-announcements/fda-approves-first-COVID-19-vaccine (accessed on 27 September 2021).
14. Baden, L.R.; El Sahly, H.M.; Essink, B.; Kotloff, K.; Frey, S.; Novak, R.; Diemert, D.; Spector, S.A.; Rouphael, N.; Creech, C.B.; et al. Efficacy and Safety of the MRNA-1273 SARS-CoV-2 Vaccine. *N. Engl. J. Med.* **2021**, *384*, 403–416. [CrossRef]
15. Polack, F.P.; Thomas, S.J.; Kitchin, N.; Absalon, J.; Gurtman, A.; Lockhart, S.; Perez, J.L.; Pérez Marc, G.; Moreira, E.D.; Zerbini, C.; et al. Safety and Efficacy of the BNT162b2 MRNA COVID-19 Vaccine. *N. Engl. J. Med.* **2020**, *383*, 2603–2615. [CrossRef]
16. Dagan, N.; Barda, N.; Kepten, E.; Miron, O.; Perchik, S.; Katz, M.A.; Hernán, M.A.; Lipsitch, M.; Reis, B.; Balicer, R.D. BNT162b2 MRNA COVID-19 Vaccine in a Nationwide Mass Vaccination Setting. *N. Engl. J. Med.* **2021**, *384*, 1412–1423. [CrossRef] [PubMed]
17. Thompson, M.G.; Burgess, J.L.; Naleway, A.L.; Tyner, H.L.; Yoon, S.K.; Meece, J.; Olsho, L.E.W.; Caban-Martinez, A.J.; Fowlkes, A.; Lutrick, K.; et al. Interim Estimates of Vaccine Effectiveness of BNT162b2 and MRNA-1273 COVID-19 Vaccines in Preventing SARS-CoV-2 Infection among Health Care Personnel, First Responders, and Other Essential and Frontline Workers—Eight U.S. Locations, December 2020–March 2021. *MMWR Morb. Mortal. Wkly. Rep.* **2021**, *70*, 495–500. [CrossRef] [PubMed]
18. Maltezou, H.C.; Panagopoulos, P.; Sourri, F.; Giannouchos, T.V.; Raftopoulos, V.; Gamaletsou, M.N.; Karapanou, A.; Koukou, D.-M.; Koutsidou, A.; Peskelidou, E.; et al. COVID-19 Vaccination Significantly Reduces Morbidity and Absenteeism among Healthcare Personnel: A Prospective Multicenter Study. *Vaccine* **2021**, *39*, 7021–7027. [CrossRef] [PubMed]
19. Keehner, J.; Horton, L.E.; Pfeffer, M.A.; Longhurst, C.A.; Schooley, R.T.; Currier, J.S.; Abeles, S.R.; Torriani, F.J. SARS-CoV-2 Infection after Vaccination in Health Care Workers in California. *N. Engl. J. Med.* **2021**, *384*, 1774–1775. [CrossRef] [PubMed]
20. Daniel, W.; Nivet, M.; Warner, J.; Podolsky, D.K. Early Evidence of the Effect of SARS-CoV-2 Vaccine at One Medical Center. *N. Engl. J. Med.* **2021**, *384*, 1962–1963. [CrossRef] [PubMed]
21. WHO. Tracking SARS-CoV-2 Variants. Available online: https://www.who.int/en/activities/tracking-SARS-CoV-2-variants/ (accessed on 28 September 2021).
22. Shastri, J.; Parikh, S.; Aggarwal, V.; Agrawal, S.; Chatterjee, N.; Shah, R.; Devi, P.; Mehta, P.; Pandey, R. Severe SARS-CoV-2 Breakthrough Reinfection with Delta Variant after Recovery from Breakthrough Infection by Alpha Variant in a Fully Vaccinated Health Worker. *Front. Med.* **2021**, *8*, 737007. [CrossRef] [PubMed]
23. Dhar, M.S.; Marwal, R.; Vs, R.; Ponnusamy, K.; Jolly, B.; Bhoyar, R.C.; Sardana, V.; Naushin, S.; Rophina, M.; Mellan, T.A.; et al. Genomic Characterization and Epidemiology of an Emerging SARS-CoV-2 Variant in Delhi, India. *Science* **2021**, *374*, 995–999. [CrossRef]
24. Maltezou, H.C.; Dedoukou, X.; Tseroni, M.; Tsonou, P.; Raftopoulos, V.; Papadima, K.; Mouratidou, E.; Poufta, S.; Panagiotakopoulos, G.; Hatzigeorgiou, D.; et al. SARS-CoV-2 Infection in Healthcare Personnel with High-Risk Occupational Exposure: Evaluation of 7-Day Exclusion from Work Policy. *Clin. Infect. Dis.* **2020**, *71*, 3182–3187. [CrossRef]
25. Thorsteinsdottir, B.; Madsen, B.E. Prioritizing Health Care Workers and First Responders for Access to the COVID-19 Vaccine Is Not Unethical, but Both Fair and Effective—An Ethical Analysis. *Scand. J. Trauma Resusc. Emerg. Med.* **2021**, *29*, 77. [CrossRef] [PubMed]
26. Ledda, C.; Costantino, C.; Cuccia, M.; Maltezou, H.C.; Rapisarda, V. Attitudes of Healthcare Personnel towards Vaccinations before and during the COVID-19 Pandemic. *Int. J. Environ. Res. Public Health* **2021**, *18*, 2703. [CrossRef] [PubMed]
27. Al-Amer, R.; Maneze, D.; Everett, B.; Montayre, J.; Villarosa, A.R.; Dwekat, E.; Salamonson, Y. COVID-19 Vaccination Intention in the First Year of the Pandemic: A Systematic Review. *J. Clin. Nurs.* **2022**, *31*, 62–86. [CrossRef]
28. McEllistrem, M.C.; Clancy, C.J.; Buehrle, D.J.; Lucas, A.; Decker, B.K. Single Dose of an MRNA Severe Acute Respiratory Syndrome Coronavirus 2 (SARS-CoV-2) Vaccine Is Associated with Lower Nasopharyngeal Viral Load among Nursing Home Residents with Asymptomatic Coronavirus Disease 2019 (COVID-19). *Clin. Infect. Dis.* **2021**, *73*, e1365–e1367. [CrossRef]
29. Riemersma, K.K.; Grogan, B.E.; Kita-Yarbro, A.; Halfmann, P.J.; Segaloff, H.E.; Kocharian, A.; Florek, K.R.; Westergaard, R.; Bateman, A.; Jeppson, G.E.; et al. Shedding of Infectious SARS-CoV-2 Despite Vaccination. *medRxiv* **2021**. in pre-print. [CrossRef]
30. Moher, D.; Liberati, A.; Tetzlaff, J.; Altman, D.G.; The PRISMA Group. Preferred Reporting Items for Systematic Reviews and Meta-Analyses: The PRISMA Statement. *PLoS Med.* **2009**, *6*, e1000097. [CrossRef] [PubMed]
31. Brownson, R.C.; Fielding, J.E.; Maylahn, C.M. Evidence-Based Public Health: A Fundamental Concept for Public Health Practice. *Annu. Rev. Public Health* **2009**, *30*, 175–201. [CrossRef]
32. Munn, Z.; Moola, S.; Lisy, K.; Riitano, D.; Tufanaru, C. Methodological Guidance for Systematic Reviews of Observational Epidemiological Studies Reporting Prevalence and Cumulative Incidence Data. *Int. J. Evid.-Based Healthc.* **2015**, *13*, 147–153. [CrossRef] [PubMed]

33. Migliavaca, C.B.; Stein, C.; Colpani, V.; Munn, Z.; Falavigna, M. Quality Assessment of Prevalence Studies: A Systematic Review. *J. Clin. Epidemiol.* **2020**, *127*, 59–68. [CrossRef] [PubMed]
34. Bergwerk, M.; Gonen, T.; Lustig, Y.; Amit, S.; Lipsitch, M.; Cohen, C.; Mandelboim, M.; Gal Levin, E.; Rubin, C.; Indenbaum, V.; et al. COVID-19 Breakthrough Infections in Vaccinated Health Care Workers. *N. Engl. J. Med.* **2021**, *385*, 1474–1484. [CrossRef] [PubMed]
35. Bouton, T.C.; Lodi, S.; Turcinovic, J.; Schaeffer, B.; Weber, S.E.; Quinn, E.; Korn, C.; Steiner, J.; Schechter-Perkins, E.M.; Duffy, E.; et al. Coronavirus Disease 2019 Vaccine Impact on Rates of Severe Acute Respiratory Syndrome Coronavirus 2 Cases and Postvaccination Strain Sequences Among Health Care Workers at an Urban Academic Medical Center: A Prospective Cohort Study. *Open Forum Infect. Dis.* **2021**, *8*, ofab465. [CrossRef] [PubMed]
36. Fowlkes, A.; Gaglani, M.; Groover, K.; Thiese, M.S.; Tyner, H.; Ellingson, K. HEROES-RECOVER Cohorts Effectiveness of COVID-19 Vaccines in Preventing SARS-CoV-2 Infection among Frontline Workers before and during B.1.617.2 (Delta) Variant Predominance—Eight U.S. Locations, December 2020–August 2021. *MMWR Morb. Mortal. Wkly. Rep.* **2021**, *70*, 1167–1169. [CrossRef]
37. Geysels, D.; Van Damme, P.; Verstrepen, W.; Bruynseels, P.; Janssens, B.; Smits, P.; Naesens, R. SARS-CoV-2 Vaccine Breakthrough Infections among Healthcare Workers in a Large Belgian Hospital Network. *Infect. Control Hosp. Epidemiol.* **2021**, 1–2. [CrossRef]
38. Ioannou, P.; Karakonstantis, S.; Astrinaki, E.; Saplamidou, S.; Vitsaxaki, E.; Hamilos, G.; Sourvinos, G.; Kofteridis, D.P. Transmission of SARS-CoV-2 Variant B.1.1.7 among Vaccinated Health Care Workers. *Infect. Dis.* **2021**, *53*, 876–879. [CrossRef]
39. Jacobson, K.B.; Pinsky, B.A.; Montez Rath, M.E.; Wang, H.; Miller, J.A.; Skhiri, M.; Shepard, J.; Mathew, R.; Lee, G.; Bohman, B.; et al. Post-Vaccination Severe Acute Respiratory Syndrome Coronavirus 2 (SARS-CoV-2) Infections and Incidence of the Presumptive B.1.427/B.1.429 Variant among Healthcare Personnel at a Northern California Academic Medical Center. *Clin. Infect. Dis.* **2021**, *2*, ciab554. [CrossRef] [PubMed]
40. North, C.M.; Barczak, A.; Goldstein, R.H.; Healy, B.C.; Finkelstein, D.M.; Ding, D.D.; Kim, A.; Boucau, J.; Shaw, B.; Gilbert, R.F.; et al. Determining the Incidence of Asymptomatic SARS-CoV-2 among Early Recipients of COVID-19 Vaccines: A Prospective Cohort Study of Healthcare Workers before, during and after Vaccination [DISCOVER-COVID-19]. *Clin. Infect. Dis.* **2021**, ciab643. [CrossRef] [PubMed]
41. Teran, R.A.; Walblay, K.A.; Shane, E.L.; Xydis, S.; Gretsch, S.; Gagner, A.; Samala, U.; Choi, H.; Zelinski, C.; Black, S.R. Postvaccination SARS-CoV-2 Infections among Skilled Nursing Facility Residents and Staff Members—Chicago, Illinois, December 2020–March 2021. *MMWR Morb. Mortal. Wkly. Rep.* **2021**, *70*, 632–638. [CrossRef] [PubMed]
42. Thompson, M.G.; Burgess, J.L.; Naleway, A.L.; Tyner, H.; Yoon, S.K.; Meece, J.; Olsho, L.E.W.; Caban-Martinez, A.J.; Fowlkes, A.L.; Lutrick, K.; et al. Prevention and Attenuation of COVID-19 with the BNT162b2 and MRNA-1273 Vaccines. *N. Engl. J. Med.* **2021**, *385*, 320–329. [CrossRef]
43. Gholami, M.; Fawad, I.; Shadan, S.; Rowaiee, R.; Ghanem, H.; Hassan Khamis, A.; Ho, S.B. COVID-19 and Healthcare Workers: A Systematic Review and Meta-Analysis. *Int. J. Infect. Dis.* **2021**, *104*, 335–346. [CrossRef] [PubMed]
44. Maltezou, H.C.; Raftopoulos, V.; Vorou, R.; Papadima, K.; Mellou, K.; Spanakis, N.; Kossyvakis, A.; Gioula, G.; Exindari, M.; Froukala, E.; et al. Association between Upper Respiratory Tract Viral Load, Comorbidities, Disease Severity, and Outcome of Patients with SARS-CoV-2 Infection. *J. Infect. Dis.* **2021**, *223*, 1132–1138. [CrossRef] [PubMed]
45. Kroidl, I.; Mecklenburg, I.; Schneiderat, P.; Müller, K.; Girl, P.; Wölfel, R.; Sing, A.; Dangel, A.; Wieser, A.; Hoelscher, M. Vaccine Breakthrough Infection and Onward Transmission of SARS-CoV-2 Beta (B.1.351) Variant, Bavaria, Germany, February to March 2021. *Eurosurveillance* **2021**, *26*, 2100673. [CrossRef]
46. Lange, B.; Gerigk, M.; Tenenbaum, T. Breakthrough Infections in BNT162b2-Vaccinated Health Care Workers. *N. Engl. J. Med.* **2021**, *385*, 1145–1146. [CrossRef]
47. Sansone, E.; Tiraboschi, M.; Sala, E.; Albini, E.; Lombardo, M.; Castelli, F.; De Palma, G. Effectiveness of BNT162b2 Vaccine against the B.1.1.7 Variant of SARS-CoV-2 among Healthcare Workers in Brescia, Italy. *J. Infect.* **2021**, *83*, e17–e18. [CrossRef] [PubMed]
48. Schulte, B.; Marx, B.; Korencak, M.; Emmert, D.; Aldabbagh, S.; Eis-Hübinger, A.M.; Streeck, H. Case Report: Infection with SARS-CoV-2 in the Presence of High Levels of Vaccine-Induced Neutralizing Antibody Responses. *Front. Med.* **2021**, *8*, 704719. [CrossRef] [PubMed]
49. Strafella, C.; Caputo, V.; Guerrera, G.; Termine, A.; Fabrizio, C.; Cascella, R.; Picozza, M.; Caltagirone, C.; Rossini, A.; Balice, M.P.; et al. Case Report: SARS-CoV-2 Infection in a Vaccinated Individual: Evaluation of the Immunological Profile and Virus Transmission Risk. *Front. Immunol.* **2021**, *12*, 708820. [CrossRef] [PubMed]
50. Levine-Tiefenbrun, M.; Yelin, I.; Katz, R.; Herzel, E.; Golan, Z.; Schreiber, L.; Wolf, T.; Nadler, V.; Ben-Tov, A.; Kuint, J.; et al. Initial Report of Decreased SARS-CoV-2 Viral Load after Inoculation with the BNT162b2 Vaccine. *Nat. Med.* **2021**, *27*, 790–792. [CrossRef] [PubMed]
51. Dai, L.; Gao, G.F. Viral Targets for Vaccines against COVID-19. *Nat. Rev. Immunol.* **2021**, *21*, 73–82. [CrossRef] [PubMed]
52. Kennedy-Shaffer, L.; Kahn, R.; Lipsitch, M. Estimating Vaccine Efficacy against Transmission via Effect on Viral Load. *Epidemiology* **2021**, *32*, 820–828. [CrossRef]
53. Kustin, T.; Harel, N.; Finkel, U.; Perchik, S.; Harari, S.; Tahor, M.; Caspi, I.; Levy, R.; Leshchinsky, M.; Ken Dror, S.; et al. Evidence for Increased Breakthrough Rates of SARS-CoV-2 Variants of Concern in BNT162b2-MRNA-Vaccinated Individuals. *Nat. Med.* **2021**, *27*, 1379–1384. [CrossRef] [PubMed]

54. Walker, A.S.; Vihta, K.-D.; Gethings, O.; Pritchard, E.; Jones, J.; House, T.; Bell, I.; Bell, J.I.; Newton, J.N.; Farrar, J.; et al. Increased Infections, but Not Viral Burden, with a New SARS-CoV-2 Variant. *medRxiv* **2021**. in pre-print. [CrossRef]
55. Liu, Y.; Liu, J.; Xia, H.; Zhang, X.; Fontes-Garfias, C.R.; Swanson, K.A.; Cai, H.; Sarkar, R.; Chen, W.; Cutler, M.; et al. Neutralizing Activity of BNT162b2-Elicited Serum. *N. Engl. J. Med.* **2021**, *384*, 1466–1468. [CrossRef]
56. Xie, X.; Liu, Y.; Liu, J.; Zhang, X.; Zou, J.; Fontes-Garfias, C.R.; Xia, H.; Swanson, K.A.; Cutler, M.; Cooper, D.; et al. Neutralization of SARS-CoV-2 Spike 69/70 Deletion, E484K and N501Y Variants by BNT162b2 Vaccine-Elicited Sera. *Nat. Med.* **2021**, *27*, 620–621. [CrossRef] [PubMed]
57. The CITIID-NIHR BioResource COVID-19 Collaboration; The COVID-19 Genomics UK (COG-UK) Consortium; Collier, D.A.; De Marco, A.; Ferreira, I.A.T.M.; Meng, B.; Datir, R.P.; Walls, A.C.; Kemp, S.A.; Bassi, J.; et al. Sensitivity of SARS-CoV-2 B.1.1.7 to MRNA Vaccine-Elicited Antibodies. *Nature* **2021**, *593*, 136–141. [CrossRef] [PubMed]
58. Zhou, D.; Dejnirattisai, W.; Supasa, P.; Liu, C.; Mentzer, A.J.; Ginn, H.M.; Zhao, Y.; Duyvesteyn, H.M.E.; Tuekprakhon, A.; Nutalai, R.; et al. Evidence of Escape of SARS-CoV-2 Variant B.1.351 from Natural and Vaccine-Induced Sera. *Cell* **2021**, *184*, 2348–2361.e6. [CrossRef] [PubMed]
59. Ledda, C.; Carrasi, F.; Longombardo, M.T.; Paravizzini, G.; Rapisarda, V. SARS-CoV-2 Seroprevalence Post-First Wave among Primary Care Physicians in Catania (Italy). *TropicalMed* **2021**, *6*, 21. [CrossRef] [PubMed]
60. Costantino, C.; Cannizzaro, E.; Verso, M.G.; Tramuto, F.; Maida, C.M.; Lacca, G.; Alba, D.; Cimino, L.; Conforto, A.; Cirrincione, L.; et al. SARS-CoV-2 Infection in Healthcare Professionals and General Population during "First Wave" of COVID-19 Pandemic: A Cross-Sectional Study Conducted in Sicily, Italy. *Front. Public Health* **2021**, *9*, 644008. [CrossRef] [PubMed]
61. Magaña-Guerrero, F.S.; Trujillo, D.H.; Buentello-Volante, B.; Aguayo-Flores, J.E.; Melgoza-González, E.A.; Hernández, J.; Jiménez-Martínez, M.C.; Pérez-Tapia, S.M.; Garfias, Y. SARS-CoV-2 Seroprevalence among the Health Care Staff of an Ophthalmological Reference Centre, a Cross Sectional Study. *Ophthalmic Epidemiol.* **2021**, 1–8. [CrossRef]
62. Herzberg, J.; Vollmer, T.; Fischer, B.; Becher, H.; Becker, A.-K.; Sahly, H.; Honarpisheh, H.; Guraya, S.Y.; Strate, T.; Knabbe, C. Half-Year Longitudinal Seroprevalence of SARS-CoV-2-Antibodies and Rule Compliance in German Hospital Employees. *Int. J. Environ. Res. Public Health* **2021**, *18*, 10972. [CrossRef] [PubMed]
63. Havervall, S.; Marking, U.; Greilert-Norin, N.; Ng, H.; Gordon, M.; Salomonsson, A.-C.; Hellström, C.; Pin, E.; Blom, K.; Mangsbo, S.; et al. Antibody Responses after a Single Dose of ChAdOx1 NCoV-19 Vaccine in Healthcare Workers Previously Infected with SARS-CoV-2. *eBioMedicine* **2021**, *70*, 103523. [CrossRef]
64. Hossain, A.; Nasrullah, S.M.; Tasnim, Z.; Hasan, M.K.; Hasan, M.M. Seroprevalence of SARS-CoV-2 IgG Antibodies among Health Care Workers Prior to Vaccine Administration in Europe, the USA and East Asia: A Systematic Review and Meta-Analysis. *EClinicalMedicine* **2021**, *33*, 100770. [CrossRef]
65. Heyming, T.W.; Nugent, D.; Tongol, A.; Knudsen-Robbins, C.; Hoang, J.; Schomberg, J.; Bacon, K.; Lara, B.; Sanger, T. Rapid Antibody Testing for SARS-CoV-2 Vaccine Response in Pediatric Healthcare Workers. *Int. J. Infect. Dis.* **2021**, *113*, 1–6. [CrossRef] [PubMed]
66. Morales-Núñez, J.J.; Muñoz-Valle, J.F.; Meza-López, C.; Wang, L.-F.; Machado Sulbarán, A.C.; Torres-Hernández, P.C.; Bedolla-Barajas, M.; De la O-Gómez, B.; Balcázar-Félix, P.; Hernández-Bello, J. Neutralizing Antibodies Titers and Side Effects in Response to BNT162b2 Vaccine in Healthcare Workers with and without Prior SARS-CoV-2 Infection. *Vaccines* **2021**, *9*, 742. [CrossRef]
67. Buonfrate, D.; Piubelli, C.; Gobbi, F.; Martini, D.; Bertoli, G.; Ursini, T.; Moro, L.; Ronzoni, N.; Angheben, A.; Rodari, P.; et al. Antibody Response Induced by the BNT162b2 MRNA COVID-19 Vaccine in a Cohort of Health-Care Workers, with or without Prior SARS-CoV-2 Infection: A Prospective Study. *Clin. Microbiol. Infect.* **2021**, *27*, 1845–1850. [CrossRef] [PubMed]
68. Schieffelin, J.S.; Norton, E.B.; Kolls, J.K. What Should Define a SARS-CoV-2 "Breakthrough" Infection? *J. Clin. Investig.* **2021**, *131*, e151186. [CrossRef]
69. Tretyn, A.; Szczepanek, J.; Skorupa, M.; Jarkiewicz-Tretyn, J.; Sandomierz, D.; Dejewska, J.; Ciechanowska, K.; Jarkiewicz-Tretyn, A.; Koper, W.; Pałgan, K. Differences in the Concentration of Anti-SARS-CoV-2 IgG Antibodies Post-COVID-19 Recovery or Post-Vaccination. *Cells* **2021**, *10*, 1952. [CrossRef]
70. Doria-Rose, N.; Suthar, M.S.; Makowski, M.; O'Connell, S.; McDermott, A.B.; Flach, B.; Ledgerwood, J.E.; Mascola, J.R.; Graham, B.S.; Lin, B.C.; et al. Antibody Persistence through 6 Months after the Second Dose of MRNA-1273 Vaccine for COVID-19. *N. Engl. J. Med.* **2021**, *384*, 2259–2261. [CrossRef] [PubMed]
71. Bayart, J.-L.; Douxfils, J.; Gillot, C.; David, C.; Mullier, F.; Elsen, M.; Eucher, C.; Van Eeckhoudt, S.; Roy, T.; Gerin, V.; et al. Waning of IgG, Total and Neutralizing Antibodies 6 Months Post-Vaccination with BNT162b2 in Healthcare Workers. *Vaccines* **2021**, *9*, 1092. [CrossRef] [PubMed]
72. Shrotri, M.; Navaratnam, A.M.D.; Nguyen, V.; Byrne, T.; Geismar, C.; Fragaszy, E.; Beale, S.; Fong, W.L.E.; Patel, P.; Kovar, J.; et al. Spike-Antibody Waning after Second Dose of BNT162b2 or ChAdOx1. *Lancet* **2021**, *398*, 385–387. [CrossRef]
73. Hacisuleyman, E.; Hale, C.; Saito, Y.; Blachere, N.E.; Bergh, M.; Conlon, E.G.; Schaefer-Babajew, D.J.; DaSilva, J.; Muecksch, F.; Gaebler, C.; et al. Vaccine Breakthrough Infections with SARS-CoV-2 Variants. *N. Engl. J. Med.* **2021**, *384*, 2212–2218. [CrossRef]
74. Stephenson, J. COVID-19 Vaccinations in Nursing Home Residents and Staff Give Robust Protection, Though Breakthrough Infections Still Possible. *JAMA Health Forum* **2021**, *2*, e211595. [CrossRef]

75. Tagoe, E.T.; Sheikh, N.; Morton, A.; Nonvignon, J.; Sarker, A.R.; Williams, L.; Megiddo, I. COVID-19 Vaccination in Lower-Middle Income Countries: National Stakeholder Views on Challenges, Barriers, and Potential Solutions. *Front. Public Health* **2021**, *9*, 709127. [CrossRef] [PubMed]
76. Bolcato, M.; Rodriguez, D.; Feola, A.; Di Mizio, G.; Bonsignore, A.; Ciliberti, R.; Tettamanti, C.; Trabucco Aurilio, M.; Aprile, A. COVID-19 Pandemic and Equal Access to Vaccines. *Vaccines* **2021**, *9*, 538. [CrossRef] [PubMed]
77. Stein, F. Risky Business: COVAX and the Financialization of Global Vaccine Equity. *Glob. Health* **2021**, *17*, 112. [CrossRef] [PubMed]

MDPI
St. Alban-Anlage 66
4052 Basel
Switzerland
Tel. +41 61 683 77 34
Fax +41 61 302 89 18
www.mdpi.com

Tropical Medicine and Infectious Disease Editorial Office
E-mail: tropicalmed@mdpi.com
www.mdpi.com/journal/tropicalmed

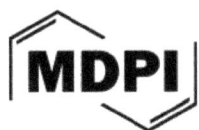

www.ingramcontent.com/pod-product-compliance
Lightning Source LLC
LaVergne TN
LVHW070229100526
838202LV00015B/2108